Health for effective living

A basic health science text for college students

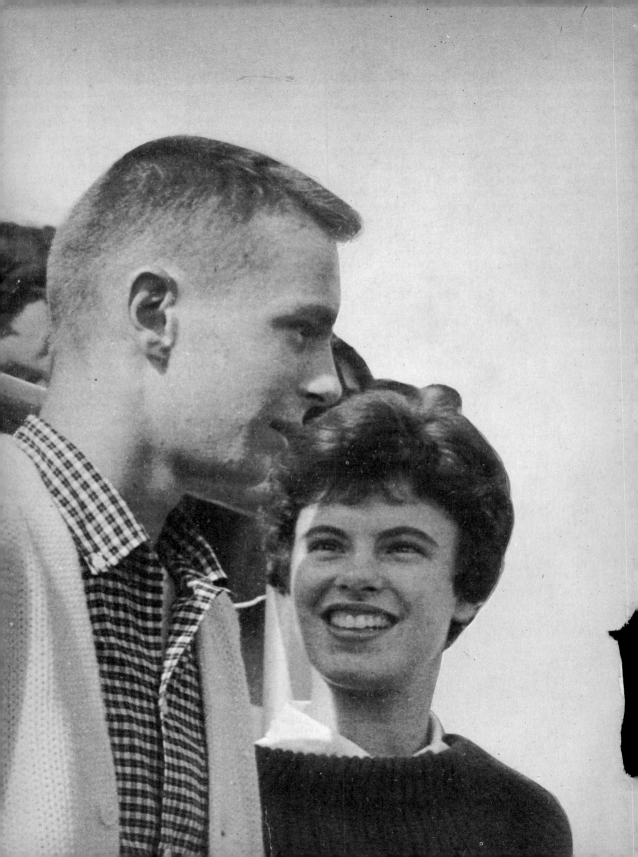

HEALTH FOR
EFFECTIVE LIVING

Third Edition

A BASIC HEALTH SCIENCE TEXT FOR COLLEGE STUDENTS

EDWARD B. JOHNS, Ed.D., F.A.P.H.A. *Professor, School Health Education, University of California, Los Angeles. Formerly a Health Education Consultant, California Community Health Education Project*

WILFRED C. SUTTON, Ed.D., F.A.S.H.A. *Associate Professor, School Health Education, University of California, Los Angeles*

LLOYD E. WEBSTER, M.A., F.A.A.H.P.E.R. *Director of Health Education, Los Angeles County Schools. Formerly Associate Professor of Health Education, University of Southern California*

Adviser and Consultant **Walter H. Brown, M.D.,** *Professor Emeritus, Stanford University. Formerly Professor and Acting Dean, School of Public Health, University of California*

Foreword by **Bernice Moss, Ed.D.,** *Professor of Health Education, University of Utah. Editor, NEA-AMA, Health Education, 1961*

McGraw-Hill Book Company, Inc.
New York / San Francisco / Toronto / London / 1962

II   32553

 This book is set in Intertype Century Schoolbook, a typeface based on the original letter form Century Roman, designed in 1895 by Linn Boyd Benton.

CREDITS FOR PHOTOGRAPHS

PART TITLES. Pages 34, 100, 172, 298, and 444: Shelton from Monkmeyer.

CHAPTER 1. Page 4: top and bottom, Richard Szladowski; center, Stanley Troutman. Page 6: left, Richard Szladowski; right, Stanley Troutman. Page 7: Richard Szladowski. Page 9: top, Richard Szladowski; center and bottom, Stanley Troutman. Page 22: top, H. Lee Hansen, courtesy of Los Angeles City College; center and bottom, Stanley Troutman. Page 23: Stanley Troutman.

CHAPTER 2. Page 58: left, H. Armstrong Roberts; right, Merrim from Monkmeyer. Page 59: top, H. Armstrong Roberts; center, Hays from Monkmeyer; bottom, Max Tharpe from Monkmeyer. Page 62: left top, Hays from Monkmeyer; left center and bottom, National Association for Mental Health; right top, Ford Foundation by William Simmons; right bottom, Shelton from Monkmeyer.

CHAPTER 3. Pages 72 and 73: Stanley Troutman.

CHAPTER 4. Pages 110 and 111: Gary Kline, Stanford University Quad.

CHAPTER 5. Pages 136 and 137: Robert Berenson.

CHAPTER 6. Pages 156 and 157: Robert Berenson. Page 168: top and bottom, Kodak, Inc.; center, Merrim from Monkmeyer.

CHAPTER 7. Page 198: left top, Gillette Safety Razor Company; right side, Cleanliness Bureau. Page 199: left top and right bottom, Cleanliness Bureau; top right, A. Devaney, Inc.; bottom left, Merrim from Monkmeyer.

CHAPTER 8. Pages 210 and 211: Stanley Troutman; bottom right, Alec Waterhouse, Jr.

CHAPTER 9. Page 224: top, Merrim from Monkmeyer; center and bottom, Stanley Troutman.

CHAPTER 10. Page 260: American Medical Association. Page 269: top and center, Food and Drug Administration; bottom left and right, Robert Berenson. Page 288: top left, Chas. Pfizer & Co., Inc.; top right, Blue Cross and Blue Shield; center, Health Insurance Plan of Greater New York; bottom, Kaiser Services, Oakland, Calif.

CHAPTER 11. Page 322: left side, Hochman from Monkmeyer, Dr. F. Heinmetz, General Biological Supply House, National Tuberculosis Association, Society of American Bacteriologists, Robert Berenson; right side, Air Force Academy, Jean Ewing, U.S. Public Health Service, U.S. Forest Service, Robert Berenson. Page 323: left side, *Food Engineering,* McGraw-Hill Medical Department, U.S. Public Health Service, Stanley Troutman; right side, Fred Thompson, McGraw-Hill Text-Films, U.S. Public Health Service. Page 335: Stanley Troutman.

CHAPTER 12. Page 357: Ford Foundation by Homer Page and William Simmons. Page 376: top, Godsey from Monkmeyer; center and bottom, American Cancer Society. Page 377: American Cancer Society.

CHAPTER 13. Page 397: Alcohol Research Clinic, State University of Medicine, Brooklyn, N.Y. Pages 412 and 413: Pix Incorporated.

CHAPTER 14. Page 426: left top, Hays from Monkmeyer; right side, H. Armstrong Roberts, Ford Motor Company, Standard Oil Company. Page 427: National Safety Council, American Red Cross, National Safety Council, United Nations.

CHAPTER 15. Page 452: Santa Monica City College; U.S. Department of Health, Education, and Welfare; 4-H Clubs; U.S. Department of Agriculture; McGraw-Hill Text-Films; Los Angeles City Health Department by Soibelman; Los Angeles County Tuberculosis and Health Association. Page 453: Los Angeles County Tuberculosis and Health Association; Lionel Freedman, courtesy of the Greenwich Hospital, Greenwich, Conn.; Thelner Hoover, Los Angeles City Health Department; American Cancer Society; U.S. Public Health Department; American Red Cross. Page 454: Los Angeles County Tuberculosis and Health Association.

CHAPTER 16. Pages 488 and 489: United Nations Children's Fund.

CHAPTER 17. Page 500: National Aeronautics and Space Administration. Page 504: Official U.S. Air Force Photos. Page 505: Boeing Airplane Company.

FOREWORD

The protection, maintenance, and improvement of the health of its students has long been an accepted objective of the American college or university. Basic to the realization of this objective is the instruction of the students in the principles and practices of healthful living. Freshman or sophomore courses in health education (hygiene) are generally available and frequently required, and some such courses are now organized on the upper division level as well.

Health for Effective Living has been written to meet the needs of students enrolled in these courses. The approach of the authors indicates a keen recognition of the present-day needs and interests of college students and of the nature of the college and the wider communities in which students live. The emphasis given to problems of emotional and social adjustment is indicative of the trend toward guidance of young people in the areas of major concern to them. Here is where the text begins—not with cells, organs, tissues, bones, and blood. An honest attempt is made to assist students with their life adjustment problems, to supply them with scientific information, to build improved attitudes, to stimulate effective behavior, and to encourage better all-round living.

While emphasizing the emotional and social adjustment of college youth, the text does not neglect important basic concerns in body maintenance and protection, such as nutrition, balanced daily living, and protection against disease, accidents, and drugs. The inclusion of challenging information in these and other areas makes for balance and for adequate consideration of all important health problems which college students face or in which they indicate a need or an interest.

Another emphasis is noteworthy: the inclusion of information concerned with the college health program, with the community, state, and national approaches to group health protection and improvement. The role of the college student as a participating citizen on his campus and in his community is effectively developed.

It is of interest that in the third edition the authors have demonstrated a concern for current health problems, including the new dimension of health in space.

Students who pursue the text, and who participate in other meaningful learning activities, should develop broader understandings and appreciations of the social responsibilities of citizens in the interest of a vigorous and healthy commonwealth. This is a need in the nation today.

This book contains a challenge to students and to their instructors. It represents a new and more functional approach to a basic concern—that of building healthy, happy, effective citizens in a democracy.

BERNICE MOSS, Ed.D.,
Professor of Health Education,
University of Utah, and
Editor, Joint Committee on
Health Problems in Education,
NEA-AMA, Health Education, *1961*

ix

TO THE INSTRUCTOR

Recent scientific discoveries, as well as political, social, and international events, have guided us in preparing the third edition of *Health for Effective Living*. Constructive suggestions from numerous instructors and students and our own augmented experience with college students in health education have also helped to shape this new and extensively revised edition.

Our specific purpose is to provide a basic health science text for college students that is functional. This edition, like its predecessors, is written as a guide for students and instructors studying together the essential factors for producing and maintaining health and effective living.

Our philosophy of health education also remains the same. This philosophy is based upon the conviction that college students can enrich their lives through health education experiences. It is based upon the staunch belief that health behavior can be changed favorably through teaching that results in the acquisition of new understandings of scientific health information and the formation of positive health attitudes and health practices.

In *Health for Effective Living* the emphasis is upon the application of scientific health facts and principles that relate to living a better life, rather than on a reorganization of familiar anatomical and physiological information. Such material is included only to the extent that it enables the student to understand specific health education areas.

Our concepts are in keeping with the recommendations of the 1956 National Conference on College Health Education, which recognized health education as a vital part of education for *all college students*. These concepts are further substantiated by the point of view and discussion of 25 health education authorities who met in the Health Education Planning Conference at Highland Park, Illinois, October 10–12, 1959. The views of the conferees are presented in the report of the conference entitled *Guidelines for Health Education: A Suggested Plan for Action*. The conference was sponsored by the American Association for Health, Physical Education, and Recreation, and the report is distributed by the Association.

Although the major features of this book, which have proved effective in the previous editions, have been retained, a thorough revision and rewriting was necessary. This edition provides an up-to-date, pertinent, and valuable book for both instructors and students as we enter the first stages of the Space Age. Readers will discover that the revision entails much more than a new cover and format.

Two important modifications are apparent in the organization of the book. First, the former two beginning chapters have been streamlined into one introductory chapter. This chapter provides the student with an orientation in health education in the form of guides for effective living in college, including a description of college health resources. Second, a new concluding chapter has been added. This chapter, entitled "Health in Space," is concerned with the health problems of those who are exploring space as well as the effect of space explorations on the health of individuals and groups.

The organization of the major health content areas, the greatest portion of the book, has been kept intact. The plan was based on extensive study of the health needs of college students by one of the authors. Of course the events of the times, with their inherent stresses and problems, along with new scientific findings, have led to the inclusion of new health material in each of the areas. As a result, new material is presented in each chapter, and is particularly evident in the discussions of APHA concepts about health, the family cycle, pinning, care of the new baby, food additives, radiological health, civil defense plans, highway safety, and the new organization of the USPHS.

The illustrations, too, have been carefully revised. The best pictures from the second edition, those which clearly told their story, have been retained. However, new picture stories, line drawings, charts, and graphs have been added to make a more completely illustrated text.

The lists of suggested student activities that appeared in former editions have been eliminated. Such lists and other instructional and learning materials now comprise a new study guide to accompany the text. *Health for Effective Living,* the five McGraw-Hill text-films correlated with the book, the revised instructor's manual, and the study guide to accompany the text now constitute a comprehensive college health education packet.

Every effort has been made to allow for flexible use of the book and its accompanying materials, in accordance with the specific needs and interests of students in a particular college or university. We firmly believe that adequate coverage of health topics, not a skimpy treatise, should be provided for the college student, now and in the future. Sufficient material is included for a three-unit, semester course or for a four-unit course—two units each semester. Content can be selected for a two- or a one-unit course, as decisions are made with regard to the most imperative needs and interests of students. Some suggested patterns for specific situations are given in the instructor's manual. The activities in the study guide offer other clues for selection.

In addition to its use as a text for an organized course, this book can serve as a resource in a core program of instruction and as a personal guide for the student in self-study. It also may prove valuable for reference in one's personal library.

In view of these varied situations, and in keeping with the present trends in health education, *Health for Effective Living* is designed to assist the student in believing, as well as questioning wisely; it is designed to help the student understand himself, to stimulate an exploratory and creative attitude toward living, and to help him achieve wholesome health behavior.

We wish to acknowledge our gratefulness to the many persons who were most helpful in the development of the first and second editions as well as to those who contributed to this third edition.

We extend our sincere appreciation to the following health education authorities who critically reviewed our manuscripts or book and gave constructive criticism, support, and encouragement to the extent that preparing the third edition was a much easier task: Dr. Elena Sliepcevich, Director of the Bronfman School Health Education Study, (AAHPER) NEA, and Professor of Health Education, The Ohio State University; Dr. Wesley Staton, Professor and Chairman of Health Education, Colorado State

College, Greeley; Dr. Charles Richardson, Assistant Professor of Health Education, and Dr. Donald Boydston, Chairman, Department of Health Education, Southern Illinois University; Dr. Mary Beyrer, Associate Professor of Health Education, The Ohio State University; and Dr. Richard K. Means, Associate Professor, Health Education, Temple University.

Our particular thanks are extended to the following city college instructors for their helpfulness: Miss Doreen Abbott, Pasadena City College; Miss Mary Elizabeth Marshall, Long Beach City College; Miss Carol Nilsen and Mr. Edward B. De Groot, Santa Monica City College; and to our UCLA Health Education faculty: Dr. Ruth Abernathy, Dr. Ethel Bell, Dr. Joy Cauffman, Miss Orsie Thomson, Dr. Raymond Snyder, and Mr. John Fodor. Dr. Donald S. MacKinnon, Director, and Dr. Gertrude T. Huberty, Associate Physician, UCLA Student Health Service, continued to provide expert advice and counsel, for which we are most grateful.

Sincere appreciation is expressed to the following for reviewing special parts of the book: Representatives of the Food and Drug Administration; Mr. Glen L. Herstine, Supervisor, Space Thermodynamics and Nuclear Science Section, Missiles and Space Systems Division, Douglas Aircraft Company, Inc.; Dr. Kenneth H. Sutherland, Los Angeles County Health Officer and his staff; Mr. Roger Plaisted, Director of First Aid and Water Safety, Los Angeles Chapter, American National Red Cross; Dr. Leonard J. Dolton, Director of Health Education, National Dairy Council, Chicago, Ill., formerly Director of Dental Health Education, Southern California State Dental Association; Miss Marie A. Wall, Consultant in Hearing and Vision Education, Los Angeles County Superintendent of Schools' Office; and Mr. Donald Billam-Walker, Executive-Director, Honolulu Better Business Bureau.

We wish to acknowledge the United States Public Health Service and the American Association for Health, Physical Education, and Recreation for the privilege of attending and participating in the National Institute on the Science of Health Education, National Institute of Health, Bethesda, Maryland, as well as the Southwest Regional Institute. Both meetings, designed for college health instructors, were beneficial in making available the latest scientific health information.

Miss Jean Paty, Director of Health Education, Hawaii State Health Department, and Mr. J. Albert Torribio, Director of Health Education, Los Angeles City Health Department, provided new materials and assisted competently in our up-dating of health information.

Mr. Stanley Troutman and Mr. Richard Szladowski of the ASUCLA Photographic Department were most cooperative in photographing several of the new picture series, as were numerous college students who participated.

Special thanks go to our UCLA health education students who critically appraised the second edition and offered sound student opinion with regard to making the third edition more valuable to the consumer.

We again pay tribute to our wives—Bertha Johns, Merriom Sutton, and Grace Webster—for their continued valuable assistance in the preparation of the revised manuscript and for their constant encouragement and understanding.

To the publishing companies cited in the text we gratefully acknowledge permission to quote and reproduce materials.

EDWARD B. JOHNS
WILFRED C. SUTTON
LLOYD E. WEBSTER

TO THE STUDENT

This basic health science text is designed to help you to live a more effective life in our democratic society. It is built on our experience with college students and our belief that you can improve the essential factors that produce and maintain health. It is our firm conviction that basic health education can do much to help you in your efforts to favorably change your health behavior, with assistance from your family group, or your living group, and with the valuable guidance of your instructors.

The book is concerned with some of the determinants necessary for behavioral change, such as knowledge of scientific facts and principles, the formulation of sound personal goals, and understanding of the social pressures, customs, and traditions of college students. Other factors include the individual's own personal perceptions, growing out of his past experience, and his readiness and willingness for behavioral change, as well as opinion information received from home, church, and school, from peer groups, and from radio, television, newspapers, and magazines.[1]

[1] AAHPER, *Guidelines for Health Education: A Suggested Plan for Action*, Health Education Planning Conference, Highland Park, Illinois, October, 10–12, 1959, pp. 18–19.

The discussion in Chapter 1, on effective living in college, begins where you are now. It describes the college scene in the Space Age. Then a modern point of view on health is presented, to give you an understanding of basic concepts of health and the factors that influence health. The characteristics of a health-educated individual are outlined, to serve as guides for you in formulating goals—goals that can be achieved partially during the course and partially as you progress through your college years.

The discussion moves on to health problems of college students. These may be similar to problems you have or that you may soon face. The needs underlying these problems serve as the foundation for the college resources which are organized to protect, maintain, and improve your health. A brief description of the resources of a college community are presented so that you may be aware of the services, facilities, and educational activities available for your use. Opportunities for you to participate in and utilize these resources are discussed and illustrated.

The remaining chapters of the book provide scientific health information, and discuss factors that influence health and effective living.

HEALTH EDUCATION FILMS

The following 16-mm sound motion pictures are especially recommended for use with this book as they are correlated with particular chapters.

MAKING LIFE ADJUSTMENTS

A story of one student making both personal and social adjustments as he faces common problems of college students. Specific problems include lack of motivation and self-direction, emotional immaturity, and inadequate human relationships. CHAPTER 3.

QUACKS AND NOSTRUMS

A story based on the activities of the modern quack preying on the uninformed public. Clearly described are the organizations and agencies designed to protect the consumer from fraudulent health products and practices. CHAPTER 10.

CHOOSING A DOCTOR

The story shows how a family in a new community learns the importance of early and careful choice of a physician. This is brought home to the young married couple after an emergency forces hasty selection of an unknown doctor. CHAPTER 10.

SHOULD YOU DRINK?

This film discusses the importance of self-analysis in determining the part alcoholic beverages will play in each person's life. It analyzes motives for abstention, moderate drinking, and excessive drinking. CHAPTER 13.

COMMUNITY HEALTH IS UP TO YOU

This film shows how the health of a community depends on the collective action of its people, and how the people themselves can initiate action for solving their various health problems through a Community Health Council. CHAPTER 15.

Prints of these films may be rented from local film libraries or purchased from Text-Film Department, McGraw-Hill Book Company, Inc.

CONTENTS

Orientation in health education

It is apparent that you as a college student are interested in yourself as a person, in the way you live at college, and in the way you expect to live in your community after graduation. Most college students have a deep regard for their families and are developing a growing sense of responsibility toward their communities. They are not interested in "health for health's sake" or in "blood and bone hygiene," but this is only natural and normal. You, and other students, want to gratify your basic needs, such as to love, to be loved, to belong, to be recognized, to be independent, to have worthy goals, to have fun out of life, to get well when you are ill, to reproduce your kind, and to nurture your young. These are all aspects of good health and effective living.

Many of these fundamental needs remain the same. For example, you must always have food, water, and oxygen to survive. But many of your current problems, which may be considered as needs to be satisfied, do change, just as your environment changes. These problems must be faced during your college career, and they have an effect on your health and your life in college. Let us look, for example, at the environmental scene on your campus.

The college scene in the Space Age

The present college scene is a panorama that is constantly changing. It may include a beautiful campus with well-kept and artistically landscaped grounds and buildings and spacious acreage; or the campus now may be increasingly crowded with new buildings and parking facilities. The physical setting of colleges and universities is taking on new shapes and new hues as enrollments double, triple, or even, in some cases, quadruple, during this period of tremendous population increase.

Regardless of the psychological effect of the physical setting, steps are more than likely being taken to make your college environment a healthier and safer place to study, work, recreate, and live. Such efforts should include provisions for health services and health education, essential facets of an organized college health program for your benefit and protection.

In the Space Age there are bound to be changes in the ways people act and react in their environment. The new college scene undoubtedly depicts changes in human relationships, in institutions, and in personal and group values and goals. Such changes create new problems and new pressures, which must be solved and equalized; for example, now competition to enter and to stay in college is keener. The pace of everyday living is accelerated, with accompanying tensions. The social life of the campus, an important part of college life, brings the student into contact with the opposite sex, and dating, love, marriage, and preparation for parenthood are of real concern to many students.

Automation makes push-button living more real than was even thought possible a few years ago. Having a car at college provides easier transportation but cuts down on walking as an important type of physical activity. Faster and better transportation makes the intermingling of peoples more commonplace than in the past. Also, there are today more foreign students enrolled in our colleges and universities. Likewise, there is a trend toward establishing American campuses abroad. We are assuming more responsibilities for international health than in previous years. This is important, since disease-producing organisms know no boundaries.

Scientists on the campus and elsewhere are conducting research on ways and means to explore outer space. Newspapers, television, and radio report continuously on new rockets, missiles, satellites, and other space objects. Consequently, space terminology is a necessary part of our vocabulary. Problems of outer space, including health problems, are of interest to us all. Space exploits may affect our health, even as the employment of atomic power has created radiation and other problems that affect our lives. The attempts to conquer space may even change our concept of the wider community, which at present includes the local area in which we live, the state, the nation, and, to some degree, the world; in the future perhaps it may include outer space as well.

New scientific discoveries, particularly

in medicine, are so numerous as to be almost commonplace; yet there is a great lag visible between scientific knowledge and usage by both college students and the general population. The U.S. Public Health Service [1] reported in 1961 that every year medical research produces new, lifesaving knowledge. Because of the recent discoveries it is now possible to

> Cut Cancer Deaths
> Prevent Some Heart Disease
> Reduce Mental Illness
> Lessen Physical Handicaps
> Save Eye Sight
> Wipe Out Tuberculosis
> Prevent Polio
> Keep Teeth From Decaying

Many handicaps occur and many unnecessary deaths result because the available knowledge is not fully used. It is still a major problem to motivate people to accept and apply scientific information. There is a need for health education to provide scientific information, including knowledge of valuable service re-

sources, development of positive attitudes for effective living, and ways of facing problems and making wise decisions about health matters pertaining to the individual, the family, and the community.

To present the foundation of college health education, discussion in this chapter has been organized around the following questions:

What are the basic concepts about health, and health for effective living?

What health factors influence health and effective living?

What are the health problems of college students, shown from statistics and from research studies of health needs and interests?

What are the characteristic student goals of a health-educated college student?

What resources are essential in the college environment to meet these problems?

How can the student utilize these resources?

Concepts about health

Historically, the term *health* is derived from an old Anglo-Saxon word *haelth,* meaning the condition of being safe and sound, or whole. For many years this historical definition was lost because of the common belief that health was, in essence, freedom from disease. Health as a relative condition, state, or quality still has various meanings and interpretations for different people.

To the man on the street health may mean that he is not sick. The youngster may see it as washing his hands and face or brushing his teeth. To the mother it implies a happy family. To the coed it may refer to the way she looks, the way she feels, and the dates she gets. To some college men it is closely aligned with body build and skills derived from

physical education and athletics; to others it is the ability to spend long periods solving a problem in the laboratory.

To the quack doctor health results from the patient's buying that "best bottled health-winning nostrum" or habitually using "organic irrigations" for a fee payable in advance. To the physical culturist it is a "body beautiful," exhibiting rippling muscles gained through performing a set of prescribed systematic exercises. To the physiologist it is the product of the normal function of cells, organs, and systems. To the family physician it means constant supervision and care, utilizing the most modern medical services, including health guidance and periodic examinations, and the best equipment and facilities to ensure happy, zestful living of the total family.

To the person who has lost his health

[1] Public Health Service, *The Costly Time Lag,* Publication 813, U.S. Department of Health, Education, and Welfare, Washington, 1961, p. 2.

4

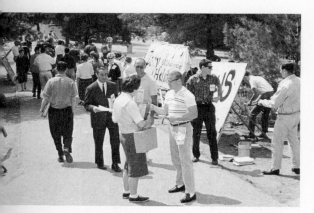

College life, from beginning to end, is a sum total of many activities.

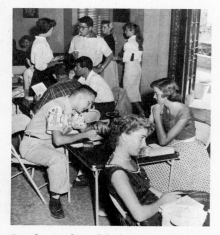

For the student, life begins with registration—and what a bewildering maze it is!

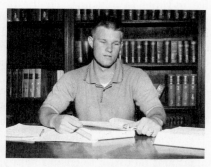

It is a time for seeking and gaining knowledge through study and intellectual discipline.

it is the most priceless possession of all. As Sir William Temple wrote: "Health is the soul that animates all the enjoyments of life, which fade and are tasteless without it." Franklin P. Adams stated that health is the thing that makes you feel that *now* is the best time of the year. To the person who has lost his money, health is his one hope. To quote an old Arabian proverb: "He who has health has hope, and he who has hope has everything." Disraeli once pointed out the significance of health to the state and nation in the statement, "The public health is the foundation upon which reposes the happiness of the people and the strength of the nation."

In 1961 the American Public Health Association published a report of a "Broadened Spectrum of Health and Morbidity." [2] This spectrum is visualized in four levels of public health concern and effort: (1) Mortality, (2) Serious morbidity, (3) Minor morbidity, and (4) Positive health. Each level will be described briefly:

Level 1: Mortality deals with the first essential of public health, which is to conserve life, as in the case of fighting deadly plagues and famine. Level 2: Serious morbidity refers to efforts to prevent, control, and reduce chronic illness. The prevention and control of accidents is a recent example. The treatment of streptococcal diseases for prevention of rheumatic fever is an older example. Level 3: Minor morbidity concerns are apparent in countries such as the United States that are far advanced in public health. Efforts are directed toward alleviation of minor illness such as the common cold, digestive disturbances, effects of smog, states of personal tension, and impairment of social relations. Level 4: Positive health. To reach this stage,

[2] Roscoe P. Kandle, "Report of the Chairman of the Technical Development Board to the Governing Council 1959-60," *American Journal of Public Health,* 51:287–288, February, 1961.

levels 1, 2, and 3 must have been met. It is at this point in which a society is applying social efforts by helping all persons toward a constructive and wholesome state of health in a safe and pleasant environment that longevity and happiness are promoted.

The authors believe that it is this last level toward which health education can be effectively directed and to which it can make a large contribution. Certainly it plays a part in each of the first three levels. However, its greatest function is the promotion of positive health for all.

The World Health Organization[3] defines health as "a state of complete physical, mental and social well-being and not merely the absence of disease or infirmity." This definition is important because 54 nations reached international agreement on it at the first World Health Assembly in 1948. It is the most widely accepted definition today.

Many of the above concepts or expressions of feelings about health are sound. Some are only partially true. A few are unscientific but represent common opinion. Such statements, along with the widely accepted but traditional definition by the World Health Organization, led the authors to attempt a more functional definition of health.

A MODERN DEFINITION OF HEALTH

Health is the quality, resulting from the total functioning of the individual, that empowers him to achieve a personally satisfying and socially useful life [22, 33]. This definition reflects the meaning of the old English term pertaining to the wholeness of the individual. It expresses health as a state of well-being, a dominance of positive or favorable adaptations, resulting from the interaction of the individual and his environment.

[3] Constitution of the World Health Organization, p. 3, from *Chronicle of the World Health Organization,* 1:29–43, 1947.

A point of view about health for effective living is derived from the above definition. Its key concepts are the unity of the individual, health as a quality of life, achievement of a personally satisfying life, and achievement of a socially useful life.

THE UNITY OF THE INDIVIDUAL

The individual responds to his environment as a whole. Sufficient scientific evidence points to the fact that he lives as a total being. He is made up of cells, organs, and systems, but they are so interrelated and integrated that he functions as a complete unit. That which affects one part brings about changes in others. The concept of psychosomatic medicine is based on the belief in this unity of the organism. Psychosomatic medicine is not a new field of medicine, designed as a cure for man faced with new health problems peculiar to the twentieth century. Actually, it is a medical approach that considers the patient as a whole person rather than as one with a specific localized disease. This approach unifies the physical, mental, and social factors producing health. All these factors are considered in treating a patient who has a disease. Psychiatrists have shown that a number of bodily disturbances are due to emotional causes. Fear of a disease can be so strong as to incapacitate a person from his daily activities, even though no disease organism is present; or the ideas he builds up about his own body may cause him great physical distress. These disturbances interfering with his quality of living are diseases just as much as are the common cold, influenza, and pneumonia.

There is no such thing as separate physical, mental, or social health. Each is an aspect of the whole, as the derivation of the term "health" implies. For purposes of discussion, physical and mental health may be considered separately, but in function they are inseparable. They are interrelated, integrated

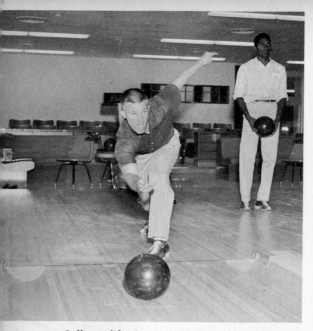

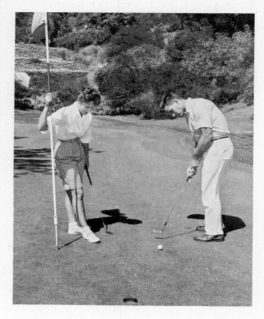

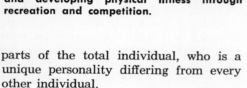
College life is a time, too, for continuing and developing physical fitness through recreation and competition.

parts of the total individual, who is a unique personality differing from every other individual.

HEALTH AS A QUALITY OF LIFE

The *quality of life* resulting from total functioning denotes a positive outcome of the art of fine living. This is *effective living*. The word "effective" is in keeping with the definition of health. According to Webster's *New Collegiate Dictionary, effective* means "producing a desired effect and being ready for service or action." The phrase "quality of life" implies that the person utilizes to the fullest his innate powers and all his capacities for living. Effective living results from the individual's functioning in a variety of life activities, including physical, mental, social, and spiritual experiences. What a person does—his work, his play, the food he eats, his sleep and rest, his loves, his hates, his successes, and his failures—all play a part in determining the quality of his life, or how effectively he lives. His daily experiences serve to mold his health; his present actions assist in building his future health

status or, conversely, tend to impair it. Today, emphasis is on the quality as well as the length of the life span.

ACHIEVEMENT OF A PERSONALLY SATISFYING LIFE

Personal achievement means effective action, through daily experiences, in reaching the goals established by the individual. This indicates that health is not a gift but rather something earned through personal actions.

Best action results when we obtain the facts about a problem, make sure of their accuracy, develop a deep belief in the significance and validity of this knowledge, and then use knowledge and belief as a basis for action. Our formula for action, then, is [4]

$$Scientific\ knowledge + positive\\ attitudes = best\ action$$

In health education this means that we must acquire facts regarding the factors that determine health, develop wholesome health attitudes, and demonstrate sound health practices to enrich our lives.

A personally satisfying life contributes

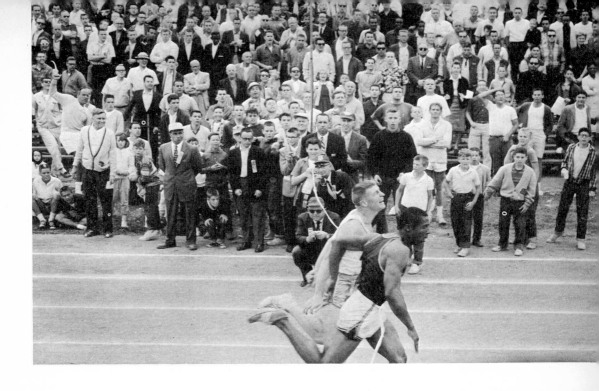

to effective living, that is, to being happy and at the same time useful. It denotes the ability to adjust to one's own environment—to fulfill individual responsibilities within the family group, to develop wholesome attitudes toward life, and to control emotions; it implies freedom from disease, health practices of personal cleanliness, immunization against disease, competent medical and dental care, and avoidance of accidents. It means a balanced program of life activities, including work, play, love, and faith.

ACHIEVEMENT OF A SOCIALLY USEFUL LIFE

The culture influences effective living. In a democracy, each individual is entitled to reach his fullest development and to live an effective life regardless of race, religion, political belief, or economic situation. Health in the cultural setting, however, means more than personal satisfaction or pure self-gratification. It involves the lives of others as well as one's own life. Health involves the home, the neighborhood, and the larger community.

Democratic group action is illustrated by the fight Americans are waging against heart disease, cancer, poliomyelitis, venereal disease, blindness, and many other diseases and defects. It is demonstrated by citizens' groups working together to assure the building of a community hospital; by the permanent civil defense program in a community; or by the response of college students to the blood bank in time of emergency. Community health endeavors extend from a health committee meeting in the smallest village to the World Health Assembly of the World Health Organization.

In a democracy the individual has the right to live effectively but he must accept the responsibility for helping provide the same right to all others. Whether he knows it or not, he changes his behavior as a result of participating in community activities. He changes in the interaction process. Furthermore, he has the opportunity, as well as the responsibility, to help shape his environment. In this respect, the individual's health potential is multiplied when he joins a group interested in health problems.

Effective living in society implies that the individual makes a contribution to society. He functions best when he is working for a cause greater than himself.

The individual is living more effectively when his attention is directed to others rather than when it is focused entirely on himself [33].

Factors influencing health

For a better understanding of health and health education it is desirable to discuss the essential factors that influence health. These are interrelated factors, which contribute to the total functioning of the individual. For the purpose of study they are categorized as hereditary and environmental factors. The significant environmental health factors are presented in terms of basic health needs, which have been determined from research studies.

HEREDITY

Heredity contributes to effective living the innate endowment for health given by one's parents. It plays an important role in determining the uniqueness of each individual and his particular health status. Good heredity implies a sound constitution, a well-developed body, and normal intelligence. Effective living signifies that the individual is utilizing all his innate capacities to the fullest extent. He cannot change his heredity; no activity of the body cells can affect the germ cells. However, guidance from competent counselors can assist him to make the most of his endowment. Further discussion of heredity is found in Chapter 2, pages 45 to 47.

ENVIRONMENT

The total environment consists of all the external influences from conception to death. Our food, shelter, and clothing; cultural patterns, including language, customs, traditions, beliefs, superstitions, and taboos; mass media such as television, radio, newspapers, popular magazines, and scientific journals—all affect our daily actions. The physical environment, especially climate and geography,

also exerts an influence on our lives and sets limits on activities and achievements.

Environmental activities are all the experiences engaged in by the individual. These are the experiences that determine the way one lives, which to a large extent produces the quality of one's life and the degree of effective living. Experiences can be classified as physical, mental, social, and spiritual. They include all daily activities and all health practices. Selection of wholesome experiences and participation in a balanced program of life activities exert a positive influence on the quality of life.

Mental health factors. To be healthy psychologically and emotionally requires an understanding of one's self image, one's mental assets and liabilities and basic life goals. An individual's adjustment pattern is determined by his fundamental personality structure. The total integration of the individual results from making intelligent personal and social adjustments while engaging in life activities.

Personal adjustments include adjustments to one's environment, such as accepting and making the best of one's own body, accepting responsibility and making adjustments within the family group, controlling emotions, and developing wholesome attitudes toward life. Satisfying basic mental health needs, such as those for affection, recognition, and independence, is a specific example. Meeting needs does not mean mere conformity. The highest levels of adjustment are those requiring critical judgments, value discriminations, creativity, and initiative.

Social adjustments include adaptation to the physical, social, and cultural environment. Achieving success in the significant areas of living and making a contribution to society are examples of the highest type of social adjustment.

Family health factors. The family is the basic unit in our society. Therefore, each individual has a responsibility to play successfully several roles in the family-life cycle. The way we carry out these responsibilities definitely influences our health and effective living. Family-life roles include the following:

Being sincere, communicative, and sociable and acquiring status in relationships with family members.

Being able to make satisfactory heterosexual adjustments, understanding one's sex role, and being able both to express and to control emotions.

Selecting the right marriage partner.

Making intelligent adjustments during marriage or if one does not marry.

Becoming, when married, an interested, responsible, and effective parent able to guide and direct the development of children.

Being a good and strong parent is more difficult than ever before because of our changing times and cultural patterns.

Factors of body maintenance and care. A well-developed, physically fit body is one of the most essential of health needs; yet our American way of life is not conducive to a high degree of physical fitness. Each person should be able to perform the day's activities without becoming unduly fatigued and still have an adequate reserve to meet any emergency that might arise. President Kennedy, in his article, "The Soft American," [4] described

[4] John F. Kennedy, "The Soft American," *Sports Illustrated*, 13:16–17, Dec. 26, 1960.

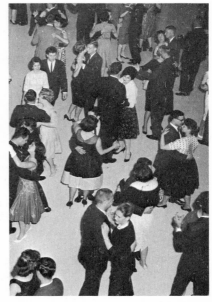

Social activities add needed balance to successful college life.

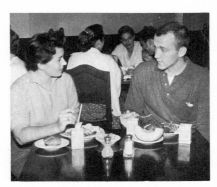

Eating well is essential to enable the student to carry out his academic and social responsibilities.

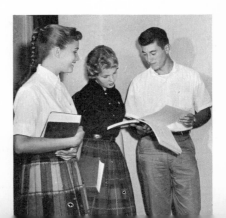

Sharing work and pleasures with others is a part of every student's college education.

the decline of physical strength and ability of young Americans. Specifically, he wrote:

For physical fitness is not only one of the most important keys to a healthy body; it is the basis of dynamic and creative intellectual activity. . . . In this sense, physical fitness is the basis of all activities of our society. And if our bodies grow soft and inactive, if we fail to encourage physical development and prowess, we will undermine our capacity for thought, for work and for the use of those skills vital to an expanding and complex America.

It is known that regular exercise increases the circulation, improves respiration, increases endurance, and helps develop muscle tonus. It assists in removing wastes, aids in keeping down the cholesterol content of the blood vessels, and contributes to total body health.

Good posture, sound dental health practices, proper elimination of body wastes, and good grooming are all aspects of maintaining and caring for a healthy body.

Nutritional factors. Eating a balanced diet is an essential life activity. Because of the absolute necessity of nutrition to life and health, it is considered here as a separate health-producing factor. A balanced diet provides the cells of the body the essential nutrients for three main purposes: (1) for growth and repair, (2) for regulation of body processes, and (3) for a source of energy. The right kinds of foods—milk, eggs, vegetables, fruits, meat or fish, cereal, and whole-grain or enriched bread—in proper balance provide the nutritional needs of the body and markedly affect the quality of life. Also, proper foods aid in regular elimination of body wastes.

Improper nutrition is a health problem in the United States, but not for lack of food. Rather, a large proportion of our population is undernourished because the food eaten is not of the proper quality and is not in proper balance. Overweight is also a major problem. Much improvement can be made in the nutritional practices of individuals and groups.

Consumer health, including professional health services. This factor consists of: wisely purchasing health products, adequate medical and dental care, and applying health education to all consumer health activities. Health services range from preventive to curative measures, including health guidance, periodic health examinations, recording of health histories, and clinical, surgical, and hospital care. Health education should enable one to understand the role of professional services in effective living, select competent health advisers, discover how to secure continuous medical supervision and care, and determine ways and means to pay for health products and professional services. Great strides in solving the nationwide problem of providing competent professional health services for both the individual and the group are being made, and will be made in the near future.

Freedom from disease and accidents. Although this factor is no longer considered as total health, it is a vital aspect of health. Modern control of communicable disease is one of man's great achievements and has done much to increase effective living and longevity. Metropolitan Life Insurance Company [5] reports life expectancy at birth in the United States among its policyholders to be seventy years. Influenza, pneumonia, tuberculosis, and the venereal diseases still have not been completely eliminated, and there is much yet to be accomplished in disease prevention and control. The chronic and degenerative diseases, heart disease, cancer, and other top killers are still unconquered. Examples of intelligent health practices to increase effective

[5] Metropolitan Life Insurance Company, *Statistical Bulletin*, June, 1960, p. 2.

living include building resistance to disease through a balanced program of physical activity, adequate sleep and rest, proper diet, and scientifically proved immunizations; avoiding sources of infection; seeking prompt medical and dental care, including regular medical and dental examinations; and taking plenty of time to recover when disease strikes.

Accidents in the home, on the highways, and in industry constitute an unsolved problem. Living effectively yet safely in present-day society is definitely an art that must be learned.

There is great opportunity for improvement, personally and in the community, with respect to freedom from disease and accidents, through better health education.

Stimulants and depressants as factors affecting health. Stimulants and depressants continue to be major factors relating to personal and community health as new evidence of their effects is made available by research.

Former Surgeon General Leroy E. Burney, M.D., of the U.S. Public Health Service, in a statement on "Smoking and Lung Cancer" in the Nov. 28, 1959, issue of the *Journal of the American Medical Association;* Malcolm H. Merrill, M.D., Director of the California State Department of Public Health, in the June 1, 1959, issue of *California's Health;* and Herman E. Hilleboe, M.D., Commissioner, New York State Department of Health, have all summarized the data from the research studies. Dr. Hilleboe's Bureau of Cancer Control sets forth general conclusions as follows: [6]

The evidence indicates that persons who smoke cigarettes increase their chances of developing lung cancer. There is no evidence to contradict this conclusion. This does not

mean that cigarette smoking is considered to be the sole or essential cause of lung cancer or that it may not require other causative factors or act in conjunction with them. The role of air pollution, exhaust from cars, trucks, and buses, and other irritants remains to be established. . . .

From the practical standpoint we believe there is already enough evidence incriminating cigarette smoking to justify advising the public that the available evidence is consistent with the view that cigarette smoking is one of the causative factors in lung cancer and that stopping cigarette smoking may therefore be a means of lowering the incidence of lung cancer.

Alcohol is a depressant—not a stimulant, as some persons believe. It depresses the cerebral cortex, the most sensitive part of the brain. When the cortex is affected, tensions subside, self-consciousness disappears, and inhibitions are removed. Alcohol relaxes many persons who use it moderately. At the same time memory, reasoning, responsible behavior, and conscience are affected adversely. When alcohol reaches the lower brain centers, speech becomes thickened and coordination is poor. Its use is dangerous when it is uncontrolled or habitual. Overdrinking is cited as a leading factor in the increased divorce rate. The worst consequence of even moderate drinking is its direct relationship to traffic accidents. The National Safety Council reports that a drinking driver is involved in 30 per cent of fatal traffic accidents [21].

Certain drugs have most serious effects on health. Marihuana, the hypnotic drug, is the steppingstone to heroin addiction. Heroin is a habit-forming drug, with effects similar to those of morphine. There is temporarily great elation and loss of the sense of pain; for a while the user is at complete peace with the world. But in three to six hours the addict needs another dose and this is a continuous process. Nothing is more silent and sinister than drug addiction; nothing is more difficult to cure. The addict is a sick person—physically, mentally, and mor-

[6] Herman E. Hilleboe: *"Cigarette Smoking and Lung Cancer,"* Bureau of Cancer Control, New York State Department of Health, pamphlet distributed outside New York State by Health Education Service, Albany 1, N.Y., 1959.

ally. Unfortunately, the greatest number of drug addicts are teen-agers or young adults.

Community health factors. Major health problems that affect individuals and groups together become the concern of the total community. Most health factors that relate to the individual also relate to the community. Community organization, the process of uniting individuals and groups to solve common problems, is the focus of community health education. Most communities have available health services provided by a city, county or state health department (the official agency); education, services, and research from voluntary health agencies (such as the American Heart Association, the American Cancer Society, and the National Tuberculosis Association); professional associations, for example, the county medical and county dental societies; and coordinating agencies, such as coordinating councils and welfare planning councils. Citizen participation assists the officials of these many health resources in their fight to eradicate disease and defects and to promote better health.

Health problems, needs, and interests

Health problems can be identified by various means. Three procedures are presented here: first, there are some interesting and rather startling statistics, to illustrate specific health problems; second, the results of investigations of the health needs of college students are summarized; third, a selection of questions most frequently checked in a study of student health needs and interests is discussed.

SELECTED PERTINENT HEALTH STATISTICS

Did you know that: A study of Cornell University students revealed that 96 per cent of students require medical care during one to eight semesters of their academic career [25].

A fantastic number of young people suffer from various forms of mental disturbance. It is estimated that 16 per cent of all new admissions to state mental hospitals are patients between 16 and 29 years of age. (U.S. Public Health Service, May 4, 1959.)

Mental illness afflicts one person in every ten. (National Association for Mental Health, 1959.) The mentally ill fill half the nation's hospital beds.

(*The Costly Time Lag,* U.S. Public Health Service, No. 813, 1961.)

Approximately one college student in five is married, and 93 per cent of all Americans are or will be married. (Bowman, *Marriage for Moderns,* 1960.)

Money and children are the two most common areas of disagreement between husband and wife. (Blood and Wolfe, *Husbands and Wives,* 1960.)

Maternal mortality has dropped 55 per cent in ten years. Now maternal death occurs once for every 2,700 live births. (*Monthly Vital Statistics Report,* Annual Summary for 1959, Part 2, Vol. 8, Aug. 12, 1960.)

Dental caries affects almost 100 per cent of America's youth. (U.S. Public Health Service, May 4, 1959.) The average American has lost half his teeth by the time he is 40. (*The Costly Time Lag,* U.S. Public Health Service, No. 813, 1961.)

Poor vision and blindness together rank fourth in the list of disabilities in the United States. (U.S. National Health Survey, *Health Statistics,* April, 1959.)

Nearly 6 million persons in the United States have some degree of hearing impairment. Hearing loss is the No. 1 physical impairment. (U.S. National Health Survey, *Health Statistics,* 1959.)

An estimated six out of ten Americans make frequent use of laxatives. (Hook, *Today's Health,* October, 1960.)

Girls in the 13–20 age group demonstrated the least favorable nutritional status of subjects in a nationwide study. (Morgan, *Nutritional Status, U.S.,* 1960.)

Most American families at present are not able to pay for modern medical care. (Strauss, "Can We Afford to Be Healthy?" *Harper's Magazine,* July, 1960.)

Some 50,000 cases of infectious venereal disease are reported annually for the group under 20 years of age. (U.S. Public Health Service, May 4, 1959.) In 1960 an increase of 11.4 per cent occurred in the 15–19 age group. (American Social Health Association, February, 1960.)

Almost three out of five acute conditions are respiratory. (U.S. National Health Survey, *Health Statistics,* Series B, No. 18, June, 1960.)

About 70 million persons in the United States have one or more chronic conditions. (U.S. Department of Health, Education, and Welfare, *Indicators,* January, 1961.)

One out of every thirteen men aged 20 or over is an alcoholic. (O'Hollaren and Wellman, *California Medicine,* 89:129, August, 1958.) Approximately 4¼ million men and ¾ million women in the United States are alcoholics. (Keller and Efron, *Quarterly Journal of Studies on Alcohol,* 19:316, June, 1958.)

Eighty-six per cent of juvenile drug addicts are between 18 and 20 years of age. (U.S. Treasury Department, Bureau of Narcotics, Dec. 31, 1958.)

Injuries in colleges and universities may occur in a ratio as high as one to six students, according to an accident survey. (Dvorak, reported by Richardson [25].)

Research has established that at least 5,000 lives could be saved annually if occupants were not thrown from motor vehicles when accidents occur and that the severity of injuries experienced in motor vehicle accidents is lessened when occupants are restrained by safety belts. (*Public Health Reports,* April, 1960.)

Pollution of the nation's waters by municipal and industrial wastes is currently regarded as a national disgrace. (*Today's Health,* March 1961.)

In 1960, malaria continued to be a constant threat to more than 1 billion people. (*World Health,* March-April, 1960).

There is one certainty concerning protective shelters. Under existing conditions of nuclear possibilities a total artificial environment created well underground would provide safety. (*Consumer Reports,* January, 1962.)

These sample statistics point up some basic problems, which will be discussed in more detail in the following chapters.

HEALTH NEEDS AND INTERESTS OF COLLEGE STUDENTS

Data are presented by many authorities on the needs and interests of college students [7, 30, 31]. Needs relating primarily to *mental health*—problems of adjustment to self and others—are most frequently reported. These needs can be summarized as follows [30]:

Lack of adjustments in home and family relationships

Lack of motivation and self-direction

Unfavorable relationships with others

Inadequate emotional adjustment

Tensions resulting from conflicting moral codes

Tensions associated with the academic program

Tensions associated with economic adjustments

Tensions associated with problems of housing and transportation

Tensions associated with disparity between individual goals and a student's capacity to achieve them

Worry about personal health

Problems resulting from poor attitudes concerning mental illness

These mental health needs are not

separate and distinct. Many needs arise from a combination of factors, and sometimes one problem may lead to another and in this way involve several needs. Adjustment to these needs is considered in detail in Chapters 2 and 3.

The area of family-life education, hereafter referred to as *family health,* and the use of stimulants and depressants are high on the list of students' interests. College students are involved in establishing good relationships with the opposite sex. Petting and premarital sex relations are immediate problems that many college students have difficulty in solving satisfactorily. Some students are confused because of the lack of accurate information; others, because of conflicting moral codes regarding sex relationships. Most college students are vitally concerned with laying the proper foundation for a successful marriage and a happy home of their own. They feel the need for assistance in this matter.

The use of *alcohol* is sometimes a problem. Students coming from homes where alcohol has not been used and associating with other students who accept its use must resolve the conflict between the moral code established in their homes and that practiced by other members of the college group.

The time required for studies, work, and social activities results in the piling up of class assignments unless the student plans carefully. When this happens, some students begin to use *stay-awake drugs* for long periods of time in order to cram for exams and to complete other work. Occasionally, a student, because of emotional tensions, finds it difficult to sleep and makes use of sleep-inducing drugs. In either case—stay-awake drugs or sleep-inducing compounds—a vicious habit may be started.

Since *ill health* is a liability, each student needs to reduce the number and severity of the conditions that cause it. Information gathered from health service records provides some insight into the problems of concern to the general college student [30]. Colds and other common respiratory infections are the most frequent cause of students' seeking the assistance of health service personnel. Skin disorders resulting either from infections or from dietary inadequacies also cause many to seek treatment through the college health service. Problems associated with vision and with hearing difficulties cause some to call for a physician's service, though there is evidence that more individuals should be under medical care for the prevention and treatment of such troubles.

The increase in the number of students requiring medical care after busy school weekends and holidays and near the end of the semester indicates that *chronic fatigue* is a problem. Nutritional insufficiencies are found to be a contributing factor in the poor health status of such students in a number of cases.

Failure to plan effectively for adequate rest, relaxation, sleep, and leisure-time activities is commonly suggested by students as the reason for a general rundown physical condition. A student who is active in the social life of his college finds that careful planning is necessary in order to provide for adequate rest, along with the time required for studying and for leisure-time activities. A high percentage of students at some time find that their programs are out of balance, and the effect on their general health becomes quite apparent to them.

Of the more *serious communicable diseases* that attack the college age group, tuberculosis is a major problem. Medical science and education have been partially successful in reducing the seriousness of this disease. Tuberculosis may be further reduced in prevalence and severity through improved and intensified case finding, development of effective immunization procedures, and the application of specific drug treatment.

In the general population, the age group that includes college students has a comparatively high venereal-disease rate. College students as a group do not contract venereal diseases to the extent that the same age group in the general population does. However, any sexually promiscuous individual is a possible source of venereal infection. Therefore, these diseases are a problem to some college students. Another communicable disease, infectious mononucleosis, is of sufficient concern to be referred to as the "college student's disease" by health service personnel.

Although the *chronic and degenerative diseases* do not become an immediate problem to most college students, some individuals in this group have malignant growths, diabetes, nephritis, heart disorders, or rheumatism, as well as other diseases. In addition, the parents of college students are in the age groups more frequently affected by such disorders. The individual whose parents or other relatives have cancer, heart disease, or diabetes needs accurate information about these diseases. Otherwise, all the false information that exists about them, and the many poor attitudes toward them, may create persistent problems.

College students who eat all their meals at one of the college- or university-regulated food services are likely to be offered a *well-balanced diet*. The offering of well-balanced meals does not ensure, however, that the students make wise selections. In addition, many students eat their meals in restaurants or other public eating places where they may not be offered foods that provide all the nutrients needed by the body. College students, generally speaking, are well fed; few of them show extreme deficiency symptoms. Many students, on the other hand, are operating at a level below their achievement potential because of insufficiencies in their diet.

Dental health, a major health problem in the total population, is also a problem to college students. In a study of health needs of college students the poorest health practices were those relating to dental health.

Because of the impending selection of a mate, the hereditary transmission of characteristics or traits becomes a concern for some students. The individual who is concerned should seek help in securing accurate information to solve personal problems of this type.

The individual student is confronted with the need for *selecting competent health services,* particularly if the college health services are limited in scope. The influence of advertising makes it difficult to evaluate effectively the many health products offered for sale. Some of these products are harmless, the only ill effect being felt in the pocketbook. Others, however, are harmful to a particular person. The widespread use of laxatives, painkillers, and vitamin preparations illustrates the need for improved understanding in this area.

Students need assistance in overcoming postural problems or difficulties associated with *body mechanics.* Since remediable defects of this type can have a pronounced effect on the individual, psychologically as well as physiologically, their detection and correction are beneficial. Many corrective or adapted programs are carried on by the physical education department, working closely with medical personnel.

Poor muscular coordination is a severe health problem for some students because it leads them to restrict their participation in many group activities. Such an individual may limit his physical activity to the extent that his health is affected, or he may develop unhealthy attitudes.

Accidents continue to play an important role as a cause of disablement or death. Students have accidents in living quarters on and off campus, in vehicles used for transportation to and from classes or for recreational purposes, in physical education activities, and in the college buildings. To some degree, partial disablement resulting from an accident affects nearly every student at one time or another during his college career. Fortunately, for the majority this disablement is temporary.

The health concerns of college students can be summarized under the following headings: [7]

Mental health

Family health

Healthy body developed through a balanced program of physical activity, rest, and relaxation

Dental health

Nutrition

Consumer health (health products and services)

Communicable diseases

Chronic diseases

Stimulants and depressants

Safety and accident prevention

Community health

HEALTH INTERESTS DETERMINED BY CUSHMAN-BENNETT HEALTH PROBLEM CHECK LIST

An example of identifying health problems by means of a check list is the Cushman-Bennett study of specific health problems of high school seniors and college freshmen [7]. From the investigators' research with 199 questions covering personal and community health, a list of pertinent problems was formulated, based on student needs and interests.

The following are some examples selected from the check list:

Mental Health: What qualities are characteristic of the mature adult? What signs and symptoms indicate that one is poorly adjusted? How can I avoid worry?

Preparation for Marriage: What are the important things to consider in selecting a marriage partner? How far should one go in petting and necking? What are the early signs of pregnancy? What hereditary factors should be considered by a young couple before marriage?

Body Maintenance and Care: How does one develop good posture? Is there anything I can do to prevent skin blemishes? How can I reduce tooth decay?

Alcohol, Smoking and Drugs. Can people addicted to drugs such as heroin be cured? How does alcohol affect one's ability to drive? Are there good reasons for not smoking?

Nutrition: What is a safe way to lose weight? Can a poor diet make me tire more easily and become fatigued?

Consumer Health: When one moves to a new community how does one make a wise selection of a doctor and dentist? What kind of health insurance should I buy?

Communicable Disease: How can one prevent tuberculosis and upper respiratory diseases such as the common cold, flu, and pneumonia?

Degenerative Disease: What can one do to reduce the possibilities of cancer? Heart disease? Hardening of the arteries?

Safety and First Aid: What first-aid procedures should I be able to carry out? What is the best method of artificial respiration?

Community: What services should be provided by a good local department of health? What measures can the community take to protect its citizens against acute and chronic diseases?

These questions, which were those most frequently raised by students participating in the investigation, may be of help to you. They may suggest for you particular interests that you have or may want to develop in each of these health education areas. An attempt is made to answer these and other questions in subsequent chapters.

Characteristics of a health-educated individual

Behavior characteristics, in the form of specific goals to be achieved, have been

formulated from a study of the health problems of college students and their needs and interests. These characteristics are outlined to indicate the health knowledge, attitudes, and practices of a college

[7] Wilfred C. Sutton, "Determining the Health Needs of College Students," unpublished doctoral dissertation, University of California, Los Angeles, 1954.

student who assumes responsibility for his own health and for that of his family and that of his community.

Some of these characteristics you have attained already; others may be incorporated into your own program of action as you finish a part of this book and a part of the health education course or when you have finished the book and completed the course; still others may become a part of your personal health program in later years. These characteristics are presented to help determine action for better health and more effective living. They also indicate the health information to be found in subsequent chapters. They are organized under three headings: (1) personal living, (2) personal-social relations, and (3) community relations.

PERSONAL LIVING

The student:

Is developing a consistent and unified outlook on life—a philosophy of life; expresses several attainable major goals and has a plan for achieving a useful life centered in work, play, love, and faith.

Is achieving status as a person through growth in independence.

Understands his own health assets and liabilities; appreciates health appraisals, including periodic health examinations and screening tests; is willing to improve when positive changes can be made.

Keeps himself in good physical condition through a balanced program of exercise, recreation, rest, and sleep.

Selects food wisely, using a guide such as *A Daily Food Guide* to assure a balanced diet as well as a variety of foods for pleasure.

Establishes a regular habit for elimination of waste products.

Views his body as a medium of self-expression; increases his poise through good posture; dresses appropriately for occasions and seasons; attempts to make his own appearance as attractive as possible, exemplifying personal cleanliness.

Shows vitality with reserves of energy and power while participating in activities.

Has a feeling of achievement resulting from participation in life activities.

Understands his sex role; both expresses and controls emotions.

Makes intelligent decisions on the use of drugs, tobacco, and alcoholic beverages.

Knows reliable sources of health information and appraises health information according to basic criteria, e.g., education and experience of the author, scientific accuracy of content, and underlying motivation.

Selects health products wisely to save money and also to safeguard health.

Distinguishes between sound medical practice and quackery.

Is aware of the dangers of self-medication.

Takes advantage of immunizations as a means of protection against disease.

Recognizes the common danger signals of disease and is prompt in seeking medical attention when they appear.

Takes time to recuperate after illness or accident occurs.

Protects himself against dental caries by regular brushing of the teeth, proper nutrition, and periodic visits to dentist.

Attempts to do things the right way—the safe way; is a careful, considerate driver and an alert, intelligent pedestrian.

PERSONAL-SOCIAL RELATIONS

The student:

Has status in family relations.

Has status with his fellow students of both sexes through his effective participation in several groups.

Is sincere, communicative, and sociable, entering heartily and with enjoyment into social activities.

Is considerate and helpful and is growing in his concern for other people, their plans, successes, and failures; is willing to sublimate personal desires for the larger concerns of the groups to which he belongs.

Makes satisfactory heterosexual adjustments.

Understands the importance of having a family physician and dentist as personal health advisers for his own and his family's protection and care.

Understands the importance of a medical-care plan for himself and his family.

Knows how to select a health adviser of the type that can best assist him and his family.

Takes care of others as well as himself in unfamiliar surroundings—e.g., water, fire, or forest—or in emergencies.

Helps maintain a safe, orderly home.

COMMUNITY RELATIONS

The student:

Knows the health resources of the community—official, voluntary, professional, and commercial.

Expresses an interest in promoting effective living in his own environment.

Is beginning to participate effectively in the health activities and projects of social institutions—the home, the school, and the community; e.g., participates in group discussions of common college and community problems, becomes a member of college health and safety committees or councils.

Reports frauds and suspected frauds in writing to nearest bureau of the Food and Drug Administration or to the Better Business Bureau.

Reports to authorities environmental hazards in college neighborhood and community, such as broken pavements or poorly lighted streets.

Appreciates the health professions as careers that are personally and socially useful.

College health resources

The foregoing discussions point out the significance of health education, health services, and a healthful environment. It is now pertinent to consider the resources provided by the college and/or the community to promote, protect, and maintain the health of students and to meet their health needs.

SPECIFIC HEALTH ACTIVITIES AND SERVICES

Each health resource comprises a number of activities and services designed to meet the health needs of students, referred to previously. Together the activities and services of the health resources constitute the college health program.

To develop an understanding of these resources, the following questions are raised for your consideration:

How can I improve my health status?

How am I protected against communicable diseases at college?

What do I do when I catch a cold, break out with a rash, or develop a high fever?

How can I protect myself against chronic diseases, such as cancer, heart diseases, and nephritis?

What do I do if I develop a severe pain in the abdomen, the chest region, or some other part of the body?

How can I correct a physical defect while at college?

To whom do I turn for assistance if problems pile up on me and seem to overpower me?

To whom should I turn for premarital and marital scientific information?

To whom can I refer a fellow student who shows signs of becoming a disturbed person?

How do I know whether I am following the right vocational pursuit?

Why should I develop understanding about health education?

How can I keep physically fit and maintain a sound academic schedule?

How can I develop physical skills for future participation in sports?

What are my responsibilities as a citizen in the college environment?

How can I contribute to making the college campus a better community?

THE COLLEGE HEALTH PROGRAM: ORGANIZATION OF HEALTH RESOURCES

Every college or university has a number of health resources, which provide opportunities for students to develop their maximum potentialities and which establish procedures for the health protection of students, faculty, and other personnel.

Not all colleges are able financially or in terms of personnel and facilities to incorporate all phases of an ideal health program. It is encouraging, however, to report that better college health programs are increasing. Perhaps in the near future every college will have a complete program that adequately meets the needs of each individual student. Credit for efforts toward this goal must be given the professional associations, such as the American College Health Association and the American Association for Health, Physical Education, and Recreation, and the voluntary health agencies, particularly the National Tuberculosis Association. These associations and agencies are interested in the college health team and serve as a stimulus to those persons who comprise it. Improved programs in educational institutions are the results of their coordinated professional efforts.

The factors determining the type and extent of the program in each educational institution include the size, location, and financial resources of the institution; the composition of the student body, i.e., the number of day students and dormitory students and the number of married students; the professional health personnel employed; and the community health resources available. The focus in this chapter is on the health resources of the college community.

The significant health resources on the campus that contribute to health promotion and the protection of the student comprise the college health program. These resources may include:

A health committee or council
College health service
Health education
Healthful college living (environmental aspects), including environmental sanitation, study facilities, counseling and guidance center, and student housing
Physical education
Off-campus community health resources

Because of varying factors that determine the program, no one common pattern of organization exists throughout the country. Several colleges and universities have established an administrative division for each of the following: health education, healthful college living, and health services. Some combine the three under health education and health services. Others combine health education and physical education, with health services separate. The activities within these components of the program range from no specifically planned health education and only minimum first aid or emergency care to a complete array of health education experiences and environmental health procedures, and health services with medical care and hospitalization. A part of this varied program includes a well-organized counseling and guidance service along with a diversified program of physical education and recreational activities. The community health resources with their many activities supplement and support many of these college functions in a complete program.

Health committee or council. The college president, as the chief administrative officer, is responsible to the board of trustees for the health program. It is common practice for the president to delegate responsibility for the program to a director and/or a faculty health committee or council. Such a committee or council frequently is organized to serve as a planning, problem-solving, coordinating, and recommending body. Recommendations are made to the president for the conduct of the program.

Some colleges and universities have a health coordinator as the administrative officer responsible to the president. In others the president, a vice-president, or a dean coordinates functions that are performed by several departments. In such cases the director of health service and the director of physical education, among others, would each report to the administrative officer.

It is common practice for the committee or council to work with faculty and student groups to identify the current major health problems facing the students and the college. Then a priority rating is given these problems. A plan of action is developed for each problem. The facts are assembled and interpreted. Recommendations are then sent to the president, who makes the necessary decisions and implements the recommendations. Problems may range from removing a safety hazard on the campus to hiring additional health personnel or establishing new health education courses in the college curriculum.

The success of the program is enhanced when there is adequate representation of persons on the committee or council from the significant health resources, when there is clarification of lines of authority, when there is coordination of functions among the many departments contributing to the program, when there is opportunity for students to share in the development of the program, and when each faculty member assists in meeting the health needs of students.

Cooperation and support by the administration, faculty, nonacademic personnel, students, and community leaders working together in a team effort makes possible a functional college health program.

Health service. A college health service may function as a medical office, an infirmary, a student hospital, or a student health service. Despite the variation in form, the function is to determine student health needs and find ways and means to meet them.

The following are essential activities and services:

Appraising the health status of all students. This means assessing the health needs of students through health histories, screening tests for vision and hearing, chest X rays, chest photofluorograms for tuberculosis, medical examinations including urinalysis, eye, ear, nose, and throat examinations, and dental and psychological examinations. Some colleges and universities require that appraisals be made by family physicians. Others provide these as a student health service function.

Encouraging and advising the student on ways to correct remediable defects. Defects are corrected if possible; otherwise, students are referred to private physicians, local clinics, or other resources as the cases demand.

Following up on the correction of defects and the examination findings.

Controlling communicable disease, including protection of the student through immunizations, such as those for smallpox, typhoid, poliomyelitis, and influenza. Some student health services place the responsibility for obtaining immunizations on the student.

Providing medical treatment of ambulatory patients. This service may be restricted to emergency care only, with limited diagnosis and treatment, or it may include complete diagnosis and treatment. Some modern student health services now provide adequate clinical care for the ill as a part of their own function or as a coordinated and cooperatively conducted function with medical schools and clinical consultants situated in the local community.

Providing dental care. The present trend is to include dental care, at least emergency dentistry, as well as medical care.

Providing hospitalization for students needing bed care.

Providing health education through health guidance and medical counseling.

Classifying students with physical and mental defects and recommending the appropriate academic work load and physical activities.

Providing mental health and psychiatric care, comprising both prevention and clinical treatment.

Cooperating with other departments to provide a safe, healthful environment.

Many student-health-service activities involve health guidance or counseling. More students come to the health service with personal problems such as chronic fatigue than appear with tuberculosis, anemia, heart disease, glandular disturbance, or other organic disease.

Medical and dental examinations provide information essential in determining health status. The family physician keeps a complete health history with detailed information about the individual and the other members of his family. The function of the medical doctor in treating one who is ill has long been accepted, but his function as an adviser who helps prevent illness and maintain optimum health is too frequently overlooked. The entrance examination by the college physician—or the family physician, as is the practice in some institutions—provides the health personnel of the college or university with basic information beneficial in health protection and maintenance. It is the individual's responsibility to make the most of the opportunities provided by the health service personnel. A new trend is to require health examina-

tions for faculty members and other employees as well as for students.

College physicians may find a student attempting to do something which does not interest him or for which he has no aptitude. They may recommend that a student change his course or major field. With the aid of his counselor this change may be brought about. Many students are able to stay in college by having their load lightened or receiving valuable advice to relieve worry or anxiety. The student who is not sleeping at night may find a consultation with a doctor at the health service most valuable. Proper interpretation of defects found during the entrance or periodic medical examination may relieve needless worry due to lack of understanding of the condition. Advice on premarital and marital health is given students by the staff when it is requested.

In some colleges and universities health services are financed entirely by general funds; in others, by a special health service or medical fee paid for in tuition fees or included in student fees. Still others use an insurance plan plus one of the above-mentioned methods. It is a wise health service policy to provide the student with the experience of participating in a prepayment plan for medical care. This practice, carried over into later years, serves to protect his health and that of his family.

Student health services in every college and university may not satisfy all the above objectives adequately; however, the majority of institutions are striving for complete programs and are rendering a high quality of service. The trend throughout American colleges and universities is to give greater attention to student medicine to meet the needs of adolescents and young adults. Student medicine bridges the gap between pediatrics and internal medicine, which implies the care and treatment of adults [18].

The staff of the student health service varies considerably with the size of the institution. The staff may consist of one or more nurses, of one or more nurses and a part-time physician, or of one or more nurses and at least one full-time physician. Full-time physicians are found at two out of every ten, 20 per cent, of college health services. Part-time physicians are associated with more than half the colleges. More than two out of ten colleges have no physician on the health service staff.[8]

The college or university health service is the center around which the effective health program revolves. Its educational activities and medical services contribute immeasurably to meeting the health needs of students.

Health education. Health education may be defined as *the process of providing learning activities which favorably influence knowledge, attitudes, and practices relating to individual, family, and community health.*

Health education, which is one of the behavioral sciences, sometimes is referred to as the *applied science of healthful liv-*

[8] Norman S. Moore and John Summerskill, *Health Services in American Colleges and Universities, 1953,* Cornell University Press, Ithaca, N.Y., 1954.

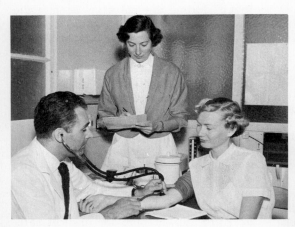

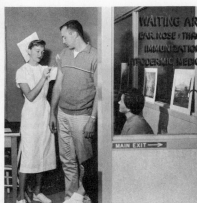

The student health service, another important resource for students, is available for health appraisal . . .

and health protection.

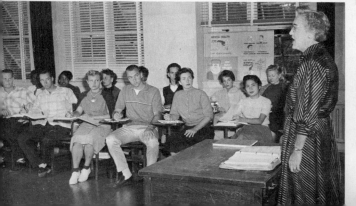

College health education, an important phase of the college health program, assists students to make wise decisions for effective living. Acquiring scientific information about health problems and their solution is one aspect of health education.

ing, and rightfully so. It is not a pure science, for it draws much of its content from the basic sciences, such as anatomy, physiology, bacteriology, medicine, and another applied science, public health. Health education is not composed of all these sciences added together; rather it derives from them the purposeful applications that particularly pertain to more effective living. Certainly, health education does not deal with the treatment of disease or defect as does the science of medicine. On the contrary, it is vitally concerned with educating people to live healthfully, to prevent disease, and to

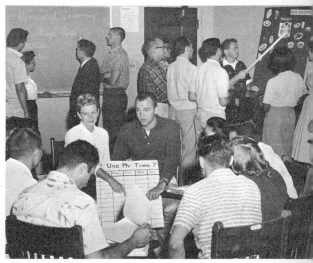

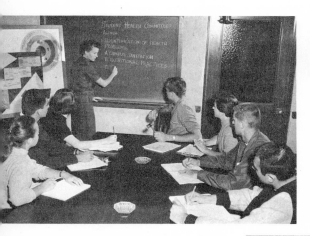

Positive health attitudes and health practices can be developed through problem-solving experiences, including small group discussions and individual and group projects . . .

and through participation in student health councils or committees.

Health guidance is often the best type of health education.

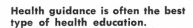

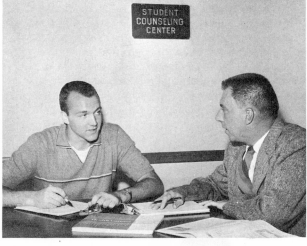

take intelligent action when disease or defect occurs. Health education is not synonymous with anatomy, physiology, or bacteriology. These basic sciences form its foundation. More specifically, it results from what is known about health and the factors that promote, maintain, and improve health. These factors have already been discussed.

Education, psychology, educational psychology, and sociology furnish the insights, theories, and activities that assist the individual to change his behavior for more effective living in his environment. Health education is not something done to, or for, someone; neither is it the memorizing of health facts. It is the provision of opportunities for individuals and groups to participate in experiences for healthful living. This means engaging in activities that give meaning and purpose to people's lives, aiding them in achieving personal and social goals through effective action.

Health education experiences occur in many situations in your college environment. For example, health education takes place in the student-health-service office when the doctor discusses the results of the medical examination with the student. It takes place in the gymnasium when the physical education instructor discusses with the student the selection of physical activities to suit his needs or considers with him a problem such as improving his posture. It takes place in class when the student is engaged in problem-solving situations such as analyzing his own daily diet or when he participates in a field trip to the local health center to study the protective health services of the community. Health education becomes effective when the student through self-direction applies his learning to everyday living situations. An example of such application is seen when the student living in a fraternity house rearranges his study desk to receive maximum daylight as well as adequate artificial illumination.

Since health education is an academic field, it is an essential part of the college and university curriculum. This applied science of healthful living is first studied in a foundation course. Common titles for such a course are Personal and Community Health, Principles of Healthful Living, and College Health Education. The contents of the course are based on the needs and interests of the college student.

After completing the basic course, the student is encouraged to enroll in advanced courses, such as Family Relations (or Marriage and the Family), Mental Health, Advanced Nutrition, Social Psychology, Culture and Personality, Consumer Education, Community Control of Communicable Disease, Epidemiology of Chronic Disease, Safety Education, School Health Education, Child Health, Industrial Health, and Rural Health.

Health education is an important part of the total college curriculum and is a major administrative division of the college health program. Health education experiences are utilized by each division in a way unique to that division. Health education through physical education is an example.

Healthful college living. Numerous specific activities, services, facilities, and interpersonal relationships contribute to environmental health. All these together constitute healthful living in the college community. The impact of the environment on the student is the theme of this whole chapter. In the organization of a college health program certain specific activities are established to promote healthful college living.

The following paragraphs consider some aspects of the environment with which the student should be familiar. They make a significant contribution to his health.

Environmental sanitation on the campus involves control of the drinking-water and milk supply; the food in eating halls, restaurants, and soda fountains; garbage disposal; water in the swimming pools; health protection of food handlers; housing; building maintenance; and insect and rodent control. Recently added to these functions is the supervision of radiation on the college and university campus. Radiologic monitors now detect radioactive isotopes and other sources of radiation that affect safety.

These control functions constitute a major aspect of the college health program. Responsibility for such controls rests with a faculty public health committee, the student health service, a campus health officer, or a campus sanitarian, or it is assumed by the local public health center in the community. Environmental control standards are available from the U.S. Public Health Service, Office of Education and Bureau of Standards, Department of Health, Education and Welfare, Washington, and from the American Public Health Association, the professional association for public health workers.

The student has opportunities to help keep the environment safe and sanitary by taking care of his immediate surroundings. He follows safety precautions, removes unsafe objects, and exercises care in cleaning his room and study area. He properly disposes of leftover food and waste material. He takes part in class and group projects for improving the sanitation and safety of the college or university environment.

In order to make the most of his opportunities, a college student spends many hours in the *classroom,* the *laboratory,* and the *library.* An ideal physical environment for learning is provided by a classroom or laboratory that is properly lighted to assure a minimum of eye fatigue, adequately heated and ventilated to promote physical and mental efficiency, correctly equipped with chairs and tables to fit the individual student, and decorated with colors both pleasing and soothing to the eye. The same characteristics

are needed in the study rooms in the library.

A student should leave the classroom and laboratory each day with an increased understanding and appreciation of the subject matter, a challenge to discover and understand the significance of topics being discussed, and a feeling of satisfaction with his own contribution to the group. Desirable environmental conditions can contribute greatly to these objectives. The student therefore plans carefully for each class session. He strives to seat himself where he is able to see and hear, in order to receive information, and where he can be seen and heard, in order to contribute to the discussion. If he is assigned a seat that is not conducive to hearing and seeing, he takes time to discuss the situation with the instructor.

The mental tone of the classroom and laboratory is likewise important to a healthful environment. Student-instructor relations should be friendly yet objective. There must be a continuous attempt to explore and clarify values. The student feels free to ask intelligent questions about the instructor's statements. Student progress in understanding, appreciation, attitudes, and skills is evaluated.

A student may find it difficult to determine his vocational goals because he may not comprehend clearly the personal traits required for success in a specific vocation or because he may have an erroneous conception of his own personal qualifications. The *counseling services* of a college are established to help solve such problems. An opportunity is provided for determining through appraisal of capacities, aptitudes, and interests whether or not a student is likely to attain certain vocational goals. The counseling personnel cannot be expected to determine by testing and through interviews that a student will become an outstanding doctor, lawyer, engineer, teacher, or businessman, but they can determine whether he has the qualifications for success in a particular field.

You, as a student, owe it to yourself to become informed about available counseling services and to take advantage of the assistance offered. A counseling center provides services to students with educational, vocational, and personal-social-emotional problems. These services include admission counseling, orientation activities for new students, educational counseling, vocational testing and guidance, financial counseling, housing information, counseling on religious matters, social activities, health services, and other personal and social aid. There exists a close relationship among the counseling service, the student health service, and the physical education and other departments, since all are vitally concerned with health guidance.

Whether one lives in a fraternity or sorority house, a dormitory, a club, a rooming house, a room in a private house, or at home, one's *living quarters* affect health and efficiency. For example:

Good lighting can decrease eye fatigue, headaches, nervousness, and irritability.

Bright, cheery surroundings have a definite psychological uplifting effect.

Proper heating and ventilation reduce the likelihood of contracting respiratory diseases, such as colds, sinusitis, and pneumonia.

Adequate space in living quarters prevents the spread of a number of communicable diseases.

Properly equipped and arranged quarters, with intelligent use of appliances, prevent many home accidents.

College or university authorities concerned with housing for students are giving attention to the requirements for good housing as well as to the deficiencies that lead to substandard housing. Standards for the quality of good housing are controlled by the campus public health officer or committee or by the local health department in the community.

Some aspects of an individual's living quarters are beyond his control. He can report unhealthful conditions or make suggestions for improvement, but in most instances, if his suggestions are not carried out, he can only change his residence. There are, however, a number of factors of environmental sanitation that the student himself can control. It is with these factors that the following discussion is concerned. One of them is *lighting*.

The unit of measurement of the intensity of light is the foot-candle, which is the intensity of illumination on a perpendicular screen 1 foot away from a standard candle. Proper illumination for eye health and comfort can be attained by having sufficient intensity of light, 30 foot-candles, on the visual task. Additional foot-candles are recommended for close work. The quantity of light is assured by having lamps of sufficient wattage to provide the proper intensity. The local electric-light company will send a representative to measure the light in one's living quarters. Light meters also can be obtained from the college or university maintenance division, from the campus public health officer, and from the sanitation division of the local health department.

Freedom from glare is a basic principle of proper illumination. All lamps should be provided with shades deep enough to cover the bulbs, and lights should be properly placed so as to avoid glare. Semi-indirect lighting fixtures give a soft, glareless light that is well diffused throughout the whole room. Light contrasts are avoided by having sufficient light in enough places throughout the room. Reading by a lamp that is the only source of light in the room is a frequent cause of eye fatigue because of the constant adjustment and readjustment necessary when the eyes glance from the printed page and back again. Approved study lamps have a large part of the light directed to the ceiling as well as on the study desk. Ceiling fixtures are designed for light to be reflected down from the ceiling rather than projected directly down from the fixture. The combination of study lamps and ceiling fixtures assures proper distribution of light and eliminates dark and bright spots in the room. The color of the walls is also important for balanced lighting. Better reflective value and consequently more even distribution of light occur when the ceilings are painted a dull white, cream, or ivory, the walls are light pastel colors, and the furniture is light-colored with a dull finish. One factor that is quite controllable by the student is the direction of light on the visual task. He must arrange floor lamps, table lamps, and study lamps of all types so that he is not facing the light. Light should come over his left shoulder if he is right-handed, and over his right shoulder if he is left-handed, to avoid shadows on the work.

The student has some control over heating and ventilation. Frequently, this is only a matter of being aware of the situation. Artificial heat is necessary when the natural temperature is 68°F or less. It is important that a temperature of 68 to 72° be maintained for comfort and general good health. Overheating is common in the winter season. Discomfort results from an operating temperature over 75°.

Proper ventilation with sufficient air exchange reduces bacterial concentration in the air and disperses body odors and odors from cooking or heat sources. An air exchange of 10 cubic feet per person per minute is an adequate standard [9]. This is obtained automatically in cold weather by normal leakage through doors, windows, ceilings, and walls. In other seasons, the student can make use of windows, transoms, fans, and air-cooling systems. This procedure merely requires good judgment.

Noise has a definite effect on personal efficiency, particularly on study and sleep. Noise is measured in decibels. A decibel is a unit of measurement of sound similar to the foot-candle of light. It is the ratio of the sound measured to the smallest distinguishable sound. Noise surveys have shown that the average noise level for homes varies from 22 to 45 decibels and should not exceed 50 decibels [9]. Much can be done in the construction of modern buildings to reduce noise. If the student's living quarters are noisy, he should first determine whether the noise is from a temporary source that can be stopped. If not, his recourse is to rearrange his study schedule, avoiding noisy periods, or to move to a different location.

The student should realize that adequate space in sleeping rooms is necessary in controlling communicable disease. Three feet between cots gives the necessary 50 square feet of floor area to prevent spread of communicable disease [9]. Staton[9] found an increase in acute upper respiratory conditions in a study of college students sleeping in rooms with less than 50 square feet of floor space per person. Ceiling heights should be 7 feet 8 inches to 8 feet.

The student can do much to prevent accidents from electric shocks, burns, gas poisoning, and falls. He can see that all live conductors are placed in such a way as not to be exposed to contact. He can check to be sure metal enclosures of electric appliances are well grounded. He knows that wall switches are dangerous if touched by a person in a bathtub or shower. He can be careful with portable appliances to make sure that no one comes in contact with the appliance and with a plumbing or gas pipe simultaneously. He knows that carbon monoxide poisoning from gas heaters has caused many deaths, and he understands that to prevent such poisoning it is necessary to have proper vents to flues. He also knows it is unwise to use an unvented heater in a bedroom when one is asleep

[9] Wesley M. Staton, "Relationship of Occupancy and Adequacy of Student Housing to Incidence of Acute Upper Respiratory Conditions," *Research Quarterly,* 27:229–234, May, 1956.

or likely to fall asleep. He should avoid smoking in bed and should be careful how and where he disposes of cigarettes.

The above examples point out some of the responsibilities of the college or university administration, the faculty, and the student, who together help create and maintain a safe, healthful environment.

Physical education. Although physical education is usually administered in a separate department from health services or other divisions of the college health program, it, too, plays an important role in enabling the college student to live an active, satisfying, effective life. Physical education is concerned with the total development of the student through physical activities.

Participation by the student in physical education activities under the guidance of well-prepared leaders contributes significantly to his health through the development of organic fitness and psychological strengths. It provides experience in democratic citizenship, skills, and appreciation for leisure-time pursuits. Such experiences are vital for women as well as for men. Every college student's life is enriched through participation in physical education activities, particularly in dancing and in indoor and outdoor sports. The student achieves the following objectives through this division of the college health program [13, 19, 20, 22]:

The ability to see himself as he is through self-appraisal of his capacities and limitations.

An appreciation of, and responsibility for, a healthy body.

Skillful performance in a number of activities providing fitness in terms of strength, endurance, and reserve power.

Skills in physical activities to provide continuing recreation in later years.

An understanding of the importance and need for rest and relaxation.

Leadership ability, as well as apprecia-

tion for the talented performance of others.

Ability to participate cooperatively and effectively in group activities.

Emotional control and release of emotional strains and tensions.

Achievement of a normal physical condition by remedying defects correctable through physical activity.

An appreciation of physical activities as a participant and as a spectator.

The physical education department carrying out the above objectives includes the following components: instructional courses in physical education on a required and/or elective basis, adapted or corrective activities, a teacher-education program for physical education majors, recreational activities, and, in a number of institutions, intercollegiate athletics.

A unique guidance function is performed in physical education through the informal personal-social relationships between the faculty members and students. These relationships are due to the nature of the activities, the method of conducting the activities, and the interest of well-qualified physical education instructors in the welfare of students. By means of this guidance function, physical education supplements and complements the other divisions of the college health program.

It is through the personal-social relationships with students that the physical education instructor is able to cooperate with the student health service in observing, screening, referring, and following up the student with a health problem. The adapted or corrective program, supervised by health service and physical education personnel on an individual-need basis, serves as an important means of correcting remediable defects. This cooperative phase of the program also provides a medium for carrying out the classification of activities according to the findings of the student's medical examination. For example, the student who is appraised as "healthy" may participate in any or all of the physical education activities that are offered him. However, the student who has a serious defect is necessarily restricted to certain activities.

Physical education contributes to health education through guidance in such student problems as conditioning, preventing infection, cleanliness, bathing, and adjusting to the opposite sex. The permissive, democratic atmosphere in a physical education class in which the instructor promotes personal security, self-reliance, and social acceptance among the students is in itself an example of the contribution to a healthful environment. Other examples include the continuous effort for safety and sanitation of fields, gymnasiums, and locker rooms; the safety precautions in conducting activities; and a morale factor. This factor results from the participation in, and appreciation of, skilled performance in physical education, including intercollegiate athletics. Skills developed in carry-over sports are valuable assets for continuing recreational activities in future years.

College physical education offers a variety of activities carefully selected and organized to assist the student in his total personal and social development.

Off-campus community health resources. Off-campus community health resources supplement and support the college health program, and their activities are considered a part of the college environment. In turn, college health resources contribute to the community health program. This reciprocal relationship may be compared to a modern freeway with traffic flowing in both directions. A detailed consideration of community health activities is presented in Chapter 15. A study of these resources reveals many possible contributions that can be made to the college health program.

Opportunities for student participation. A student becomes a bona fide citizen of the college community when he is officially enrolled. As a citizen he is not only concerned about his own life, but because his life is affected by others and by his surroundings, he assumes civic responsibilities for the improvement of his community. The college citizen assists in making the college community a healthier environment.

The faculty and administration are aware of the importance of student participation. They see the student's assumption of civic responsibilities in college as a value that carries over into adult life. They view the well-educated individual today as one who personally adjusts well to his society and is consistent in his efforts to contribute to the improvement of his social order. Their beliefs in student participation are based upon sound principles of democracy, the psychology of learning, and the objectives of education.

Opportunities for student participation vary from campus to campus. The following discussion illustrates a few of the specific activities organized in some colleges or universities or types that could be developed with sound faculty-student planning.

One of the most common current opportunities for student representation and participation is through the health committee or council. Such activities are now carried on in numerous colleges and universities throughout the country.

Three plans are prevalent. The first is a plan in which student representation occurs on the faculty health committee or council. This may be an over-all committee, planning and coordinating the entire college health program, or it may be concerned with only one facet of the program, such as health education or health service functions.

A second plan is to have student representation pertaining to the college health program on the student governing board. For example, one or more members of the student legislative council, responsible for student government as a whole, may be concerned with the health program.

A third plan, considered superior to the first two, is the organization of a special student health committee or council composed of students only. Some groups prefer a faculty adviser as ex officio member. This body is relatively free from faculty domination. On the other hand, with a faculty sponsor it is closely coordinated with a similar faculty committee, which approves student plans and recommendations and aids in implementing them into action.

The Director of Health Services at Stanford University, California, has stated publicly on several occasions that a 12-member student advisory committee has been invaluable to him in promoting public relations for the student health service, improving operational procedures pertaining to range and types of services and to financial policies, and obtaining new facilities.

Other authorities believe that students should have a voice in deciding the type of services provided, the cost of services, the payment, the hours during which services are available, and the manner in which students are received, cared for, and discharged.

Students share many opportunities to participate in health education activities. Several institutions have students engaged in planning with curriculum committees. They participate in the task of constructing new or improved courses, prescribing health education courses as requirements or electives, or adding health experiences to courses in related fields such as education, science, home economics, nursing, and sociology.

Other opportunities are found within the courses themselves. In such instances there is instructor-student planning to decide the health needs and interests of the class; a priority basis for studying

health education areas; and types of student activities, such as individual health appraisals to determine health status with individual interpretation, individual projects such as analysis of the student's own diet, daily program, exercise program, social activities, and medical-care plans, field trips to campus and community health resources, and a study of environmental health and safety problems and hazards.

Several examples of student participation in activities to improve the environment have been mentioned, but innumerable other examples exist. Students may take part in improving the food service, drinking-water facilities, sleeping and studying quarters, washing and bathing facilities, provision of facilities for maintaining total physical fitness and providing recreation. Additional examples may be found in interpersonal relationships within the college community. These include the previously mentioned instructor-student relations, doctor-patient or nurse-patient relations in the health service or community, administrator-student relations, and—by far the most frequent—student-student relations among both men and women. The establishment and enforcement of rules of conduct by the students themselves is a specific example of creating good interpersonal relations.

Student groups are most proficient in studying and bringing about improvement in traffic safety and parking problems. Health education classes can make a scientific study of lighting, heating, and ventilation problems and present pertinent proposals for improvement. Student groups can bring about beautification and cleanliness of the campus through well-planned campaigns. Presentation of the college health program in orientation periods, as a part of class activities of health education courses, is another example.

In the planning, conduct, and evaluation of the college health program and its resources, activities, and services, there are many opportunities for student participation. Each program is enriched by planning for such participation and by determining the degree to which it takes place. These range from activities where there is complete responsible decision by the students to those where there must be complete control by faculty and administration. The premise upon which student participation is based is that the student is a citizen of the college community.

Summary

College students are interested in themselves, their way of life, their families, and their communities. They are not concerned with "health for health's sake" or "blood and bone hygiene" but rather with satisfying their own needs and interests.

While basic needs do not change, new problems and pressures appear and must be resolved and equalized. The college scene in the Space Age illustrates changes occurring in the college environment.

A major problem is the failure to apply knowledge available from medical discoveries to provide for effective living. The authors think that health education can help solve this problem. The foundations for college health education are presented in this chapter, setting the stage for the content of subsequent chapters.

Modern health concepts are presented, from the views of the man in the street to the American Public Health Association's "Broadened Spectrum of Health and Morbidity"; also presented are definitions of health, formulated by the World Health Organization and by the authors. The authors' view of health for effective living is given. This includes a formula for changing behavior:

Scientific knowledge + positive health attitudes = best action

Factors that influence health and effective living are described in brief summary statements. These factors include mental health, family health, body maintenance and care, nutrition, consumer health, communicable and chronic disease, safety, stimulants and depressants, and community health. In addition, the health problems, needs, and interests of college students, as indicated in research studies, are identified and briefly discussed. There appears to be a definite similarity between the health factors and the problems, needs, and interests of students. The characteristics of a health-educated individual are presented as specific goals for the student to achieve during his health education course as well as in the future. All these foundation factors help determine the content of subsequent chapters.

The foundations of college health education also determine, to an important degree, the kind and scope of health resources made available on the college campus to promote, protect, and maintain the health of students.

The many and varied health resources within the college environment are organized into a college health program. A health committee or council, along with a director, coordinator, or other administrative officer, provides leadership and a team approach to the program. College health services, health education, healthful college living (environmental aspects), physical education, and community health resources are the major divisions of a college health program.

Opportunities to participate as a citizen in the college environment in health planning and development occur with each health resource. The purpose of the college health program is to assist the student to satisfy his health needs and to enable him to live effectively in college and in later life.

Suggested readings

1. Anderson, Gaylord W.: "Health Education—A One-world Challenge," *American Journal of Public Health,* 50:127–133, February, 1960.

2. Bennett, Margaret E.: *Getting the Most Out of College,* McGraw-Hill Book Company, Inc., New York, 1957.

3. Bosch, Herbert M.: "Some Aspects of an Effective Environmental Health Program," *Student Medicine,* 9:150–159, December, 1960.

4. Cassidy, Rosalind: "Effective Action: The Ends for Which We Strive," *California Journal of Secondary Education,* 27:191–192, April, 1952.

5. Craig, Marjorie L., and Frances U. Everett: "Developing Health Potentialities," *Teachers College Record,* 8:429–434, May, 1960.

6. Creswell, William H., Jr.: "Health Education in the College Program," *Student Medicine,* 8:209–217, February, 1960.

7. Cushman, Wesley P., and Bruce L. Bennett: "A Health Problems Check List," *Journal of Health, Physical Education and Recreation,* 30:28–29, 64, December, 1959.

8. Dunn, Halbert L.: "High-level Wellness for Man and Society," *American Journal of Public Health,* 49:786–792, June, 1959.

9. Ehlers, Victor M., and Ernest W. Steel: *Municipal and Rural Sanitation,* 5th ed., McGraw-Hill Book Company, Inc., New York, 1958.

10. Farnsworth, Dana L.: "The Relationship of a Student Health Service to Other University Departments," *Student Medicine,* 2:4–18, October, 1953.

11. Fourth National Conference on Health in Colleges: *Proceedings: Teamwork in Meeting the Health Needs of College Students,* American College Health Association, New York, 1955.

12. Ginsburg, Ethel L.: "The College and Student Health," in *Report of the Fourth National Conference on Health in Colleges,* National Tuberculosis Association, New York, 1955.

13. *A Health Program for Colleges: Report of the Third National Conference on Health in Colleges,* National Tuberculosis Association, New York, 1948.

14. Johns, Edward B.: "Spotlight on College Health Teaching—1955," *Journal of Health, Physical Education and Recreation,* 26:29–30, 76, March, 1955.

15. Johns, Edward B.: "Forecast for the Future," *Journal of Health, Physical Education and Recreation,* 31:87–88, 116, April, 1960.

16. Joy, William W.: "Health Service Responsibility for Sanitation and Safety of Food Service," *Student Medicine,* 7:268–273, April, 1959.

17. Lantagne, Joseph E.: "An Analysis of the Health Interests of 1,000 Junior College Students in California," *Junior College Journal,* 21:429–433, April, 1952.

18. Moore, Norman S., and C. D. Darling: *Student Health and the Changing Order,* Cornell University Press, Ithaca, N.Y., 1951.

19. Moore, Norman S., and John Summerskill: *Health Services in American Colleges and Universities, 1953,* Cornell University Press, Ithaca, N.Y., 1954.

20. National Conference on College Health Education: *A Forward Look in College Health Education,* American Association for Health, Physical Education and Recreation, Washington, 1956.

21. National Safety Council: *Accident Facts,* The Council, Chicago, 1960.

22. Oberteuffer, Delbert: *Physical Education,* 2d ed., Harper & Brothers, New York, 1956.

23. Oberteuffer, Delbert: *School Health Education,* Harper & Brothers, New York, 1960.

24. Public Health Service: *Summary of Health and Vital Statistics,* Publication 600, U.S. Department of Health, Education, and Welfare, Washington, June, 1958.

25. Richardson, Charles E.: "Total College Health Programs," *Journal of Health, Physical Education and Recreation,* 30:23–24, March, 1959.

26. Rockefeller, Nelson A.: "Present-day Health Problems," *American Journal of Public Health,* 50:8–13, January, 1960.

27. Rogers, Edward S.: *Human Ecology and Health,* The Macmillan Company, New York, 1960.

28. Smith, Sara Louise: "Health Education Faces the Future," *Journal of Health, Physical Education and Recreation,* 29:31–32, September, 1958.

29. Steel, Ernest W.: *Water Supply and Sewerage,* 4th ed., McGraw-Hill Book Company, Inc., New York, 1960.

30. Sutton, Wilfred C.: "Determining the

Health Needs of College Students," unpublished doctoral dissertation, University of California, Los Angeles, 1954.

31. Sutton, Wilfred C.: "Appraisal of Health Attitudes and Practices of College Students," *Journal of School Health,* 26:125–130, April, 1956.

32. Van Dalen, Diabold: *The Health, Physi-cal Education and Recreation Teacher: An Introduction to the Profession,* Prentice-Hall, Inc., Englewood Cliffs, N.J., 1956.

33. Williams, J. F., and G. G. Wetherill: *Personal and Community Hygiene Applied,* W. B. Saunders Company, Philadelphia, 1950.

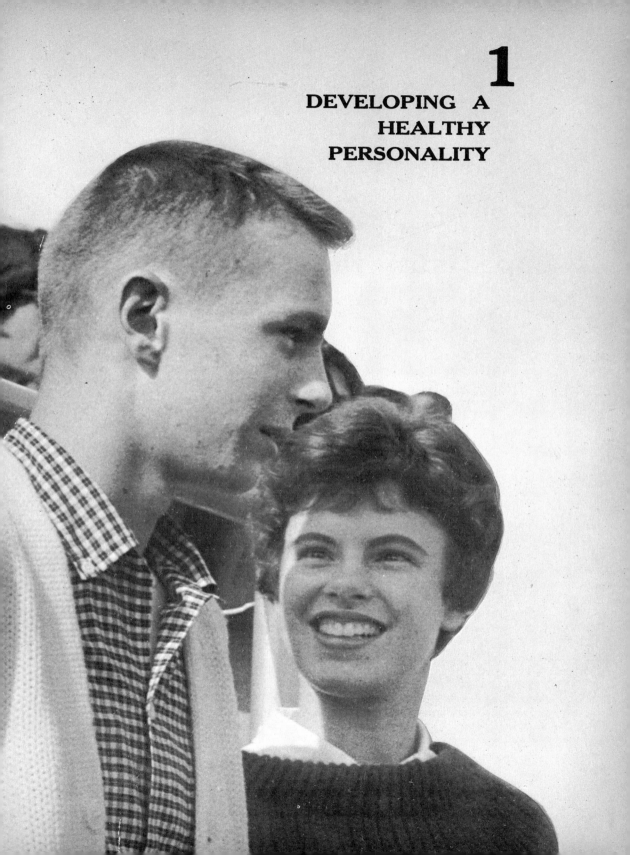

1

DEVELOPING A HEALTHY PERSONALITY

TWO

Appraising mental health

Mental Health Concepts

Theories of Personality Emergence

Foundation Factors for Mental Health

Criteria for Mental Health

Each one of us is a complex person psychologically. We are products of our past experience and of the interplay of many biological, structural, environmental, social, and cultural forces. Much of our present behavior was determined in our early childhood. Our childhood impulses, adjustments, and behavior patterns are not just extended into adulthood, but adulthood is built solidly upon our previous behavior.

To achieve a sound mentally healthy state, it is necessary to appraise the constituent factors of personality and of mental health. Such an appraisal should provide you with full understanding of the concepts of mental health, of the theories of personality emergence as they relate to mental health, of the foundation factors that influence personality and mental health, and of the principles for developing a personal mental health program. The discussion in this chapter is organized around these key questions:

What are the modern concepts of mental health?

What are the accepted theories of personality emergence that have implications for our own mental health?

What are the foundation factors that influence both personality emergence and sound mental health?

What criteria for mental health serve as guiding principles to direct our course of action?

Mental health concepts

Mental health involves the individual's everyday living and today is recognized as an important facet of his total health status. It helps maintain physical health as well as social effectiveness.

The increase in problems of mental illness evidenced in the last twenty years is due partly to the inability of the individual to understand himself and his fellow men and partly to his failure to apply the fundamental principles of mental health in adjusting to present-day society with its speed, competition, pressure, strain, and anxiety. These factors are also present in the college environment.

Mental health is a normal state of well-being, a positive but relative quality of life. It is characteristic of the average person who meets the demands of life on the basis of his own capacities and limitations [3].

MENTAL HEALTH: A RELATIVE QUALITY OF LIFE

The degree of mental health is relative, since no one has all the traits and characteristics of a healthy mental state all the time. The individual's condition, or state, of mental health is continually changing, depending upon his own actions and the factors and forces acting upon him. In appraising his physical health, the individual recognizes that he may have minor deviations from normal or temporary symptoms of ill health, such as a headache. The same is true of mental health. The individual may have a bad day, may be depressed in spirits, or may unconsciously depend upon rationalization in adjusting to a particular situation. Also, it is possible that he may deviate from normal in one particular, yet make his everyday adjustments. Such a person is not called abnormal; he is merely described as deviating in one special way. Since mental health is a matter of degree, one person may have a higher degree of mental health than some of his friends who are likewise considered normal.

NORMALITY

What is meant by *normal?* It is important to understand the term, since it is so frequently used to describe the condition of the mentally healthy individual. In one sense, "normal" is a synonym for "typical." This is a statistical use of the word, meaning that an individual is average compared with group norms. The classic example is that of the individual whose height and weight are considered normal because he is average in height and weight for his age.

A second concept refers to overt behavior judged by social standards. For example, a normal behavior characteristic of the adolescent is "showing off." It is expected at this developmental period and therefore is considered normal behavior. This same behavior in an adult would be considered abnormal.

The third concept of normality pertains to the individual's health status. The individual is well, as opposed to being sick. One may say of a student that he is small in stature for his age and he does some queer things, but he is healthy. This means that he is an active, alert person with a good color and an interest in doing things. An important element in this concept is the assumption that all normal people have problems to solve. It is when a person is overpowered by his problems that his condition deviates from patterns regarded as normal [28].

Normality, although it is only a relative term, is of considerable value in appraising mental health. The best single index of normality is the total life situation of the individual which includes his behavior while making adjustments to his family group; his inner life, exemplified by his philosophy of life, his self-confidence, and his emotional stability; his relations with friends, acquaintances, fellow students, and professors; and his efficiency in work and study [18].

DEFINITIONS OF MENTAL HEALTH

Mental health is difficult to define, and no single definition is accepted universally. The following definitions are offered as examples:

Dana Farnsworth, M.D., Director of the Student Health Service, Harvard University, defines mental health as: [1]

That state of mind in which one is free to make use of his natural capacities in an effective and satisfying manner. . . . Mental health implies a moderate amount of self-understanding, the capacity to be creative, the ability to love and to accept love, and to think in terms of other people rather than of oneself only.

Dr. Margaret Mead, of the World Federation for Mental Health, has stated: [2]

Mental health defies precise definition. Instead, it is the mid-twentieth century way in which the world is expressing our hope of what good may come from a greater knowledge of the way in which men's lives are shaped by childhood experiences, by relation with others, and by the forms of the societies in which they live.

The authors believe that mental health is aptly described in the following terms [22, 23]:

Mental health is the quality of personal health resulting from the individual's satisfaction of human needs through personal and social adjustments in his environment. In making personal and social adjustments the individual attempts to develop to the fullest extent his own unique personality through socially considerate behavior. His behavior demonstrates his ability *to face problems realistically, to make choices intelligently, to guide his emotional expressions skillfully, to work efficiently and live effectively, to find satisfaction, success, and happiness in the accomplishment of everyday tasks,* and *to contribute to the betterment of society.*

Theories of personality emergence

The constituents of personality and their relationship to mental health principles are derived from basic theories of personality development or emergence. Selected basic theories are presented for consideration.

MASLOW'S THEORY OF MOTIVATION AND PERSONALITY

A very significant theory of personality is Maslow's theory of personality maturity, which stresses motivation. His theory postulates the individual's personality emergence and continuing self-enlargement from the lower levels of growth, or attaining satisfactions, through five levels of development. The five levels

[1] Dana L. Farnsworth, *Mental Health in College and University,* Harvard University Press, Cambridge, Mass., 1957, p. 6.
[2] Elizabeth Dach, *Your Community and Mental Health,* Public Affairs Pamphlet 263, Public Affairs Committee, Inc., New York, 1958, p. 21.

comprise his hierarchy of needs, in which the satisfaction of higher-level needs is founded on the adequate satisfaction of lower-level needs. The first level includes the basic physiologic needs, such as food and sex; the second, the need for safety from external dangers; the third, the need for love and affection from others; the fourth, the need for self-esteem and the respect and esteem of others; and the fifth, the need for self-realization through achievement [8].

Physiologic needs. Physiologic needs are the starting point for motivation. The need to maintain physical well-being and to satisfy the tensions caused by hunger, thirst, fatigue, sex-stress, lack of sleep, and physical pain are physiologic needs. Maslow thinks that physiologic needs are the most prepotent of all needs. For example, a person who lacks one or more of these basic satisfactions would desire the fulfillment of these needs more strongly than that of any higher-level need. A hungry person desires food more than the satisfaction of some higher-level desire. If these basic needs are not satisfied, all other needs are nonexistent. A hungry person organizes all his body capacities to satisfy the hunger, and the desire to buy a new pair of shoes or an automobile becomes secondary. The extremely hungry person can think or dream only about food; his concept of utopia is a place where he can devour lots of food.

Fortunately, in our culture extreme hunger occurs most infrequently. When these physiologic needs are satisfied, at once higher needs emerge; when the next level of needs is met, others become dominant. This is Maslow's *hierarchy* of needs. The organism is dominated by, and its behavior is motivated to satisfy, unmet needs.

Safety needs. When physiologic needs are satisfied, the safety needs emerge. These desires also dominate, only to a lesser degree than physiologic needs. All the capacities of the individual may be organized to serve for safety purposes, including safety from destructive forces and from threats of injury. Living safely may be the person's strongest desire. The importance of satisfying the safety need can be seen more clearly in children than in adults. Adults have learned to inhibit this reaction, but infants do not inhibit it at all. A child frantically clinging to his parents shows them in their role as protectors. Children in our society for the most part seek a safe, orderly, predictably organized environment protected and shielded by parents. Children in such a world express dangerous reactions to objects or situations much the same as adults do. Most adults have their safety needs adequately satisfied because they have few dangers to fear. The need is felt, however, when illness strikes, in the event of injury, during war, or when natural catastrophes occur. People now are becoming more concerned about safety because accidental death and injury are increasing. A neurotic person may demonstrate safety needs much as a child does. He may continually fear a great catastrophe or the end of the world. He usually responds as a mentally healthy person would respond to an emergency.

Love needs. When physiologic and safety needs are met, the love, affection, and belongingness needs emerge. These needs are apparent when a sweetheart, wife, husband, or children are absent. They may be expressed in the longing for friends or in the hunger for affectionate relations with people in general. Included in this level also is the desire for a place and acceptance in a group.

In this category of needs, sex and love are not considered synonymous. Sexual behavior includes sex, love, and affection. Love needs are concerned with both giving and receiving love. Love and affection in our society are bound by many restrictions and inhibitions. The thwarting of love needs has a strong relationship to maladjustment, according to clinical studies.

Esteem needs. Most persons in our society need self-esteem, self-respect, and respect from others. These needs are classified by Maslow into two groups: desires for strength, for achievement, for adequacy, and for independence; and desires for recognition, for importance, for attention, and for a reputation, or prestige. Satisfaction of esteem needs makes possible feelings of self-confidence and worth, including the feeling of being useful and necessary. The thwarting of self-esteem needs leads to feelings of inferiority and discouragement and to compensating behavior.

Need for self-actualization. When all the previous needs are satisfied, the need for self-actualization emerges, an ongoing process driving the individual to accomplish his lifework. This is a high-level need, expressed by the teacher when he teaches, by the artist when he paints, by the musician when he plays or sings, by the doctor when he cures disease and cares for his patients, and by the successful housewife and mother. Continuous satisfaction of this need leads to ultimate happiness. It is not a life of leisure that brings about happiness, but rather a life in which the individual achieves what he wants. For a college student this implies the importance of setting life goals, of choosing the right vocation, and of receiving the best preparation for his chosen lifework.

Maslow believes that the majority of people appear to satisfy the basic needs in the order that has been described. However, he makes the point that there are always exceptions so the hierarchy is not absolutely fixed. For example, some persons may feel that self-esteem is more vital than love. They may seek self-assertion for love rather than for self-esteem itself. Some innately creative persons appear to have a drive to create as a basic satisfaction rather than as a part of self-actualization. Some persons who have experienced life only at a low level may be satisfied in life by merely obtaining sufficient food. Our hoboes and some chronically unemployed persons fall into such a category. Some exceptions to the hierarchy occur when persons have extremely high social standards, high ideals, or high values. These persons reverse the hierarchy when they are willing to give up anything for the sake of a particular ideal or value.

Maslow's theory includes the belief that persons whose basic needs have been satisfied throughout their lives, especially in their earlier years, develop an exceptional power to withstand the thwarting of needs. This condition results, he thinks, because such persons have developed strong, healthy character structure as a result of basic need satisfaction. They can, without much difficulty, weather disagreement or opposition. They can go against public opinion and can stand up for their own convictions, even at great personal cost. It is those who have loved and been loved and who have many deep friendships that can stand out against hatred, rejection, or persecution.

Maslow thinks the basic needs are more often unconscious than conscious, although they may be either. With the majority of people, physiologic needs are unconscious. It is possible that unconscious needs may be changed into conscious ones by appropriate psychological procedures.

Although not all behavior is determined by basic needs, the evidence indicates that some behavior is highly motivated, some is weakly motivated, and some is not motivated at all. However, all behavior is determined, although it may not be determined by motives, or by motives alone. In adjustment, or field, theory, which will be discussed later, behavior is seen as determined completely

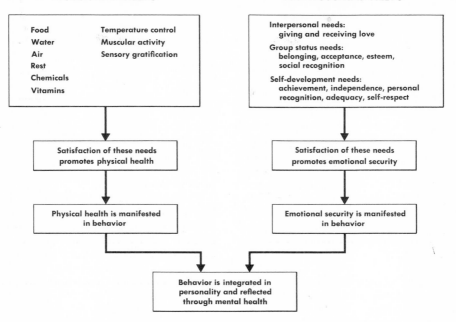

The integration of biological and psychosocial needs. (Adapted from Louis Kaplan, *Mental Health and Human Relations in Education,* **Harper & Brothers, New York, 1959, p. 233.)**

by the field, or by external stimuli, such as in the association of ideas [20].

Gordon Allport, in his book *Becoming* [1], strongly supports Maslow and his theory of motivation of personality. Allport contends that one of the most striking characteristics of a psychologically mature person is that he seeks to *become* something more than he is. He holds that the quality or level of striving is the most important single aspect of an individual's personality. He views the psychologically mature person as one who is much more concerned with where he is going than with where he has been. He also believes that adulthood is built on childhood. It is a time in which there can be an ever-increasing realization of higher-level potentialities for future achievement. Such assumptions underlie the concepts of health education and the belief that college students can change their health behavior to provide for more effective living.

THE TRAIT THEORY OF PERSONALITY

The trait approach to personality is a relatively simple theory, in that a list of qualities or traits describes or distinguishes one individual from another. Each trait is so distinct that it can be evaluated and studied experimentally. A trait is considered to be a permanent aspect of a person's behavior or experience, which can be identified clearly enough to show the uniqueness of one person in relation to another.

Smith[3] has selected 25 traits to illustrate this approach:

DRIVE TRAITS. Activity, sensory awareness, and sexuality

[3] Henry Clay Smith, *Personality Adjustment,* McGraw-Hill Book Company, Inc., New York, 1961, p. 31.

TEMPERAMENTAL TRAITS. Emotionality, optimism, and expressiveness

PERCEPTUAL TRAITS. Thinking extroversion, speed of closure, and flexibility of closure

SELF TRAITS. Self-extension, self-confidence, and self-insight

VALUE TRAITS. Economic, religious, scientific, aesthetic, and liberal values

PROBLEM-SOLVING TRAITS. Ambition, emotional control, orderliness, and intelligence

HUMAN-RELATIONS TRAITS. Gregariousness, dominance, warmth, and conformity

Not all psychologists agree upon any list of traits. Such agreement may come after further research and experimentation.

THE STRUCTURAL APPROACH, A PERSONALITY THEORY

The structural approach to personality emergence is concerned with the internal organization of behavior. It is based on the assumption that man is a biological organism and that he acts and reacts as an organized whole. It emphasizes the balanced, interdependent aspects of the personality structure, permitting one to see the parts in relation to the whole or total personality. Advocates of the structural approach emphasize the internal organization of personality and deemphasize the environment in which the personality makes adjustments. Freud's psychoanalytic theory is one type of structural approach. He viewed the *id*, the *ego*, and the *superego* as central features of personality structure. The id comprises all the psychological parts present at birth and is the biological side of personality. The ego represents the psychological workings. Whereas the id identifies the mind, the ego distinguishes between things in the mind and things in the environment. The ego is a secondary process in which realistic thinking takes place; also, it formulates and tests need satisfaction.

The superego is the social side of personality. It serves as the moral judge of whether behavior is right or wrong. For example, control of the sexual impulses of the id, which might be condemned by society, is a typical function of the superego.

The structural approach views the individual personality as a whole, unique in its own structural attributes [32].

THE ADJUSTMENT APPROACH

The adjustment theory of personality emphasizes not only internal structure but also the structure of the environment in which the individual must adjust. The adjustment approach is frequently referred to as the field approach. Emphasis is given to the unity of the individual's behavior and the environment in which it takes place, and the adjustment that occurs between these forces is stressed. Simply stated, the adjustment approach gives equal attention to internal and external forces.

Personality may be described by the ways in which certain kinds of adjustment are made. *Adjustment* describes the ways in which a person endeavors to solve his frustrations, internal problems, and interpersonal conflicts and to meet the demands of a situation or of society. Adjustment is the product of an individual's experiences during the process of development.

Adjustments may be on a low level—in fact, they may resemble psychoneurotic behavior—or they may be on a high plane, characteristic of maturity. The highest levels of adjustment are those requiring critical judgment, value discrimination, creativity, initiative, and daring.

The authors' view, in this health education text, is that *life is a continuous process of adjustment, in which the individual arrives at satisfactory relationships between his own needs and interests and the demands of society*. Satisfactory adjustment leads to a well-adjusted personality and a mature person.

REINFORCEMENT THEORY

Dollard and Miller believe that all behavior, both normal and abnormal, is learned through the interaction of four basic elements: drive, cue, response, and reinforcement [32]. _Drive_ is defined as a strong stimulus impelling action, such as physiologic needs provide. _Cue_ is a strong stimulus that determines what response an individual makes and when and where it will be made. The bell that signifies the end of a class period is an example of a cue; at least, it is a cue for the instructor to end his lecture. _Response_ is the action that is performed in reaction to cues. The actual closing of the lecture is the response. Other responses would include the students closing their notebooks, gathering up their books, and walking out of the room. _Reinforcement_ is any event that strengthens the tendency of the response to be repeated. The important part of reinforcement is that it results in the prompt reduction of the strength of the drive. For example, a person learns that taking an aspirin relieves a headache. When he has another headache, he readily takes an aspirin to relieve the condition without any hesitation or fuss.

A person also may learn a response that reduces a strong fear. Dollard and Miller assume that behavior, including emotional problems, can be learned or solved through the complex interaction of the four basic elements. They further contend that such learning will bring about changes and improvement in behavior. The reinforcement theory attempts to explain personality as the cumulative product of what the individual learns during his life [32].

SHELDON'S CONSTITUTIONAL THEORY

Sheldon differs from a number of personality theorists because he gives heredity a central role and stresses the importance of heredity factors in personality development. His theory of constitutional psychology was developed during his studies of college students. He photographed 4,000 or more students nude and then categorized his subjects by body type. The result was three body types: _endomorph, mesomorph_, and _ectomorph_. The types are called after the embryonic cell layers from which different body tissues develop. These body types are described in more detail in Chapter 7, pages 176-178.

Each dimension in Sheldon's classification is rated on a 7-point scale from 1 to 7. The first rating refers to endomorphy, the second to mesomorphy, and the third to ectomorphy. An individual rated 7+1+1 is extremely fat with little muscle; one rated 1+7+1 is extremely hard and muscular with no fat; a 1+1+7 rating indicates an extremely thin, tall, and delicate individual.

After his physical classification was formulated, Sheldon postulated a temperamental component related to each physical component: _viscerotonia_ related to endomorphy, _somatotonia_ to mesomorphy, and _cerebrotonia_ to ectomorphy. Temperaments were also rated on a similar 7-point scale.

According to Sheldon's theory, personality is centered around the viscera, especially the digestive tract. An individual with a temperament rating of 7+1+1 is extremely viscerotonic: he would have a general love of comfort, sociability, food, people, and affection. An extremely somatotonic person, with a rating of 1+7+1, is aggressive, noisy, courageous, active, and dominating. One who is cerebrotonic is secretive, self-conscious, and afraid of people.

Other investigators have found less correlation between physique and temperament than Sheldon did, but he is given credit for devising a system that demonstrates the relationship between the genes and personality. His work indicates the need for further research on this relationship [32].

UNCONSCIOUS VERSUS CONSCIOUS MOTIVES

Authorities in the science of personality differ over the importance of unconscious and conscious motives. The psychoanalysts consistently emphasize unconscious factors as major determinants of the most central elements of human behavior. The opposing position is that there is no unconscious motivation, that all behavior results from rational motives when the individual is aware of his actions. This view is less apparent now than in the past. Others accept the existence of unconscious motives but insist that these determinants operate only under exceptional situations, such as in extreme stress or where there is mental disorder, and that these occur only when ordinary modes of behavior have failed. Another current theory holds that both conscious and unconscious motives are important and emphasizes a balance of these motives [17].

There are several meanings for "unconscious." Ordinarily, we think of being "unconscious" as meaning the condition of being under the influence of anesthetic drugs or of having a brain concussion. It must be remembered that "unconscious" also refers to habitual or automatic action. We are unconscious of many of our idiosyncrasies, such as running a hand through the hair to smooth out a lock, scratching the head, beginning a conversation with "ah," or coughing nervously during a telephone conversation. We are entirely unaware of these behaviors but they are most apparent to others.

Memory is part of the unconscious. The attempt to recall a name that has been temporarily forgotten calls upon the unconscious. Putting off an unpleasant task without really meaning to do so is unconscious behavior.

"Unconscious" and "subconscious" are used frequently as synonymous terms. Subconscious thought is uncontrolled thinking. It refers to vague, unclear, and not fully realized thoughts, desires, and actions. Subconscious thinking takes place in our semidream and dream states as in daydreaming and reverie.

Of course, *conscious* refers to our usual daily activities, in which our attention is concentrated. We are fully aware of our conscious behavior. Our mental capacities are concentrated on achieving our goals. These activities include the freely acknowledged, the socially acceptable, the logical, and the relevant behavior.

The psychoanalyst delves into the subconscious behavior of a patient in order to develop a clearer and better balance between the conscious and subconscious. By doing so, he is able to help an individual understand himself more clearly and behave more rationally. It is thought that improper relationships between the conscious and subconscious are important causes of nervousness and troubled thoughts and feelings. Such actions lead to overemphasis on fantasies, daydreaming, and unpleasant emotional behavior. Psychoanalysis assists in restoring a normal relationship between the subconscious and the conscious [34].

Foundation factors for mental health

Mental health is based upon not one but many factors. The basic factors are the total make-up of the individual as a biological organism, i.e., his interrelated physical, emotional, and mental traits; the influences of the environment, including the society in which the individual finds himself; and the interaction process between the individual and society—the experiences by which the individual influences other people and is influenced by them. This is the process by which one learns and develops into maturity. The individual, within his biological limits, develops into his eventual personality on the basis of his experiences.

The developing person is sometimes

spoken of as the *self*, a unique personality. This personality is a composite of the biological self, the social self, and the self ideal.

The *biological self* is determined largely by hereditary endowment. The *social self* develops from the individual's interaction with his environment. The *self ideal*, superself, or psychological self is the individual's conscious or unconscious concept of his own behavior, including what he aims to be and do. Psychoanalysts term these aspects of the self the id, the ego, and the superego, as previously stated. These interrelated selves have a direct bearing upon the individual's mental health.

For the sake of simplicity in understanding the foundations of mental health, the basic factors have been broken down into common terms. Some of these major factors are heredity, physical factors, and the fundamental social forces—the home and family, the school, the neighborhood, and the community.

HEREDITY

Heredity provides the raw material, the potentialities of the individual, and tends to set limits for his mental health. Good heredity in itself does not ensure mental health, but the exact role of heredity in mental health is not yet fully known. It is known that heredity accounts for innate potentialities of the individual.

Hereditary traits are transmitted from parents to offspring by means of determiners of heredity called *genes* (see Chapter 6, page 158). The individual's heredity is determined when the sperm and the egg unite to form the zygote, a new individual. The exact number of chromosomes characteristic of human beings was formerly thought to be 48. More recently cells have been described with 46 chromosomes. It is generally accepted that most human cells contain 46 chromosomes. However, when two chromosomes fail to separate, one cell has an extra chromosome and the other one less.

If these survive and continue to divide, clinical abnormalities result. For example, Mongols are found to have 47 chromosomes. Whatever the number of chromosomes, they are arranged in pairs. The single cell normally contains 23 from the egg cell and 23 from the sperm cell, making the total of 46. The rodlike chromosomes contain the genes, which are the determiners of heredity.

When the cell begins to divide, the chromosomes line up along the center of the cell nucleus and divide also, making 46 pairs. This means that there are two cells with the same sets of chromosomes and identical sets of genes. The germ or sex cells contain only 23 chromosomes, since these cells pass through a stage in which their chromosomes split apart; this leaves only one of each pair. The two single germs cells from the sperm and egg combine to make new pairs in the zygote, which then contains 23 pairs of chromosomes, or 46 chromosomes altogether.

Each cell has the same hereditary material as the original fertilized egg. The genes provide the functional potentialities of the individual. The offspring has inherited potentialities for growth, appearance, intelligence, personality, and the like.

The genes are not contained in a vacuum. Their effects are influenced by both the internal and the external environments of the individual. Any trait or characteristic of the individual, therefore, including intelligence and personality, results from the interplay of both heredity and environment. Primarily it is capacity that is inherited, such as a capacity for thinking, feeling, and acting. How that capacity is utilized depends upon environmental influences.

The part heredity plays is clearer for physical than for mental traits. There is no doubt that one's physical features are inherited. As Scheinfeld[4] points out,

[4] Amram Scheinfeld, *The New You and Heredity*, J. B. Lippincott Company, Philadelphia, 1950, p. 87.

"Making faces happens to be one of the most interesting jobs done by genes . . . your size and shape are pretty closely determined by your genes." Since each individual is different from all others, it is obvious that individuality results from the genes. Genes may combine in a great variety of ways and with only minor differences. The present problem is to discover how important these differences are with regard to specific functions. For example, it would be helpful to know which traits enable one individual to live more effectively than another.

Much remains to be learned concerning the inheritance of specific mental traits. Present evidence indicates that the mental potential or native intelligence is hereditarily determined and that the environment determines the extent to which this potential is realized. Studies on identical twins compared with fraternal twins show the importance of heredity. There is evidence that when an individual is well motivated and has ample opportunity, intelligence quotients can be slightly improved. Similarly, an unfavorable and culturally impoverished environment may limit the extent to which mental potential is developed and utilized. It is also true that damage to the brain resulting from injuries or disease may lower mental capacity.

There is no doubt that superior mental traits are found in those persons with superior hereditary endowment. Lorge,[5] of Columbia University, states:

Superior intellectual ability is not a miracle. It is as natural as superiority in height or weight. Basically it is genetically constituted, but what the superior individual will do with his intellect will certainly be conditioned to a large degree by his environment and his education.

Genetic studies also show a hereditary basis for special capacities such as musical, artistic, and mechanical ability.

Fortunately for mankind, the mechanism of heredity works in such a way that most persons are normal (that is, within a normal range). Hereditary defects are generally recessive, while normal traits are dominant. There are a few exceptions; e.g., the rare disease Huntington's chorea is caused by a single dominant gene. This disease results in complete degeneration, finally terminating in death. There is no known cure.

In most cases there is insufficient evidence of the precise role of hereditary factors in mental illness. What evidence there is indicates that most mental illnesses are not directly inheritable. It is apparent, however, that heredity may predispose a person to development of a particular type of mental illness, such as schizophrenia or manic-depressive psychosis, when he is placed under excessive stress. It is possible, too, that heredity plays a contributing role in psychopathic personalities and in the psychoneuroses, such as compulsive neurosis, anxiety neurosis, and hypochondriasis.

Heredity plays an important part in producing many of the mentally defective or feeble-minded—idiots, imbeciles, and morons. It is often a factor in convulsive seizures. The term *epilepsy* (meaning "seizure") is applied to a chronic nervous disorder usually characterized by convulsions. Most authorities agree that epilepsy is not inherited directly but that a tendency or susceptibility to some types of epilepsy may be inherited. Epilepsy is discussed further in Chapter 12, pages 387–388.

A summary of Scheinfeld's [6] report of the effect of heredity on mental disorders, in which there is widespread agreement of authorities, is as follows:

1. Schizophrenia possibly may develop in an individual with an inherited predisposition coming from *both* parents through recessive genes.
2. Manic-depressive psychosis as a tendency probably is a function of partly

[5] As cited by Scheinfeld, *ibid.*, p. 383.

[6] Amram Scheinfeld, *The Human Heredity Handbook*, J. B. Lippincott Company, Philadelphia, 1956, pp. 131–142.

dominant or irregularly dominant genes, as well as of other "key" genes which mutually influence each other.

3. Huntington's chorea and Pick's disease (cerebral atrophy) are transmitted through a single dominant gene.

4. The neuroses are largely environmentally conditioned but there possibly may exist a hereditary predisposition in the selectivity of the symptoms.

5. Feeblemindedness is positively correlated statistically with parental IQs, and some evidence exists that recessive-gene inheritance may be a contributing factor.

Implications for the college student derived from the available data on heredity in mental health are as follows:

It is important for the individual to know his own hereditary limitations and potentialities.

Of even more vital concern is maximum, or at least greater, utilization of his potentialities. Good material has made many football coaches successful in the public eye. The greatest coaches from the viewpoint of the coaches themselves are those who have the ability to get the most out of their players, the material at hand. Improving mental health may be viewed as a parallel: almost everyone can further develop his potentialities, since few persons today are living up to capacity.

It is wise for the college student contemplating marriage to choose a mate of sound heredity and to know his own hereditary history as well as that of his mate.

Much research is needed to determine further the effect of heredity on mental abilities and specific traits.

Finally, the extent to which the individual's potentialities are developed depends upon the other foundation forces, particularly the environment and personal behavior. Heredity is but one factor in the development of personality.

PHYSICAL FACTORS

A brief analysis of the physical factors involved in mental health will help clarify the foundations upon which personal and social adjustment rests. In this discussion it is important not to lose sight of the premise of the total individual functioning as an integrated unit. A major portion of this book is devoted to physical health and the reciprocal influence of the mental and physical aspects. Chapter 7, Maintaining a Healthy and Attractive Body, contains a more detailed account of the total physical aspects of effective living.

From the available data it is apparent that physical health factors significantly contribute to mental health. The development of a wholesome, pleasing personality, resulting in a well-adjusted individual, depends on this foundation of physical health. An erect posture, a winning smile, color in the cheeks, and a feeling of exhilaration promote a sense of personal security and have a marked influence on other people. Strength, good looks, and robust health provide a social advantage in the development of personality characteristics.

A feeling of physical well-being makes possible intellectual alertness, enthusiasm, a good disposition, a desire to live, to achieve, and to be happy. Not all individuals in good physical health have good mental health; however, in most cases the better the physical health, the better also the mental health [3]. There is evidence that mental vitality is improved by physical health. Intelligence itself is not improved, but the motivation and drive through which the individual applies his intelligence are increased, bringing about added intellectual efficiency.

We can remember easily that our own mental health is poor when we are physically tired from hunger, overwork, or loss of sleep. Sick people, particularly the chronically ill, have a harder time making life adjustments. Data show that vitamin deficiencies lead to poor health and consequent personality problems. For example, vitamin B deficiencies result in restlessness, anxiety, and a quarrelsome attitude. In pernicious anemia, a deficiency of red corpuscles produces characteristic symptoms of apathy, irritability, depression, and anxiety. Persons suffering from serious physical defects tend to have similar problems of adjustment, though there are exceptions. On the other hand, the individual who follows a balanced regimen of food, drink, elimination, bathing, physical activity, work, sleep, rest, relaxation, prevention of disease, and correction of defects is more likely to have good mental health.

The nervous system. You, as a living person, are always active to some degree, continuously transforming food into energy and directing that energy into activity. The nervous system mobilizes and directs the energy created by metabolism. All human activity, therefore, has a neural basis. The 10 billion or more neurons making up the nervous system are divided into two principal parts: the *central nervous system,* composed of the brain and the spinal cord; and the *peripheral nervous system,* made up of the cranial and spinal nerves and the specialized set of peripheral nerves, the autonomic system. The functions of the nervous system consist in coordinating, integrating, inhibiting, reinforcing, facilitating, and associating. It is continually converting stimulation into activity and controlling and guiding the energy developed within the body.

The brain and spinal cord act as the central station of what might be called the vital communication center handling innumerable experiences. The *cerebrum,* the frontal and the largest single part of the brain, controls learned behavior. It enables the individual to sort out stimuli from the environment and to reflect, reason, judge, and think. Consciousness, intelligence, memory, insight, and interpretation of sensations are its functions.

The central nervous system is the integration center of organic function.

Many, if not all, bodily processes, such as digestion, skin eruptions, and heart action, may be influenced by thoughts and anxieties, which are produced by central nervous system action.

Reflexes enter into all bodily activities, and life itself depends upon such vital reflexes as breathing. A reflex is a simple innate response to a specific stimulus. A good example is the patellar tendon reflex. The physician tests this reflex during a routine medical examination to check a person's neural activity. The scratch reflex is an example of a reflex involving the total organism. Reflexes are altered by influences from high centers and are altered by reflex activity of the spinal cord. Limping because of a nail in the shoe is such a reflex action. The nail stimulates pain receptors, which produce a flexion reflex [36].

The *central nervous system* as a whole provides different levels of learning, enabling the person to acquire habits and skills which, once learned, may be used over and over again. This makes learning continuous.

The *autonomic nervous system* controls the functioning of bodily organs, the heart, lungs, digestive tract, and glands. In turn, this system is divided into the *sympathetic* and *parasympathetic* systems. The sympathetic nerves speed up function or drive the organism, and the parasympathetic slow down or act as a brake on the individual's activities. The cerebrum has no control over the autonomic nervous system; for example, the heartbeat cannot be speeded up or slowed down at will. The sympathetic system strengthens and accelerates the heartbeat, constricts arteries and raises blood pressure, slows peristalsis (wave-like contractions in the wall of the alimentary canal), dilates passages such as the bronchial tubes, makes for easier breathing, and increases basal metabolism.

The functions of the sympathetic nervous system are illustrated when there is fear. Fear reactions are actually the effect

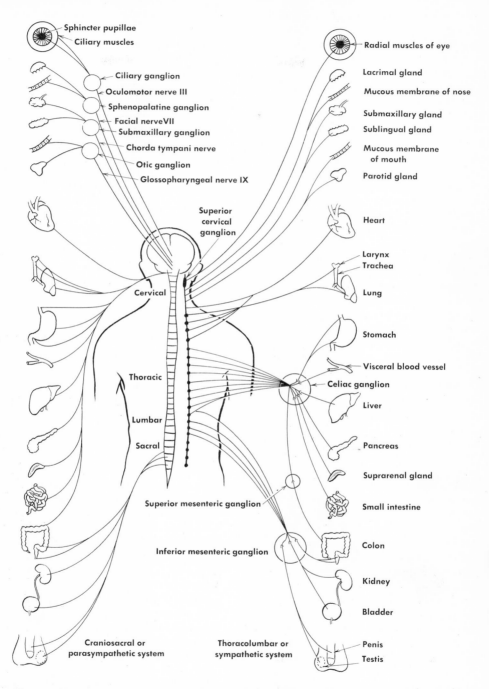

The autonomic nervous system showing its two divisions: the craniosacral or para-sympathetic, and the sympathetic. (Adapted from Russell M. DeCoursey, *The Human Organism*, McGraw-Hill Book Company, Inc., New York, 1961.)

of sympatheticoadrenal functions. The mouth is dry because the saliva is produced only in a thick and viscous form. The pupil of the eye dilates because muscles are under control of the sympathetic nervous system. The heart increases its rate. The blood pressure also increases, and there is constriction of the peripheral blood vessels in some parts of the body. Peripheral vasoconstriction is what makes one appear pale and wan, with a cold skin. Perspiration is due to the response of the emotional sweating areas, which include the palms of the hands, the soles of the feet, the armpits, and the groin. Digestion stops as the muscular contraction, peristalsis, for the whole gastrointestinal tract is inhibited.

The sympathetic nervous system goes all out in emergency situations. It also goes into concerted action when the individual is in temperature extremes, hungry, involved in intense exercise, or in pain or suffering from bodily injury [36].

The parasympathetic system, on the other hand, weakens and slows the heartbeat, dilates arteries and lowers blood pressure, speeds peristalsis, constricts passages such as the bronchial tubes, but has no effect on basal metabolism. These nerves have an antagonistic effect on the organs innervated in some instances; in others there is no antagonism.

Local reflexes are responsible for many parasympathetic effects. Eating produces an increased quantity of saliva and hydrochloric acid and stimulates peristalsis. Many forms of parasympathetic function result from excitement. In such instances, peristalsis and secretion of hydrochloric acid again are increased. Increased hydrochloric acid secretion is considered to be a major cause of stomach ulcers [36].

A stimulus received by the individual may set off reactions in the central nervous system without much action of the autonomic; contrariwise, the autonomic may be stimulated without much control from the central nervous system. A stimulus may set off reactions in both systems.

The autonomic nervous system is intimately related to the endocrine system. Together they regulate most internal functions and serve to maintain homeostasis. Both functions are necessary to maintain the internal environment.

The autonomic nervous system nerve fibers liberate chemical substances at their terminal endings. The organs they stimulate react to these chemicals and to chemicals from the blood stream. For example, the vagus nerve stimulates the liberation of insulin from the islets of Langerhans in the pancreas. In turn, the insulin facilitates the responses of organs with parasympathetic innervation.

The nervous system can connect any sense organ or part with any group of muscles. It also can strengthen and distribute the impulses from any stimulation so that all the muscles are called into action. This function is called *facilitation*. This is similar to the head of the communication center talking to all the employees at once, calling on them for support and concerted action.

Conversely, the central nervous system, corresponding to the executive's office, can handle communications from all the employees. Impulses arising from many different sense organs at the same time may be *coordinated* and *integrated* so that the executive puts into effect a single action. In addition, these communications may be sent to the central office with certain impulses *inhibited* while others call for appropriate action. This is a canceling out of impulses. The opposite function is *reinforcement,* in which some impulses are strengthened by others.

A further significant function of the nervous system is its *associative* function. The central office changes with every impulse that is handled by it. In this way, improvement occurs. Past experience affects the present, and the present affects future actions. This means the individual can recall past experiences, bring the past to bear upon the present, and plan for the future action. The neuron patterns of the moment determine the perceptors and hence our thoughts and activities. The nervous system enables the individual to retain information and experiences, to acquire new knowledge and skills, and, in general, to improve his behavior.

Endocrine glands. The endocrine glands are small, ductless glands often referred to as *glands of internal secretion.* Their secretions, called *hormones,* flow directly into the blood or lymph stream. No gland acts independently; each has a supplemental function. One gland may stimulate or inhibit the function of another. When one gland does not function properly, because of defect or disease, the effect may be felt on other glands, with a consequent effect on the total body. Such a pathologic condition is called a *functional disease.*

The bodily functions affected most by the endocrine secretions are growth and development, metabolism, sex, and the coordination of smooth muscle activity relating to the autonomic nervous system. Table 2.1 summarizes the endocrine glands and their primary functions.

The regulatory function of the endocrine glands is to maintain constancy of the internal environment. *Homeostasis,* or the maintenance of a steady state, is essential to normal functioning. When this steady state is not maintained, the individual's behavior is affected abnormally. Energy output and drive as well as temperamental differences may be influenced by thyroid activity. In women, changes in mood are associated with

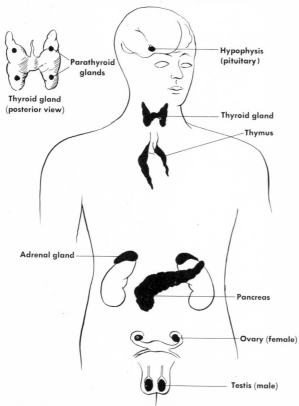

Parathyroid glands

Thyroid gland (posterior view)

Hypophysis (pituitary)

Thyroid gland

Thymus

Adrenal gland

Pancreas

Ovary (female)

Testis (male)

Diagram indicating the endocrine system of the human body. (Adapted from Russell M. DeCoursey, *The Human Organism,* **McGraw-Hill Book Company, Inc., New York, 1961.)**

Table 2.1 The endocrine glands*

Gland	Location	Hormones secreted	Apparent function
Adrenal: Cortex	Top of kidneys	Hydrocortisone, cortisone, sex hormones	Aids in regulation of metabolism of water and salts (sodium, potassium, chlorine)
Medulla		Epinephrine (adrenalin)	Similar to autonomic nervous system; appears to aid in time of emergency
Gonads: Ovaries	On each side of uterus in female	Estrogens Progesterone	Secondary sex characteristics; reproductive functions
Testes	Scrotum in male	Testosterone	Secondary sex characteristics
Islets of Langerhans	In pancreas	Insulin	Regulation of carbohydrate metabolism
Parathyroid	Imbedded in thyroid	Parathormone	Regulation of calcium metabolism
Pineal	Below cerebrum	Unknown	Not clearly demonstrated
Pituitary (Hypophysis)	Beneath brain, in depression of sphenoid bone		
Anterior		ACTH, thyrotropic hormone, growth hormone, gonadotropic hormones	Regulating effect on other endocrine glands; regulation of growth and development; regulation of ovarian cycle in female
Posterior		Vasopressin, oxytocin	Antidiuretic (decreases the excretion of urine); oxytocic effect (contraction of uterine muscles)
Thymus	Upper chest	Unknown	Not clearly demonstrated
Thyroid	Each side of trachea and joined in front	Thyroxin	Regulation of metabolism; growth and development

Source: Based on Russell M. DeCoursey, *The Human Organism*, 2d ed., McGraw-Hill Book Company, Inc., New York, 1961; and Arthur C. Guyton, *Textbook of Medical Physiology*, W. B. Saunders Company, Philadelphia, 1956.

Disorders due to malfunction

Hypofunction: Addison's disease
Hyperfunction: acceleration of sexual development
No known disease entities

Hypofunction: underdevelopment of secondary sex characteristics

Hyperfunction: sexual precocity

Hypofunction: diabetes mellitus
Hyperfunction: (rare) low blood sugar concentration

Hypofunction: tetany
Hyperfunction: increased calcium concentration in blood; loss of muscle tone

Malfunction of other endocrine glands
Hypofunction: retarded development (dwarfism)
Hyperfunction: giantism or acromegaly

Hypofunction: diabetes insipidus

Hypofunction: infants—cretinism; adults— myxedema, simple goiter
Hyperfunction: increased metabolism, toxic goiter

* Includes only the more commonly known hormones, primary functions, and most common disorders.

endocrine secretions pertaining to the menstrual cycle. The endocrine glands exert a powerful influence on the total individual, including both physical and emotional functions.

Hormones are produced by the body in relatively small amounts. The effect, however, of a minute amount of a given hormone can be extensive. Current findings relative to hormones and their effect on the human organism are incomplete. The extreme potency of these substances, combined with incomplete information about their effects, makes the use of hormone preparations dangerous unless prescribed by a qualified medical person. It is highly advisable to use such preparations only on the advice of a physician. Anyone reading the "popular" articles about hormone preparations should do so critically. Cortisone, ACTH (adrenocorticotropic hormone), insulin, and the other hormones can effect unbelievable improvement in the health of individuals if used properly, but they can do great harm if used improperly.

Metabolism. Mental health also depends on body mechanisms that maintain an appropriate chemical balance. When the body metabolism, which regulates this balance, is upset in some way, a mental disturbance may result. The underlying causes of metabolic changes are still not clearly understood. However, present research studies indicate that such disturbances can be treated to some extent by chemical means. For example, the release of epinephrine (adrenalin) by the adrenal gland is subject to control both by nerve impulses and by chemicals brought to the gland by the blood. In the nervous system itself the nerve cells transmit signals from one cell to the next and finally to the body cells that activate the nerves. Transmission of signals across the junction between two nerve cells (the synapse) is controlled to a large degree by two substances, epinephrine and acetylcholine. It has been determined experimentally that acetylcholine excites transmission and epinephrine inhibits it. These two chemicals working counter to each other have a regulatory effect on the nervous system. An excess of inhibitory substances may cause a mental disturbance; so may an excess of an exciting substance. The metabolism of the body normally regulates both the production of the opposing chemicals and their destruction, usually by enzymatic action, to maintain a proper balance. If excesses should develop, however, it is possible to treat this condition by administering chemical drugs; for example, the tranquilizing drugs counteract the inhibitory effect of excessive epinephrine [19]. See pages 94 and 95.

The action of epinephrine, as described above, may seem unusual. It is explained by the fact that this inhibiting effect in communications first occurs in exaggerated activity. Then, when there are excessive amounts present, epinephrine acts as a depressant or inhibitor, not as a stimulant. This effect is similar to that of alcohol on the body. When alcohol is consumed, the effect is a depressant action, not stimulation.

Epinephrine also has a self-limiting effect. When it rises to an abnormally high level in the blood stream, production is automatically slowed down because communications are slowed down. The level of epinephrine in the adrenal gland is reduced because of lack of stimulation by the nervous system.

Action is the major purpose of nervous system function, through adjustment of the individual to his environment. The highly complex structure of the brain permits complicated activity to occur. Its function makes possible the storing up of knowledge. Through action we are able to live, to protect ourselves, and to prolong life and maintain security. In well-adjusted mental life, sensations, feelings, and thoughts lead continuously to purposeful action. Sensations serve as signals to inform us that it is time to do certain things. Feelings for persons make us act with them

or for them. In either case they lead to action. Emotions enable us to run faster, strive harder, love more—all of which make action possible. Memory, thought, and imagination enable us to act more wisely and to live happier lives [34].

Homeostasis. Homeostasis is the relative constancy, or maintenance of equilibrium, of internal physiologic conditions. The body's automatic efforts maintain a constant state of the blood stream, including the water, salt, protein, calcium, and oxygen content, the acid-base balance, and the temperature. Man's internal temperature is kept relatively constant through homeostasis. A homeostatic function occurs when lactic acid is injected into the blood stream and eliminated through the kidneys until equilibrium is restored. When the water balance in the blood is upset, a "thirst drive" is set in motion so that the individual will act to maintain this needed balance. Equilibrium is achieved both through internal mechanisms and through outside assistance.

Psychosomatic relationships. Psychosomatic relationships include more than psychosomatic medicine; they include all interrelationships between mental activity and body functions. Commonly, the term is used to describe physical disorders of mental origin or specifically influenced by mental activity. Not only medicine but psychology as well is concerned with psychosomatic problems. Another term—*somatopsychic*—may be needed to describe the opposite effect, that of body functions on mental activity. Physical fatigue and prolonged wakefulness are examples. The use of drugs, alcohol, tobacco, coffee, and tea produces effects on the body, which, in turn, affects the mind.

Psychosomatic medicine is concerned with the mind-body relationship because the mind can influence the state of the body to produce illness. Psychosomatic relationships differ greatly with different people. Some individuals have a nervous system that easily upsets the function of their internal organs. Others have a nervous system that does not disturb normal organic functions. These people may be even-tempered and calm, rarely becoming excited about events. They appear to take life in stride and are perfectly well year in and year out. Still other persons have stormy and violent emotions and are easily stirred up over small matters. They are frequently tense and jittery and demonstrate varying moods both up and down. Some of these emotional tides may be the result of internal secretions of a chemical nature from one of the endocrine glands.

Knowing that some of anyone's troubles may be psychosomatic may be helpful. When a person is suffering from a psychosomatic condition, the fact that he realizes this helps both him and the doctor to correct the condition. Also, discussing personal fears with someone else—the doctor, a friend, or a relative—may be most helpful. Finding a way to relieve the tension or strain, such as changing a course or a program or moving from poor living quarters, may help considerably. Acquiring the best professional help is most important [2].

The dynamics of growth and development. The psychological development of young people is such that few individuals, if any, mature without facing physical, mental, or emotional problems. All normal children follow a generally similar continuous sequence of growth; yet each child follows his own pattern and his own time schedule as he progresses through various stages. Such progress to maturity is not always a pleasant trip. Growth may occur as a spiral, with a child making progress upward and then dipping downward to an earlier stage before going upward to reach a still higher level. There are many hurdles along the way. Learning to walk, for instance, is a real developmental achievement, but it leads to new problems as well as new interests. The same is true in mental development. As an individual becomes

able to imagine and anticipate a future pleasure, he also becomes able to worry about the future. A gain in ability carries with it increased responsibility. As children and young persons meet the demands of development, maturation, and socialization at their own rate of progress, they also develop the functional capacities and personality that manifest their unique patterns. When growth is most rapid or, conversely, when it slows down perceptibly, emotional problems are more common and more apparent.

Growth does not automatically bring about an improvement of behavior. The growth process may seem to create new problems or aggravate old ones. A child does not leave one growth stage completely when he enters another; he keeps old ways of behaving, although his new mannerisms and actions tend to obscure his old behavior. The child retains part of the infant's behavior, and the adolescent has some childish characteristics in his behavior.

Children with good inheritance and home environment are expected to go through a rapid growth period during their preschool years. This is followed by a latent period in middle childhood and a growth spurt during puberty. Adolescence is a period of reorganization, a period of re-forming the personality in a new world. The early teens are disturbing years, as young persons are experimenting with new feelings and new roles. When given understanding and guidance, the adolescent can handle his conflicts and attain a reasonable degree of integration in the late teens.

Development is enhanced when adults, particularly parents, are able to identify the emergence and recession of a stage of development and know when to provide aid and encouragement and when to leave the child alone. Adults should remember that each child has his own rate of growth and cannot be unduly pressured to achieve another pattern. Good support and wise guidance from parents and other adults aid materially in solving the temporary problems of young persons, enabling them to emerge through the growth process as mentally healthy individuals [12].

SOCIAL AND CULTURAL FACTORS

Social factors are the individual's *environment*, the society in which he lives, and the *interaction process*, his social functioning with other persons. Of special importance is his ability to make adjustments in social situations and with other people as he participates in everyday activities. These social forces affect the individual's mental health. The environment in which the individual finds himself from birth influences him in a variety of ways. From his own particular environment he gains his social heritage. The stimulation he receives, the knowledge he acquires, the skills he develops, the interests he utilizes, the attitudes he forms, the habits he establishes, the values and goals he develops— all are shaped by his environment. He enters this society, which is already established; so he learns to adapt to it and acquire from it the content of his behavior.

From birth, the individual is a part of society. He soon notices a few people, who in turn notice him. He uses his equipment —sense organs, muscles, and nervous system—and begins to integrate what he sees with what he does. Interaction takes place when the infant, using his equipment, perceives and responds to others, who are perceiving and responding to him in ways that are characteristic of the culture. By this medium the individual gradually changes himself. He learns, he develops a unique personality, and he participates in his society.

The human personality emerges and is modified not only by the influence of parents, teachers, administrators, employers, and workers but also by existing social patterns. Cultural as well as physiologic factors influence personality emergence. The demands of a culture help mold the personality of its members.

Social patterns are quite responsive to new circumstances and change. The United States is a society in transition, with changing conditions calling for new and greater adjustments. These changes may be seen in rapid developments in science and technology, new types of industrialization and urbanization, the still great cultural lag between the availability of scientific information and its utilization by the citizenry, changing community and rural-urban patterns of living, changes in institutions and in social organization, increased leisure time, changing physical resources, and the timeless disasters of nature, including forest fires, floods, tornadoes, and cyclones.

Adjustment to cultural change may be resisted because persons fail to understand the nature of the new social patterns and also because they are not fully aware of the implications of new circumstances for their daily living. Following old traditions may impede the adoption of new social patterns.

More and more, however, it is now being recognized that social patterns can be understood and adapted to socially desirable goals that have a significant effect on the mental health of society. The provision for health and social services, the organization of industry, and the administration of the government must be considered in reference to the needed change in society. A mentally healthy society calls for not only better understanding of opportunities to improve social patterns but development and implementation of effective plans to alleviate human frustration and bring about better social adjustment. The ultimate goal of mental health is a social one, that is, to help men live more effective lives with their fellows [35].

The home and family. The first developmental experiences take place in the home or family. Investigations have shown that young children learn to pattern their behavior after that of their parents. In most cases, both boys and girls are closer to the mother during the first ten years than to the father. The mother contributes to mental health by giving the child affection and security and by guiding his development efficiently and effectively. The child reflects the mother's fears and her ideas of right and wrong [18]. Reports of college students describing their mothers indicate that the mother contributes to mental health when she is gentle, agreeable, and even-tempered. Conversely, the mother tends to cause insecurity when she is nervous, tense, self-centered, and insecure. Mothers affect their children adversely when they are overprotective, reject the child emotionally, are domineering, are unreasonable or inconsistent in disciplinary practices, have favorites among their children, and are not well-adjusted themselves, with a resultant reflection of their frustrations in their children. The mother plays an important role in establishing ideals, attitudes, and practices of extreme significance in making adjustments.

The father as a provider generally has less contact with the children, though his role seems to take on greater importance as the children grow older. This is especially true if the father takes time to share his life with his family, if he shows interest in the development of his children, plays with them, works with them, shares their joys and troubles, is just in his discipline, and becomes an ideal in the eyes of his children.

Brothers and sisters, often referred to as *siblings*, also influence the development of mental health in the family. Often older children, as well as parents, provide affection, security, and guidance for younger children, assisting them in establishing ideals and values. Negative influences result if older children dominate and create feelings of insecurity through constant friction. Sibling rivalry is a definite factor in emotional development.

Evidence from studies shows that broken homes produce a larger percentage of children with adjustment problems than do stable homes. However, not all broken homes result in maladjusted children. A home with one understanding parent is often superior to one in which

there are two parents who are in constant conflict, creating an atmosphere of discord.

A good home is one in which there is:
Genuine affection for each member
A harmonious relationship between parents
Parental understanding of the needs and interests of the children
Parental assistance in helping children to realize their needs and interests
Consistent, firm discipline
Opportunity for children to participate in responsible activities, engage in play and recreation, and invite friends into the home

Stevenson [7] states that "the family is the social capsule in which feelings develop, and therefore it becomes the most potent force in shaping the mental health of everyone." No other unit meets the basic human needs more directly than does the family. The family in its ideal form is a miniature democratic society. It provides the setting, the stimulation, the emotional support, and the guidance that enable the child to make successful personal and social adjustments.

The school. The school is the chief continuing and supplementing institution where individuals develop sound mental health practices. The school provides experiences to develop the total individual through self-realization, human relationships, economic efficiency, and civic responsibilities. School experiences are designed to enhance growth and development, stimulate learning, and develop good behavior patterns. This calls for pupils to participate in an enriched curriculum, under the guidance of well-adjusted teachers and administrators, in a wholesome environment. To achieve the purposes of the school, the experiences comprising the school curriculum are designed to meet the following fundamental individual needs [13, 35]:

[7] George S. Stevenson, *Mental Health Planning for Social Action*, McGraw-Hill Book Company, Inc., New York, 1956, p. 213.

A feeling of personal worth

Social competence in winning acceptance from associates

Physical satisfactions necessary to the well-being of the body

Freedom to play and to accomplish purposeful tasks

Developing interests and activities providing social values

The experiences in school, in addition to experiences in the home, determine, to a large degree, one's sense of personal worth. The result of school work is not always positive from a mental health standpoint. Self-realization is achieved only to the extent that successful adjustments are made and satisfactory progress results. On the other hand, if the school experiences cause many emotional stresses, do not provide affectional responses, and offer few chances for success, there is likelihood that the individual will adjust by using socially undesirable defense mechanisms. The pupil is expressing feelings of insecurity, anxiety, or frustration if his conduct in school takes the form of antisocial destructive behavior or if he shows withdrawal or regressive tendencies.

Social growth outside the family is developed to a great extent in school. The feeling of personal acceptance which one acquires lays the groundwork for socializing with others. The individual learns to respect the rights, feelings, and property of others in school. He learns to win the approval of his associates and to feel secure in the presence of others.

The school shares with the home in the development of social and cultural values. The attitudes and habits that become the attributes of mature adults are determined to a large measure through school experiences. The school exerts a dominant influence in the formation of attitudes and practices relating to customs, morals, politics, sex, marriage, and principles of living in general. These attitudes, whether positive or negative, are instrumental in determining the effectiveness of the behavior of the individual in society.

The school contributes to sound mental health, assisting in preventing behavior disorders, when it provides:

Respect for the pupil as an individual

Regard for the whole personality as an integrated unit

An enriched curriculum of activities, cooperatively planned, meeting the needs and interests of pupils

Extraclass activities, a part of the curriculum, such as dramatics, clubs, athletics, and recreational pursuits, for the development of broad interests

Developmental tasks for each student, allowing some freedom in accomplishing the tasks

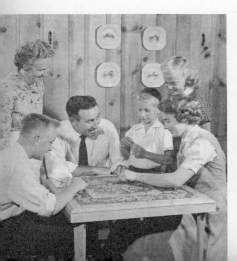

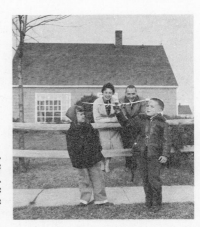

Beginning in early childhood, the foundations of mental health are established in the experiences of an individual as part of the family.

Tasks adjusted to the level of development
of each student

Activities that develop habits of cooperation, an attitude of civic responsibility,
and a creative approach to life

Well-adjusted teachers and administrators

Individual and group counseling

A wholesome environment for pupils and
school personnel

In addition to the above preventive
measures, the school attempts to identify
children with problems and refer those
with behavior disorders to child guidance
clinics. The school attempts to provide
well-adjusted classroom teachers; specially prepared teachers in health education, family-life education, and counseling;
and psychologists and psychiatrists in
child guidance centers. Also, the existing
mental health resources of the community
are utilized to carry out this corrective
health service program.

The Delaware public schools, working
with the Delaware State Society for Mental Hygiene, have organized classes in
human relations, which in actuality are
direct teachings in mental health.

This project, initiated and led by H. E.
Bullis, centered around three textbooks
entitled *Human Relations in the Classroom.* They provide teachers with essential materials for mental health lessons.
The goals of this direct teaching are to
help school children: make decisions, accept responsibilities, profit from their mistakes, bring their fears out into the open
by discussing them, develop self-acceptance, face reality, and look forward with
interest to the future. The success of the
project in Delaware led to its spread to
other states [12].

Other planned programs in mental
health education are organized in a number of schools throughout the United
States. The Forest Hills Village Project
and the Ojemann Project illustrate such
programs. In the Forest Hills Village Project, a team of clinicians from the University of Toronto taught the principles of
mental health to the teachers in the

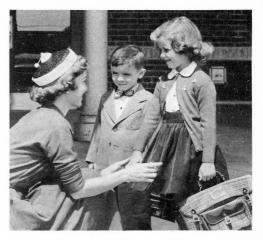

The process of personality emergence
has already begun. Gradually horizons broaden, and adjustments to
new situations must be made.

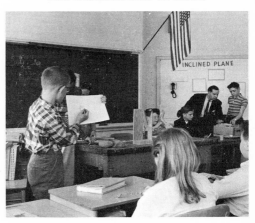

From the family environment a child
takes his place in the school environment . . . and in the community.

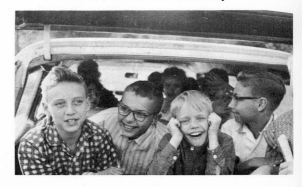

schools. In turn, the teachers conducted human relations classes with their children for one hour per week in grades five through twelve. These are permissive discussion sessions in which the children talk about their problems. The administrators and teachers are pleased with the discussion sessions, which serve as group therapy sessions.

The Ojemann Project, developed at the University of Iowa, is an attempt to integrate human relations education into the public school curriculum. Instruction is planned in such a way that pupils are prepared in the basic principles of mental health and apply the principles in their daily behavior. Results of the instruction in grades one through twelve showed that children improved in their understanding of human relationships and in their attitudes toward themselves and others [12].

Every school program must be developed to assist students to satisfy their basic needs of love, acceptance, security, projection, independence, faith, guidance, and self-control. These are the needs of children as defined by the National Association for Mental Health [26].

The community. Dr. Robert H. Felix, Director of the National Institute of Mental Health, U.S. Public Health Service, has stated: [8]

Mental health begins with people—first in people's thinking of their own needs, then in extending this consideration to those within the family circle and finally, to those in the community at large.

The community provides the environment in which the individual achieves his stature as a personality and in which his family lives and grows. The individuals in the family develop not only through the interpersonal relations within this group but also through participation in community activities. The community may influence personality emergence either positively or negatively. A community will

influence its members negatively when there is constant strife and unhappiness in its populace, when there are families destroyed and children deserted because of emotionally unstable parents unable to find needed assistance, and when there are people merely existing in quiet despair. Some communities seem to have the essential resources but lack leadership to develop community mental health programs.

On the positive side, there are communities, and there should be many more, that can provide adequate jobs and have residential sections, busy stores, an abundance of churches, sufficient recreation centers, and well-planned and well-functioning mental health programs, all of which provide residents with a good home, a lifework, a sense of belonging, and contentment necessary for the mentally healthy state.

The constituents of successful, functioning community mental health programs include the realization that each community is unique and that there is no one formula to bring about action for better mental health. A good starting place in developing a sound program is to make an inventory of mental health needs and evaluate available mental health resources. A study of the community, with professionals and lay persons working together, can be worked out by taking one area of need at a time and making the task a possible and practical one. Leadership will have to be mobilized to bring about action. A local health council, a voluntary health agency, a professional health society, civic and fraternal groups, or citizens at large can provide the necessary leadership. A representative group of citizens, including professionally trained mental health workers, health educators, and citizens, can work out ways to gain necessary community support.

The survey would provide the necessary facts, and a representative group would make action possible. No doubt, the survey would identify such problems as the lack of professional personnel in mental

[8] Reported by Elizabeth M. Dach, *Your Community and Mental Health*, Public Affairs Pamphlet 263, Public Affairs Committee, Inc., New York, 1958, p. 2.

health, lack of mental health education, misunderstanding of mental health goals, lack of funds, existing stigma of mental illness, need to strengthen family groups, need for mental health services to provide for counseling, early detection, diagnosis, and treatment, and, finally, need for accepting the mentally ill as useful citizens after treatment.

The representative group would be able to inform people that mental health services in the community include not only those in clinics and hospitals but also such resources as churches, schools, health agencies, courts, law-enforcement agencies, and community centers.

The group or council might bring about better coordination between the mental hospital, if one is present, and the health department, the welfare department, and other health agencies. It might find ways to secure professional workers to improve diagnosis, treatment, and rehabilitation. Also, it might utilize volunteer workers, who can contribute significantly to the program [5].

Citizens, as individuals or as members of groups, can render valuable service in the following roles: [9]

PROMOTER. Encouraging the development of local services

ORGANIZER. Setting up a mental health association or committees

LEADER. Joining local study or action groups as a clinic or agency board member

TABOO BREAKER. Replacing poor attitudes with understanding

VOLUNTEER. Helping in hospital, clinic, or local group

LAY EDUCATOR. Helping others to learn the facts

SUPPORTER. Supporting legislation and appropriations

ENCOURAGER. Writing and visiting patients and families

RECOGNIZER. Honoring service well done

GIVER-JOINER. Supporting local groups

Criteria for mental health

The criteria for positive mental health, derived from clinical experience, careful observation, and research studies reported in the literature, serve to guide us in understanding mental health and to direct our own course of action. The criteria presented here are selected from Marie Jahoda's study of the writings of well-known authorities in the field [10]. Her *Current Concepts of Positive Mental Health* is the most comprehensive and authoritative study devoted specifically to positive concepts. Concepts relating to mental illness are omitted purposely.

In her study to determine the psychological meaning of various criteria for positive mental health, Jahoda arrived at six categories:

Attitudes of the individual toward himself—the *self image*

The degree to which a person realizes his potentialities through action—*growth, development, and self-actualization*

Unification of function in the individual's personality—*integration*

The individual's degree of independence of social influences—*autonomy*

How the individual sees the world around him—*perception of reality*

The individual's ability to take life as it comes and master it—*environmental mastery*

To understand fully positive mental health concepts some of the specific criteria relating to each category must be considered.

THE SELF IMAGE

Authorities agree that healthy attitudes toward one's self are basic to good mental health. Such attitudes include self-acceptance, self-confidence, and self-reli-

[9] William G. Hollister, *An Overview: Providing Better Mental Health for Our People, An Introductory Manual for Mental Health Workers*, at 10110 Parkwood Terrace, Bethesda 14, Md., 1956, p. 6.

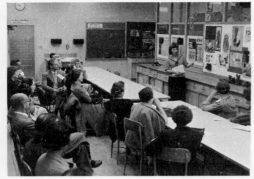

In the important process of understanding a child, adults must often receive guidance, which may even shape a new understanding of themselves . . .

for mental health is a concept which applies to individuals of every age

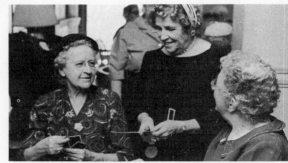

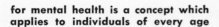

. . . in every situation.

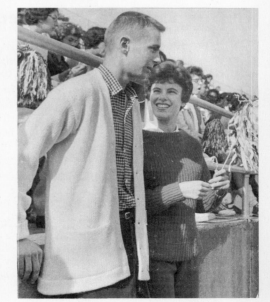

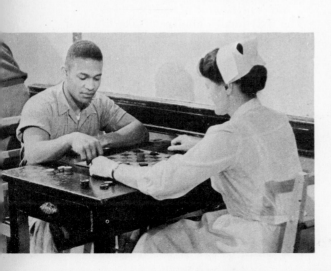

ance. Self-acceptance means that the person has learned to live with himself. He has some insight into his motives and desires as well as into his weaknesses and strong points. He is able to evaluate his own behavior and his own strengths and weaknesses. He can laugh at himself and at his own mistakes. He accepts his own human make-up without feeling real concern; yet he tries to improve himself.

Self-confidence, self-esteem, and self-respect imply that the person has ability to succeed. He believes he will do reasonably well in whatever he undertakes. He solves his problems largely by his own initiative and effort. He neither overestimates nor underestimates his abilities. He feels able to meet the demands of daily life.

It is well to realize the self image does not imply being self-conscious of every act or purpose. It does, however, indicate the importance of being one's self and possessing the ability to survey objectively one's own capacities and goals. This calls for both objectivity and reason on the part of the individual.

A sense of identity or the sentiment of self-regard in the mentally healthy individual is an integrative aspect of the self concept. This is an ability to see himself as a total person to the extent that he knows who he is and what he does. A sense of identity provides the student with assurance as he seeks friends, particularly those of the opposite sex, and assumes leadership roles. It is definitely a characteristic of the mature individual.

Self-adjusted applies to the individual who likes and respects himself and can enjoy himself in the process of living while pursuing his goals. It means that he is free from serious and disturbing internal conflicts, persistent worries, and pathologic guilt feelings [4]. The self image is one of the important sources of motivation of all behavior. It is of primary significance in both personal and social behavior because we are prone to respond to others in the manner in which we regard ourselves. Behavior is a function of the individual's conception of his perceptual field, or the events in which he participates. We respond to any stimulus situation by the way we interpret its meaning within our own frame of reference. The pattern of life an individual chooses to live is one compatible with his self image. Each individual strives both consciously and unconsciously to maintain a consistent view of himself.

The self image affects social adjustment, too. For each individual responds to any social situation and to others in the social setting on the basis of the way he feels about himself. We like others to the extent that they help us to like ourselves [4]. Respect for instructors is based on this principle. The confidence and stimulation given by an instructor encourages students to achieve their goals and, in some instances, to progress beyond their expectations.

GROWTH, DEVELOPMENT, AND SELF-ACTUALIZATION

The degree to which a person realizes his potentialities through action is an ongoing process, which can be described as attaining *self-realization,* or *self-actualization.* This process includes the positive self image previously described, motivational drives, and the maximum development of the individual's basic mental and physical faculties. From the motivational point of view, self-actualization includes growth motivation leading to the development of potential capacities and talents and also to the carrying out of a mission in life or to vocational accomplishment. As described previously in connection with Maslow's theory of motivation, self-actualization signifies the condition in which an individual is working for a cause greater than himself. It leads to the striving for and attainment of goals higher than the satisfaction of basic needs. The striving for and the attainment of these goals mean a richer life. The increase of health information, the development of

DEVELOPING A HEALTHY PERSONALITY

new and wholesome health attitudes, and the establishment of positive health practices that can result in more effective living are all parts of self-actualization. Formulating and making reasonable progress toward well-defined, realistic goals enables one to attain self-realization.

INTEGRATION

Although integration is a part of the self image and the self-actualization concept, it is sufficiently important to be discussed separately. Integration means the interrelationship of all parts, processes, and attributes. It is best described as the unity of the organism—the individual as a total being. Jahoda's study found that integration as a criterion for mental health involved particularly a balance of psychic forces in the individual, a unifying outlook on life, and resistance to stress.

The *balance of psychic forces* means a balance of the ego, superego, and id or of unconscious, preconscious, and conscious behavior. This balance in the healthy personality is flexible. The ego may function strongly, but occasionally it may be brought under central control, with domination by the id or the superego.

Flexibility of action also appears to be a characteristic of the healthy state and an essential aspect of integration.

A *unifying philosophy of life* is also part of integration. The mature person develops a philosophy of life that gives meaning and purpose to his daily activities. This does not mean a philosophy that is written out or spoken in a certain few words; rather, a person's actions, his participation in events, his religion—all these may demonstrate his philosophy of life and indicate that he has achieved a place for himself in the world. In addition, long-range goals, as a part of the philosophy of life, are a unifying factor of personality and of good mental health. Leading authorities agree that a unifying outlook on life is a significant characteristic of mentally healthy persons.

Research studies indicate that a person's ability to *resist stress* is an essential characteristic of sound mental health. This does not mean that all tension, anxiety, frustration, or unhappiness are avoided. The criterion for a healthy state is the ability to cope with stress. This means that a person has resilience of character, or *ego strength,* to satisfy his needs, but when he is blocked in need satisfaction, he is able to adapt and find new ways to bring satisfaction. For example, when he is unsuccessful in a particular pursuit or venture, the mature person has strength enough and is confident enough to bounce back and find a new way to success. He can face anxiety without disintegration. Having experienced anxiety about a situation, he is better able to cope with the danger. In general, the individual must have strong enough personality organization or feelings of security to stand and withstand tension without becoming panicky.

AUTONOMY

Gaining independence, developing self-determination, or *autonomy,* is a valuable characteristic of mental health. Autonomy means that the individual can accept or reject from a selection of environmental factors. An autonomous person is one who is capable of conforming to the dictates of society but at the same time is secure enough to be free to choose whether to conform or not. In another sense, an autonomous person is able to organize his personality in such a way that the events of his life are brought under his own jurisdiction and control; yet he is able to work for, and become a part of, a cause greater than himself.

PERCEPTION OF REALITY

Another criterion of mental health is a person's perception of reality, or his view of the world around him. When he sees what actually is in his environment and acts accordingly, this perception is an important aspect of mental health. The ability to perceive correctly contrasts with the psychotic's inability to perceive reality. What we see is accurate and objective if others who are mentally healthy also see the same conditions. The mentally healthy person will be willing to, and actually does, seek to prove that what he sees is also perceived by others. A mentally ill person would assume correctness without testing his beliefs.

The perception of the feelings and attitudes of others is of concern to a mentally healthy individual. He has regard for the inner life of others, or *empathy* with them, which is a type of social sensitivity.

ENVIRONMENTAL MASTERY

Jahoda found that reality perception and ability to master the environment were the criteria for mental health most frequently selected by authorities. In relation to the mastery of the environment, the emphasis appeared to be upon achieving success in significant areas of living and upon ability to adapt or adjust to the environment.

Jahoda breaks down environmental mastery into the following specific qualities: [10]

(1) the ability to love; (2) adequacy in love, work and play; (3) adequacy in interpersonal relations; (4) efficiency in meeting situational requirements; (5) capacity for adaptation and adjustment; and (6) efficiency in problem-solving.

Ability to love, in the psychological literature, means sexuality. Sexual gratification experienced with a love mate of the opposite sex is one of the chief signs of a healthy personality. This concept tends to make sex less obsessive.

The ability to hold a job, have a family, keep out of trouble with the law, and enjoy the usual opportunities for pleasure are characteristics that indicate environmental mastery and success in *love, work, and play.* Health educators who hold this premise would advise a daily program of health practices to promote healthful living with regard to nutrition, excretion, sleep, rest and relaxation, and physical activity. They might suggest that mental health is proportionate to physical health.

Authorities agree that *interpersonal relations* are important for mental health. This means an ability to get along with other people and refers to ways in which members of a family interact to achieve common goals. It denotes ability to work with another person or persons for mutual benefit. The mentally healthy individual understands the motives and problems of other people. He is able to give, as well as to receive, love and affection in the family and in friendship relationships.

The way an individual meets the *requirements of a situation* is a criterion of positive mental health. Since situations differ so widely, three situational requirements have been suggested as guides: (1) establishing appropriate relations with authority, which, in a college situation, means the instructor; (2) establishing appropriate relations with peers; and (3) acquiring knowledge and skills. To the degree that the individual meets these three requirements effectively he exhibits good mental health. The degree of mental health of the instructor is evaluated by these same requirements, with the substitution of the appropriate authority figures. Jahoda clearly points out in her study the difficulty in controlling every situation or in meeting all situational requirements. She indicates that this criterion can only be adhered to when there is agreement on the reasonableness of the requirement.

One's capacity for adaptation and adjustment is basic to sound mental health. *Adaptation* implies that a workable arrangement between reality and the individual can be achieved by changing either or both through individual initiative. Adaptation conveys the idea that a healthy person can change his inner balance of mental forces as well as his external environment.

Adjustment is the product of the indi-

[10] Marie Jahoda, *Current Concepts of Positive Mental Health,* Basic Books, Inc., New York, 1958, p. 53.

vidual's experiences during the process of development. Each person adjusts through his unique personality, which includes his own assets and liabilities. An individual makes an adjustment when he attains a satisfactory relationship between himself and his environment and/or between his needs and interests.

Adjustment has been mentioned previously in the discussion of field, or adjustment, theory; it is discussed in more detail in Chapter 3, Making Life Adjustments.

The literature indicates that *problem solving* has two connotations: one is related to success, since success means the ability to solve problems, to find a solution; the second refers to the process of problem solving. In this second sense, problem solving is the ability to identify a problem and attack it realistically. Jahoda believes that participation with appropriate feelings in the problem-solving process, with a direct approach to the problem, indicates a mentally healthy state regardless of whether the problem is solved. Problem solving is an important criterion for mental health. This health education text assumes that problems can be attacked and better solutions found so that life is enriched.

HAPPINESS

The authors add happiness as an additional criterion for mental health. They believe this characteristic of personality should be included among the criteria of mental health. The well-adjusted individ-

ual enjoys life. His experiences are, for the most part, pleasant ones. Happiness is the by-product of resolving conflicts and attaining goals. A happy person enjoys human contacts, gets along well with people, and is enriched by such associations. On the other hand, chronic unhappiness is a symptom of maladjustment.

MENTAL HEALTH PRINCIPLES

The authoritative criteria of mental health and some applications derived from foundation factors of mental health may be restated as principles. These general principles may assist us in developing a mentally healthy state:

Realize that all human behavior is motivated by needs.

Behave and adjust in ways that tend to satisfy needs.

Develop an objective self image and promote self-regarding attitudes.

Strive for self-actualization, or self-realization.

Try to achieve integration, a unified, integrated personality structure resulting from the interrelationship of all parts, processes, and mental faculties, a balance of psychic forces.

Develop autonomy by gaining independence of action and orientation toward becoming.

Perceive reality accurately and objectively, free from inner distortion.

Develop the ability to master life as it comes, to cope with interpersonal relations and group belongingness, and to achieve happiness in life.

Summary

Each of us is a complex person psychologically. We are products of our past experiences and of many biological, structural, environmental, social, and cultural forces. We are concerned to reach the highest level of our personality potential so as to achieve a sound mentally healthy state.

Mental health concerns the individual's everyday living throughout life. The increased problem of mental illness in our society is due to the inability of the individual to understand himself and his fellow men and to his failure to apply the principles of mental health in adjusting to present-day society with its stresses or strains. The basic factors and forces for developing mental health give insight and understanding for successful personal and social development.

Mental health is defined as the quality of personal health resulting from the individual's satisfaction of human needs through personal and social adjustments in his environment.

The foundation factors of mental health include the total make-up of the individual as a biological organism, the influences of the society in which the individual finds himself, and the interaction process between the individual and society: the experiences by which the individual influences other people and is influenced by them. Heredity is the foundation force that provides the raw material, the potential of the individual, and sets the limits for mental health.

Physical factors contribute significantly to the well-adjusted individual. Mental vitality is improved by physical health.

Social factors pertain to the individual's environment and the interaction process. The social factors that influence the development of mental health are the home and family, the school, and the community. The family situation provides the setting, the stimulation, and the guidance for personal and social adjustment. The school is the chief continuing and supplementing institution in which individuals develop sound mental health practices. More and more the community is found to be significant in developing mental health, particularly in relation to the individual's ability to fulfill the responsibilities of his family, demonstrate efficiency in his chosen vocation, and accept social responsibilities in his neighborhood and in his local community. The community also provides supplementary services in addition to creating a healthy atmosphere for its families.

Each member of society assists in establishing and maintaining the social order by what he knows, thinks, feels, and does; also, each member responds to the social order that he himself has helped to establish.

Criteria for developing a mentally healthy state include formation by the individual of positive attitudes toward himself—the development of the *self image;* realization of individual potential through action—*growth, development, or self-actualization;* unification of the function of personality—*integration* of mental capacities; independence or *autonomy;* objective *perception of reality* from social influences, and the ability to take life as it comes and master it—*environmental mastery.* These criteria and applications from the theories of personality emergence underlie the general principles of mental health.

Suggested readings

1. Allport, Gordon W.: *Becoming,* Yale University Press, New Haven, Conn., 1955.
2. Alvarez, Walter C.: *Live at Peace with Your Nerves,* Prentice-Hall, Inc., Englewood Cliffs, N.J., 1958.
3. Bernard, H. W.: *Toward Better Personal Adjustment,* 2d ed., McGraw-Hill Book Company, Inc., New York, 1957.
4. Bonney, Merl E.: *Mental Health in Education,* Allyn and Bacon, Inc., Boston, 1960.
5. Dach, Elizabeth: *Your Community and Mental Health,* Public Affairs Pamphlet 263, Public Affairs Committee, Inc., New York, 1958.
6. Farnsworth, Dana L.: *Mental Health in College and University,* Harvard University Press, Cambridge, Mass., 1957.
7. Glasser, William, M.D., *Mental Health or Mental Illness?* Harper & Brothers, New York, 1960.
8. Gorlow, Leon, and Walter Katkovsky: *Readings in the Psychology of Adjustment,* McGraw-Hill Book Company, Inc., New York, 1959.
9. Hollister, William G.: *An Overview: Providing Better Mental Health for Our*

People, An Introductory Manual for Mental Health Workers, at 10110 Parkwood Terrace, Bethesda 14, Md., 1956.

10. Jahoda, Marie: *Current Concepts of Positive Mental Health,* Basic Books, Inc., New York, 1958.

11. Kallmann, Franz J.: "The Genetics of Human Behavior," *American Journal of Psychiatry,* 113:496–509, 1956.

12. Kaplan, Louis: *Mental Health and Human Relations in Education,* Harper & Brothers, New York, 1959.

13. Katz, Barney, and George Lehner: *Mental Hygiene in Modern Living,* The Ronald Press Company, New York, 1953.

14. Lane, Howard, and Mary Beauchamp: *Understanding Human Development,* Prentice-Hall, Inc., Englewood Cliffs, N.J., 1959.

15. Lehner, George F. J., and Ella Kube: *The Dynamics of Personal Adjustment,* Prentice-Hall, Inc., Englewood Cliffs, N.J., 1955.

16. Lemkau, Paul V.: *Mental Hygiene in Public Health,* 2d ed., McGraw-Hill Book Company, Inc., Blakiston Division, New York, 1955.

17. Lindzey, Gardner (ed.): *The Assessment of Human Motives,* Grove Press, Inc., New York, 1960.

18. McKinney, Fred: *Psychology of Personal Adjustment,* 3d ed., John Wiley & Sons, Inc., New York, 1960.

19. Marrazzi, Amedeo S.: "Messengers of the Nervous System," *Scientific American,* 196:87–94, February, 1957.

20. Maslow, Abraham H.: "A Theory of Human Motivation," in Gorlow, Leon, and Walter Katkovsky: *Readings in the Psychology of Adjustment,* McGraw-Hill Book Company, Inc., New York, 1959.

21. Maslow, Abraham H.: *New Knowledge in Human Values,* Harper & Brothers, New York, 1959.

22. Menninger, Karl A.: *The Human Mind,* 3d ed., Alfred A. Knopf, Inc., New York, 1951.

23. Moore, Bernice M., and Robert L.

Sutherland: *Family, Community, and Mental Health: Profiles of Community Action,* The Hogg Foundation, Austin, Tex., 1950.

24. Murphy, Gardner: *Human Potentialities,* Basic Books, Inc., New York, 1958.

25. National Association for Mental Health: *Mental Health Is 1, 2, 3,* The Association, New York, 1951.

26. National Association for Mental Health: *What Every Child Needs,* The Association, New York, 1954.

27. Opler, Marvin K.: *Culture and Mental Health,* The Macmillan Company, New York, 1959.

28. Redl, Fritz, and William W. Wattenberg: *Mental Hygiene in Teaching,* Harcourt, Brace and Company, Inc., New York, 1951.

29. Scheinfeld, Amram: *The New You and Heredity,* J. B. Lippincott Company, Philadelphia, 1950.

30. Scheinfeld, Amram: "Heredity and Mental Illness," *Today's Health,* 34:22–23, 52–55, May, 1956.

31. Scheinfeld, Amram: *The Human Heredity Handbook,* J. B. Lippincott Company, Philadelphia, 1956.

32. Smith, Henry Clay: *Personality Adjustment,* McGraw-Hill Book Company, Inc., New York, 1961.

33. Stevenson, George S.: *Mental Health Planning for Social Action,* McGraw-Hill Book Company, Inc., Blakiston Division, New York, 1956.

34. Strecker, Edward A., Kenneth E. Appel, and John W. Appel: *Discovering Ourselves,* 3d ed., The Macmillan Company, New York, 1959.

35. Thorpe, Louis: *The Psychology of Mental Health,* 2d ed., The Ronald Press Company, New York, 1960.

36. Wenger, M. A., F. N. Jones, and M. H. Jones, *Physiological Psychology,* Henry Holt and Company, Inc., New York, 1956.

37. Wolf, Anna, and Margaret C. Dawson: "What Makes a Good Home," The Child Study Association of America, Inc., New York, 1958.

THREE

Making life adjustments

Chapter 1 pointed out that making satisfactory life adjustments to ensure a mentally healthy state is more important in the Space Age than ever before. It is true not only of the problems and pressures in society at large but particularly so in the highly competitive environment of the present college campus.

Previous discussion has given you a background for understanding the meaning and make-up of mental health. In describing the foundation factors, the point was made that mental health, like physical health, is a unifying quality to be achieved. In both cases, heredity plays its part. The important thing is to make the most of heredity by intelligent participation in life activities. This means making personal and social adjustments to satisfy needs as they relate to yourself, your family, your college, your community, and your widening environment of total society, including, in the near future, outer space.

A basic aspect of mental health is knowing how to adjust appropriately and how to apply this knowledge in everyday situations. Satisfactory adjustment of motives can lead to better mental health and also can prevent serious frustration, anxieties leading to nervous breakdowns, and other maladjustive behavior.

This chapter is designed to help answer the following questions:

What is the adjustment process, and how are satisfactory adjustments made?

What are the common mental health problems facing college students that can help them identify their problems and develop self-understanding?

How do we adjust to the stress of everyday situations?

What are the common adjustment reactions or mechanisms?

How do personality maladjustments develop?

What are the serious personality maladjustments, and how can they be prevented?

How do we develop greater maturity?

Where or to whom can we turn for assistance in making life adjustments?

What are the constituents of a sound mental health program that can serve as a guide in developing a personal program?

The adjustment process: an overview

A simple description of a most complex process shows the sequence in the process of adjustment as well as the principles involved [23, 30]. See diagram below. The process may be described as follows:

Human behavior is motivated by needs, problems, desires, and goals.

Some needs are easily satisfied and some adjustments readily made. However, blocks often occur in both our internal and external environments.

As a result of blockage, frustration and conflict occur. Incompatible needs, methods, goals, and traits all may cause conflict.

When motives are blocked, emotional tension is produced. A person feels tense and uncomfortable.

We tend to select patterns of adjustment that show the least possible conflict. Often the behavior selected may be inappropriate for the development of maturity and mental health.

The feeling of frustration, the intensification of needs, and varied responses may overcome obstacles.

Satisfactory responses reduce tension, satisfy motives, and permit adjustments. Sound mental health is the result.

Other responses must be readjusted when

The sequence in adjustment.

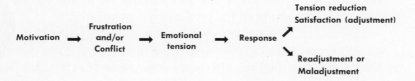

new goals are chosen, when a choice is made between several goals, when goals are reorganized, and when readjustment occurs.

Some behavior is unsatisfactory in that motivating conditions are not removed. Tension is not reduced and conflict still exists. In many instances we learn to avoid these activities and to select more suitable patterns. Some behavior produces immediate satisfaction but later on causes conflict and anxiety, with increased tension. Readjustment is necessary in such instances to eliminate unsatisfactory reactions.

Consistent use of unsatisfactory behavior may lead to maladjustment, with both minor and serious consequences. This occurs when blocking is disruptive to the personality. Such behavior is exhibited when we get rattled, lose our control, fail to think straight, and are willing to use any adjustive reaction to relieve our situation.

The prevention of maladjustment through readjustment and satisfying behavior is basic to sound mental health.

THE DYNAMICS OF ADJUSTMENT

Application of the dynamics of the adjustment process is developed in the remainder of this chapter. Applications include the following:

Identifying the problems facing the college student

Understanding and selecting appropriate reactions to stress

Understanding adjustive reactions and the common defensive mechanisms, which are both helpful and detrimental to adjustment

Noting and applying the principles of adjustment to make satisfactory adjustments

Studying the behavioral maladjustments

Knowing the sources of help in preventing or solving mental health problems

Considering the principles of mental health as guides to a personal mental health program

Mental health problems of college students

An initial phase of the adjustment process is realizing that behavior is caused. From the discussion in Chapter 2 and the description of the adjustment process, we learned that motives are driving forces that direct behavior until we respond in such a manner as to satisfy them. Motives include not only conscious desires for accomplishment but also the unconscious physical process, which creates tension until the motive is satisfied or reduced [23].

This understanding of the causes of behavior is important not only in seeing the initial stage of the adjustment process but also in learning to change health behavior for better mental health. For one must understand the causes of old behavior and remove or readjust them in order for new behavior to occur. The realization of causes can permit development of new motives, changing how we feel and what we do in a particular situation about our health. The realization of what determines our behavior begins with an examination of the mental health problems of college students.

The following analysis of adjustment problems of college students is derived from research studies in which college students themselves reported their problems and from authorities in the mental health field who have presented their views of student problems [4, 6, 11]. The problems exemplify the forces motivating student action. This discussion leads to the next step in the adjustment process: solving the problems.

COMMON MENTAL HEALTH PROBLEMS REPORTED BY STUDENTS AND AUTHORITIES

These problems have been identified:

Failure to relinquish home and family relationships

Renouncement by students of parental and home situations

Lack of motivation and self-direction (poorly defined goals, lack of personal drive and ability to accomplish tasks, disparity between goals and capacity to achieve them)

Lack of a definite choice of career

Lack of social adjustment (social inferiority or superiority, antisocial behavior)

Lack of emotional adjustment (emotional immaturity expressed in overstimulation, fears, anxieties, and the like)

Sexual relationships (maintaining standards and codes, inadequate sexual adjustment)

Desire for marriage when circumstances make it impossible or difficult

Scholastic difficulties (pressure of making grades)

Desire for athletic attainment when one has limited physical health and abilities

Uncertainties about military service

Lack of economic adjustment (lack of opportunity to earn sufficient money, and unwise spending of funds)

Inability to adjust to housing and transportation conditions (lack of adjustment with large groups of individuals in dormitories, clubs, fraternities and sororities, and other housing groups; inability to withstand strains of commuting long distances with poor transportation facilities)

Poor health conditions

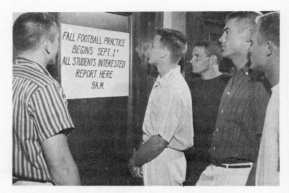

Most students want to use their abilities in a satisfying way. This young man, who is interested in many things, joined a group reading the fall announcement . . .

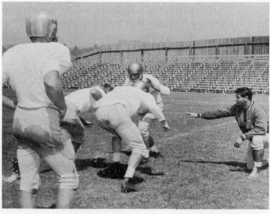

and was motivated to join the football team. He enjoyed the game and the association with his teammates . . .

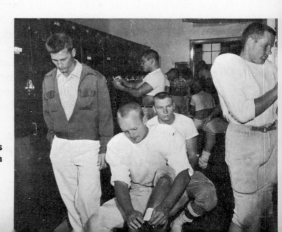

but he could not make the grade and was dropped from the squad. Feeling the tension of frustration . . .

he modified his behavior. His concern with what was going on around him and his need for status in the college community brought him to the staff of the college paper . . .

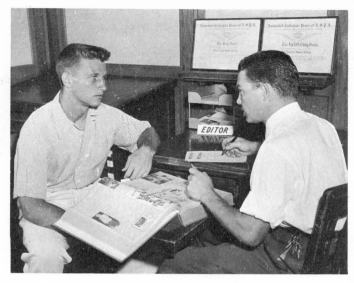

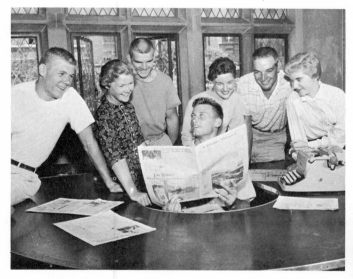

where his interests could be used. He developed new relationships and channeled his athletic interests toward a sport he could enjoy throughout his life.

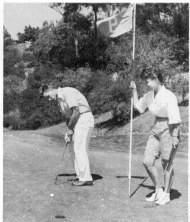

MENTAL HEALTH PROBLEMS OF COLLEGE STUDENTS REPORTED BY PSYCHIATRISTS

A Committee on the College Student of the Group for the Advancement of Psychiatry has identified the common mental health problems or areas of adjustment as follows:

Dependence-independence relationships

Emotions of love and hate

Problems of sexuality

The need for security, adequacy, and prestige

Development of standards and value systems

A brief description of these problems and their meaning and application to the college situation is presented [8, 11].

Dependence-independence. Based upon previous experiences and acceptance of responsibility, the mature college student is capable of exercising sound judgment. He is now on his own, perhaps for the first time. This is all the more reason why he should be treated as an independent person. Of course, not all students have had the same background and experience, and some cannot assume complete responsibility, particularly when it is thrust upon them suddenly. Some students demonstrate their independence by behaving in antisocial ways such as destroying property, being rowdy, and showing no concern for another's right to study. Others follow all rules to the letter and display quiet submissiveness. Still others strike a happy medium in achieving maturity through independence. For those who have not had experience in accepting responsibility for themselves and others, college may be their first and best proving ground.

Love and hate. The ability to love and be loved was previously identified as a basic need of all persons and an important facet of the healthy personality. Attaining love and respect is necessary at college and even in an academic atmosphere. Socializing on the campus, dating, even going steady and becoming engaged seem to be enhanced in college. In some instances, colleges and universities appear to be matrimonial centers. On the other hand, the need to express love can meet with rejection. Rejections from social groups—clubs, fraternities, and sororities—and from individuals of the opposite sex call for life adjustments that sometimes tax the strongest personalities.

Hate may be expressed toward a member or members of a social group, toward the faculty, or toward the administration. Sometimes such feelings are warranted; however, learning to control hatred and finding ways to express more constructive emotions is a genuine mark of maturity.

Sexuality. Properly controlling the sex drive is one of the most significant problems facing college students. The development of biological maturity for sexual activity before social and economic conditions enable its mature fulfillment presents an important problem. In addition, various communication media place undue stress on sexuality as a part of the culture. Free expression of sexuality presents certain problems for the college student, and total suppression presents others. Sexuality, as an example of application of the principles of adjustment, is discussed in Chapter 4, pages 112–117.

Need for security, adequacy, prestige. Developing esteem and self-actualization is most essential during the college years. College life offers many opportunities for gaining social prestige, political power, and athletic superiority, which may strengthen an individual's personality or, in many cases, lead to a false set of values. Overemphasis on intellectual attainment to the exclusion of social and athletic ability may lead to similar difficulties. However, college activities present opportunities for strengthening self-confidence, for intellectual accomplishment, for demonstrating integrity, for creative thinking and problem solving, for developing social attributes, and for athletic achievement. They afford opportunities to broaden cultural interests and to develop spiritual security and a sense of civic responsibility. These qualities assist the student in his further progress toward maturity and a successful adult life.

Development of standards and value systems. A basic purpose of colleges and universities is to prepare students to attain optimum intellectual development and to maintain high standards of conduct. At the same time, to permit the growth of value systems, students must be helped to engage in activities that will bring about their own high standards and values. Problems exist for each individual student in achieving these educational goals.

Farnsworth [11] thinks that the indirect influences of college life exert a powerful force on developing standards and values. He believes that side remarks and ridicule of cherished beliefs as well as the sincerity, tolerance, and understanding demonstrated by faculty and upperclassmen exert a significant negative or positive effect on the student. Through his experience as a psychiatrist working with college students, Farnsworth[1] has found that the following general situations may interfere with effective personality functioning in those persons who in their earlier years need help:

1. Parental discord and friction. . . .
2. Rigidity of thought, behavior, and emotional expression in those with whom the growing person has had close and intimate contact.
3. Inconsistent or absent discipline.
4. Relative lack of masculine attributes in the father and feminine traits in the mother.
5. Teaching, by direct and indirect methods, of distorted or squeamish attitudes toward body functions at an early age.
6. Living in a neighborhood where the preponderance of influences are harmful

and sources of conflict and stress numerous.
7. Inadequate mental ability in comparison to other members of the family, even though quite good in comparison to the general population.

The problem of emotional instability is also a serious one for the student. An individual with this personality characteristic has to spend much of his time defending himself against real and imagined threats. In addition to wasted energies, his behavior is such that he may become unpopular with persons close to him and with others who condemn his actions.

Understanding one's self. Identifying problems is part of understanding one's self and knowing one's self better. Self-analysis and self-searching are part of mature behavior. They also are characteristic of the individual who is making perfectly good adjustment. Our actions do not always satisfy us completely. Mistakes and temporary setbacks raise such questions as, Why did I do that? How can I avoid social slips? What are my assets? Can't I do better than I have been doing? How can I improve myself?

Many problems may be merely symptoms or minor difficulties. Self-analysis may be enough to tell us that our present trouble is physical—fatigue, poor nutrition, or insufficient sleep. It may be due to finances, which we can or cannot do something about but which may cause a modification of behavior. It may be the result of an unfavorable comparison with another person, being snubbed by someone we like, or being let down by a friend. Self-understanding may help us to understand others, to accept them, and to learn how to deal with minor conflicts. More serious problems and conflicts call for assistance from persons prepared to help us. How to deal with these problems, how to make suitable adjustments, and how to know whom to call on for help are discussed later in this chapter [23].

Other problems from the above lists will

[1] Dana L. Farnsworth, *Mental Health in College and University*, Harvard University Press, Cambridge Mass., 1957, pp. 51–52.

be discussed and dealt with further in this chapter as examples of the adjustment process. These discussions may prove valuable to you by demonstrating that you are not the only person who has problems. Most students are confronted with the problems outlined above. Some may be major problems for particular students. Some students may have several of these problems woven together, which need to be resolved. To others they may all be minor and of small concern. The two sets of problems may help you identify more clearly your own particular problems.

The important thing is not that a person has problems but that he knows how to face them and how to act in order to solve them. The following discussion is designed to assist each individual in attacking his own problems.

Satisfying needs

We showed in Chapter 2 that the individual establishes a satisfactory relationship with his environment when he makes steady advancement toward meeting his needs. The fulfillment of needs results in healthful, effective living. When needs are not met, the individual functions ineffectively and unsatisfactorily; in fact, he is uncomfortable. People's actions are an indication of their attempt to satisfy their needs. Some persons are happy, successful citizens who enjoy life, and others become misfits, troublemakers, alcoholics, and sociopaths. These are a few examples of mentally disturbed persons.

FRUSTRATION

An individual is not always successful in satisfying all his needs in all situations. Generally speaking, the individual is motivated to gain his desires and demands. However, in attempting to satisfy his needs he may meet a barrier or an obstacle, which causes frustration. *Frustration is the thwarting of desires or needs brought about by factors which interfere with normal and immediate adjustment of the individual. It may be due to the individual himself, to life situations, or to society.*

If frustrations are due to the individual himself, these are referred to as *internal* frustrations; they may be the result of defects, illness, injuries, or fears. If the frustrations are *external,* they may arise from various life situations involving finances, education, employment, and other factors. External frustrations also may be the result of society's control through the individual's contact with social mores or his interaction with social groups. For example, some groups do not approve of marriage outside their own group. An example pertaining to the college campus is the tradition in some colleges requiring

Schematic representation of the results of frustration of desires and demands. (Adapted from Louis P. Thorpe, *The Psychology of Mental Health*, The Ronald Press Company, New York, 1960, p. 79.)

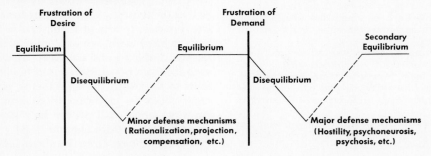

freshmen to wear special costumes as a means of identification. Such restrictions may be frustrating to some individuals seeking to achieve their own personal goals.

The individual generally reacts to frustration or stress by attack, withdrawal, or compromise forms of behavior. These may be accompanied by emotional reinforcements, such as hostility, fear, and anxiety [7]. Reactions to stress frequently result in an act of hostility with emotional tension present. Expressions of hostility range from minor reactions, such as swearing, throwing away the golf club after a bad shot, or spreading gossip about a person, to such aggressive acts as fist fighting and even murder [18]. The more intense the frustration, the more intense the emotion. When frustration becomes a threat to the integrity of the ego, fear and anxiety are aroused. In such situations, the individual's reactive behavior utilizes more and more the defense mechanisms, many of which are socially disapproved. Each person has a frustration or stress tolerance. The ability to tolerate frustration depends upon the feelings of security and personal worth. When stress exceeds the individual's tolerance limit, he undergoes various degrees of personality disorganization. Adjustment depends on the individual's ability to withstand a strongly frustrating situation or many mild barriers, such as disappointments in everyday life, without becoming disorganized.

In considering frustration it is helpful to distinguish between needs classed as desires and those classed as demands and to understand the behavior resulting from the blocking of satisfaction of each type of need. A *desire* is a need for a temporary satisfaction of a rather minor nature, which the individual would like to have though he can well get along without it. A *demand,* however, is a basic need. If this need is not fulfilled, the resulting tension leads to maladjustment. When the demand is satisfied, the result is personal security and mental health. A schematic

drawing of these results is presented in the accompanying diagram. See page 76.

CONFLICT

Frustration occurs when basic motives are thwarted. When basic motives oppose each other, the individual must choose between them in deciding upon a course of action. The state of tension occurring before the course of action is decided upon is called *conflict.*

All conflicts involve frustration. The stronger the motives, the more severe is the frustration. Time is a factor that often makes resolving a conflict difficult. In some circumstances, more than one motive might be achieved; however, the individual usually acts at once in only one direction. Most conflicts are easily resolved and result in only minor frustration. The choice of a life vocation often arouses a conflict in college students. A more frequently occurring conflict, however, concerns the satisfaction of sexual desire. Should one marry before finishing college, engage in premarital sexual relations, practice masturbation, or sublimate the sexual desire by participating in socially accepted activities?

Conflicts may be conscious or unconscious in nature. The majority of conflicts resulting in disordered behavior are unconscious and therefore beyond the individual's awareness. Such conflicts are associated with feelings of insecurity, feelings of guilt, or contradictory tendencies, such as love and hate of the same person. At this point, it is important to note that every person, including the well-adjusted individual, has frustrations and conflicts. Even in Paradise or Shangri-la, conflicts or frustrations occur when human beings are present. But the well-adjusted individual lives with these disturbances without experiencing serious symptoms of maladjustment.

All behavior involves conflict to a certain degree. Almost every situation tends to call for a variety of responses, which cannot all be made at once. In many cases, first one, then another of these responses becomes dominant so that adjustments are made easily. When the degree of conflict is intense, the responses may produce hesitancy, tension, vacillation, or complete blocking. These responses indicate that a more intense degree of conflict is present [16].

Reaction to stress

Stress is the threat to the fulfillment of basic needs, to the functioning of the nervous system including homeostatic functioning, and to growth and development [13]. Stress relates to biological as well as to psychological aspects of behavior. Psychologically, stress means stimuli that are likely to produce disturbance in most individuals. It refers to a continuum of stimuli. At one end of the continuum are stimuli or cues that have meaning only to a single person or to few persons and seem quite trivial. At the other end are stimuli definitely threatening to the vital functioning of the individual, particularly to the mental mechanisms by which he copes with problems and situations.

Stress can be spoken of as a *stress situation,* which contains stimuli that, because of their potential effect, could threaten the individual but do not because of his adaptative capacity.

PSYCHOSOMATIC CONDITIONS

In some individuals, when there is inadequate release of tension caused by excessive stress, functional body disorders, called *psychosomatic disorders,* develop. Psychosomatic disorders are symptoms of ill health stemming from psychological factors. The symptoms are due to severe emotional stress and are commonly called *tension symptoms.* Emotional disturbances may affect any organ in the body and thus produce pain and discomfort.

Psychosomatic symptoms include chronic fatigue, aches and pains, digestive disorders, disturbances of eliminative functions, genitourinary disorders, and cardiovascular dysfunction. The most common specific symptoms are headache, neckache, backache, palpitation of the heart, pain in the region of the heart, tightness in the chest, tightness in the throat, choking sensations, loss of appetite, vomiting, indigestion, constipation, diarrhea, frequent urination, tiredness, weakness, and dizziness. Several common illnesses, notably bronchial asthma, migraine, ulcers, and colitis, are primarily psychosomatic in origin.[2]

[2] Barney Katz and George Lehner, *Mental Hygiene in Modern Living,* The Ronald Press Company, New York, 1953, p. 136.

Adjustment to stress. Personality development (emergence) determines motivational patterns. Motivational pattern and stress jointly determine reaction to stress, which will include ego defensive mechanisms if the stress is ego-involved. (Adapted from James Coleman, "Types of Adjustive Reactions," in Gorlow and Katkovsky, *Readings in the Psychology of Adjustment,* McGraw-Hill Book Company, Inc., New York, 1959, p. 329; originally from Coleman, *Abnormal Psychology and Life,* Scott-Foresman and Company, Chicago, 1956.

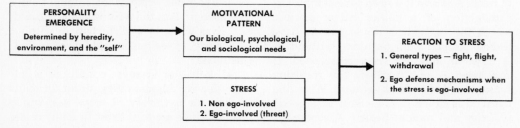

PERSONALITY EMERGENCE	MOTIVATIONAL PATTERN	REACTION TO STRESS
Determined by heredity, environment, and the "self"	Our biological, psychological, and sociological needs	1. General types — fight, flight, withdrawal
	STRESS	2. Ego defense mechanisms when the stress is ego-involved
	1. Non ego-involved	
	2. Ego-involved (threat)	

In psychosomatic conditions pain may originate in the brain, but it is referred to other parts of the body, such as the abdomen. Such conditions may be due to fear, anxiety, or other forms of tension.

Individuals differ greatly in their emotional reaction. Some persons can have the most trying and fearful experiences with little or no emotional response. Others react violently to their anxieties. Some persons have a nervous system that seems to affect the functions of their internal organs, such as "tying the stomach in knots" or causing complete loss of appetite. Others feel no fear or threat of fear. Emotion also can elicit symptoms of disease that may be present in the body but latent except under severe emotional stress.

Alvarez reports a case of a man who only suffered from ulcers in several instances of emotional stress: when the girl he loved refused him; when the same girl actually did marry him in a large social wedding; and when he lost his money in a stock-market crash [1].

Selye's theory of stress postulates that almost any disease can be caused by emotional tension. He points out the function of the pituitary and adrenal hormones in combating stress and warding off threats to body processes. He indicates that in our competitive life our glands help us adjust to stress by producing excess hormones. Finally, after constant exposure to stress, this defensive system may break down. He cites stress as a factor in hardening of the arteries, in high blood pressure, and in inflammatory diseases, such as arthritis. He definitely lays the blame for obesity on stress, especially in certain persons. At the same time, he states that loss of weight is one of the most apparent consequences of chronic stress.

Selye views stress as the great equalizer of activities within the body, acting to prevent "onesided overexertion." He cites the example of having to change hands when carrying a suitcase. Local stress, indicated by muscle fatigue, acts through the nervous system to suggest a change of hands [29].

Selye further indicates that stressful activity prepares us for rest and sleep. On the other hand, emotional stress before going to bed or which wakes a person during the night is a cause of insomnia.

Alton Blakeslee[3] reports that one-third of all human illnesses, from the common cold to cancer, apparently are definitely related to reactions to troubles or crises in our lives. Illnesses for many people occur in clusters just when they are having the most social, economic, or domestic troubles.

Psychosomatic disorders may be corrected when the individual understands how the condition occurs and after he realizes the importance of seeking guidance from a clinical psychologist or psychiatrist. Generally, such competent assistance is necessary in order to eliminate the causes of the emotional stress. A medical doctor may be of help also.

NERVOUS BREAKDOWNS

A nervous breakdown may occur at almost any time when tensions are great and the individual has an inborn tendency to nervousness. A breakdown may be due to overwork, studying too hard, lack of sleep and rest, too much emotional pressure, or too much needless worry. A cold, the flu, or physical fatigue may produce an extreme nervous condition. Dr. Alvarez has two rules for reducing tension [1]: "1. Do one thing at a time; 2. do not set a time limit on when it is to be finished." He also passes on some very good advice that he received from his friend, Dr. Austen Riggs, for relieving the suffering of the worried [1]: "(1) Ask yourself, is this *my* problem? If not, leave it alone. (2) If it *is* my problem, can I tackle it *now*? If a person can get right at it and settle it, he should do so. (3) If your problem can be settled by an expert in some field, go quickly to him and take his advice."

3 Alton L. Blakeslee, "Today's Health News," *Today's Health*, 36: 11, August, 1958.

Adjustive reactions

Adjustive reactions are best understood when two sets of factors are considered: the total personality of the individual and his specific life situation [7]. In general, individuals follow rather definite principles in their attempts to adjust to actual or potential stress in the satisfaction of needs.

Adjustive reactions can be categorized by the three ways that individuals adjust: by attack, withdrawal, or compromise.

ATTACK

In adjusting by *attack* we attempt directly to remove the barrier to our goal through increased effort or through a varied approach. Attack reactions may be either constructive or destructive. In many instances of direct action we are bound to be unsuccessful; the frustration remains and, with it, irritation, pain, and unpleasantness. We may attach these reactions to objects or to persons, either or both, that become obstacles. This calls forth emotional reactions, especially hate or hostility. When hostility is present the reaction may be largely destructive. Stealing, destroying property, assault, sexual misbehavior, and setting fires are examples of hostile reactions [7]. Hostility toward authority or power figures may be inhibited to the extent that it is not outwardly manifest. Hostility may be shown in physical or verbal behavior, in fantasies, or in competitive physical activities.

FLIGHT, WITHDRAWAL, AND FEAR

Many animals adjust to their environment through simple *withdrawal*. Man is no exception. From infancy we learn to withdraw from dangerous situations, particularly from those in which we are threatened by fear. Withdrawal may include not only physical withdrawal but also inhibition of dangerous internal desires, abandonment of goals, or restriction of threatening situations. Fear involves a definite tendency to flight. However, anxiety may be aroused, and this complicates the picture. Stress arising from anxiety leads to apprehension and general vagueness and uncertainty.

COMPROMISE

Perhaps our most common way of dealing with conflicts is by *compromise*, since many situations cannot be resolved by direct attack or withdrawal. Compromise means accepting substitute goals, aspirations, or ethical standards through modification of the original objective. In order to get our way we may have to compromise, although our original objective is modified. An unemployed person facing starvation for himself and his family may resort to stealing, when otherwise

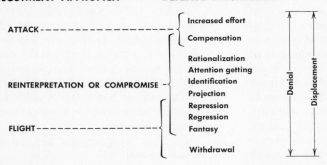

ADJUSTMENT APPROACH   DEFENSE MECHANISM

ATTACK − − − − − − − − − − − − − { Increased effort
                                    Compensation

                                    Rationalization
                                    Attention getting
REINTERPRETATION OR COMPROMISE − { Identification
                                    Projection

                                    Repression
                                    Regression
FLIGHT − − − − − − − − − − − − − { Fantasy

                                    Withdrawal

Denial   Displacement

Diagram illustrating adjustment approaches of defense mechanisms. (From George F. J. Lehner and Ella Kube, *The Dynamics of Personal Adjustment*, Prentice-Hall, Inc., Englewood Cliffs, N. J., 1955, p. 113.)

he would be completely honest. Hate, fear, and love are emotional reactions which also relate to compromises.

COMMON ADJUSTMENT MECHANISMS

The individual develops a number of techniques to overcome frustration and conflict during the process of adjusting. These adjustment mechanisms are devices used to reduce tension by achieving an indirect satisfaction of a need. They are learned forms of behaviors, used quite unconsciously, and are considered common practices in everyday life. They help the individual make temporary adjustments because they protect him from threats to his security. He uses them when he feels he must defend himself to others because of his failure, or the possibility of his future failure, in a situation. They are a means of justifying his actions and saving face.

Defensive mechanisms used occasionally are not harmful to the personality. Whether they assist the individual in making good life adjustments or lead to maladjustive behavior depends upon the specific type of mechanism and its intensive effect on the individual and upon the extent to which the individual learns to depend on one or more of them in making adjustments.

The adjustment mechanisms lead to maladjustment when they interfere with objective self-analysis and when they prevent a direct attack on a problem by concealing its true nature. A number of the common adjustment mechanisms are described in the following paragraphs [7, 30, 34].

Compensation is a means of achieving satisfaction in a roundabout way. It may be the exaggeration of a desirable trait to reduce a feeling of inferiority resulting from an undesirable trait. Handicapped individuals who have achieved greatness illustrate this characteristic; for example, the late President Franklin D. Roosevelt became a great leader despite a physical handicap. Compensation may be noted

in students who are not intellectually brilliant but who make up for this by studying harder so that they still achieve scholastic success. Sometimes students who lack physical prowess and have weak muscles exercise more diligently than others to strengthen their physical condition. Another example is the girl who is not naturally pretty, but makes herself attractive and smart looking by taking special care of her hair, her skin, and her clothes.

Many compensations of this kind are stimulated by our present highly competitive society. One is constantly compared with others by status, by achievements, and by possessions. Compensation that leads to strong motivation in achievement is adjustive. When such motivation leads to increased anxiety or takes antisocial forms, it is judged to be harmful.

Dissociation is the segregation from consciousness of certain components of the mental processes, which then function independently. For example, dissociation may separate ideas from their natural and appropriate feelings. It also serves as a device by which the individual can satisfy contradictory motives, which would lead to conflict if allowed to operate simultaneously. Our present-day attempt to lead a normal existence in chaotic world conditions is an example of mild dissociation.

Egocentrism is an exaggerated attempt to increase the importance of the self. Such behavior may range from temper tantrums to swimming the English Channel to gain publicity and public attention.

Fantasy consists in unreal activities that have meaning and existence only for and within one's self. It indicates, directly or indirectly, the problems faced, and its primary goal is escape from reality. In fantasy the individual achieves his goals in substitute fashion. In fantasy, we imagine that we are a chorus girl, a movie actress, a football star, or the owner of a lucrative business. This is nonproductive fantasy based on wish-fulfilling activity. Using creative imagination is an example of productive fantasy. The soap operas, magazine stories, and some novels permit escape from one's own status and identification with hero or heroine. The ability to escape into a fantasy world temporarily has adjustive value. It is dangerous when escaping into a dream world becomes easier and easier when the going gets tough.

Identification is hero worship—identifying one's self with persons or institutions that represent ideal qualities. Collecting autographs of famous persons is an example. Other examples include using the reflected glory of a football team and enjoying the social prestige of fraternity and sorority membership to enhance feelings of adequacy and worth. Alumni identify themselves with their colleges. They, as well as others, enjoy identification with their occupation, membership in exclusive clubs, large bank accounts, and sporty cars. The individual basks in the desirable attributes of the groups or institutions with which he is identified. Almost everyone uses such identification to some degree. It is beneficial so far as it builds up a sense of worth and helps reduce frustrations. There is potential danger in identifying ourselves too completely with the adventures and achievements of heroes. Loss of personal identification and the complete acceptance of some famous personality is a characteristic in some psychotic reactions. In such reactions a person may believe he is Napoleon, George Washington, or former President Eisenhower.

Negativism is persistent opposition to efforts made to aid or improve the individual. This device is common in children, but it occurs in adults as well. A person who is contradictory, stubborn, or rebellious exhibits negativism. The patient who refuses to follow his doctor's orders or the advice of his family also illustrates this mechanism.

Projection is the denial of one's own weakness by shifting a problem or the blame for a situation to other persons. An executive discharging a subordinate to cover up his own mistakes is using projection. We also defend ourselves against our repressed guilt feelings by projecting them to others. Dishonest or immoral individuals are quick to condemn such tendencies in others. They may justify their behavior because others have the same tendencies, or they may use projection to protect themselves from moral lapses.

Some forms of projection are used by all of us every day. It is easy to blame the golf club for a poor golf shot; the housewife burns the dinner and blames the stove; the student flunks an exam and blames the professor. In this sense, projection provides a good ego defense. In its extreme form projection is a central quality of paranoia. A mental patient may be obsessed by socially unacceptable sexual ideas and accuse others of having given him the ideas.

Rationalization is finding reasons to justify actions or conditions in our own eyes and in the eyes of other persons. For example, a person may buy a new car with the excuse that the tires of his old car are worn smooth. Actually, he needs new tires, not a new car. Rationalization helps us justify what we do and believe and helps soften the letdown when we have unattainable goals. Buying the new car illustrates the first aspect. The second aspect refers to the "sour grapes" and "sweet lemon" mechanisms. In the "sour grapes" reaction we might say, if we didn't buy the car, that a new car is not worth having this year because they cost more than they are worth. The "sweet lemon" attitude is an extension of "sour grapes": we did not buy the new car because of its many disadvantages but because our old one has so many good points and runs so well that losing money by trading it in would be foolish.

Rationalization is operating when we search for reasons to justify behavior or ideas, when we are unable to recognize inconsistencies and have to justify them, and when we become emotional when rationalizations are questioned, for this threatens us [7, 13].

Regression is a return to a former, somewhat primitive, and rather childish type of reaction. Examples of regressive reactions are furnished by the tennis star who throws his racket against the net when he receives an adverse decision or by the college student who leaves school and returns home because life is simpler there.

Repression is a tension-producing mechanism. It is a process of selective forgetting, in which the individual unconsciously tries to forget those aspects of his past or present behavior that may cause pain or discomfort. He fights to hold his desires down or pretends they do not exist. He feels one way and acts another. An illustration of repression is given by the marine who has undergone many unpleasant experiences and seen many horrible sights on the battle front but who represses his thoughts of these events, refusing to review them for himself voluntarily. It is a mechanism in which an individual represses feelings of horror, shame, guilt, or humiliation.

Repression sometimes takes the form of behavior and feelings exactly opposite to the repressed tendency. For example, the alcoholic driven by the desire for alcohol represses his desire and gives temperance lectures. Repression plays a positive role in controlling dangerous desires and minimizing painful experiences. However, it is damaging when used to an exaggerated degree or when it protects the individual from problems he should face realistically.

Sublimation is the expression of a desire in a way that is useful and acceptable to society and overcoming frustration by striving for success in other situations. An illustration is provided by the college student who sublimates his sexual urges in socially accepted activities, such as athletics, dances, and parties.

Some psychologists believe that basic drives can only be repressed, not sublimated, and that sublimation does not take place completely. The traditional view presented in the example holds that sublimation utilizing bodily energy in constructive activities reduces tension built up by frustrated sexual and other drives. Constructive activities also keep the individual so busy that he has no time to dwell on the frustration. The degree to which sublimation does occur has both individual and social value.

Substitution is a kind of compensation. The individual reduces tension by changing from a frustrated activity to one that is more easily accomplished. An illustration would be substituting journalistic achievement for athletic prowess, or vice versa.

Sympathism is a technique by which the individual, to avoid facing a problem or an obstacle, tries to gain attention and receive expressions of concern over his difficulties. An example is the college student who fails a course and then seeks the sympathy of others to explain the failure, which in his mind was due to unfair treatment given him by the instructor.

Transference is an attachment to a person similar to another person to whom one is already attached. For illustration, if a person to whom one is introduced resembles a friend, one tends to be attracted to this new person.

Withdrawal is the avoiding of unpleasant situations by retiring from them or evading them. The student who continually secludes himself, preferring solitude to socializing with others who are participating in the usual college activities, is an example. Such a person feels that he avoids all danger of failure in connection with these situations. He makes an indirect adjustment by not facing his problem.

ATTITUDE OF SOCIETY TOWARD ADJUSTMENT MECHANISMS

The value of the different defense mechanisms varies considerably. Some have beneficial effects, as they actually help the individual to solve a problem, to maintain his ego, and to uphold his status in a group. Others are of little value, and still others are dangerous because they prevent a positive approach to everyday situations. The adjustment mechanisms are classified according to their degree of desirability and social approval [19]:

Most desirable (socially approved) adjustment mechanisms: compensation, rationalization, substitution, sublimation.

Less desirable (socially tolerated) mechanisms: identification, projection, egocentrism, sympathism, regression, dissociation, repression, transference.

Least desirable (socially disapproved) mechanisms: negativism, fantasy, withdrawal.

It is important to point out that even the least desirable mechanisms may be used by all of us on occasions. For example, everyone should be able to say "no" and take a negative stand on some issues. This is not negativism. The person who exhibits negativism almost always says "no"; he rarely, if ever, sees the positive side. He refuses to solve the problems confronting him because of his negative approach. He makes it a point to demonstrate to others that he cannot be made to do things he does not want to do. Or he may gain personal satisfaction from turning people down just to spite them.

Fantasy or daydreaming is a mechanism everyone uses at some time. This may be helpful when it permits an individual to withdraw temporarily and relax from the tensions of our modern life. Some daydreaming enables one to make useful plans, thereby achieving future goals. Furthermore, the individual who possesses creative imagination may become the scientist, the inventor, or the novelist. Daydreams become harmful and socially disapproved when one resorts to them continuously and they become more satisfying than regular daily experiences. Such practice leads a person to lose contact with the world about him; he lives in a dream world of hallucinations and delusions of grandeur.

Withdrawal may be helpful when an individual is so involved in a situation or with a problem that he cannot make an objective decision at the time. When he withdraws for a while and then comes back to face his task, he may see all aspects of the problem or a point he had overlooked previously and then can make a wise decision. Withdrawal is least desirable and tends to lead to maladjustment when the individual continually retires within himself so that he seeks seclusion and avoids his responsibilities. Such behavior is dangerous to his personality because he fails to meet his needs.

The defensive mechanisms are either adjustive or maladjustive, depending upon their intensity and their frequency of use.

Guidelines for making adjustments

The basic principles of successful human behavior become guidelines in meeting everyday problem situations. These principles, resulting from the adjustment sequence, are summarized briefly.

Every individual has fundamental physical, or organic, and psychological, or ego, needs. Needs motivate behavior. They must be satisfied or removed; otherwise tensions leading to maladjustment are generated. Generally, needs are not easily satisfied because of the conditions in the situation or in the mind that block their direct satisfaction. Therefore, frustration and conflict exist naturally and normally. To overcome frustration and conflict, the individual varies his behavior, selecting that which is most integrating and unifying. This behavior is based on influences from his total past development and reflects his total self. His modified behavior resolves the frustration and conflict. In solving the problem, adjustment takes place, resulting in personal security and mental health [7, 11, 16, 23]. Reactions indicating adjustment are shown in the diagram on page 88.

The ways in which life adjustments are made are summarized as follows: [4]

Use abilities and capacities with satisfaction and enthusiasm.

Do one's share in worthwhile group activities.

Get along well with people, whether or not they are superiors.

Meet situations involving stress with constructive ideas and the will to succeed.

Try to solve difficult problems or complete difficult tasks in spite of obstacles.

Do not permit daydreaming or wishful thinking to take the place of genuine accomplishment.

Be tolerant and understanding of the needs and desires of associates.

Give as well as receive assistance and favors.

These principles of adjustment can be illustrated by a description of the actions of a college coed. Katherine Jamison was a college sophomore. Although not a beautiful girl, she was careful of her appearance and was considered attractive. Her budget for clothes was limited. She did not complain but selected with care what she was able to purchase so that she always looked well-groomed.

She liked to play tennis and badminton and to swim, bowl, and skate and enjoyed other activities. As a consequence she had a good appetite and slept well. She ate a balanced diet and avoided overeating. The doctor told her at her last medical examination that she was in fine physical condition. However, he warned her about doing too much and becoming overfatigued. She heeded his advice and added an hour's sleep to her daily schedule.

Katherine was a good student. She was not brilliant. However, by organizing her work and daily activities, she found adequate time for study. She listened attentively in class, kept up in her assignments, and received satisfactory grades.

Her mother and father loved her very much and gave her a feeling of security at home. Yet they urged her to attend college away from home. While she was in high school, they had given her freedom and expected her to assume responsibilities in the household. They continued to do so even when she came home from college on visits. Her parents insisted that she make her own decisions. They would help her find out both sides of the question; the rest was up to her. She got along well with her older brother and sister despite the fact that they teased her continually. She soon learned to "dish it out" too.

Katherine realized her faults as well as her good points. She had discussed her faults with her mother, who showed her that her fine qualities far outweighed her shortcomings. She was well liked in her neighborhood. At one time she helped a neighbor whose daughter was seriously hurt in an accident.

Katherine was popular with college men. They liked to date her. She was good company, danced well, and was a fluent conversationalist but also a good listener. She could have a good time without wanting to go to places her date could not afford.

Since she liked people, she became interested in student-body activities. She ran for sophomore representative to the student executive committee but was defeated. In her campaign she made many new friends and had several interesting experiences. Although she was disappointed by her defeat, she decided that it was good experience and that she would try for office again after she became better known.

Katherine was a well-adjusted girl from a good home that provided her personal security. She was a healthy, normal coed. She liked to do things. As a result she had many accomplishments which gave her personal satisfaction. She had a num-

[4] Katz and Lehner, op. cit., p. 62.

ber of good friends, both men and women. She liked people, and they liked her. She not only desired recognition in socially accepted ways but wanted to contribute to the welfare of her group and her college. She generally was successful in what she undertook, yet could adjust when she was unsuccessful.

Maturity and adjustment

The individual develops from relatively unorganized behavior to organized and structured behavior. He is motivated toward goals or purposes within his environment. From the environment or within himself, barriers or rival motives arise, causing frustration and conflict. Conflict brings a necessity for choice between two different lines of action. A shifting back and forth may occur before a decision is made between the two existing tensions. The individual uses various adjustment mechanisms to resolve his conflicts. As a rule, he uses the socially desirable defensive mechanisms. As his behavior becomes more and more patterned, he achieves new goals and develops the capacity to work for remote goals. He gains self-control and self-management. He develops interests and wholesome attitudes and habits. He achieves a wholeness or balance of emotions and desires. Through his actions he gains in effectiveness and becomes a mature individual.

DEVELOPMENT OF INTERESTS, ATTITUDES, AND HABITS

Basic human needs are not the only aspects of behavior that influence the individual's growth into maturity. Interests, attitudes, and habits are also significant.

Interests. An interest implies the recognition of a need. An interest also refers to the special attention the individual pays as he is directed toward activity. The activity may relate to an object, an area, or persons in the environment. Such activity brings about pleasure and satisfaction, and consequently it increases motivation. The value of interests lies in their significant effect upon the life of the individual. For example, interests that lead the individual to active participation rather than to a passive role are more desirable, since greater personal development results. Also, interests in activities that stimulate the individual to create and discover bring about greater personal development than do passive activities.

Many interests are temporary in nature. They change as people age, and they differ from person to person. Greater satisfaction comes from more enduring and lasting activities. The more enduring interests often lead to vocational choices as well as recreational pursuits. In addition, activities that can be shared with others bring about development to a greater degree than do those performed alone. Interests are preferred which develop personality through increased understanding and the shaping of wholesome attitudes and practices.

As the individual matures, his interests increase. The infant is interested primarily in food, sleep, and affection. The mature person seeks out the many activities within his environment. Some environments restrict interests, and others broaden them. Anderson proposes a specific interest-classification system. He organizes life interests as follows [3]:

Manipulation and construction activities, illustrated by the child's interest in toys and the adolescent's construction of objects and machines

Sports and athletics, in which children, young persons, and adults develop muscles, improve coordination, and make personal and social adjustments

Outdoor life, exemplified by camping as practiced in the youth organizations, such as the Boy Scouts and Girl Scouts, exemplified for adults in hunting, fishing, and traveling

Clubs and social groups, such as ski clubs, service clubs, fraternities, and sororities

Stories, reading, and literature interests, such as the child's interest in pictures and stories about objects and animals, the adolescent's interest in fiction, later on leading into religious and philosophical material and ranging from incidental appreciation to professional activity in reading and writing

The comics or serial stories in newspapers and magazines

Motion pictures

Radio and television

Acting and the theater

Music

Dancing

Artistic activities

Hobbies

Religious endeavors

Interests provide a means of releasing tensions, realizing new satisfactions, projecting one's inner life outward, seeing one's self in a new perspective, and obtaining needed companionship. Interests are vital to the development and maturity of the individual, as they enable him to acquire new attitudes, habits, and traits along with increased ability to make personal and social adjustments.

Attitudes. Attitudes are defined as tendencies to respond either positively or negatively toward persons, objects, or situations.[5] Attitudes are composed both of ideas and of emotional factors. They are the result of many experiences involving points of view and feelings. They are the by-product of a situation rather than a response resulting from direct stimulation. For example, the late President Franklin D. Roosevelt influenced many persons' attitudes through his speeches, not so much by what he said as by the manner in which he said it. Since attitudes are important in influencing behavior, they become a powerful force in the individual's development and his growth into maturity. A person develops negative attitudes, such as prejudice and bias, as well as positive attitudes, in the form of attachments and loyalties to individuals, objects, and ideals.

Home life shapes attitudes in the closely knit family association. The examples set by parents aid in attitude formation. Parental control, love, and affection and family social activities have a powerful effect on attitudes. Important, too, in attitude development are relationships with associates of both sexes. The social life of the community exerts a potent influence on the development of attitudes. Advertising in the newspapers and magazines, over the radio, and on television is specifically directed toward shaping attitudes of children, youth, and adults. School experiences are planned by teachers, students, and parents with a primary purpose of modifying beliefs and attitudes.

On the national and international level, political attitudes play a major role. In a democracy, there is little attempt to control attitudes through the state. The process of attitude formation is based on the intelligence of each individual. It is an educational approach in which there is a free exchange of ideas. Decisions are arrived at through rational processes, after weighing the evidence on both sides of an issue. Individual self-directive behavior, leading to the optimum development of the individual, and civic participation in solving problems are the desired results, not indoctrination by the state on preconceived principles directed by a selected few. The individual's critical evaluation, by the problem-solving method, of health information gained from various communication media—radio, television, newspapers—is an illustration of the mature shaping of attitudes in a worthwhile manner.

Attitudes represent behavior in a suspended state.

[5] Clifford T. Morgan, *Introduction to Psychology*, 2d ed., McGraw-Hill Book Company, Inc., New York, 1961, p. 112.

Habits or practices. The individual is largely a creature of his habits. The well-adjusted person has established a set of habits that permit him to perform his everyday tasks with ease and efficiency. Old habits tend to guide him unless he himself breaks the old and develops new ones. It is still possible even at the college age to develop new habits, though it is much easier to develop good habits during early years.

Habits are a type of learned behavior so often repeated that the action becomes automatic, calling for little or no attention. "Habits are any response actions which may be initiated by a particular set of stimuli and terminated by a particular reaction." Habits are not static; rather, they are in a constant state of change. For this reason, the development of wholesome practices for improved mental health is possible if the individual so desires, that is, if he exerts conscious control over his actions. New habits can be established by following these steps [4]:

Clearly state the purpose of the new habit.
Plan how this habit can be carried out.
Begin the new plan vigorously.
Do not permit any exceptions to the new habit, particularly at first.
Continue to perform the new habit.

Old habits may be broken by applying the same method; however, an old habit must be replaced by a new, improved habit so as to direct attention to another interest and not permit indulgence in the old habit. The mature, well-adjusted individual exerts conscious control of his emotional behavior by rational processes. By such action he is able to change old habits for new, improved ones and to develop habit patterns that aid in the development of sound mental health and more effective living.

DEVELOPMENT AND CONTROL OF EMOTIONS

It has been pointed out that when the individual is under stress, he experiences feelings of tension and excitement called *emotions*. Uncontrolled emotions characterize the early stages of adjustment. They tend to decrease as the individual acquires the ability to satisfy his needs.

Emotion is characterized as a "stirred-up" state. A condition may result in which the individual becomes so excited in an emergency situation that he is unable to act; conversely, he may be stimulated and keyed up to rise to new heights in his particular activity. Emotions may give him the most satisfying feelings or bring about trouble and disaster. Fear, anger, love, and jealousy are typical emotions.

Fear. Fear is an emotion that is often present when frustration and conflict occur. It is characterized by dread or expectation of harm. Fear is in reality an internal state of readiness to fight or run away from whatever threatens. Typical minor fears are lack of confidence and fear of the dark. Such fears often are passed on verbally from generation to generation.

Reactions indicating adjustment. (Adapted from Barney Katz and George Lehner, *Mental Hygiene in Modern Living,* The Ronald Press Company, New York, 1953.)

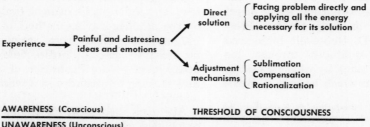

New research points out that few if any fears are innate. Fear almost always is learned. Fear of the dark is conditioned either from actual experience or from stories heard in childhood. Anxiety is a type of fear resulting from the unknown or unpredictable. It usually arises from conflict and frustration. Experience and education aid in reducing this type of fear, as motives become more easily directed and satisfied.

Worry. Worry is a form of anxiety. It may express itself in a variety of ways, for example, insomnia, a vague feeling of restlessness, indigestion, hyperacidity, overconscientiousness, or obsessions or compulsions varying from minor disturbances to more severe ones.

An anonymous writer has developed a worry table indicating what people generally worry about in our times.

	Per cent
Things that never happen	40
Things over and past that couldn't be changed by all the worry in the world	30
Petty worries	10
Needless health worries	12
Real legitimate worries	8

Worry may be a symptom of mental conflict or of insecurity. In such cases, the feelings must be relieved, or the worry persists. Worry can be relieved by adjustment to the problem at hand, by a direct attack, or by formulating a definite plan to solve a problem. Talking or writing about his fears, worries, and anxieties often relieves the individual from the resulting disturbing factors. This aids him in regaining his equilibrium. Attaining experience, improving skills, and developing interests assist the individual in adjusting to these emotionalized reactions.

Inferiority feeling. An inferiority feeling is an emotional state of mind. The person believes he is a failure or is different from others physically, mentally, or socially.

Often a feeling of inferiority differs from an actual inferior state measured by objective standards. In many instances an inferiority feeling is due to frustration in one's social setting. Such feelings are best adjusted by understanding one's self, by observing that most persons have similar feelings, by achieving success, or by admitting inferiority in one field and transferring to another field where success can be achieved. Self-confidence is the opposite of fear, anxiety, and worry. The self-confident person faces his fears because he has made adjustments in personal and social relationships. He has gained success where he naturally excels and has extended his efforts into other areas, achieving new goals.

Love. Love is an emotion of attachment and affection for other persons and objects. In normal development, love begins with self-love, spreads to an affection for parents, then to affection for persons of the same sex, and finally to an affection for the opposite sex. This development may be interrupted by circumstances at any stage along the way. Some individuals never progress beyond the stage of interest in which homosexual attraction is dominant. In the development of the love emotion a cycle prevails. First comes idealism, then disillusionment. Out of these stages there is a gradual development of true values. Many individuals when their love ideals are shattered never permit themselves to engage in further social interaction of this type. These persons do not progress to the heterosexual stage and marriage. A more detailed discussion of this emotion is presented in Chapter 4.

GUIDES FOR CONTROLLING EMOTIONS

In controlling emotions the following principles will help [3, 23, 28]:
Strive to understand fears, anxieties, and worries. Information relative to the emotion and to the cause of the emotional response is often helpful. If one knows

the situation bringing about the response exhibited and what the adequate response should be, behavior can be redirected. As previously suggested, some of the disturbing elements can be eliminated by meeting the emotions objectively, by talking about the fears and anxieties, or by writing about them. With the disturbing elements eliminated, the individual often has a new perspective and sees new ways to face these feelings.

Realize that emotions are stirred by the emotional responses of others. If one understands the fact that it is a first reaction to exhibit emotion in response to the emotions of others, this tendency may be restrained and emotional control will result.

Keep emotions isolated or in context with a situation, not allowing them to affect general behavioral responses. Emotional control keeps emotions segregated and concerned only with their original stimulus. Thus if a specific fear arises because of a disturbing event, it is not permitted to become a major problem and cause general inferiority feelings.

Do not worry over past mistakes. Approach new situations with confidence. Emotional adjustment comes through profiting from mistakes or failures, with a "comeback" in new situations. Brooding over past mistakes and defects only permits poor past behavior to influence present and future conduct. The well-adjusted individual has the ability to "come back," for he lives in the present and the future, not in the past.

Use direct positive action in controlling emotions. Get at the basis of the conflict immediately. Determine what caused the real trouble. See your instructor, your boss, or your father or mother. Talk the situation through instead of withdrawing and worrying over it.

Become reassured after the removal of emotional conditions. When the basic condition is understood and a plan of action has been formulated to remedy the situation, self-reassurance or reassurance by a friend gives added confidence and a greater chance of success.

Observe friends who meet emotional stress with calm and collected behavior. They can help one to meet similar conditions.

Maturity involves improvement in controlling emotions. Emotional reactions accompany stages in the process of adjustment. As individuals mature, experience and skill are gained in progressing from emergency reactions to skilled behavior.

Energy and enthusiasm are positive aspects of emotions and must be retained to make life adjustments.

Emotional maturity is reached when the individual develops a sound set of values, self-confidence, a sense of personal worth, and a sense of humor. Emotions may be helpful to the individual [28] when they:

Provide a stirred-up state that brings out reserves of energy.

Cause expressive changes, such as joy and tender feelings.

Remove inhibitions, permitting ideas to be acted upon which otherwise might be stultified.

Emotions may be detrimental when they:

Cause irrational action.

Impair motor skill.

Block mental processes.

Restrict the range of desirable activity and experience.

Impair health.

Personality maladjustments

Personality maladjustments result from inability to meet life needs. Variations in adjustment seem to differ primarily in degree rather than in kind [34]. Some of the minor personality maladjustments, such as inferiority feelings, feelings of insecurity, and nervous states, have been discussed. These minor deviations are characterized by feelings and tensions, for the most part are not serious, and are often only temporary in nature, with a return to well-adjusted behavior a real possibility. However, if not corrected, they may lead to greater degrees of maladjustment and serious mental disorders. Such maladjustments also may result from disease, accidents, heredity, shock, intoxication, endocrine dysfunction, or continuous presence within the environment of frustration, conflict, and threats to security. These disorders are characterized by definite observable symptoms indicating the presence of emotional tension, with resultant loss of personal efficiency.

The major personality maladjustments are not of great concern to college students because of their low incidence within this select group. However, an understanding of these disorders is important from a preventive aspect and from the point of view of the total mental health problem in the general population.

Those suffering from the major mental disorders are classified as psychoneurotics, psychotics, psychopathic personalities (sociopathic or character disorders), and mental defectives. For reference to each of these classifications see Suggested readings Nos. 7, 18, 22, and 24.

PSYCHONEUROSIS

Psychoneurosis, or neurosis, is a partial separation from reality marked by eccentric behavior. Such a mentally ill person is commonly called a *neurotic*. The two terms "psychoneurosis" and "neurosis" are now used synonymously, although "psychoneurosis" is more widely employed, to avoid confusion with medical terms relating to neurologic conditions [34]. A psychoneurosis is a behavior disorder due to emotional tension resulting from frustrations, conflicts, repressions, or marked insecurity. It is a form of adjustment, usually to an overwhelming anxiety. The psychoneurotic individual finds it difficult to meet his needs, his social obligations, and the demands of daily living, since his efficiency is limited by his emotional state.

However, he still maintains some adjustive capacity within the limits of his social structure [34].

Psychoneuroses can be prevented by parents who understand and assist their children in solving their problems, particularly those related to fears, dislikes, and aversions. Treatment and correction of the psychoneuroses can be secured and achieved by psychotherapy, such as interview therapy and psychoanalysis.

The psychoneuroses may be classified into five forms: hysteria, psychasthenia, neurasthenia, anxiety, and hypochondriasis [34].

Hysteria. Hysteria is an adjustive state in which the thwarted individual resolves his emotional conflicts by developing physical disease or disability symptoms. The symptoms developed are such that it is temporarily impossible to return to the troublesome situation. They resemble the symptoms of organic disease or disability, yet no bacteria, lesions, unusual chemical reactions, or defects are present. For example, a student may develop a headache, stiff neck, convulsions, or other conditions to escape from a situation with which he can no longer cope. Actually, hysteria is a functional disorder of the personality due to emotional disturbances.

Psychasthenia. Psychasthenia comprises the phobias, obsessions, and compulsions. A phobia is a specialized type of obsession in which there is an intensified unreasoning fear of some object or situation within the environment. When a person shows undue fear of an object or situation where there is no apparent danger, he is exhibiting a phobia. The more common phobias are fears of high places, open places, closed places, crowds, noise, light, darkness, thunder, lightning, storms, pain, disease, and sharp or pointed objects. Most of these fears do not interfere with personal and social adjustment. No emotional reactions occur if the individual restrains and restricts himself to the limits imposed on him by his phobia. It is when he becomes confronted by the fear-producing object or situation in such a way that a disturbed emotional state occurs, such as a panic, that the phobia becomes detrimental to his adjustment. Although most phobias are a result of childhood experiences, they are more commonly found to occur in adult life.

Obsessions are characterized as persistent repetition of undesired thoughts or acts. Consistently worrying about finances, ill health, or death, is an example of obsessions. An obsession is abnormal when it is so strong as to interfere with everyday activity and one's personal and social adjustment.

Compulsions are acts that an individual does wthout knowing why he does them. Common compulsions are kleptomania, the compulsion to steal; pyromania, the compulsion to set fires; and the handwashing compulsion. A person with this last compulsion feels compelled to wash his hands again and again even when they are clean.

The phobias, obsessions, and compulsions are the individual's way of protecting himself against stress and anxiety by transferring his guilt feelings to an object, act, or thought [22].

Neurasthenia. Neurasthenia, or nervous exhaustion, is a classification of ailments due to stress and strain. It refers to anxiety reactions, psychosomatic conditions, combat fatigue, or stress reaction. The common symptoms exhibited are general lack of energy to the extent of chronic fatigue, depression, irritability, and inability to concentrate. Emotional tension brings about physical symptoms of tired feelings, physical weakness, little appetite, headaches, and bodily aches and pains. Worry over these symptoms causes increased tension, which in turn aggravates the physical symptoms [18, 34].

Anxiety neurosis. Anxiety neurosis is a condition accompanied by irrational fear, worry, and a sense of doom. The person exhibits fear in situations where there is no possibility of harm's befalling him. He may fear that he will lose his friends or his money, that he will meet with an accident, or that he is going to die. Such an individual usually shows the same organic symptoms as the neurasthenics but with the addition of intense fear. For this reason the anxiety state is considered one step worse than neurasthenia. Common characteristics are morbid dread and indecision. Anxiety neuroses probably are caused by intense feelings of insecurity, inferiority, or guilt or by a combination of all three.

Hypochondriasis. Hypochondriasis is a condition in which the individual exhibits great concern about his health. He is overanxious about his bodily organs and their functions, particularly those affected by emotional conditions as well as by organic disease. Heart disease, kidney disease, and ulcers are commonly feared. The hypochondriac's symptoms and suffering are greatly overestimated by himself. By an exaggeration of his condition, the individual gains sympathy and attention, which bring a feeling of security. The hypochondriac is often a health faddist looking for special diets or remedies, which he thinks will improve or restore health.

PSYCHOSES

The psychoses are serious mental disorders. They are commonly referred to in lay terms as *insanity*. A psychotic person is one who is not able to face reality and therefore is unable to meet his obligations to society. His whole personality is affected. His behavior may be such that he injures himself or other persons. The majority of psychotic persons are acutely ill and are committed to mental hospitals.

The behavior of some mentally ill individuals combines the symptoms of both psychoneurosis and psychosis. In some cases there can be no clear line of demarcation. Usually, however, a differentiation can be made, as the psychotic reactions are more severe, affect a greater part of the personality, and are more dangerous to the individual as well as to other persons [7, 18].

The psychoses may be classified into organic, toxic, and functional types.

The organic psychoses. An organic psychosis is a major disorder of personality due to some physical or structural condition. All persons in this group are afflicted with brain disease or brain injury. The brain injury is for the most part responsible for the failure of the individual to adjust to his environment. Examples of conditions in this category are senile psychosis, which is the result of softening of the brain and hardening of the arteries, and paresis, caused by advanced syphilis.

The toxic psychoses. This type of psychosis displays two symptoms: a *disorganization* of time, of place, and of the individual's own personality; and *hallucinations* ranging from mild to extreme, producing great anxiety. Examples are alcoholic psychosis and psychoses from drugs. Alcohol has a toxic effect on the central nervous system, which is demonstrated by the emotional responses, the functional activities, and an effect on the nervous tissue. Alcoholic persons have some unmet need or hidden mental conflict that alcohol temporarily satisfies. While intoxicated, a person is actually mentally ill; his behavior during this time is psychotic. However, because of the rapid recovery from this condition in some cases, the individual is not usually thought of as psychotic. It is the chronic drinker who suffers from hallucinations, delirium tremens, and loss of memory. Drug addicts, such as those who use morphine, find that the intellectual faculties are affected much more than the physical condition. The action of alcohol and drugs may eventually result in some form of brain injury.

The functional psychoses. In this class of psychosis the brain appears normal, but a malfunctional condition exists within the individual. Two common examples of the functional type are schizophrenia and manic-depressive psychosis. For further information and description of other psychoses, see references 7, 18, 22, and 34.

Schizophrenia (dementia praecox) is the most common and the most important severe mental disease, especially from a social standpoint. Approximately 50 per cent of all patients in state mental hospitals are schizophrenic, and for every one in a mental hospital there is probably one in a less disturbed condition cared for by relatives in a private home. A great many criminals, prostitutes, and hoboes suffer from schizophrenia [24]. While the well-adjusted individual is an integrated unit, the schizophrenic person lacks integration between thinking and feeling. The result is a complete withdrawal from human relationships. Such persons commonly are referred to as *shut-in personalities.* They show in their disorganization of personality a loss of interest in former activities. Also, they exhibit preoccupation and fantasy about sex, religion, money, or bodily functions, finding an illogical or unreal solution for their overemphasized problems. Hallucinations often support their illogical beliefs. Delusional experiences frequently occur about health, strength, or power. Frequently there is loss of feeling for others—in fact, complete disregard for social living, exhibited in a breakdown of habits of cleanliness and thoughtfulness.

Manic-depressive psychosis is a type of mental illness in which the individual is disturbed in the way he feels about life and his experiences. His feelings are intensified and overemphasized to the point where his judgment and behavior are affected. Depression or elation becomes set, lasting as long as months or years. Although the name of the illness refers to alternating moods, there are cases in which only one mood appears; such conditions are called *manic-depressive manic* or *manic-depressive depressed*. In the majority of cases there is a period of excitement and overactivity followed suddenly by a period of depression. The opposite order is seen less frequently. The period of depression usually lasts longer than the excited state. In most cases, chronic manic-depressive patients spend the last years of their lives in hospitals in a worried, despondent, unhappy state.

MENTAL ILLNESS IN THE COMMUNITY

According to a 1960 report from the National Association for Mental Health [6] at least 1 person in every 10 had some form of mental or emotional illness which was serious enough to require treatment for full recovery. It was estimated that 1 out of 12 Americans would be hospitalized for mental illness during some period in their lifetimes. The evidence was conclusive that half of the hospital beds throughout the country are used for the mentally ill. Also, it was estimated that 14,100 young people between fifteen and twenty-four years are admitted to public mental hospitals yearly for mental illness.

The Association's report classified mental hospital admissions as follows:

Kinds of illnesses	Per cent and ages of patients, years	
Schizophrenia	23	15–35
Senile psychosis and cerebral arteriosclerosis	21	Mainly 60 and over
Involutional psychosis	6	Mainly 45–60
Manic-depressive psychosis	5	Mainly 35–50
Severe alcoholism	13.7	Mainly 25–55
Personality disorders other than alcoholism	6	Mainly 15–35
Psychoneuroses	9	Mainly 25–45
Mental deficiency	2.3	Mainly 15–45
Other disorders	14	

[6] *Facts About Mental Illness,* National Association for Mental Health, New York, 1960.

TREATMENT OF MENTAL ILLNESS

Great strides are being made in the treatment of the mentally ill. Psychiatrists are using with considerable success various kinds of treatment for serious mental illnesses. Individual therapy is effective to gain rapport with a patient and then to influence him favorably. Group therapy is valuable, using such media as recreation, art, music, painting, and dancing. Electric therapy is administered frequently in depressive types of mental illness, where the patient feels unworthy or has guilt feelings. Surgery may be necessary in some cases although psychosurgery or lobotomy is now seldom used. Stereotaxic surgery is proving successful to some extent as a new surgical method. This consists of operating with an electrode through an opening in the skull to destroy certain nerve cells identified as responsible for the mental disturbance.

Hypnosis, the trance or sleeplike state, under the direction of competent psychiatrists and psychologists with special training in this art, can prove to be valuable therapy for mental illness. It can serve as supportive therapy as well as a way of overcoming resistance in reconstructive therapy. Hypnosis can be valuable as a device to bring out hidden facts that the person is unable or unwilling to tell about in a conscious state. It may be used to penetrate the subconscious mind, facilitating dreams and the restoring of forgotten memories. Hypnosis may be dangerous when used for the purpose of stage entertainment by a hypnotist without thorough knowledge of psychodynamics.

The comparatively new psychiatric drugs are receiving widespread use in the treatment of mental illness in the United States and Europe. These are called *tranquilizing drugs* because of their calming effect on the patient. They make possible psychotherapy for even the severely disturbed patients by reducing their anxieties, enabling them to appear much more normal and assisting the psychiatrist in establishing effective contact with them. The administration of these drugs as a common practice has opened up a new era, referred to as the *biochemical era.*

There are three major tranquilizing drugs, with many more in the experimental stage. Each one varies in its effect on the individual. Chlorpromazine (trade name Thorazine) is useful in suppressing the delusions of paranoid patients, as it relieves deep-seated anxieties of chronic mental disease. Reserpine (Serpasil), an alkaloid from the root of a plant called *Rauwolfia serpentina,* is similar to chlorpromazine but less rapid and more sustained. It is most helpful with patients whose speech is unintelligible and those who maintain a peculiar rigid posture for long periods of time. The best known of another class of tranquilizers, referred to as *muscle relaxants,* is called meprobamate (Miltown, Equanil). The muscle relaxants affect the nervous system to relieve tensions without impairing the higher thinking capacities of the individual.

The tranquilizing drugs offer the hope that the cost of caring for mentally disturbed persons will be reduced markedly. They reduce substantially the number of patients who need to be hospitalized, permitting many to be treated in the community, at a clinic, or in a psychiatrist's office. Also, more patients may be able to be released after shorter periods of hospitalization.

There are drawbacks and disadvantages to the tranquilizing drugs too. Large doses are dangerous for their physical effect on the body and because they can cause certain serious side effects with some persons. For example, chlorpromazine or reserpine may lower the blood pressure and may cause tremors, gastric disturbances, and skin eruptions. In addition, there is danger of these drugs being taken without proper supervision. Under the supervision of a physician most side effects can be controlled by such measures as adjusting the dosage, combining agents, and varying the drugs. With good medical supervision, side effects are not serious enough to prevent an individual from using a needed drug. On the other hand, self-dosage without the advice of a physician is a dangerous practice. Much further research and study, along with more rigid controls, are necessary to make biochemical treatment completely safe and effective. This new approach to the treatment of mental illness may prove in the future to be one of the greatest of medical discoveries.

With good care and treatment 7 out of 10 patients can leave mental hospitals partially or totally cured.

Professional assistance

Personality maladjustments, either minor or serious, are not a disgrace. They can happen to anyone, and they do occur more often than is realized. Most deviations are temporary and cause no permanent damage if discovered early. In most instances, such conditions develop gradually, sending out warnings in advance. The majority of persons with adjustment problems can be helped to lead happy, normal, useful lives. The important fact is that mental illness demands prompt care just as does physical illness. To know where to turn for assistance when a person needs help for himself, a member of his family, or a friend is the first step in making necessary adjustments.

When the student is confronted with a minor problem while at college, he can immediately contact the counseling center, the student health service, or a member of his family. It is more than likely that the counseling center will have a clinical psychologist trained and experienced in counseling techniques and skilled in handling personal-social-emotional problems. The counselor will refer serious conditions needing medical attention to a qualified psychiatrist. If the student prefers to talk with his own physician or the college physician at the student health service, this medical adviser can provide necessary assistance. When the problem is a serious one, the physician is an excellent person to recommend a qualified psychiatrist. A psychiatrist is a medical doctor with specialized training in the prevention and treatment of emotional disturbances and mental diseases. He has had experience in a mental hospital or a mental health clinic.

If as a citizen in the community an individual is faced with such a problem, the logical person to consult is the family physician. Again, the physician will recommend a reputable clinical psychologist or psychiatrist if one is necessary.

The student or the citizen who does not have a family physician can consult the local mental health clinic or mental health association, the local public health department, or the state department of mental health for qualified assistance.

Beware of the quack or charlatan and the advertising self-appointed specialist. Psychological cultists are prevalent everywhere, preying on the uninformed public.

Formulating a personal program for mental health

Undoubtedly, the college student has been following some type of mental health program for a number of years. It may have been sound or unsound, according to modern principles. It may have been planned intelligently or followed haphazardly. The chances are better than even that the program has been a good one because the college student has attained various goals and made many successful adjustments, resulting in a high degree of maturity. However, many desires, wishes, and goals are yet to be satisfied. A four-point personal program for mental health is suggested to enable the student to continue making successful life adjustments and to ensure improved personal and social relationships:

Understand mental health—its basic factors and forces, including the personal and social adjustment process.

Study and appraise mental health principles.

Plan and replan a course of action for happier, more effective living.

Apply mental health principles to life experiences.

DEVELOPING AN UNDERSTANDING OF MENTAL HEALTH

A fundamental assumption of this chapter is that the college student understands the basic factors involved in the personal and social adjustment process. The student is aware that mental health is not a mysterious process but is the result of his everyday living in the home, in college, on the job, or in other community activities. He knows that he can do something about shaping his own thinking, feeling, and doing to live more effectively. He realizes that heredity has set limitations for him. He understands his environment with its particular mores and its stresses. He learns what his capacities are. He is aware of his assets and liabilities. He is assured that he has many unique abilities upon which he can capitalize. Also, he knows that most persons in our society are not utilizing their maximum capacities.

Insight into the adjustment process further enables the student to understand that it is natural for many of his goals to be attained with little or no difficulty.

On the other hand, many goals are difficult of achievement, with frustration and conflict present as desires and wants are blocked. He realizes that some of these are blocked temporarily and that other barriers are permanent. In either case, new adjustments or readjustments are required. It is apparent to the student that the majority of his problems can be solved successfully by appropriate behavior, utilizing wholesome, purposeful experiences. He uses several of the mental or defense mechanisms occasionally for achieving adjustments, but he recognizes that he does use them. He makes sure they are not used excessively or to the extent that they become habitual. They do not inhibit his ability to face reality in making adjustments. For example, when a life problem occurs, he faces it realistically and applies all his attention and energy in working out a solution.

As the student gains a clearer understanding of mental health, he has greater opportunities to apply its principles in his everyday living in home, college, and community activities.

STUDY AND APPRAISAL OF MENTAL HEALTH PRINCIPLES

Some fundamental principles of mental health are reviewed and presented in the form of *guidelines* for effective living. These can be studied and considered by the student for incorporation into his own mental health program. The following specific suggestions or guides have been derived from a number of authorities in the field of mental health [4, 19, 23, 34]:

Have a practical plan for achieving a successful life centered in work, play, love, and faith. Develop your philosophy of life. Have several major attainable goals, and enjoy working toward them.

Keep yourself in good physical condition through a balanced program of physical activity, rest, wholesome diet, proper elimination, and personal cleanliness.

Gain confidence through making sure of some small successes and a few major ones.

Face your troubles, worries, and fears. Do what you can about them; then direct your efforts to more pleasant things. Gradually do the thing you fear. Time and experience aid in the solution of problems. Remember that time heals.

Find desirable ways to express disturbing emotions rather than repress them. Attempt to determine why you go off at a tangent. Know yourself. Control your emotions.

Feel the importance of dedication to a significant cause which is greater than yourself. This dedication may be to your family, your girl or boy friend, or your chosen vocation.

Adopt a wholesome attitude toward sex. "Love, but love wisely." Remember that sex functions when in keeping with the standards and mores of society are a source of rewarding satisfactions contributing to personality development.

Cultivate a variety of active interests. Special interests, such as sports and hobbies, are examples.

Cultivate a sense of humor. Admit your own mistakes, and be able to laugh at yourself for some of your "boners."

Accept criticism impersonally, and profit by it. Avoid brooding over past mistakes. Turn the next opportunity into a successful accomplishment.

Enjoy a social life with both sexes. Acquire a few close friends and companions with whom you can share your successes and problems.

Maintain a sensible independence. Gain independence from parents, but maintain your love and respect for them.

Accept responsibility with a willing spirit when given a job to do.

Find moments in each day to relax completely. Find serenity; avoid strain. Cultivate periods of contemplation, meditation, and appreciation as well as active participation.

Get along with others. Learn to live in

your environment, getting along with yourself, your family, your neighbors, and your community.

Do the best you can. Do not try to reach all your goals at once. Do not try to do better than your best. Be satisfied with making some progress if it is the best you can do.

After carefully reading these precepts for sound personal and social adjustment, and thinking them through, the student can use them as a check list to evaluate his own situation.

PLANNING AND REPLANNING A PROGRAM FOR HAPPIER, MORE EFFECTIVE LIVING

Meeting health needs and interests requires the student to take time to consider and chart his desired course of action and life activities. This means deciding what he wants to accomplish in life, what values he believes in, what principles he is going to follow, and what course of action will enable him to attain his goals.

The student who plans his own program feels more secure in himself. He knows what he wants, where he is going, and how he is going to get there. Temporary blocks do not discourage him because he is able to replan in view of new situations, modifying his goals if necessary to meet the changing situations, but making successful adjustments. His goals are in harmony with his needs and interests. They are not too remote, nor are they above or below his capacities. He substitutes planning for worrying. He is achieving an integrated, purposeful life.

The student's program based on his own needs and interests is a well-balanced program in terms of life activities. The student's goals formulated in relation to the major areas of life activities should include social, political, religious, educational, industrial, and recreational aims [26]. It is the responsibility of every mature individual to participate in activities in each of these areas. He may be more active in some areas than in others, but a balanced program, which is what he strives for, should include a real interest in each.

APPLICATION OF THE PRINCIPLES OF MENTAL HEALTH

An understanding of the principles of mental health is important to better personal and social adjustment, but actually it is only a beginning step toward improvement. It is only when the principles become guides to action that real achievement occurs. It is paramount that the principles give intelligent direction to the student's own life activities. Only the student himself can shape his life the way he wants to live it. Only he can make life adjustments to find the happiness he seeks. It is well to remember Henry Drummond's remarks regarding the pursuit of happiness: "Half the world is on the wrong scent in the pursuit of happiness. They think it consists in having and getting and in being served by others, but it consists in giving and in serving others." To follow the precepts of mental health takes persistence and fortitude, but applying these principles to everyday living can bring about happier, healthier, more effective living.

Summary

The discussion of making life adjustments is based upon the principles of personality emergence developed in Chapter 2. In order to understand fully how to make satisfactory adjustments, the process of adjustment is presented. A simple description of the adjustment process indicates that human behavior is motivated by needs, desires, goals, and values. These motives must be satisfied or removed; otherwise, tensions leading to readjustive behavior or to maladjustment are generated. Generally, needs are not easily satisfied because of the conditions within the situation or the mind that block their direct satisfaction. Therefore, frustration and conflict exist naturally and normally. To overcome frustration and conflict the individual varies his behavior, selecting that which is most integrating and unifying. His modified behavior resolves the frustration and conflict. When he solves his problem, adjustment takes place, resulting in personal security and mental health.

The dynamics of adjustment and the essential factors in the adjustment process are discussed in considerable detail. The remainder of the chapter is organized to develop these factors. The common problems facing the college student are identified. They include gaining independence, controlling the emotions of love and hate, controlling the sex drive, satisfying the need for security, adequacy, and prestige, and developing standards and value systems. The individual's reactions to stress are described.

The adjustive reactions, the common defense mechanisms by which we frequently demonstrate fight, flight, or compromise, are outlined and classified with examples. Guides for adjustment are expressed in a summary of the ways in which satisfactory adjustments are made. Guides for controlling emotions in general are given to assist the student. Suggestions also are included for developing one's personality potential and becoming a mature individual.

Since maladjustments are common in our society and are becoming an increasingly greater health problem, the minor and major maladjustments are described. These include the common psychoneuroses and psychoses. The sources of professional assistance for mental health problems are described. These include the professional services provided for the student with mental health problems through the counseling center or the student health service. Expert assistance and advice may be obtained from the psychiatrist, a medical specialist in the prevention and treatment of emotional disturbances and mental diseases; from the physician; and from the clinical psychologist trained and experienced in counseling techniques and personal-social-emotional problems. Such services can be depended upon for needed help, as opposed to those of quacks or charlatans.

Finally, a four-point program for developing a personal mental health program is provided. This program summarizes the mental health principles for application to life experiences and may be used to help the individual student make his own satisfactory life adjustments and achieve a sound mentally healthy state.

Suggested readings

1. Alvarez, Walter C.: *Live at Peace with Your Nerves,* Prentice-Hall, Inc., Englewood Cliffs, N.J., 1958.
2. Anderson, Camilla: *Saints, Sinners, and Psychiatry,* J. B. Lippincott Company, Philadelphia, 1950.
3. Anderson, John E.: *The Psychology of Development and Personal Adjustment,* Henry Holt and Company, Inc., New York, 1949.
4. Bernard, H. W.: *Toward Better Personal Adjustment,* 2d ed., McGraw-Hill Book Company, Inc., New York, 1957.
5. Bonney, Merl E.: *Mental Health in Education,* Allyn and Bacon, Inc., Boston, 1960.
6. Carrol, Herbert A.: *Mental Hygiene, the Dynamics of Adjustment,* 2d ed., Prentice-Hall, Inc., Englewood Cliffs, N.J., 1956.
7. Coleman, James C.: *Abnormal Psychology and Modern Life,* 2d ed., Scott Foresman and Company, Chicago, 1956.
8. Committee on the College Student, Group for the Advancement of Psychiatry: *Considerations on Personality Development in College Students,* Report 32, May, 1955.
9. Engel, Leonard: *New Trends in the Care and Treatment of the Mentally Ill,* National Association for Mental Health, New York, 1959.

10. English, Oliver S.: *Emotional Problems of Living,* W. W. Norton & Company, Inc., New York, 1955.

11. Farnsworth, Dana L.: *Mental Health in College and University,* Harvard University Press, Cambridge, Mass., 1957.

12. Felix, R. H.: "Your Mental Health," *NEA Journal,* 48:9, January, 1959.

13. Glasser, William, M.D., *Mental Health or Mental Illness?* Harper & Brothers, New York, 1960.

14. Gorlow, Leon, and Walter Katkovsky: *Readings in the Psychology of Adjustment,* McGraw-Hill Book Company, Inc., New York, 1959.

15. Hollister, William G.: *An Overview: Providing Better Mental Health for Our People, An Introductory Manual for Mental Health Workers,* at 10110 Parkwood Terrace, Bethesda 14, Md., 1956.

16. Hunt, J. McVickers: *Personality and the Behavior Disorders,* The Ronald Press Company, New York, 1944, vols. I and II.

17. Kaplan, Louis: *Mental Health and Human Relations in Education,* Harper & Brothers, New York, 1959.

18. Katz, Barney, and George Lehner: *Mental Hygiene in Modern Living,* The Ronald Press Company, New York, 1953.

19. Katz, Barney, and Louis P. Thorpe: *Understanding People in Distress,* The Ronald Press Company, New York, 1955.

20. Lane, Howard, and Mary Beauchamp: *Understanding Human Development,* Prentice-Hall, Inc., Englewood Cliffs, N.J., 1959.

21. Leeper, Robert Ward, and Peter Madison: *Toward Understanding Human Personalities,* Appleton-Century-Crofts, Inc., New York, 1959.

22. Lehner, George F. J., and Ella Kube: *The Dynamics of Personal Adjustment,* Prentice-Hall, Inc., Englewood Cliffs, N.J., 1955.

23. McKinney, Fred: *Psychology of Personal Adjustment,* 3d ed., John Wiley & Son, Inc., New York, 1960.

24. Milt, Harry: *Basic Facts about Mental Illness,* Scientific Aids Publications, New York, 1959.

25. Milt, Harry: *How to Deal with Mental Problems,* National Association for Mental Health, New York, 1960.

26. Morgan, Clifford T.: *Introduction to Psychology,* 2d ed., McGraw-Hill Book Company, Inc., New York, 1961.

27. Murphy, Gardner: *Human Potentialities,* Basic Books, Inc., New York, 1958.

28. Saul, Leon J.: *Emotional Maturity,* 2d ed., J. B. Lippincott Company, Philadelphia, 1960.

29. Selye, Hans: *The Stress of Life,* McGraw-Hill Book Company, Inc., New York, 1956.

30. Smith, Henry Clay: *Personality Adjustment,* McGraw-Hill Book Company, New York, 1961.

31. Stevenson, George S.: *How to Deal with Your Tensions,* National Association for Mental Health, New York, 1958.

32. Stevenson, George S., and Harry Milt: *Tensions and How to Master Them,* Public Affairs Pamphlet 305, Prentice-Hall, Inc., Englewood Cliffs, N.J., 1960.

33. Strecker, Edward A., Kenneth E. Appel, and John W. Appel: *Discovering Ourselves,* 3d ed., The Macmillan Company, New York, 1959.

34. Thorpe, Louis P.: *The Psychology of Mental Health,* The Ronald Press Company, New York, 1960.

35. Welfare Planning Council, Los Angeles Region: *Los Angeles County Surveys Its Mental Health Services,* The Council, Los Angeles, 1960.

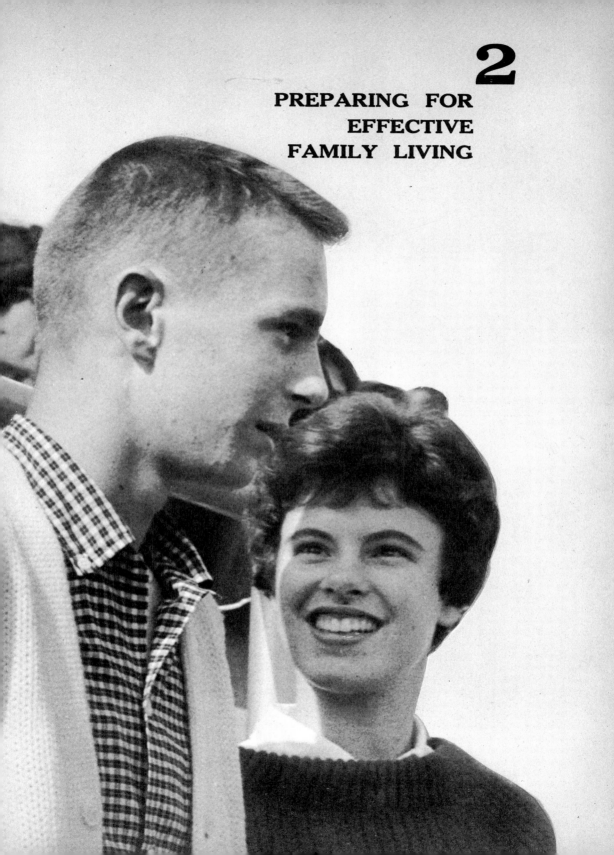

2

PREPARING FOR EFFECTIVE FAMILY LIVING

Choosing a life partner

Your preparation for the responsibilities of your own family during the college years or soon thereafter occurs through dating and courtship activities leading to selection of a life partner and to marriage. It also presupposes that you understand your role in marriage, the problems of adjustment, and the important responsibilities of parenthood. No doubt you have some knowledge of, and experience in, dating. Possibly you have some understanding of other topics in the natural progression of family life processes. You may be married and also a parent.

Regardless of your status, the natural sequence of events in family life is worthy of review and further study. These events satisfy the most basic needs and the areas of most intense interest, according to all available data regarding both men and women college students. Choosing a life partner is obviously one of the most common goals of students. The factors relating to the emergence of the total personality and the ability to make life adjustments, described in Chapters 2 and 3, are applicable to this discussion. The mature individual finds it easier to make wise decisions in choosing a mate and becoming a parent than does an immature person. However, further maturity may be gained through this developmental process. Many individuals do not use mature judgment in selecting a mate. As a college president once said, "You wouldn't pick a horse out by moonlight, but you choose a life partner that way."

The individual seeks a life partner from within his field of eligible persons. In so doing, whether consciously or unconsciously, he attempts to choose a person who he believes will assist him in satisfying his physical and psychological needs.

It is especially desirable to have numerous contacts with members of the opposite sex before choosing a partner. This affords an opportunity to test personalities and make emotional and intellectual appraisals, which helps each member separately and both together to prove or disprove their mutual suitability.

The necessary preparation for successful marriage and parenthood is not something recently attained in high school. It is a product of the continuous growth process of the individual from birth to adulthood. Some of these past events, as well as future ones to be predicted, may be visualized in an analysis of the family cycle.

The discussion in this chapter is organized to aid you in answering some questions pertinent to the wise choice of a husband or wife:

How may I predict events through the family cycle?

How does one gain understanding of the opposite sex?

How does dating aid in selecting a life partner?

What are desirable qualities to look for in a lifetime partner?

How does one make satisfactory sex adjustments?

What is love?

How does one know when love comes along?

What appraisals should be made when a couple is in love?

How important is the courtship and engagement period in preparation for marriage and parenthood?

The family cycle

The life activities discussed in this part of the book, and mentioned specifically as well as implied throughout the entire text, are part of a family-life cycle in which we all participate. We are aware that families are quite diverse in their make-up and that there are many kinds and varieties in locations throughout the world. The family represents the basic structural group or unit of society regardless of race or locality —whether it is located in cities, towns, or suburban areas, on farms, or in isolated, faraway places.

Duvall,[1] in her family-life studies, has noted that the one thing all families have in common is the family cycle. It may be used for a better understanding of our family roles and for help in reaching important decisions. It is helpful to the students of family life and researchers studying the long view of family living.

The family-life cycle interests all of us because we are all part of it and will continue to be as we grow older. Each family

[1] Evelyn Duvall, *Family Development*, J. B. Lippincott Company, Philadelphia, 1957, pp. 3–5.

grows and lives out its life cycle in its own unique way.

Duvall [2] recognizes and depicts the family-life cycle as consisting of eight stages:

Stage I. Beginning Families (married couple without children)

Stage II. Childbearing Families (oldest child, birth to 30 months)

Stage III. Families with Preschool Children (oldest child, 2½ to 6 years)

Stage IV. Families with School Children (oldest child, 6 to 13 years)

Stage V. Families with Teenagers (oldest child, 13 to 20 years)

Stage VI. Families as Launching Centers (first child gone to last child's leaving home)

Stage VII. Families in the Middle Years (empty nest to retirement)

Stage VIII. Aging Families (retirement to death of one or both spouses)

The family cycle is based upon the successive patterns clearly visible in the continuity of family living from their beginning to their end. The cycle is similar to the various stages of growth of the individual. Certain predictable factors are apparent at a particular stage or can be viewed together in the total cycle.

Families begin when a young couple is married and a home is established. Even though the husband and wife are only a couple, they become the "beginning family." They serve as potential parents before the children arrive, and then they are a "childbearing family." The middle-aged or aging couples are still families. In many instances they have grown children and probably grandchildren, so they continue to function as family members even after their own children have homes of their own.

The cycle becomes continuous as a typical family progresses through the sequence of stages. Even before one family has completed its cycle, its children have been launched to develop their own family. Some family members may see a family-life cycle start a second and third time as their children marry and raise

their own children, who marry and have children while the elder members who began the cycle are still alive [12].

A woman's life may be outlined as follows, according to Duvall, who used the norms of American society based on the U.S. Census data of 1950. The woman comes into her *family of orientation* at birth, she starts school at six, enters her teens at thirteen, and marries at about twenty. At this point she leaves her family of orientation and enters her *family of procreation*. A predicted profile of life for an average woman may be broken down into five short phases of approximately seven years, which can be described as young womanhood, the childbearing years, the school-age children's years, teen-agers' years, and the launching-center years, when the children leave home. From the reproductive point of view, a woman spends the first twenty years growing up and preparing to have children, the next twenty-five years bearing and rearing children, and the last thirty years alone with her husband [12].

The family-life cycle can be used to present a profile for the life of a man also. Each man has particular ages and stages in his life cycle. Again taking an average situation, a man can anticipate spending most of his adult life as a husband and father. He and his wife may spend the first two years or so as a couple before the first child is born; after his last child has married and left home, he probably will have a period of fifteen years as a member of a couple again. He becomes a young man in the second decade of his life, and in his third he more than likely becomes a father. In his forties he will have children and teen-agers and can expect to launch these teen-agers into lives of their own. In his fifties and sixties he may expect to have relatively quiet years in his family. He then will be alone with his wife, but he must anticipate his role as a grandparent. The chances are good that he will leave his wife a widow, dying several years before she does. This possibility implies making

[2] *Ibid.,* p. 8.

plans for life insurance, retirement bene-fits, and housing for the later years of life [12].

This cycle has several implications for selecting a life partner. One can examine the cycle to see the types of responsibility one's mate will have to assume, the periods of time that you may be together as a couple, other periods of time spent in child-bearing and rearing, as well as the time a woman may have to spend alone as a widow. The age of the life partner may influence this to a greater or less degree than the average indicated by Duvall. The family-life cycle makes it important for you to do some critical thinking about your life, how you want to spend it, and with whom.

Mutual understanding between the sexes

One of the common problems for both youths and adults is getting along with the opposite sex. It is well to remember that learning to get along with people be-gins at home. The same qualities that en-able one to adjust in the home make it easy to adapt socially. Some examples of these social qualities are acting naturally, having something interesting to talk about, being interested enough in others to be a good listener, encouraging others to talk about their interests, expressing appreci-ation for kindnesses, showing considera-tion for others, understanding the behavior of others, and being friendly. The effect a person has on others, that is, how he makes them feel toward him, is a significant fac-tor in his ability to get along well with them. In many instances, this involves sub-jugating one's own interests in order to express a genuine interest in, and concern for, those of friends. A major factor in-volved is understanding the variations that exist between men and women. There are fundamental differences between the sexes apparent in terms of body build, functions, and behavior. Regardless of these differ-ences, the sexes are complementary to each other.

Studies do not confirm the concept that women are the weaker sex [38]. Actually, they are ahead of men in most phases of growth and development. Puberty occurs in girls two years earlier than in boys. Girls are approaching physical maturity at twelve or thirteen, as evidenced by their developing feminine figures. This earlier development also is apparent in the social transition stage. Girls tend to possess a social drive in which sex urges are more general and more easily satisfied than is true of boys. Some of these satis-factions, both physical and psychological, are found in contacts with the same sex. Slumber parties, tea parties, and fashion shows illustrate activities based on this interest. Girls do become interested in boys at this time. For this reason, the girl faces social problems, including boy-girl relationships, before she has the same amount of preparation as boys in mental development, education, and experience. It is characteristic at this point for one girl to become interested in boys while her very best friend of the same chronologic age has not developed this interest. Often friendships between girls are broken off because of this difference.

Boys, on the average, show their rapid growth between the ages of fifteen and twenty. They possess a sex drive directly concerned with the primary sex organs. The sex drive is satisfied by means of or-gasms through nocturnal emissions, mas-turbation, and, to a lesser degree, other sexual experience. The adolescent boy is greatly concerned with his voca-tional or professional choice. Much of his thinking is directed toward his vocational future. The girl, too, may have to make good on a job; however, this usually is a temporary situation until marriage. Dur-ing the teens, romances have more seri-ous implications for girls than for boys.

On the other hand, a boy gives less serious thought to his "love affairs." In the later years of high school and early years of college many girls find male classmates too young to be important to them socially.

Metabolism studies show that the male is more powerful and active physically, whereas the female adapts to the rapid changes called for by menstruation, childbirth, nursing, and menopause. It is general knowledge that man exceeds in muscular strength. Men adjust to extremes in physical exercise better than women, that is, to a variety of activities at high and low activity levels. Women adjust to temperature changes more readily than do men. Women are said to be 2° cooler than men; at least the thermometer must be raised 2° higher before women "glow." Therefore, men perspire more quickly. Women, on the other hand, withstand cold better, usually because of the insulating tissue below their skins and their more adaptable metabolic adjustment [38].

Men require more food calories than do women. A normally active man weighing 143 pounds needs 3200 calories a day, while a woman of 121 pounds similarly engaged requires 2300. This accounts for the complaint that "men are always hungry." The fact that women, in general, eat less than men yet still gain weight is a discouraging problem for many women.

Women have more sickness, with less serious results. Men have less sickness, with more serious consequences. Women are more likely to admit illness and to see a doctor sooner. Women have more operations than men. Women can stand more suffering than men. Contrary to previous beliefs, more women become mentally ill than men. It now is established that the most frequent victims of mental disease are the young, the old, and the female. Chances for good mental health are best for the middle-aged male.

Statistics show that women have a greater life expectancy than men at all ages. In addition, their gains in longevity have been greater. The life expectancy of white females at birth in 1900 was three years more than that of white males. "In 1957, the expectation of life was 72.5 years for white females and 66.3 years for white males, a difference of more than 6 years." [3]

A general social problem exists in the sex ratio, which has changed from a more or less even distribution of males and females to a shortage of prospective husbands in most parts of the United States. This is particularly true when comparing mating groups, older males compared with younger females. The average difference in age between husband and wife is approximately three years. Distribution of marriageable males further complicates the problem, since the ratio of men to women is not distributed equally over the country. In the farming and industrial sections there is an excess of men, whereas in large cities and centers of population an excess of women exists.

There is conflicting evidence as to differences in personality traits between sexes. Differences exist because of their varied functions and pursuits. Women demonstrate their emotions more readily than men. Menstruation, childbearing, and menopause are associated with more marked emotional high and low peaks. Women seem to be more expressive, have higher esthetic and religious values, and have greater warmth in their human relationships; men are more dominant and self-confident and have higher scientific values. But individuals differ from group patterns, whether male or female. It is not a case of all women being one way and all men another.

Biologically speaking, men have greater sexual freedom simply because such freedom does not affect their lives to the same extent as it does the lives of women.

[3] *Vital Statistics, Special Report, National Summary,* U.S. Department of Health, Education, and Welfare, 50:216, July 28, 1959.

Woman does not seek sexual experience as does man. She seeks love, which is a fulfillment of her motherhood urge. Woman's primary interest in man centers in her being courted, pursued, captured, loved, and protected. Man may be bent on many feminine conquests, but only one wife. The wife, generally speaking, is the one he loves and protects and also the one for whom he works. Along with more freedom for the man goes the greater responsibility for support and protection of his family. This is a paramount feature in the man's role as a family member.

Although differences between the sexes do exist, neither is superior or inferior. They differ by nature in structure and function. Each is dependent upon the other in accordance with their differences. In this sense, the sexes complement each other. Mutual understanding and cooperation are required for happy associations and for complete functioning as integrated personalities.

Dating

Since you probably have dated often in high school, you may assume that information about dating is of little importance. It may be well to remember that college dating has some points of difference. Many of the activities are the same, but the conditions of college life are quite different from those in high school. Also, the functions of dating at this level differ from those in high school. Although the college community is a miniature society, in the case of dating it represents a rather artificial setting compared with society in general. The majority of students fall in the eighteen to twenty-one or twenty-two age group. This may be beneficial for selecting a life partner of the appropriate age. On the other hand, the college setting may provide some barriers to dating and mate selection. For example, in some institutions there is an unbalanced proportion of men to women. Some colleges and universities may have too many women or too few; more often there are too many men and too few women. Greater artificiality occurs in colleges for men or for women only. In many instances, students enter the college scene as complete strangers, which necessitates making new friends in order to date [10].

Your dating depends upon how you feel about yourself, your attitude toward the opposite sex, how socially expert you are at making friends, and how well you function in mixed groups and in intimate associations.

Some students find it easier than others to get dates. The difficulty may be the imbalance of the sex ratio, but in many instances part of the difficulty is with the individual himself. It may help to know that most women and men have social handicaps, most of which can be overcome. Personal disadvantages may be changed to assets by learning the needed social attitudes and skills, whether it be developing self-confidence, carrying on pleasant conversation, accepting invitations gracefully and refusing unacceptable proposals effectively, learning to dance, sing, or get along with others, or acquiring empathy, an ability to put one's self in another's place and know how he feels. Social skills are best learned through participating in social functions. Oftentimes help is needed to bring out these social skills. Seeking such help from friends or counselors may make possible the learning of new and needed skills [10].

Dating may help to provide the necessary additional experience for understanding and adjusting to the opposite sex. Dating assists the individual in
Making friends and keeping them
Mixing socially
Having a good time

Learning objectivity in judging members of the opposite sex

Preparing for courtship

Learning to control emotions and urges

Choosing a life partner

Dating, with its inherent values, is worthy of intelligent planning. You, as a college student, might well consider the following questions:

Do I have opportunities to be friends with the opposite sex?

Is my circle of friends sufficient to provide wide acquaintanceship before marriage?

Am I able to keep friends?

Am I using my dates to appraise the desirable and undesirable characteristics of the opposite sex?

Circulation is a keynote for making friends. One does not meet people while sitting at home. Studies on dating indicate that dates are made most frequently through mutual friends, through contacts in school, at church functions, through recreational activities, at vacation areas, and at work. Planning for making friends should take into consideration places where there are opportunities for meeting members of the opposite sex. In college these opportunities are found at get-to-gether dances or parties, at a variety of informal gatherings, in groups before and after classes, at the student union or the student social center, in clubs, at athletic contests, on trips in which a number of students participate, at the library, and in classes.

Since dating is the exploration period before selecting a life partner, it is the period when the individual can "play the field" to advantage. Marriage studies have shown that young adults with many friends tend to have a greater chance for marital success than those with a very limited number of friends. In some instances when a mate has been selected at an early age, with the exploration stage omitted, a most successful marriage has resulted. However, this is not generally true. A number of friends provide a greater opportunity for selecting one who has the desirable qualities of a lifetime partner. Also, there exists a basis for favorable comparison and contrast if one has made a selection from a number of companions.

In the process of selection, keeping old friends is as important as finding new ones. Friends appreciate loyalty, dependability, and common sense, combined with an interest in the friend as a person different or unique, especially in respect to his hopes and his ambitions. Friends like a variety of interesting activities. Boys appreciate girls who are considerate of their financial status on a date. People frequently lose friends by continually bragging about their own accomplishments, by frequent references to good times on past dates, by "handing out a line," and by "gold digging." Others lose them by immediately becoming too serious, attempting right away to turn their friendship into a love affair.

Dating may be an end in itself, or it may be rated in terms of possible marriage. However, much of the emphasis during dating is upon present satisfactions rather than future needs. In a study of Michigan undergraduates, Blood found six characteristics that were considered desirable in a date: "Is pleasant and cheerful, has a sense of humor, is a good sport, acts natural, is considerate, and is neat in appearance." [4]

Studies [5, 14, 15] have shown that the following characteristics are most frequently preferred in dating partners:

Attractive appearance

Intelligent

Good listener

Good conversationalist

Emotionally mature

Dependable and honest

Willing to join a group

Makes friends with both sexes

Good manners; considerate of others

Affectionate but exhibits self-control

Ability to dance

Ambitious and energetic

[4] Robert O. Blood, Jr., *Anticipating Your Marriage,* Free Press, Glencoe, Ill., 1955, p. 24.

Going steady

There are advantages and disadvantages in going steady. If both partners have gone through the "playing-the-field" period, going steady is merely a natural step toward choosing a life partner. If, on the other hand, one or both parties are swept into going steady too soon, this experience may seriously interfere with making the right choice of a life mate. The decision to go steady is one which the individuals involved must make for themselves. It is important to weigh the evidence on both sides, using critical thinking and not merely following temporary emotional desires.

The advantages and disadvantages of going steady, as listed by authorities in the marriage field [10, 14], are as follows:

Advantages

Makes it easier to gain invitations.

Is a sure way to get to popular social affairs.

Provides personal security, particularly for insecure persons.

Is a symbol of personal achievement.

Enables a couple to get to know each other well.

Signifies a couple is in love.

Is cheaper and easier than exploring the field.

Is a preliminary to becoming engaged and being married.

Disadvantages

May mean choice of mate before maturity, before best judgment is reached.

Limits the choice of a life partner by eliminating chances for playing the field.

Fosters jealousy.

Becomes a habit and is difficult to break off.

Breaking up often causes serious emotional disturbances.

Rarely lasts into marriage, thus postponing the exploration period to the time when one should have made the choice of a mate.

Limits social experiences with different types of women and men.

Going steady in college, like dating, can be contrasted with going steady in high school. Going steady in college tends to move the couple toward informal engagement as signified by pinning or some similar symbolization before graduation. This is definitely a marriage-oriented process. Going steady certainly involves more commitment than casual dating.

Getting a friend to go steady may be just a natural process, or it may take some persuasion or subtle strategy. In the first case, going steady evolves out of a series of dates in which the partners naturally come to depend on each other, with a deeper, growing affection. In the second type, one partner either consciously or unconsciously manipulates the other individual into a welcome entangling alliance.

During the dating or friendship period, with time and favorable conditioning, the feeling of appreciation and affection for one another may logically grow and develop into love. Studies indicate that one in six or seven love affairs leads to the altar, that is, that change is the common practice during this exploratory period. Out of dating and several love affairs grows the ability to love and be loved. This is mature love.

Love changes the purpose of dating. This change occurs when one finds the companion he selects for a life partner.

Pinning

Being pinned is the stage of commitment between going steady and formal engagement. Some couples, after they are relatively far along in the going-steady stage, prefer to have their commitment to each other publicly recognized. Usually this

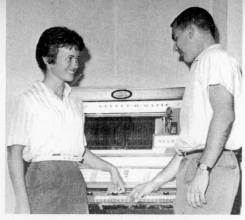

As a freshman Judy dated several boys. When she met Brad, at the beginning of her sophomore year, she knew he was "someone special."

Being together, whether for an informal snack of root beer and pizza or on a dress-up occasion, became increasingly important and meaningful.

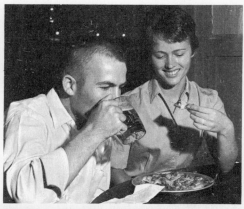

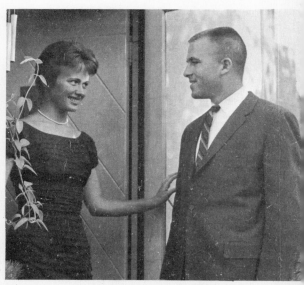

The week before Thanksgiving Brad chose a special date to ask Judy to wear his club pin to signify that they were going steady. Judy was delighted to accept, although she knew that Brad planned to transfer to State, a college 200 miles away, at the beginning of the second semester.

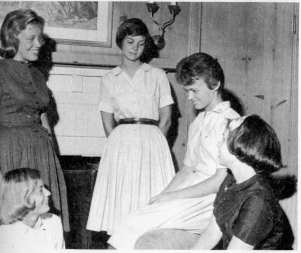

The excitement of being "pinned" delighted Judy. It also made her seem more mature and sophisticated in the eyes of her friends. The time for Brad's departure for State still seemed a long way off, and Judy consoled herself with the thought that she would see him on week ends.

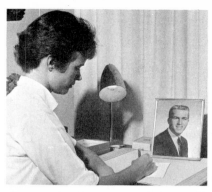

But soon Brad was gone. At first Judy devoted her free evenings to writing Brad, dutifully.

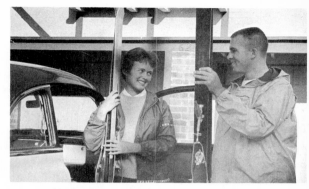

And she lived for the week ends when he could visit. The fun of being with him seemed worth all the lonely, dateless evenings in the dorm. But because of Brad's heavy academic schedule at State, the week ends of being together seemed few and far between.

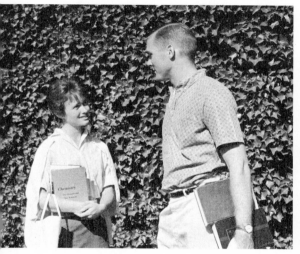

Judy grew restless and was sometimes despondent until one day Bob, tall, handsome, and a letterman, asked for a date. Judy said "no"—out of loyalty to Brad.

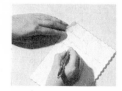

Nevertheless Bob's request for a date pleased and confused her. The question "to date or not to date" while pinned to someone else was one that had to be resolved, and Judy decided to write to Brad openly, honestly asking his opinion about the situation. Had the question already arisen in his mind too? Was he dating other girls?

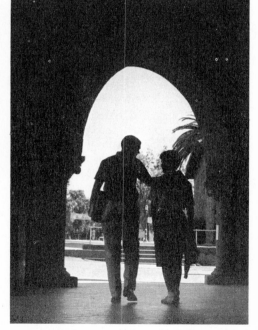

How seriously were Judy and Brad committed to each other by the symbolic act of "pinning"? This, of course, was the underlying and most important question. There is no ideal answer to this question. The solution will depend on the two individuals involved and on their own evaluation of their relationship.

means that the man gives his girl his fraternity or club pin. In a sense this is a trial engagement. In this stage the promise to marry is not fixed and permanent and perhaps is less important than in a formal engagement. This is a period for testing compatibility and the love commitment. Sometimes friends are responsible for pinning. When a couple acts as though they are engaged, their friends urge them to make a public announcement.

A pinning ceremony can be very beautiful and have a great deal of sentimental significance to the couple as well as to their friends. For example, frequently a dinner is given at either the fraternity or sorority house in honor of the couple. This is followed by a "pinning ceremony," which includes the public announcement, with the young man pinning his pin on his girl's sweater or dress. A serenade, with "sweetheart" songs and his fraternity and her sorority songs, adds to, and ends, the ceremony.

In some instances, instead of a pin, the girl receives a ring to wear around her neck. On some campuses it is traditional that when the wedding day has actually been set but the ring has not yet been purchased, the girl's pin and the man's pin are chained together to indicate an even closer relationship and commitment.

One of the problems of pinning is for both parties to understand just what it signifies. It is essential that both parties reach a mutual understanding of this point. Does it mean merely a formal announcement of going steady? Does it imply greater petting and sexual privileges? Is it actually a natural step leading to formal engagement and marriage? Proper communication of thought and understanding to make this point clear greatly increases the significance of pinning [14, 28].

Adjustment to the sex drive

Sexual adjustment is part of the individual's total development into maturity. The maturation of the sex organs, sex characteristics, and sex drives directs the individual along the pathway of development to adult attitudes and maturity. Sexual maturity helps to bring out what is best, most generous, and most constructive in the individual's life.

Sex is a basic drive upon which both race preservation and personal happiness depend. As a drive properly controlled, it becomes a powerful force aiding personal and social adjustment. From a positive point of view, it leads the young away from dependence on their parents and toward independence and the responsibility of loving, supporting, and caring for a family. In this respect, sex is a powerful, constant stimulus toward mature attitudes. If sexuality does not evolve properly, the whole process of growth and development is influenced negatively. Too much repression of sex tends to impair freedom and ease of functioning to the extent that mating and sexual satisfaction are not attained. On the other hand, too much sexual freedom can interfere with normal adjustments in love and mating functions to the degree that sexuality remains on an infantile level, as a desire for play and personal pleasure only. Disturbances in sexual development can lead to personal and social maladjustments.

The sex drive is a natural aspect of life which needs to be both understood and controlled. It should be considered squarely and frankly as a meaningful and respectable part of life. The goal of the sex drive is biological sexual maturity —the capacity to love, mate, reproduce, and care for the young. However, sex has more than reproductive functions; it is a factor in a happy family life, which is a partnership with a sharing of interests and ideas, mutual acceptance of responsibilities, self-realization, and love.

In our culture, a person matures sexually years before he can establish a home and, according to social standards, give expression to his sexual impulses and desires. For his own good and for the good of society, he is expected to conform to the conventions within the culture. This means that the sex drive must be controlled if it is to become a positive force in the development of the personality. The requirement for self-control is not unreasonable when one remembers that any great power or drive has to be controlled or its creative force becomes a destructive menace, as illustrated by atomic power. The value of the drive depends upon how well its potentialities are understood and how skillfully it can be managed [25].

According to Kraines and Thetford,[5] self-control implies these elements:

Understanding one's impulses, both as to their function and normalcy and also as to their potentiality for good or harm.

Conscious setting up of values or goals which one wishes to attain both as a person with particular desires and drives and as a member of society with definite obligations and responsibilities.

The willingness and the requisite will power to postpone and, if need be, renunciate immediate gratification for future satisfactions.

Self-control motivated from within the individual is more effective than that resulting from outside forces. This implies that the student has the right to know as much as possible about his own sexuality if he is to exercise control and if he is to make his own sexual adjustment in relation to the demands of society. He needs to know what is expected of him and why.

[5] S. H. Kraines and E. S. Thetford, *Managing Your Mind*, The Macmillan Company, New York, 1949, pp. 199–200.

He needs to become familiar with ways and means of exercising control. Briefly, he needs to understand the structure and function of reproduction (see Chapter 5, pages 144-149), the emotional factors basic to developing mature sexual attitudes toward loving and mating (see Chapters 3 to 6), and the basic problems related to the sex drive.

UNDERSTANDING SEXUAL BEHAVIOR

The premise has been established that an understanding of the basic problems relating to the sex drive is fundamental to developing self-control and self-direction. The aspects selected for discussion here because of their pertinence to the adjustment of the college student are petting, premarital sexual relations, nocturnal emissions, masturbation, and homosexuality.

Petting. Petting is the modern term for a practice that always has existed: sexual expression through physical contact, ranging from kissing and fondling to direct sexual stimulation stopping short of sexual intercourse. It may be classified as the sincere expression of genuine love and affection and as a means of deliberate sexual stimulation through exploration and excitation of the other person, at the same time inviting gratification in return. Petting of the first sort is an important phase of the true art of love. It is a part of the technique of arousal, love play, which brings about the mutual relationship and feelings preliminary to the sexual act. It is preparation for mating.

Petting of the second type, ranging from "light" to "heavy," is a general experience of youth. Light petting is stroking of the hair, the face, or the arms and hands. Heavy petting includes caressing or fondling of the body of either or both participants; usually, this includes the caressing or fondling of the breasts and genital organs of the girl.

The problem of petting is to keep it within bounds. Without self-control, owing to its progressive nature, it frequently will lead to sexual relations. If one decides to pet, some decisions should be made immediately. How far shall one go? Is it worth the resultant tensions? Pleasure to one person may mean a series of unfortunate consequences for another. For example, the dangers of pregnancy, abortion, and venereal infection may be involved even if *some* degree of self-control is used. On the other hand, some authorities maintain that petting guarded by self-control serves as an educative experience and is a step from immaturity to the full maturity of the heterosexual stage, serving as an outlet for energies and desires, as well as a stimulator of desire [5]. It is well to remember that the principle of fair play is involved, that petting affects not only one's self but the partner as well. The girl, who normally is slower to respond to such stimulation, may easily arouse the passions of her companion. She places him in a highly emotional state without realizing what she has done.

Since each case is different, no specific rules can be stated. It is important, however, to know what petting is, what kind is involved, where it leads, and what the consequences are. Then a person may decide for himself whether or not to practice it in a particular situation.

Premarital sexual relations. If there is any problem that must be faced squarely by the college student, it is that concerning premarital sexual relations. It is important to consider the issues involved and then to arrive at an independent decision, weighing the satisfactions against the natural risks. The decision may rest on the personalities of the couple, their emotional constitutions, and their social situation. This decision, however, should be based on critical thinking, not emotional rationalization.

Promiscuity is one of the most important social problems with which society must cope. Waggner [6] illustrates this point when he says:

Many of the revelations of recent sex studies are symptoms of an ailing society. But let us not confuse the ailment with the desired state of health, or change the temperature scales on the thermometer to make the fever normal.

The case for premarital sexual relations can be summarized briefly. Some authorities believe that such relations temporarily solve the problem of sexual desire and relieve tensions built up by this desire. They provide temporary physical pleasure. In some cases where there is strong sexual drive, they may prevent personality strains and possible distortions. However, in the majority of cases premarital relations create more problems than they solve.

The reasons for abstinence are good ones. Society sanctions sexual relations as a vital part of the art of love, an expression of deepest affection, in the marital partnership. It considers sex as a sacred thing. No scientific studies to date, only the rationalization of young people, give evidence that premarital sexual experience makes for better adjustment in marriage.

The House of Delegates of the American Medical Association, the British Social Hygiene Association, the American Social Health Association, and others have collected data which prove that continence and chastity are not harmful to health.

The risks involved in premarital sexual relations always must be considered. One cannot ignore the possibility that pregnancy will result. Even with the increased knowledge of birth control, medical authorities agree that there is no perfect contraceptive. Particularly is this true under the usual hurried, inconvenient circumstances of premarital relations. If the woman becomes pregnant, will she have

[6] Walter H. Waggner, "Must We Change Our Sex Standards? A Symposium," *The Reader's Digest,* 32:1–6, June, 1948.

the baby or submit to an illegal, induced abortion? The first choice is tragic for more than one person. Illegitimacy is a condition that no rational person would intentionally bring upon another human being. On the other hand, abortion is one of the greatest risks to life and health, with terrific psychological as well as physiologic effects. There also is mental anguish for the woman who has had sexual experience and merely thinks she has become pregnant. Worry may upset the menstrual cycle, causing her period to be late or even missed. In this condition, it is easy for her to rationalize the use of drugs and nostrums which, though they would not necessarily have induced an abortion, will often cause severe illness. She may even become the prey of an abortionist who will perform an operation even though she is not pregnant. It is a good health practice to see a physician and have an examination for pregnancy regardless of marital status.

Premarital relations may lead to venereal disease. Two factors are important in regard to such diseases: (1) they rank high among the reportable communicable diseases; (2) it is difficult and, in some cases, impossible to tell from outward appearances whether or not they are present. It is true that the incidence of venereal disease is low among college students as compared with the general population. However, some college students do have contacts with prostitutes and "pickups" and this of course increases the danger of such infection.

It is well to remember that mental conflicts, particularly worry, guilt, and fear, affect the peace of mind of both parties, especially of the woman. Emotional reactions often result even if pregnancy, illegitimacy, and venereal disease are avoided. Premarital intercourse, with its worries and fears, may result in an attitude about intercourse which prevents the individual from establishing normal sexual relationships in marriage.

The problem for young people becomes extremely difficult if they are unable to marry when they are ready to do so. Guilt complexes may result from indulging in premarital sex relations when couples are by necessity postponing marriage, though many couples who are not able to marry nonetheless refuse to practice premarital sexual intercourse.

A number of authorities in the field of marital relations believe in early marriage as one practical solution to the problem. If the couple have grown into mature love, are fit—physically, mentally, and socially—to marry, and have carefully considered the responsibilities involved, it is better that they should marry. Early marriage, from eighteen to twenty-five, is far superior to promiscuity and delinquency. In many instances, an early marriage necessitates financial assistance from both sets of parents, if they are in a position to help. Financial assistance by parents is merely a return to the early days of America, when a newly married couple were given a few acres of land, a team and a wagon, a house, and the like, to give them a start. Both the scholastic and the marital records made by young veteran student families provide proof for the soundness of the early-marriage concept.

Nocturnal emissions. Nocturnal emissions, or "wet dreams," are the result of psychic stimulation during sleep and are considered normal in the male. Little attention has been given to the fact that similar orgasm (climax of feelings resulting from sexual stimulation) during sleep is not uncommon in the female, particularly in the older and sexually more experienced female. This does not involve ejaculation (discharge of semen) as is the case in the male. Kinsey reports, in his study of the college group, that 99 per cent of men who go to college experience nocturnal emissions at some time in their lives [21]. The single men at the college level derive about one-sixth of their total sexual outlets from this source. Some individuals report a feeling of tiredness or weakness after a nocturnal emission. There are no serious aftereffects.

Masturbation. Masturbation is the attainment of sexual gratification by the deliberate self-stimulation of the genital organs. It is an undesirable sexual outlet belonging to a phase of development that can be outgrown by attaining complete sexual maturity and using other, more socially accepted, means of sexual adjustment. Kinsey found in his sample that at some time in their lives most of the men and over half of the women had used self-stimulation [21]. Masturbation can become an obsessive habit before puberty, at the time erotic responses are developing rapidly, and when orgasm is possible. In the adult, chronic masturbation may be a defense against defeat, and as such, becomes a mechanism of substitution for more mature satisfactions. While it may provide temporary physical relief, it does not give full emotional gratification. As a result, it may leave one with a sense of frustration and self-condemnation. It is of pathological significance when it interferes with heterosexual relations or when feelings of fear and guilt lead to personality conflicts.

Through the years masturbation has been blamed as the cause of ills ranging from pimples to insanity, including loss of manliness, feeble-mindedness, genital cancer, and many other such conditions. There is agreement today that the physical effects of masturbation are not fundamentally different from those of any other sexual activity. There is no objective evidence that the manual act itself has a definite detrimental effect on physical or mental health or sexual virility. False notions about the effect of masturbation cause undesirable influences on the personality. Many mental disturbances occur as the result of conflicts, such as feelings of guilt, inferiority feelings, fear of social disgrace, or worry about condemnation of such activity. The relationship

between masturbation and sociosexual adjustments still remains to be determined. In some cases, masturbation may be so sexually satisfying that the individual does not desire to engage in sexual relations during marriage. This condition is considered a deviation from normal living. In situations in which a youth already has a serious emotional problem, his attention may be focused on masturbation to the extent that he neglects his interests in school, recreational activities, and associations with the opposite sex.

Some students believe that "telling" characteristics, for example, thinness of stature, eye expression, facial blemishes, and curvature of the jaw, indicate to society that they are guilty of masturbation. There is no scientific base for such beliefs.

Bodily sensations occurring after an orgasm cause anxiety in some young people. Needless fear can cause the symptoms of any highly emotional state. It is the emotional state, not the physical act, that is disturbing to the individual.

As an autoerotic practice, masturbation focuses the individual's attention and affection upon himself rather than upon a member of the opposite sex. The most satisfying adjustments in marriage are concerned with the interests of one's life partner rather than those devoted to one's self.

Masturbation may or may not affect adjustment to marriage later in life. Many persons who have had strong habits of masturbation have adjusted to marriage successfully. However, in some cases this is more difficult, since the individual has adjusted to one type of sex habit and must face new adjustments in marriage.

McKinney believes that the following suggestions are helpful in dealing with masturbation as a habit [30]:

Understand that masturbation is practiced by normal persons who overcome it, that it is not limited to abnormal persons, that its physical consequences are negligible, and that its undesirable effects on personality are worry, disgust, feelings of guilt, and undue self attention.

Understand that a habit or attitude so strong as one related to the sex urge cannot be changed in a short period of time and also that some regression may take place.

Participate in social and physical activities with your own and the opposite sex (clinical studies indicate that masturbation is resorted to most frequently in moments when individuals are lonesome, depressed, blue, and not enjoying socializing with others.)

Participate in extracurricular activities, since they satisfy most of the dominant human motives and distract attention from one's self.

Understand that masturbation may be a sign of insecurity and that such realization and participation in social activities may relieve anxiety and help one gain self-assurance and acceptance by others.

Homosexuality. Homosexuality is a condition in which erotic interest is felt, or sex relations are experienced, between members of the same sex. Usually, homosexual acts include manipulation of the genital organs—interfemoral coitus, for example—to achieve sexual gratification. The three well-known theories as to the cause of homosexuality are that it is due to an inherited tendency, that it is a result of conditioning or maladjustment, such as unsatisfactory social relations with members of the opposite sex, and that it is due to a sex-hormone imbalance. The causes are complex and difficult to ascertain; it is probable that any or all of these may be involved as multiple factors.

Kinsey's findings show that 37 per cent of the total male population has had at least some overt homosexual experience, while 4 per cent of white males are exclusively homosexual throughout their lives [21]. Homosexual experience is less frequent among women than among men,

19 per cent of women reporting such experience [22]. Kinsey advocates the use of a three-point scale of heterosexual, bisexual (heterosexual and homosexual), and homosexual. He emphasizes how misleading is the tendency to consider an individual homosexual simply because he is known to have had a single experience with another individual of his own sex. Many persons in the population have had such experiences and then have developed normal heterosexual adjustments in later life [21].

Homosexuality is not confined to one or two lower social levels but occurs in varying degrees at every social level and among persons in every occupation and of most ages.

SATISFACTORY SEXUAL ADJUSTMENTS

Heterosexual adjustments, through social contacts and experiences with members of the opposite sex, indicate maturity of development from childhood experiences to adulthood. This development does not occur without many conflicts and frustrations. Two environmental conditions are essential for successful adjustment: (1) an environment in which there is a sufficient number of members of the opposite sex of appropriate age, intellectual status, and personality adjustment to give the individual an opportunity to select congenial companions and to have pleasurable social contacts with them; (2) an encouraging, sympathetic, and helpful attitude on the part of parents and other adults.

The fundamental attitude leading to maturity is shown in an ability to enjoy giving more than receiving and an interest in, and love for, the marriage partner, children, friends, a profession, and hobbies. By properly developing self-discipline, the student is able to achieve self-development, personal maturity, and adjustment. Such maturity makes it possible for him to attain his highest goal—that of contributing to the betterment of society.

Love, a prerequisite for happy marriage

What is love? Do we know when love comes along? Does love last? These are difficult questions; yet they must be answered when we are preparing for family responsibilities.

WHAT IS LOVE?

The poet Shelley gave a definition of love when he described it as "that profound and complicated sentiment which . . . is the universal thirst for a communion not merely of the senses, but of our whole nature, intellectual, imaginative and sensitive."

Love is a basic need or drive from childhood to old age. With love one grows and develops naturally and happily. Without it the individual may become frustrated and unhappy. The affectional responses begin in childhood. Children must receive love in order to give it. If the child is accepted and his individuality respected, he learns to love and be loved. If he is neglected, excluded, or repulsed, he attempts to defend himself, protecting his ego, but remains unsatisfied. Satisfaction may come later through affection from friends and sweethearts.

Love is more than possessiveness. It is not making another person over into one's own image. It is not dependency, nor is it self-sacrifice, though love usually requires sacrifice. Investigators have established that a person must qualify for love by loving himself if he expects to love others.

Robert H. Felix,[7] Director of the National Institute of Mental Health, Washington, defines self-love in this way: "One has a feeling of dignity, a feeling of belonging, a feeling of worthwhileness, a feeling of adequacy—yet a healthy sense of humility."

ROMANTIC LOVE

Romantic love is the pattern of love behavior characterized by thrill and excitement. It is a type of love made popular in many modern songs, movies, radio programs, and television plays, and it constitutes the American love ideal. It is based on the premises that one's ideal mate does exist, and will appear at the right time; that love is the mysterious attraction of two people for each other, a spontaneous recognition of one's ideal partner; that the future success of the marriage is assured by finding one's ideal mate, the one and only; and that nothing should stand in the way of love, not even wealth, position, education, or religious or racial differences. Romantic love is well expressed and characterized in the words of Robert Bridges, the poet, when he said, "Love is the fire in whose devouring flames all earthy ills are consumed."

The elements of romantic love are part of, but not all of, total or mature love. These factors must be considered as important in the selection of a life partner. However, it is essential to keep in mind that romantic love is only one phase of the love necessary for sound marital adjustment.

MATURE LOVE

Mature love leads to a happy and satisfying marriage. Erich Fromm states, "To love a person implies caring for and feeling responsible for his life, not only for his physical existence but for the growth and development of all his human powers."[8] Mature love is what holds a family together. It is the love a wife has for her husband even when he comes home irritable and cross from a hard day at the office. It is the husband's love for his wife even though she prepares a poor meal.

[7] Reported by Howard Whitman, "Science Discovers Real Love," *This Week Magazine*, June 4, 1950, p. 20.

[8] *Ibid.*, p. 4.

It is the couple's love for each other that persists even when the money saved for a new home must be applied on a young son's emergency operation.

Mature love before marriage is a synthesis of many factors, including the following:

An understanding of each other's personality

A recognition of each other's needs and feelings, such as companionship and sexual needs, and a desire to meet them

An expression for each other of the finest qualities, such as tenderness, unselfishness, loyalty, self-sacrifice, sharing, and mutual responsiveness

Mature love contains some of the elements of romantic love, but it is built upon a firmer base. It is more complete, more permanent, and more enduring. Therefore it provides security and personal worth for both partners. Mature love is total love based on the realities of everyday family living [9].

Fromm [9] believes that the deepest need of man is to overcome his aloneness. He thinks that mature love overcomes man's sense of isolation while permitting him to be himself.

In such love the paradox occurs that two beings become one and yet remain two. . . . Love is active, not passive; it is a "stand in," not a "falling for." Love is primarily giving, not receiving.

By giving, Fromm means the productive character of an individual's giving by which he experiences strength, wealth, and power. It is the giving not of material things but rather of whatever is alive in a person—his joy, his interest, his humor, and even his sadness. Fromm is referring to the type of giving that brings something to life in another person. One gains from this kind of giving because it reflects back on the giver. Such giving makes the other person a giver also.

Infantile love follows the principle "I love because I am loved"; mature love follows the

principle "I am loved because I love." Immature love says "I love you because I need you." Mature love says "I need you because I love you." To love somebody is not just a strong feeling—it is a decision, a judgment, a promise. Love is not the result of adequate sexual satisfaction, but sexual happiness—even knowledge of so-called sexual technique—is the result of love. . . .[10]

Fromm develops another important concept when he states that we frequently think love means the absence of conflict. He thinks this is not true. Two persons in love are bound to have conflicts. In mature love they can communicate with each other from the center of their existence and do not try to avoid basic issues. When real conflicts are honestly faced, clarification results and both persons emerge with more strength and knowledge. Love makes this possible, and such action is a part of mature love.

Cavan cites seven sides of enduring love, which give strength to love and lead to a good marriage:

Involvement of the total personality

Sexual attraction

Fellowship

Other-centeredness

Mild idealization

Mutual respect

Pleasure and satisfaction

These qualities may develop slowly. Therefore, time should be allowed for their full development before marriage [10].

Prescott describes the roles of love in human development with a series of hypotheses, which need to be tested in the future but which serve as guides with the information at our disposal. His hypotheses are as follows [34]:

Being loved can afford any human being a much needed basic security.

Being loved makes it possible to learn to love one's self and others.

Being loved and loving others facilitates success such as that found by belonging to groups—winning roles in group activities.

Being loved and loving in return facilitates

[9] Erich Fromm, "The Art of Loving," *Coronet*, 48:156, July, 1960.

[10] *Ibid.*, pp. 157–158.

identification with parents, relatives, teachers, and peers.

Being loved and loving facilitates adjustment to situations that involve strong unpleasant emotions.

Love not only aids adjustment but helps prevent maladjustment as well.

DOES ONE KNOW WHEN LOVE COMES ALONG?

There are still many people who believe in "love at first sight." Landis[11] found:

When 735 college students were asked whether they believed in "falling in love at first sight," 34 per cent of the men and 50 per cent of the women said they did not; but 39 per cent of the men and 34 per cent of the women said they did. The rest were undecided.

Love probably begins as a reaction to good looks, good clothes, popularity, and physical attraction. It may arise out of an inner feeling, for example, at a dance or sitting close to someone in an automobile. This is the natural sex attraction of men and women. However, this physical attraction is merely the starting point in love; it is not love itself. Love encompasses additional qualities of personal attachment over and above the sexual drive. It is manifested in one's whole personality, ways, qualities, patterns of thought and action, tenderness, devotion, sympathy, understanding. Such love is not blind; it is conscious and free. Love is developed by two people's discovery of mutual interests and goals, by their companionship and congeniality based on similar personality traits or complementary ones.

Distinguishing between infatuation and love aids in answering the question, Do we know when love comes along? Infatuation may come suddenly, but love takes time. Infatuation can be based on one or two traits (usually including sex appeal), whereas love is based on many traits. In

infatuation the person is "in love with love," whereas in love the person is in love with another person. In infatuation the other person is thought of as a separate entity and employed for self-gratification. In real love there is a feeling of identity with the other person. Infatuation produces feelings of insecurity and wishful thinking, whereas love produces a sense of security. In infatuation one suffers loss of ambition and appetite, whereas in love he works and plans to please the other person. The physical element is much more important in infatuation than in love. Infatuation may change quickly, but love lasts [5, 14].

DOES LOVE LAST?

The enduring kind of love comes to the fore when romance wears off. Daily attention and sympathetic understanding are needed for love to grow and become permanent. This daily process of loving, successfully practiced by both man and woman, is the answer to the question, Does love last? Such love calls for a real partnership, with both partners working at the job continuously. One person alone cannot make it succeed. Both must practice attitudes of thoughtfulness, tolerance, and cooperativeness to develop the companionship that makes love last. Both must avoid nagging, faultfinding, greediness, selfishness, the attitudes of boredom, uncooperativeness, and inconsiderate actions. The partnership then is based on satisfying companionship, exemplified in the motto, "A family that plays together stays together." Indeed, lovers must be true friends to make love last, believing that it takes more than romantic love to guarantee a successful marriage, but that no marriage can be a happy association without love. Love lasts when it is mature love—when it expresses concern for the partner's happiness and well-being, when there is a "we" feeling and a sense of togetherness, when there is a sharing of desires, thoughts, attitudes, and ambitions, when it is realistic, when it grows with time [14].

[11] Unpublished study by Judson Landis, reported in Judson T. and Mary G. Landis, *Building a Successful Marriage*, 2d ed., Prentice-Hall, Inc., Englewood Cliffs, N.J., 1953, pp. 45–46. Reprinted by permission of the publisher.

Courtship

Courtship is the period during which partners find out about each other. It is at this time that the couple should stop to appraise themselves, and each other, to determine whether or not their match presents elements that suggest successful marriage. It is a time to look ahead intelligently, forgetting momentarily the emotional aspects, to try to determine whether or not marriage will survive after the prenuptial ardor and interest have worn off.

APPRAISING THE PROSPECTIVE LIFE PARTNER

Perhaps more than any other point, the couple should keep in mind that love leading to successful marriage takes time to mature and develop. Such love grows best out of a happy courtship, with intelligent planning and genuine companionship.

Although the suggestions of authorities can prove of significant value in assisting a couple to know whether or not love has come along, one must remember that research studies and evaluation devices are indicators only, not mathematical equations which accurately measure the love status. Nevertheless, these appraisals serve to guide young couples.

PERSONAL CHARACTERISTICS OF A LIFE PARTNER

A number of authorities on marriage have studied personal traits that provide insight for predicting success in marriage. These should be interpreted merely as clues [8].

Are the partners:

Agreeable in basic personal habits?

Compatible in aims and ambitions?

Appreciative of each other's family background?

Socially congenial?

Able to disagree constructively, with a willingness to compromise?

Agreeable on importance of money and material things?

Agreeable on religious values to the extent of tolerating and accepting each other's divergent views and practices?

Approximately on the same level of education and intelligence?

Healthy and physically, mentally, and emotionally mature?

Intelligent about sex?

Skilled in making and holding friends?

Teammates in public and private relations?

In addition to the assessment of the positive personality characteristics in choosing a life partner, it is wise to appraise extreme behavior patterns that may make successful marriage difficult or even impossible. These characteristics are shown by the following persons [26]:

THE OVERLY POSSESSIVE PERSON. The jealous and demanding man; the clinging, very dependent and helpless woman.

THE CONTINUALLY DISSATISFIED PERSON. The man who is overambitious for unreachable goals; the woman who holds unrealistic marital and social aspirations.

THE TEMPERAMENTAL PERSON. The moody and self-centered man; the dramatic woman who views marriage as a drama and is bored by the thought of routines of housework and child care.

THE SUPERIOR PERSON. The "know-it-all" man; the woman who feels she must be a success at everything.

THE OVERMETICULOUS PERSON. The faultlessly dressed man whose personal habits are impeccable, insisting on others being the same; the woman who is a perfect housekeeper and whose drive for spotless surroundings becomes the most important goal in marriage.

THE FLIRTATIOUS PERSON. The man who prefers other feminine companionship to his prospective mate's; the woman who feels she must continually strive to attract a man, any man, despite the effect on her prospective mate.

Personality factors are of the greatest significance on both the positive and the negative side in choosing a life partner. Terman's study showed that one of the greatest dangers to marriage is the all-round unhappy temperament of one or both of the spouses [5].

The findings of the Burgess and Cottrell study on prediction of success or failure in marriage for the most part substantiate Terman's data. The following are illustrative conclusions from the study: prediction before marriage of marital adjustment is feasible; problems of sexual adjustment in marriage, with the majority of couples, appear to be the result not so much of biological factors as of psychological characteristics and of cultural conditioning of attitudes toward sex. The outstanding factors in marital adjustment seem to be affection, temperamental compatibility, and social adaptability [6].

Since personality factors are so important to marital success, lovers should find out how the prospective life partner reacts under emotional stresses or strains. *To be the right person* is more important in a successful marriage than *to find* the right person. Lovers can make it a point to discover how the prospective mate reacts to disappointments, to slights, and to reverses. Does he or she have the ability to control emotions? If not, does the partner complement or counterbalance the other in emotional control?

The factor of physical attraction definitely is present if love exists. This factor is not to be forgotten in the evaluation process, for it is a vital element. This attraction ranges from the day-by-day stages of developing love to the ecstasy of sexual relations. Sexual adjustment is primarily a matter of knowledge of sex functions and of mental attitudes, environmental influences, and time. This has been discussed more fully in Chapter 3.

APPRAISAL DEVICES

Winch [39] conducted an intensive investigation of mate selection by studying 25 young married couples. They were interviewed with respect to their needs, their life histories, and the results of a psychological projective test. The purpose of the study was to test the hypothesis that mates select each other to complement their own respective need patterns. Winch pointed out that psychoanalysts believe that *opposites attract* in mate selection, whereas sociologists' studies indicate that *like marries like*. The man in the street believes that either may happen, for he holds that opposites attract *and* that like marries like.

Winch wanted to determine what kind of person young marriageable people would meet in going about their daily routine. He postulated that mate selection is determined by needs; i.e., each individual seeks for his life partner that person within his or her field of eligibles who gives the greatest promise of providing maximum need gratification. He showed that the need pattern of each individual would be complementary rather than similar to the need pattern of the other spouse. He selected twelve needs and three general traits in developing his theory. His needs included abasement, achievement, approach, autonomy, recognition, and dominance. Some authorities in the family-life field agree with Winch's theory; many do not. This is an important research study on mate selection and opens the way for further investigations.

A more recent study based on need fulfillment resulted in Reiss's wheel theory of love.[12] In his theory, the love relationship is cyclic, similar to a wheel, and must satisfy four needs. The first step is the development of *heterosexual love relationship*. The second progressive step is called *self-revelation*. This is a feeling of ease,

12 Ira L. Reiss, "Toward a Sociology of the Heterosexual Love Relationship," *Marriage and Family Living*, 22:139–145, May, 1960.

in which the individual is more likely to reveal intimate aspects of his existence and tell of his hopes, desires, fears, and ambitions. As a result of self-revelation the third phase—*mutual dependency*—is reached. In this stage one becomes dependent on the other person to fulfill one's own habits. One needs the other person to confide ideas or feeling to and to fulfill sexual desires. Such habits tend to perpetuate relationships and are culturally determined. Without them we are lonely and frustrated. Finally, the fourth phase is *personality fulfillment*. This is fulfillment of basic needs. The four processes become one when the individual feels rapport with another; he reveals himself and becomes dependent, thereby fulfilling his personality needs. This continues cyclically, as need fulfillment was the reason for the original feeling of rapport.

In self-appraisal it may be helpful to study the factors that tend to strengthen marriage as well as those that may weaken it. These are aptly stated and classified by Cavan [13] as shown in the table below.

[13] Ruth S. Cavan, *American Marriage: A Way of Life,* Thomas Y. Crowell Company, New York, 1959, p. 142.

Favorable to happy marriage	Unfavorable to happy marriage

Positive motives for marrying:
  Love
  Desire for a home
  Common interests
  Children
  Sexual satisfaction
	Negative or escape motives:
	  Loneliness
	  Avoid parents
	  Premarital pregnancy

Positive ideal of kind of mate desired	Negative ideal, or conception of kind of mate not desired
Ideal stated as qualities of personality	Positive ideal but stated in terms of appearance, social skills
Ideal of mate based on parents stated in terms of fine qualities of either parent	Ideal based on duplication of one parent, including mate's taking the role of a parent
Each meets many needs of the mate and has his own needs met by the mate	Each unable to meet needs of mate and has few of his own needs met by mate
Needs that cannot be met in the marriage met in ways that strengthen the marriage, e.g., through friends of same sex, understanding relatives, organizations	Needs that cannot be met in marriage met in ways that weaken the marriage, e.g., through friends of the opposite sex, or destructive personal habits as excessive drinking
Happy family background or adjustment made to unhappy childhood experiences	Feelings of insecurity or distrust of marriage because of unhappy childhood
Husband and wife same age or husband only a few years older	Wife older or husband many years older than wife
Education preferably the same, or husband slightly more education	Wide differences in education
Intelligence preferably the same, or husband slightly more intelligent	Wide differences in intelligence
Many common interests, especially of the type that further home and family life	Few common interests
Acceptance of situation when interests cannot be shared and use of outside groups and organizations to supplement	Common interests that are not family centered and take husband and wife outside the home
Basic values and beliefs preferably the same	Differences and conflicts in basic values and beliefs
Any differences in marriage experience clearly understood and accepted	Intrusion of emotional "hangover" from previous marriage

Authorities from the American Social Health Association [1] believe it is possible to choose a mate properly if young people going through the courtship process can answer the following questions objectively and honestly: 1. Are you two psychologically suited? This means, Do you get along well together? Do you really understand each other? Do you have the same ideals, similar ethical standards, and mutual trust? Do you like to spend time alone together without boredom and have common interests? 2. Are you biologically suited? This means, Are you both healthy and fit? Have you checked the hereditary characteristics of yourselves and your families? Do you each feel the physical attraction necessary for a good marriage? At the same time are you able to control sexual urges, understanding the dangers of premarital sexual relations? 3. Is there a promise of economic security? This question is most important for future success. The man should at least have a job program that includes ability to support a wife and family. Both parties should understand the economic factors and agree on how money should be spent and on how to manage money carefully. Adjusting to a lower economic level until job security is achieved may be necessary. 4. Are you both really ready for marriage? If you both are mature persons, and if you fully understand the meaning of marriage and have prepared for it adequately and objectively, then you have given careful consideration to perhaps the most important decision in your life.

A religious appraisal. When couples are seeking to reach agreement on religious values, they may wish to use two appraisal scales.[14] The first scale assists the couple in determining the divergence or similarity of interest in religion on the part of each prospective partner. The second is a family scale indicating the interest of each family in religion.[15]

These two scales make it possible for young people in love to assess objectively the intensity of religious beliefs and differences. If the results show marked divergence of opinion, it is preferable to discuss

[14] James A. Peterson, *Education for Marriage*, Charles Scribner's Sons, New York, 1956, p. 151.
[15] *Ibid.*, p. 152.

Our interest in religion

	Almost no vital interest	Some interest	Much interest	A very great interest
Mine:				
My intended mate's:				

Our families' interest in religion

	Almost no vital interest	Some interest	Much interest	A very great interest
My family:				
Intended mate's family:				

these frankly and attempt to foresee and work out possible problems before marriage takes place. Studies indicate that interfaith marriages are commonly hazardous partnerships. However, many couples have found that their basic beliefs about religion are similar, and they have been able to adjust so that differences are reconciled early and serious trouble is avoided. See Suggested readings 5, 10, and 14 for additional reading on this topic.

MIXED MARRIAGES

There has been an increase in mixed marriages in recent years. Some of the factors responsible include greater urbanization, broadening of religious views, greater social mobility within the United States as well as internationally, overseas service by the armed forces, and an apparent disregard by young persons for warnings by adults of the difficulties of mixed marriage.

These marriages may be described as interfaith, interracial, international, and interclass crossings and marriages with significant differences in economic status, in previous marital status, in education, in intelligence, and in age. All marriages have some differences, but mixed marriages tend to have more extreme difference or differences than the usual marriage.

It is wise for a couple contemplating a mixed marriage to consider most objectively, individually and then together, questions such as the following, without romantic influences:

How important is the element of difference to each person?

What are all the complicating factors regarding the element of difference?

Are there strong enough bonds in addition to romantic love to provide stability to the marriage?

Is there a danger that the difference might be used by one partner to dominate the other?

What effect will the marriage have on parents, relatives, and close friends of each partner?

Can a mutually agreed upon plan for rearing children be developed before the marriage?

Any type of mixed marriage can prove to be successful:

If the partners are serious enough to make the partnership work

If they are willing to face the special problems squarely and openly together

If they have similar attitudes toward life, the raising of children, and their own recreational activities and interests

If they understand the breadwinner's vocational pursuit

If they have had sufficient experience together to assure compatibility

If each partner is highly adaptable

Studies show that mixed marriages have less chance of success and require more difficult adjustments. It should be remembered also that the element of difference may remain throughout the marriage, either unchanged or not changed significantly [5, 10, 14]. For further information, see Suggested readings 4, 10, 14, 15, 32, and 33.

Health status

Your physical and mental fitness is an important factor to be considered in the preparation for marriage and family living. No one has perfect health; therefore, one cannot expect such a degree of health from his life partner. However, it is good premarital planning to ascertain the health status of one's self and of one's prospective mate.

Health often influences the choice of a life partner. Many men and women are not attracted to persons who do not appear healthy. In other instances, a known defect or disease condition does not influence selection, and marriage takes place. When this occurs, both partners must understand the condition and accept it in order to prevent serious disturbances during marriage. Physical appearance does not tell the complete story of one's health status. Defects and disease are at times not apparent during courtship, especially in the brief, whirlwind variety.

Only on the advice of a physician should a person marry if he is afflicted by such serious conditions as acute rheumatic fever, high blood pressure, tuberculosis of the lungs, or acute or chronic kidney disease. It is important also to know that both persons are free from venereal disease.

From the standpoint of eugenics (improvement of the race), each person has the right to know if his prospective mate comes from sound hereditary stock. This protective measure can prevent the transmission of a hereditary defect and avoid the tragedy of abnormal offspring. Persons with conditions such as epilepsy, dementia praecox (schizophrenia), or manic-depressive psychosis, described in Chapter 3, should not marry unless advised by competent medical counsel. In addition, a person may be a possible carrier of a defective trait, though not showing the trait himself. One has the right to ask whether or not the prospective mate's grandparents, parents, brothers, and sisters were normal. This is important. Progressive deafness, deaf-mutism, hemophilia (a bleeding disease), cleft palate and harelip, stub fingers, and brittle bones are some of these hereditary handicaps.

The hereditary factor is the basis for controls over the marriage of close blood relations. Inbreeding results in the combination of genes to produce defective conditions such as hemophilia as well as a hereditary form of deafness. Scheinfeld believes that cousins should not marry unless the family is free of serious hereditary defects [37].

Diabetes is an example of a disease which, when present in one of the prospec-

tive partners, calls for mutual understanding. Complete understanding of the condition and wholehearted acceptance of it is necessary for proper marital adjustment. It is well to know that diabetes, in most cases, is primarily the result of an inherited predisposition. Diabetes may develop early in life or not until middle age or later. However, early recognition and treatment of the disease is helpful in making adjustments and prolonging life. Diabetic inheritance, generally speaking, is the result of two recessive genes, one from each parent. Diabetes may develop without either parent's being afflicted, but as the result of each parent's carrying a hidden recessive gene. Tests are available now to identify persons who are susceptible to developing diabetes. Further reference is made to Chapter 2, section on Heredity, and to Suggested readings 2, 6, 8, and 37.

HEALTH EXAMINATIONS BEFORE MARRIAGE

Health status is best determined by complete physical and psychological examinations. Such examinations:

Attempt to establish the state of general health.

Test the blood for syphilis and for the presence or absence of the Rh factor.

Detect anatomic defects that might affect sexual adjustment and childbearing functions.

Provide an opportunity for intimate personal counseling.

Assist in the inquiry into the family background.

Some medical examinations are complete health examinations and cover all the above items. Others are limited in scope, including only a physical examination and blood tests. Usually, the family physician is the best person to provide the *complete* health examination. Also, local health centers are assuming such responsibilities as a part of their maternal and child health or health education functions. These services from the health center, the local tax-supported public health agency, are free and of high quality. Many colleges, likewise, provide the above services as a part of their college health program through the student health service, as was indicated in Chapter 2.

Where examinations are limited to physical inspections, the student or citizen of the community may be forced to consult several sources before his health status can be appraised adequately. In addition to the physical examination in a doctor's office or a health center, useful information can be secured from the college counseling center, the marital counselor, the community family service agency, family institutes, and the like.

The state-required examinations, for the most part, include a superficial physical examination and a blood test for syphilis. Hence the prospective couple attempting to determine their fitness to marry need to go further than the law dictates.

The couple are wise to plan the examination with the family physician or with a urologist or gynecologist far enough in advance of their marriage to carry out the suggestions and requirements outlined by the health adviser. Sufficient time must be allotted during the examination to allow for frank discussion of personal questions. This is an excellent opportunity to receive authoritative advice on planned parenthood, fertility, and the like, for those who desire such information. The advice and counsel of medical and family-life education authorities are extremely important in determining fitness to marry.

The engagement period

The engagement period is a natural outgrowth of dating and courtship experiences. It is the declaration of the partners that a mutual understanding has been reached. In most cases, there is a public announcement stating their intention to marry, thus presenting to their friends notice of their serious purpose. The declaration gives the couple new status in that they are recognized as future life partners.

There is much more to the engagement than the joyful, proud announcement. It is a time for the couple to get to know each other in a more private and intimate fashion. It is a time for loving and being loved. The extent or degree of physical intimacy is a question the couple must face squarely. To be considered is the fact that conditions, though more intimate than before, are not the same as during marriage. The environment is different, and the feelings of stability and permanence are closer, yet they are not cemented as in marriage. Social approval of sexual intercourse is not the same as during marriage. Evidence from marital studies does not show that premarital sex experience enhances marital adjustment. The question of premarital sexual relations has been discussed in greater detail earlier in the chapter. All these factors indicate that the wise course to pursue is that in which intercourse is postponed until after marriage.

The late Professor Frank W. Hoffer,[16] an authority on courtship and marriage, told students at the University of Virginia:

Intimacy involves an integrating of personalities; a passionate interest in the other's ideas, hopes and aspirations; interchange of thought; respect for the other's dignity and worth. While in popular thought the physical relation is assumed to possess the greatest degree of intimacy and while this in one sense may be true, I wish to stress that the ultimate in intimacy may occur in a congenial conversation, looking at a sunset together, partaking of a meal. The sense of intimacy does not arise from mere physical contact. It is mental rather than physical.

The strongest bonds to hold the new relationship together are love and affection unselfishly expressed.

Another important aspect of the engagement period is the joint planning for the

[16] Whitman, op. cit., p. 5.

coming marriage. This is the time to double-check the choice of the partner before the life partnership begins. It offers a chance to predict, by a closer and more tender relationship, future marital adjustment. Questions concerning marital adjustment may well be raised and answered to the satisfaction of both parties; for example, when can the marriage take place? This problem becomes extremely difficult if young people are unable to marry when they are ready to do so. As has been indicated, guilt complexes may result from indulging in premarital sex relations. Many couples not able to marry at once refuse to practice premarital sexual intercourse, and

the natural result in this case, if the situation is prolonged, is the production of stresses or strains, which are bound to affect personalities. It has been stated previously that a number of authorities in the field of marital relations believe that early marriage is often a practical solution to this problem.

Other questions related to becoming better acquainted and making definite plans for the marriage may be answered if both parties complete a marriage prediction schedule (see Suggested readings 4 and 6), or James Peterson's "Analysis of Your Interaction with Future Mate" (see Suggested reading 32).

Summary

Preparation for family living is a continuous process of development from birth. However, much of this preparation takes place during the college years in the activities of dating and courtship leading to the selection of a life partner. These are activities that are a part of the over-all family-life cycle. An analysis of the family cycle assists you in gaining a perspective of total family living.

Choosing a life partner and participating in a wholesome courtship are basic factors in preparing for marriage and parenthood. In all the studies by sociologists, psychologists, and marital counselors the prime factor in choosing a life partner seems to be to find a socialized, stabilized individual with a happy temperament and a healthy personality—an emotionally mature individual. The couple should be emotionally companionable, sexually normal, and eugenically sound.

Both parties need to be able to appraise their own strengths and weaknesses and to make adjustments accordingly.

Sexual adjustment is a part of the individual's total maturation. Sex is a basic drive upon which both race preservation and personal happiness depend. Sexual maturity helps bring out what is best, most

generous, and most constructive in the individual's life. Sexual adjustment needs to be both understood and controlled.

The aspects of sexual adjustment considered include petting, premarital sexual relations, nocturnal emissions, masturbation, and homosexuality.

Erich Fromm believes that love is not the result of adequate sexual satisfaction, but that sexual happiness is the result of love. The enduring kind of love comes to the fore when romance wears off. Daily attention and sympathetic understanding are needed for love to grow and become permanent. This daily process of loving, successfully practiced by both man and woman, is the answer to the question, Does love last?

Authorities from the American Social Health Association believe that it is possible to choose a mate properly if young people going through the courtship process can answer the following questions objectively and honestly: Are you two psychologically suited? Are you biologically suited? Is there a promise of economic security? Are you both really ready for marriage?

Successful family life depends upon the

selection of the right person for a life partner. But even more important is the ability of each partner to make life adjustments so as to be the right person and thus ensure healthful, effective living in the family.

Suggested readings

1. Bacal, Jacques, and Louise Sloane: *Behavior in Courtship,* American Social Health Association, New York.
2. Becker, Howard, and Reuben Hill: *Family, Marriage and Parenthood,* D. C. Heath and Company, Boston, 1955.
3. Bernard, Jessie, Helen E. Buchanan, and William M. Smith, Jr.: *Dating, Mating and Marriage,* Howard Allen, Inc., Cleveland, 1958.
4. Blood, Robert O., Jr.: *Anticipating Your Marriage,* Free Press, Glencoe, Ill., 1955.
5. Bowman, Henry: *Marriage for Moderns,* 4th ed., McGraw-Hill Book Company, Inc., New York, 1960.
6. Burgess, Ernest W., and Leonard S. Cottrell: *Predicting Success or Failure in Marriage,* Prentice-Hall, Inc., Englewood Cliffs, N.J., 1939.
7. Burgess, E. W.: "The Marriage Prediction Schedule," in E. W. Burgess and H. J. Locke, *The Family,* American Book Company, New York, 1945.
8. Butterfield, Oliver M.: *Planning for Marriage,* D. Van Nostrand Company, Inc., Princeton, N.J., 1956.
9. Cavan, Ruth S.: *The American Family,* Thomas Y. Crowell Company, New York, 1953.
10. Cavan, Ruth S.: *American Marriage: A Way of Life,* Thomas Y. Crowell Company, New York, 1959.
11. Duvall, Evelyn M.: *Family Living,* rev. ed., The Macmillan Company, New York, 1955.
12. Duvall, Evelyn M.: *Family Development,* J. B. Lippincott Company, Philadelphia, 1957.
13. Duvall, Evelyn M.: *The Art of Dating,* Association Press, New York, 1958.
14. Duvall, Evelyn M., and Reuben Hill: *Being Married,* Association Press, New York, 1960.
15. Duvall, Sylvanus: *Before You Marry,* new rev. ed., Association Press, New York, 1959.
16. Ehrmann, Winston: *Premarital Dating Behavior,* Henry Holt and Company, Inc., New York, 1959.
17. Fishbein, Morris, and Ruby Jo Reeves Kennedy (eds.): *Modern Marriage and Family Living,* Oxford University Press, New York, 1957.
18. Fromm, Erich: "The Art of Living," *Coronet,* 48:154–159, July, 1960.
19. Good, William J.: "The Theoretical Importance of Love," *American Sociology Review,* 24:38–47, February, 1959.
20. Hacker, Helen M.: "The New Burdens of Masculinity," *Marriage and Family Living,* 19:227–233, August, 1957.
21. Kinsey, Alfred C., and others: *Sexual Behavior in the Human Male,* W. B. Saunders Company, Philadelphia, 1948.
22. Kinsey, Alfred C., and others: *Sexual Behavior in the Human Female,* W. B. Saunders Company, Philadelphia, 1953.
23. Kirkpatrick, Clifford: *The Family, as Process and Institution,* The Ronald Press Company, New York, 1955.
24. Komarovsky, Mirra: *Women in the Modern World,* Little, Brown & Company, Boston, 1953.
25. Kraines, S. H., and E. S. Thetford: *Managing Your Mind,* The Macmillan Company, New York, 1949.
26. Landis, Judson T., and Mary G. Landis: *Building a Successful Marriage,* 3d ed., Prentice-Hall, Inc., Englewood Cliffs, N.J., 1958.
27. Landis, Paul Henry: *Making the Most of Marriage,* Appleton-Century-Crofts, Inc., New York, 1955.
28. Le Masters, E. E.: *Modern Courtship and Marriage,* The Macmillan Company, New York, 1957.
29. Levy, John, and Ruth Munroe: *The Happy Family,* rev. ed., Alfred A. Knopf, Inc., New York, 1952.
30. McKinney, Fred: *Psychology of Personal Adjustment,* 3d ed., John Wiley & Sons, Inc., New York, 1960.
31. Merrill, Francis E.: *Courtship and Marriage,* rev. ed., Henry Holt and Company, Inc., New York, 1959.
32. Peterson, James A.: *Education for Marriage,* Charles Scribner's Sons, New York, 1956.
33. Pike, James A.: *If You Marry Outside Your Faith,* Harper & Brothers, New York, 1954.
34. Prescott, Daniel A.: *The Role of Love in Human Development,* reprint by The Hogg Foundation, Austin, Tex., 1959.
35. Reiss, Ira L.: "Toward a Sociology of

the Heterosexual Love Relationship," *Marriage and Family Living,* 22:139–145, May, 1960.

36. Rutledge, Aaron L. (ed.): *Courtship and Marriage Readings,* Harcourt, Brace and Company, Inc., New York, 1960.

37. Scheinfeld, Amram: *The New You and Heredity,* J. B. Lippincott Company, Philadelphia, 1951.

38. Scheinfeld, Amram: *Women and Men,* Harcourt, Brace and Company, Inc., New York, 1953.

39. Winch, Robert F.: *Mate-Selection,* Harper & Brothers, New York, 1958.

FIVE

Planning for marriage

SIGNIFICANCE OF MARRIAGE

GETTING MARRIED

ADJUSTING IN MARRIAGE

PHYSIOLOGY OF MARRIAGE

UNSATISFACTORY MARRIAGES

INDIVIDUALS WHO DO NOT MARRY

Planning for your marriage deserves as much preparation as planning for your lifework. College students in increasing numbers are finding that planning for and adjusting to marriage is no longer a future consideration. Approximately one student in five is already married and is adjusting to married life along with preparing for his vocational or professional activities. Most other students will be marrying, many in the near future. The fact that approximately 93 per cent of all persons who live to the age of fifty or older are eventually married suggests that nearly all students should be giving serious consideration to planning for successful marriage.

Some questions to be considered while planning for marriage are as follows:

What is the significance of marriage in our society today?

How can common pitfalls be avoided in planning a marriage ceremony?

What are the most common adjustments you should be prepared to make after the ceremony?

What can you do before marriage to ensure successful adjustment?

What basic information should you have about the physiology of marriage?

What are some of the problems associated with unsatisfactory marriage?

How does one adjust who is not married?

Acceptance of some definite responsibilities in the marriage partnership is a prerequisite for successful marriage. Success depends upon the best efforts of both partners, united in a deeply satisfying and worthwhile relationship. They are most likely to put forth such efforts if they enter the marriage relationship with an awareness of its significance and an understanding of the adjustments required for success.

Significance of marriage

Monogamous marriage, the accepted pattern in our society, has not become obsolete, as some persons have suggested. The 40,200,000 married couples reported in the 1960 census and the 1,530,000 marriages during 1960 indicate the need for a satisfactory marriage relationship. Blood and Wolfe, in a report on a research project involving a cross section of an entire community and including data from a representative sample of farm families, support the contention that our marriage pattern is successful: [1]

In any case, there seems to be little evidence, from the 909 wives interviewed, that American marriage as an institution is on the verge of collapse. On the contrary, as long as men and women continue to have important needs satisfied by their marriage partners, marriage is "here to stay."

To avoid an overly optimistic picture of the success of marriage in our society, it is well to remember that approximately 2,800,000 divorced persons were reported in the 1960 census and that there is approximately one divorce for every four marriages.

The marriage relationship, established for procreation and child rearing has, at least reasonably well, withstood the challenge of time. This relationship must, however, do more than merely provide for children. It must also help satisfy the individual's need for affection, belonging, sympathy, understanding, and companionship in order to help him achieve security.

There can be little doubt about the importance of marriage. People talk about it, religion sanctifies it, magazines and books record what writers think about it, lawmakers attempt to regulate it, and countless numbers of women and men continually attempt to make it successful.

LEGAL ASPECTS

Unfortunately, the legal aspects of marriage vary widely from state to state. Lawmakers are not in full agreement about regulations to provide maximum opportunities for successful marriage. The established regulations, in most instances, bear on the health of the individuals involved. It is important to be aware of the reasons for protective regulations and to promote and support requirements that ensure the best possible chance for marital success from the standpoint of both individuals and society.

Premarital physical examinations. Regulations requiring premarital health examinations for the prevention of venereal

[1] Robert O. Blood, Jr., and Donald M. Wolfe, *Husbands and Wives: The Dynamics of Married Living,* Free Press, Glencoe, Ill., 1960, p. 267.

diseases are in force in some states and not in others. All except four states require certificates showing freedom from venereal infection before individuals are permitted to marry [7].

Premarital health examinations contribute to successful marriage, especially if the examination includes more than a test for venereal disease (see Chapter 4 for additional information about premarital examinations).

Waiting period. Thirty-three states require a waiting period between the date of application for a license and the date of the marriage ceremony. This waiting period, which varies from one to five days, is required because marriages resulting from spur-of-the-moment decisions are not likely to be successful. A waiting period is, in most instances, no hardship to persons who have planned adequately for their

marriage, and it does prevent some marriages that have little chance for success.

Prohibited marriages. Nearly all states prohibit marriage of certain groups of individuals. Some states prohibit the marriage of individuals with certain infectious diseases. Insanity and feeble-mindedness are barriers, to varying degrees, in most states. The basic reason for restricting the marriage of emotionally disturbed and mentally deficient persons is their inability to fulfill social obligations. In addition, the possibility that abnormal children may result is of major significance in determining marriage restrictions.

Limitations on the marriage of blood relatives are in force in all states. The degree of relationship of persons forbidden to marry differs considerably from state to state (see Chapter 4 for health aspects of prohibited marriages).

Getting married

The actual marriage ceremony takes only a few minutes. Planning for the event may extend over a period of days, weeks, or months. This planning period provides many happy memories for the couple after the ceremony. Another phase of the family cycle is entered. A new family unit is established. This beginning is worthy of more than a spur-of-the-moment approach.

SOCIAL APPROVAL

Marriage is more than a relationship between a bride and groom. Society has a vested interest in a partnership that begins a new family group with all its opportunities and responsibilities. Social custom determines the nature of the ceremony. The desires of the couple and the approval of the social group should be considered when plans are made. The type of ceremony is important to beginning a marriage favorably. When individuals are planning their wedding, they should

take time to consider the pros and cons of different types of wedding ceremony.

ELOPEMENTS OR SECRET WEDDINGS

Elopements, in most instances, result from a desire to escape. Parental opposition, the high cost of elaborate weddings, and the desire to avoid publicity are cited frequently as reasons why couples elope. Pregnancy is another possible reason.

In the case of an elopement, friends may be offended because they are not permitted to enjoy the occasion with the bride and groom. Parents may feel that their children are unfair. All in all, the marriage partnership begins under much less favorable circumstances than if it began with a planned ceremony shared by close friends and relatives.

SECRET MARRIAGES

The secret marriage, not announced until a much later date, may give rise to unfavorable speculation. Parents are displeased because they are not informed of the plans. Marriage begins behind a screen of secrecy, which makes normal adjustments more difficult. Secrets are not always easy to keep, and sometimes the purpose of secrecy is thwarted by a slip that makes the marriage known.

Fear of censure seems to be a primary reason for keeping a marriage secret. A marriage begun in a climate of fear hardly has a fair opportunity for success. Little can be said in favor of secret marriages.

PLANNED CEREMONIES

The well-planned ceremony is more likely to be followed by satisfactory marriage. This type of ceremony indicates that the individuals have taken time to prepare for the occasion, that each is acquainted with the strong and weak traits of the proposed life partner, and that both are fully aware of the step they are taking. The marriage thus is the result of a decision based on sound thinking and not on the fancy of the moment. If the wedding ceremony is well planned, the hazards often associated with "picking a mate by moonlight" are more apt to be avoided.

Planned ceremonies, however, also have pitfalls. An elaborate wedding that leaves the bride and groom emotionally and physically exhausted launches the marriage under unfavorable conditions. An elaborate wedding may cost so much that the honeymoon and early weeks of married life are complicated by financial difficulties. The couple is fortunate if the parents of the bride (custom has delegated this responsibility to them) and/or the parents of the groom are able to pay for the wedding ceremony. Emotional, physical, and financial limitations are all factors to consider when planning the wedding ceremony.

The extent to which the church is involved in the wedding ceremony depends largely upon the religious beliefs of the bride and groom. It is wise for the couple to consider the importance of a church wedding in the light of their future relationship with the church. Studies indicate that four out of five American couples choose a religious service instead of a civil ceremony [10]. Marriages begun under the auspices of a minister, priest, or rabbi are much less frequently ended by divorce.

It is highly recommended that you plan wisely for marriage and provide a wedding occasion that can be recalled with pleasure many times during the years of married life.

THE HONEYMOON

In many ways the honeymoon is part of the process of getting married. The legal requirements for marriage are satisfied by the wedding ceremony. The honeymoon, however, plays an important role in the transition from the engaged to the married status. An expensive ship is launched with care; likewise, it is advantageous to launch carefully a life partnership of husband and wife.

The honeymoon provides the first opportunity for the partners to be with each other intimately and continuously with the approval of society. These early days of marriage may establish the pattern of relationship between man and wife. It is advisable to avoid the common mistakes made when a honeymoon is planned haphazardly.

The honeymoon is a time for activities that the partners enjoy together. In addition to providing for social activities, ample time should be allowed for rest and relaxation. For a few days the newlyweds simply enjoy the companionship of one another. It is a mistake to plan too many things and to be so busy going places that little time is allowed for enjoying each other's company.

The cost of the honeymoon depends upon finances. Like the wedding itself, the honeymoon is not supposed to use up money needed by the couple to establish the home in which they begin their married life.

The honeymoon requires, above all else, privacy. This is an occasion which calls for the newlyweds to be by themselves. The third person, relative or friend, not only is unnecessary but may jeopardize the partnership. This is a time for sharing with no one but the new mate. Intrusion upon this privacy by an outsider can do little good, and it may cause much difficulty.

For the first time these partners are completely on their own. They make their own decisions. The apron strings are severed. The success of the new partnership depends upon the ability of the partners to adjust during the honeymoon as well as in the later stages of marriage.

Adjusting in marriage

In a utopia all marriages are completely successful. Both husband and wife derive a maximum of happiness from their partnership, which in all cases is terminated only by death. It is apparent that this happy state of affairs does not always exist in our society. Many marriages are terminated by divorce. Many other marriages provide little in the way of satisfaction. Therefore, you should be aware of the adjustments necessary to assure success in your marriage.

In spite of the fact that many marriages are terminated by divorce and many others are unsuccessful, it is a rare person who does not believe that "this is for life" when the marriage vows are exchanged. Both bride and groom hope that their marriage will be a truly happy and successful lifelong partnership.

From the time the individual first begins life in this world to the time he establishes a marriage partnership, forces are at work preparing him for this experience. The actual process of getting married is only a point on his life line. He is not transformed suddenly by a ceremony that makes him a member of a marriage partnership. He does change, but the change seldom is extreme. The changes are only phases of his attempt to adjust to a new and different relationship and usually occur comparatively slowly.

The problems of necessary adjustment vary from one marriage to another. For some couples most adjustments do not involve problems, because a solution is forthcoming for each new experience. Individuals who adapt readily to such circumstances are mature persons. They are able to call upon the resources of an adequate personality and upon a wealth of individual experiences.

AREAS OF ADJUSTMENT

Authorities who have studied marriages in this country agree generally on the common areas of adjustment that confront husband and wife. Two such authorities are cited, and their suggested lists of common areas are indicated as a basis for discussion. Judson Landis, in a study on the time required by couples to attain a mutually satisfying adjustment in marriage, lists seven areas of adjustment [19]:

Mutual friends
In-law relationships
Spending family income
Social activities
Religion
Children
Sex relations

Blood and Wolfe [3] consider these major areas of disagreement in marriage:

Money
Children
Recreation
Personality
In-laws
Roles
Religion, politics
Sex

In the following consideration of adjustment the above areas are discussed, beginning with personality adjustment of one person to another.

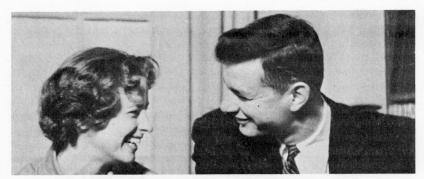

A mature couple, who love each other and have fun together . . .

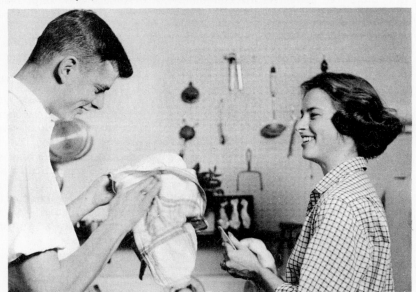

begin their marriage happy to share the work and adjustments necessary in getting along together . . .

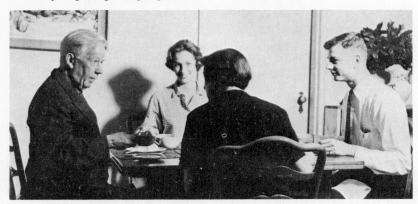

in welcoming in-laws to their home . . .

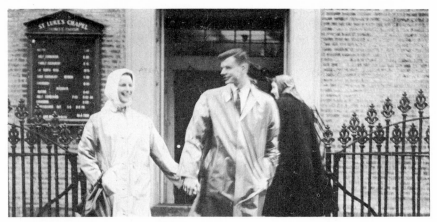

in respecting each other's religious beliefs . . .

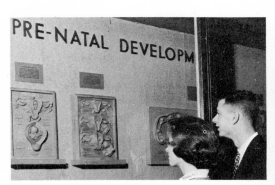

in preparing themselves for
parenthood . . .

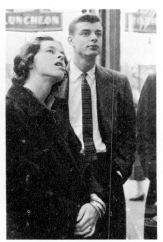

in spending the family income . . .

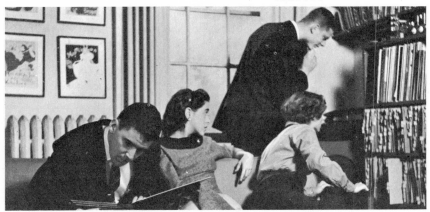

and in enriching their lives with common interests and friends.

Getting along with one another. It is advisable to begin marriage with the understanding that some conflict or difference of opinion is normal and natural. The marriage in which husband and wife are in perfect agreement at all times, on all matters, and under all circumstances is nonexistent. The task confronting the partners is to resolve differences of opinion in a mutually satisfactory manner. The desirable solution of differences enables each person to retain his own individuality and self-respect. It is in this area that the aspects of adjustment discussed in detail in Chapter 3 should be considered carefully.

A statement by Foster[2] indicates the importance of personality factors in achieving adjustment:

The majority of problems in husband-wife relationships are, basically, personality problems, essentially conflict situations between a husband and wife or other family member, and most so-called money, sex, social, or other types of problems are only symptomatic of the underlying problem.

A mature married individual respects the personality of his mate. He knows and understands those things which set the mate apart as an individual. Decisions are reached by mutual agreement. Undoubtedly, one partner exerts more influence in decisions relating to situations about which he is better informed. Even so, decisions need the backing of both persons if follow-up action is to be mutually satisfactory.

One should not be so engrossed in the big things as to forget the everyday "little things." Remembering the birthday and anniversary and failing to remember the 360-odd additional days is an example of inadequately directed attention. The words and actions that make a person feel wanted each day are the basis for a mutually satisfying relationship in marriage.

The exchange of wedding vows implies that a mate is accepted for what he is. The person who plans to reform his mate

following the wedding ceremony should avoid taking on such a task. Efforts should be directed toward finding a mate who does not need reforming. A mate should be chosen wisely and accepted for what he is. It is helpful to remember that all individuals have their limitations and that perfection cannot be expected in a mate.

Blood and Wolfe strongly point up the danger of attacks on a person's personal behavior, suggesting that such attacks hurt the ego too much to be taken lightly [3]. The damage is likely to be lasting and the threat to the marriage serious.

A sense of humor does much to relieve tensions that so easily become obstacles to successful marriage. Life is pleasant if one looks for the fun offered in everyday living.

A final point to be considered in getting along with one another is the need to reduce sources of annoyances, on the one

Table 5.1 Major areas of disagreement in urban families

Type of disagreement	Per cent tabulated *	
	Chief disagreement	Total disagreements
Money	24	42
Children	16	29
Recreation	16	30
Personality	14	28
In-laws	6	10
Roles	4	7
Religion, politics	3	4
Sex	†	1
None	15	15
Not ascertained	2	2
Total	100	168 ‡
Number of families	731	731

* Most wives typically mention two areas of disagreement, while a few mention three or four. The right-hand column shows the total of all disagreements mentioned in each category, giving a rough idea of the proportion of all couples who ever have a major disagreement in that area. The first-mentioned disagreements are used as a basis for comparison in subsequent tables.
† Less than 0.05 per cent.
‡ Total adds to more than 100 per cent because many wives gave more than one response.
Source: Robert O. Blood, Jr., and Donald M. Wolfe, *Husbands and Wives: The Dynamics of Married Living,* The Free Press, Glencoe, Ill., 1960, p. 241.

[2] Robert Geib Foster, *Marriage and Family Relationships,* The Macmillan Company, New York, 1950, p. 124.

hand, and seek areas of agreement and mutual pleasure, on the other. One of the most important steps that marriage partners can take is to recognize the need for, and the desire to improve, communication. Mature individuals are able to express their feelings and to listen to what others have to say. Anger is a deterrent to good communication, but communication serves as a means of resolving the ill will that can result from actions taken during anger. Robert Foster, who directs marriage-counselor training at the Menninger Clinic, thinks that lack of communication is the major problem in many marriages today [28].

Mutual friends. In Chapter 3 it was pointed out that an individual who makes a good adjustment is one who, among other things, has the facility for making and keeping friends. Friends continue to play an important part in an individual's life after marriage. Genuinely happy couples have at least a few close friends who are accepted and respected by both partners. Studies show that the number of friends that couples have in common is associated closely with the marital adjustment that the couple makes [12]. The need for belonging must be satisfied. Friends with whom and for whom the couple can do things are important in sat-

isfying the need for belonging. Data in the chart of the Landis study on page 141 indicate that more couples report success in achieving adjustment with respect to mutual friends than in any other area.

When a marriage brings together two individuals from different social backgrounds, they usually have different sets of friends. Each must be willing to accept at least some friends of the partner. Even more important, the partners should work wholeheartedly to find new friends who accept them as partners.

Recreation. Closely allied with the matter of mutual friends is the use of leisure time. The use of leisure time presents many possibilities for discontent, and as many opportunities for enrichment, of the husband-wife relationship. With the breadwinner in many families working less hours than in the past, there are more hours for leisure. Planning for the use of this time deserves the serious consideration of all members of the family group. Data from the Landis study show that many couples, nearly 14 per cent, never do make a satisfactory adjustment in this area. Data from the Blood and Wolfe study (Table 5.1) show that recreation rates second highest in the list of chief disagreement and total disagreements in the 731 families reported.

Table 5.2   Disagreements, by stage in family-life cycle, per cent

Disagreement	Stage in family-life cycle						
	Honey-moon	Pre-school	Preado-lescent	Ado-lescent	Postparental and retired	Un-launched	Childless couples
Money	10	28	24	23	21	23	18
Children		13	29	32	10	20	
Recreation:							
Interests	20	8	8	9	6		14
Amount	10	9	5	7	11	3	6
Personality	20	14	16	11	14	23	12
In-laws	15	8	5	2	2	3	10
Roles		5	4	4	4	5	4
Religion, politics, sex	10	4	3	3	5	2	4
None	15	11	7	10	26	22	31
Total	100	100	101	101	99	101	99
Number of families	20	130	140	101	97	65	49

Source: Robert O. Blood, Jr., and Donald M. Wolfe, *Husbands and Wives: The Dynamics of Married Living,* The Free Press, Glencoe, Ill., p. 247.

By stages in the family-life cycle (Table 5.2), combined disagreements over interests and amount of recreational activities are first during the honeymoon, second during the period of preschool children, fourth during the period of preadolescent children, and second again during the postparental and retired periods.

The happily married couple discovers activities that are enjoyed together. The pleasure derived from companionship is an essential factor in making the marriage a happy one. These same persons discover that each partner may have some activity or activities in which he participates with individuals outside the family group. It is worthwhile for the husband to play golf, go fishing or hunting, or enjoy the comradeship of other men in a service organization. Likewise, the wife profits from her association with other women in a bridge club, a service organization, a knitting or sewing group, a tennis or golfing group, community projects, or some other activity.

It is sometimes necessary, and in most instances worth the effort, for both partners to learn and to take part in new activities that can be enjoyed together. Many leisure hours are passed in company with other couples. For this reason it is important for married persons to develop skills in activities that are participated in with other couples.

Some of the activities that couples or families may enjoy either within the family or with other families are:

Sports activities, including golf, tennis, badminton, bowling, swimming, skiing, boating, hunting, and fishing

Spectator activities, including viewing theatrical performances, watching sports events, and attending exhibits of various artistic productions

Hobbies, including both collecting and making a variety of objects

Indoor activities, such as playing bridge or other group games

You can be developing skills now in a variety of such activities, in which you can continue to participate after graduation.

With many forces operating to draw members of the family away from home for their leisure-time activities, it is advisable to plan for activities enjoyed by the whole family. The family room, which is included in many homes, should be planned to provide for a variety of family-wide activities. The pleasure derived from well-planned family activities, both inside and outside the home, helps to develop happier and more secure individuals and families.

In-law relationships. When two persons marry, each of them usually acquires a set of in-laws. The relationships established with these in-laws can play a significant role in the success of the new partnership. It is well for individuals to remember that a large majority of persons are or will be in-laws. It is important for most persons to give serious consideration to their responsibilities to their own in-laws and as in-laws of other persons.

In the Landis study, more than 30 per cent of couples reported adjustment problems with in-laws, and approximately 10 per cent of couples never did achieve successful adjustment. The Blood and Wolfe study shows that in-laws account for a steadily decreasing percentage of disagreements from honeymoon on through the successive stages in the family-life cycle. Blood and Wolfe point out that the transfer of loyalties from parents to marriage partner creates a stress during the early stages of marriage, particularly for the young wife [3].

It is unfortunate that in-laws are the butt of so many jokes, because a majority of married couples make a mutually satisfactory adjustment in their in-law relationships. The steady bombardment of mother-in-law stories quite possibly causes some persons to search for reasons to be critical of their own in-laws. If one looks for something wrong, it is possible to find a basis for criticizing almost anyone.

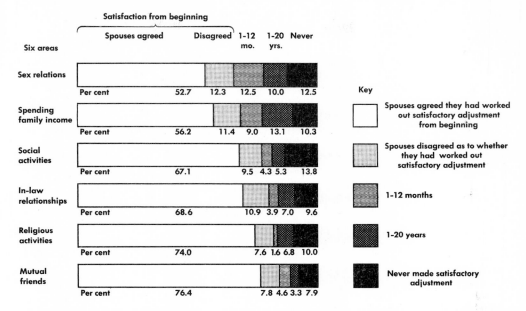

Percentages of 409 couples reporting various periods of time after marriage required to achieve adjustment in six areas. (Judson T. Landis, "Length of Time Required for Adjustment in Marriage," *American Sociological Review*, December, 1946, p. 668.)

When two persons marry, they establish their own home and expect to make their own decisions. Unfortunately, some parents are unwilling to allow their offspring to make their own decisions. It is just as unfortunate if the offspring continually turn to their parents for answers that mature persons should be able to find for themselves. Children are not expected to renounce completely their parents or other relatives as a source of counsel and guidance. It is the manner in which, and the extent to which, advice is given and sought that determines the success of in-law relationships.

Factors such as a housing shortage, husbands' being called into service, the need for additional education, and a desire on the part of in-laws to help young couples get a start sometimes lead them to live with parents or other relatives. In addition, many young couples find it necessary to have one or more of their in-laws living with them in the newly established home.

Despite the fact that it is best for newlyweds to have a home of their own without other persons in the home, many couples make a satisfactory adjustment while living with in-laws or having in-laws in the home.

Becoming a better in-law is an effective way of getting along with one's own in-laws. Acceptance and mutual respect are two of the most important factors suggested by individuals who have established good relationships with their in-laws.

Family income. Few persons are financially able to purchase all the material things they would like to have. Most families, therefore, are confronted with the problem of earning more money or determining how to spend their limited finances. The importance of money problems in married life is indicated by the fact that persons studied by Blood and Wolfe rated money as the subject of most disagreement and that 23 per cent of couples studied by Landis had not made satisfactory adjustment in regard to the spending of income by the end of the first year of marriage.

Budgeting, credit buying, insurance, and getting one's money's worth are phases of the problem to be considered. Among the specific items requiring attention is a plan for providing the best possible health protection for the family. Information in Chapter 10 is helpful for evaluating both products and services to be assured of most adequate protection for the amount of money spent.

In addition to spending the family income, the husband and wife may have to consider the matter of supplementing the income either by having the husband hold more than one job or by having the wife work outside the home. The fact that approximately one-third of married women in this country are gainfully employed outside the home indicates either that many families need supplemental income or that wives are interested in a career.

The decision whether the wife should be gainfully employed outside the home is based on long-term consideration of all factors. If a marriage of two ideally suited partners can be commenced sooner by having the wife work for a time, perhaps she should do so; this may be a better solution than postponing the marriage. For many college students the only way they can marry and continue in school is for both partners to work on at least a part-time basis.

Personal feelings regarding either temporary work or a career for the wife should be expressed by both partners before marriage. The degree to which the woman's absence affects the establishment of a happy home is of primary importance in reaching a decision.

Religion. The basic point to stress in regard to religion and marital adjustment is the need for a common interest and respect for the partner's beliefs. It is expedient to consider carefully the possibilities of differences arising from religious

preferences and practices [25]. It is advisable to reach decisions prior to marriage on situations that require agreement. The fact that 74 per cent of couples studied by Landis reported satisfactory adjustment in religious activities from the beginning of marriage would seem to indicate that many possible conflicts had been solved prior to marriage. The low percentage of disagreement attributed to religion and politics by participants in the Blood and Wolfe study tends to substantiate this point.

The extent to which religion enters into marriage can be noted by the previously stated fact that four-fifths of the marriages in this country begin with a religious ceremony. Individuals seek the sanction of the church even though the civil ceremony suffices for legal purposes.

Problems arise in relation to church attendance by the partners and by their children. If one of the partners does not attend church, is this fact accepted by the other? Does the one who fails to attend church accept the fact that Sunday is set aside for church attendance by the mate? Which church are the children to attend if the parents are of different faiths? Such problems must be met squarely. Possible disagreements should be anticipated and a solution agreed upon before the marriage vows are exchanged. Decisions should not be delayed until tensions are created by unresolved problems. Two individuals whose religious convictions are definitely in opposition may find it advisable not to marry.

There is no single answer to the problem of religious adjustment for married persons. Each couple has its own peculiar problems to solve. The solutions are more likely to be satisfactory if they are based upon respect for the partner and for his basic beliefs.

Children. The procreation and rearing of children are foundations of marriage in our society. Most parents agree that their children provide many of the happiest and most satisfying experiences of their lifetime. These same parents indicate that their children are the center of problems that create tensions between man and wife. The participants in the Blood and Wolfe study listed children as the leading area of disagreement during the pre-adolescent and adolescent stages of the family-life cycle.

Prospective marriage partners should consider the following questions:

Can we have children?

Shall we have children?

When shall we have children?

How many children shall we have?

Most couples desire children of their own. If both marriage partners do not share this feeling, they have been unwise in selecting each other as mates. Complicating the desire to have children are such factors as physical inability to have children, lack of sufficient income to provide for children, necessity for the wife to stop work because of pregnancy, and inadequate housing facilities.

Couples who have children find it expedient to agree on the way in which the children are to be handled. The greatest difficulty over children involves discipline [3]. Disagreements between parents, resulting in inconsistent parent-child relations, are difficult for the parent and for the child. Fortunately, the modern parent has resources upon which to depend for valuable assistance when the need arises. Chapter 6 provides more detailed information concerning parent-child relationships and indicates valid sources of information for parents.

Sex relations. Sex relations can serve as a strong unifying force and make the marriage relationship a richer and more satisfying experience. Unfortunately, however, there can be difficulty in achieving success in sex relations. The Landis study indicates that fewer couples report mutually satisfactory adjustment from the beginning of marriage in the area of sex relations than in any other adjustment area. The insignificant number of participants in the Blood and Wolfe study who listed sex as a major area of disagreement may be due to the fact that respondents suggested their own ideas and did not react to a prepared list of topics. The area of sex relations may have been either intentionally or unintentionally omitted.

Studies have shown that there is extreme variation in sexual capacity and desire among men and women as well as between them. There does not seem to be a specific minimum or maximum limit to normality in the sex drive. It is both unfair and unwise in a given marriage to base normal sex capacity upon averages. The difference between individuals in the need to satisfy the sex drive and the wide variation in attitudes or feelings about sexual intercourse make it difficult to evaluate successful adjustment on the basis of such factors as frequency of intercourse or the regularity with which both partners achieve orgasm. If both marriage partners feel that they are satisfied or that they have made a satisfactory adjustment, they should not be concerned with statistical averages.

Intercourse, or coitus, for the purpose of producing children to perpetuate the race has long been accepted as a normal part of married life. The concept of intercourse as a source of mutual pleasure and satisfaction and as a basis for increased feelings of security is more recent and is not yet accepted by all individuals, particularly in some religious groups. It is a fortunate individual indeed who appreciates fully the satisfaction of intimate association of husband and wife in normal sex relations. The physical satisfaction is intense and wonderful, but in reality it is insignificant when compared with the deep emotional satisfaction that comes from the love expressed when two persons not only accept but desire sexual relations as a necessary and valuable component of married life.

The rewards of successful adjustment in sex relations more than justify the efforts required for many couples to achieve it. One prerequisite for successful adjustment is a clear understanding of the sex drive and acceptance of the fact that it is normal and natural both to have the sex drive and to enjoy its satisfaction. Another prerequisite is to understand the general patterns of sex response of the opposite sex and the specific pattern associated with one's own partner in marriage. Knowing, in general, the preparations needed for achievement of orgasm or satisfaction without orgasm, the factors that influence the desire for sex relations, the physical elements of the actual act of sexual intercourse, and the terminology that makes it possible to communicate effectively is important.

This general information is not always applicable to individuals attempting to adjust. However, it does provide a background of information for a better understanding of the immediate problem. Individuals need to improve their ability to communicate to their marriage partner desires, fears, questions, and answers concerning sexual relations. They need also to respond to feelings, questions, and answers of the partner. They need to solve cooperatively those problems which can be solved and to seek assistance from a qualified physician or marriage counselor when help is required.

Petting and its relationship to premarital sex relations has been discussed in Chapter 4. Because petting is commonly frowned upon as acceptable behavior by unmarried persons, it is difficult for some adults to accept it as a normal part of sex relations in marriage. Both wife and husband need to recognize that love play, such as petting, is necessary and desirable in order for many individuals to achieve satisfaction from sex relations [12]. The relative ease with which men are aroused sexually and achieve orgasm compared with the longer time period and greater preparation required by many women makes it difficult for some couples to develop a mutually satisfying experience early in marriage. Patience and cooperative effort by both marriage partners can help to overcome difficulties.

It should be noted that some individuals have been conditioned through their own environmental influences and/or lower sexual capacity so that it is difficult for them to enjoy sexual relations. Women who are unable to achieve personal satisfaction in sexual relations can have a happy marriage and good family relationships.

Indulging in sexual intercourse prior to marriage provides an experience in sex relations that can be unsatisfactory from the standpoint of adjustment during marriage. Such factors as fear of being caught, fear of pregnancy, poor physical setting for the experience, guilt feelings, hurry, and interest only in personal gratification, which frequently are associated with premarital intercourse, provide experience that may complicate rather than foster adjustment.

The bond between husband and wife can be strengthened to a great extent by the feeling that "he is mine and I am his," which is fostered by a mutually satisfying sexual relationship. Individuals who have this feeling of belonging are more likely to be secure. Partners who are secure, who love one another, and who can depend upon this love transmit a feeling of security to their children.

An improved understanding of the physiology of sexual relations in marriage is helpful to individuals who want to work out a satisfactory adjustment. The following discussion should be helpful.

Physiology of marriage

Misinformation about human reproduction is extensive and, to say the least, unfortunate. Accurate information is important for achieving happiness in marriage. Those who know little and recognize their inadequacy will seek accurate information, but those who believe they know it all are unlikely to search for additional information.

Anatomically the male and female reproductive systems are complementary. The structure of these two systems makes it possible for the penis of the male to deposit sperm within the vagina of the female. The sperm then make their way through the female reproductive organs to fertilize the ovum and thus to produce a new life. Structurally, in all but a small minority of cases, sexual relations between male and female are free of complications. On the other hand, because of attitudes toward sexual response and misinformation about sexual relations, some individuals experience difficulty when they marry and attempt to make adjustments necessary for mutually satisfactory sexual relations.

Accurate information about the anatomy and physiology of the reproductive systems and a sincere desire to please one's partner in marriage do much to reduce difficulties in adjustment. The following

discussion provides basic information about normal function of both male and female genital systems.

MALE GENITALIA

The reproductive cell produced by the male is the spermatozoon, or sperm. The sperm cells are produced in the paired sex glands, called testes, or testicles. The male hormone testosterone is also produced by the testicles. The testicles are suspended in the scrotum, a saclike external structure behind the penis. These glands produce a sufficient number of sperm to provide 200 million to 600 million cells for each normal ejaculation, or discharge.

The microscopic, tadpole-shaped sperm are formed within the minute, coiled tubes that make up the testicle. These newly formed cells are passed along to the epididymis and thence to the vas deferens and ampulla, where they are stored until discharge.

Safeguarding the sperm. The sperm are readily affected by adverse conditions.

The male reproductive system. (Adapted from Henry A. Bowman, *Marriage for Moderns,* McGraw-Hill Book Company, Inc., New York, 1954.)

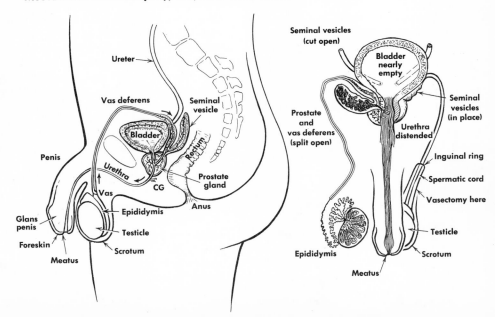

They lose their ability to fertilize an ovum (probably within 48 hours at the most) even under the most favorable conditions. The location of the testicles outside the abdominal cavity provides the lower temperature necessary for sperm formation. The male whose testicles fail to descend from the body cavity (where they are formed and go through the early stages of growth) into the scrotum is sterile unless proper medical treatment causes the testicles to move down. Normally, these glands pass down through the inguinal canal into the scrotum either before birth or soon after.

When the sperm are discharged from the vas deferens and ampulla, they combine with secretions from the seminal vesicles and the prostate gland to form the seminal fluid, or semen, which is a thick, yellowish-white, viscid fluid. In addition to providing an ideal environment for the sperm, these fluids serve as a means of transportation. The cells become activated when exposed to these secretions, and the whiplike action of the sperm's tail helps propel it when it is deposited on the surface of the vagina during intercourse.

Discharge of the sperm. The penis is composed of columns of erectile tissue that run lengthwise in the organ. In addition, the urethral canal extends the length of the penis, providing a passageway for the sperm to be discharged from the body. Even though the urethral canal also serves as a passageway for eliminating urine from the bladder, sperm and urine do not pass through the canal at the same time. During periods of sexual stimulation the penis becomes enlarged as a result of the increased amount of blood in the erectile tissue, and thus it becomes sufficiently rigid to enter the vagina during intercourse.

Continued stimulation as the head of the penis contacts the wall of the vagina during intercourse results in an orgasm. This climax of stimulation is accompanied by a series of contractions, which force the seminal fluid out through the urethral canal. Ejaculation, or discharge of semen from the penis, may occur normally while the male is asleep. Orgasm that occurs in this manner is called a nocturnal emission, or wet dream. This type of outlet for the sex drive is discussed in Chapter 4. It is important for the male approaching maturity to understand that this is a perfectly normal occurrence, along with the growth of hair on the body, appearance of a beard, deepening of the voice, and broadening of the shoulders.

Self-stimulation, or masturbation, resulting in orgasm causes a discharge of semen just the same as during intercourse or nocturnal emission. The significance of masturbation is discussed in Chapter 4.

Circumcision. It is common practice to have the foreskin of the penis freed by surgery. If this is not done, irritation and infection may develop around the head of the penis. Circumcision is usually performed within the first two weeks after birth. Surgery is easier at this early age, but it can be performed at any age.

FEMALE GENITALIA

The reproductive cell produced by the female is called an ovum, or egg. It is from this speck of protoplasm, barely visible to the human eye, that each human being develops and grows. Approximately 300 to 500 mature ova are produced by the average female during a lifetime. The maturation and release of one or more ova by the female sex glands, or ovaries, occurs approximately every twenty-eight days. The almond-shaped ovaries, which are about 1 to 2 inches in length, are located within the abdominal cavity.

Only one ovum matures or ripens during each menstrual cycle under ordinary circumstances. The reason why one particular ovary matures an ovum during any given cycle is not known. This one ovum moves to the surface of the ovary and is

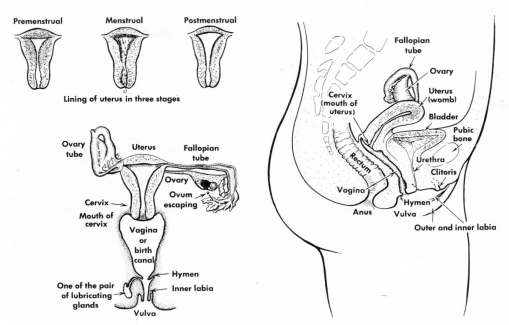

The female reproductive organs. (After a drawing by Robert Latou Dickinson, by permission from Educational Department, Tampax, Inc.)

enclosed in a saclike, fluid-filled structure called a graafian follicle. The ovum is released when the follicle ruptures. In this way the egg is freed to start on its way toward fertilization or oblivion. The release of the mature ovum is called ovulation. Mature ova are released regularly in most women for a period of approximately thirty years beginning with puberty and lasting until menopause. Ovulation may not occur during every cycle. Failure to ovulate regularly is especially true for a time following menarche, or first menstruation, and when the woman is approaching menopause. It is also true during pregnancy, when an increased production of the hormone progesterone causes a cessation of ovulation. The discovery of this function of progesterone stimulated research on substances which could be taken orally and would cause temporary cessation of ovulation. The "19-nor" steroids were developed and when used by the woman as recommended by her physician, they have proved to be highly effective in preventing pregnancy.

The mature ovum, under normal circumstances, is drawn into the open end of the fallopian tube and gradually moved down the tube toward the uterus, or womb. The uterus is a small, hollow, pear-shaped organ, which during pregnancy expands to many times its normal size as the fetus grows and creates pressure from within. At the small end of the uterus, corresponding to the location of the stem of a pear, there is an opening of about the same diameter as the lead of an ordinary pencil. The small rounded end of the uterus, called the cervix, extends into the tube-like vagina, which in turn opens to the surface of the body. During intercourse the penis is inserted into the vagina, which stretches to allow its entrance. Semen is deposited near the mouth of the uterus. From this area the sperm that survive make their way up through the uterus and into the fallopian tubes in search of an ovum to fertilize. Considering the microscopic size of sperm and the comparatively great distance they must travel if they do survive the hostile environment of the vagina, it is apparent that many sperm must be produced by the male to ensure the chance of fertilization of the ovum.

The lubricating glands of the female reproductive organs are shown in the illustration on page 147. The stimulation of love play (kissing and petting), which should precede intercourse, causes these glands to produce a fluid that aids in the insertion of the penis into the vagina. Preparation for intercourse through love play is an important aspect of good sex relations for married couples.

External genitalia. Observation of the diagram of the female genital system shows that, for the most part, the genital organs are located within the body. One of the structures located at or near the body surface is the hymen, or maidenhead. This membrane, when present, stretches across the lower part of the vagina near the external opening. The extent of the membrane varies considerably; it is negligible in many women and almost completely obstructs the opening in others. Because of its location and the nature of the membrane, the hymen is sometimes considered an indicator of virginity. It is important to understand, however, that the tissue can be broken down in other ways besides intercourse. Its absence is not valid evidence that the woman has had intercourse at some previous time.

Intercourse may be difficult or impossible if the hymen obstructs the vaginal opening. For this reason, it is wise for the woman to have her physician examine this membrane during the premarital health examination. Correction under the physician's care is a simple matter if it is necessary. This correction prior to marriage aids the couple in making a satisfactory adjustment in their sexual relations during the first days of marriage.

The labia, or folds of skin, which extend over the vaginal opening also cover the clitoris and the urethral orifice, or opening from the urinary bladder. The clitoris is the seat of much of the feeling or stimulation for the woman. Proper stimulation of the clitoris during sexual relations usually enables the woman to achieve orgasm.

MENSTRUAL CYCLE

Menstruation is one phase of the menstrual cycle. It is unfortunate that some women and men are unaware of the real significance of menstruation. The false ideas concerning this perfectly normal bodily process causes difficulty in adjustment for some individuals. The first and foremost idea to bear in mind is the fact that menstruation is not an illness. It is a normal function of the reproductive system and is one sign of female maturity. Menstruation results when the egg produced by the ovary is not fertilized and the prepared uterine lining tissue is not needed.

Some days prior to ovulation the menstrual cycle is initiated by the production of a follicle-stimulating hormone (FSH) by the anterior lobe of the pituitary gland. This hormone stimulates the maturation of an ovum. The ovum moves to the surface of the ovary and is enclosed in the graafian follicle. This follicle in turn secretes a hormone (estrogen) that causes changes in the lining of the uterus in preparation for the arrival of a fertilized egg. When ovulation occurs, the ovum leaves the follicle and the lining cells of this follicle change to form what is known as the corpus luteum. This change is stimulated by a pituitary hormone called luteinizing hormone (LH). The corpus luteum functions as a source of still another hormone (progesterone). This hormone also stimulates the lining of the uterus, or endometrium, to further its preparations for receiving the fertilized egg.

The lining of the uterus, after a period of days, is in full readiness for a fertilized egg. If the implantation of a fertilized egg has not taken place within approximately fourteen days following ovulation, the corpus luteum ceases to function. The lack of progesterone then leads to a disintegration of the endometrial tissue. The lining of the uterus gradually sloughs off, and some loss of blood occurs during the process. This passage of blood and lining cells of the uterus is menstruation. The average duration of the menstrual flow is between three and six days for most women. Variations from this are perfectly normal for some individuals, however.

Following menstruation, the lining of the uterus returns to a quiescent or resting state until stimulation by endocrine secretions initiates the cycle once again and another ovulation occurs. The average woman has a menstrual period approximately every twenty-eight days, but variation in length of time between menstrual periods is normal. For some women it is less than twenty-eight days, and for others it is longer.

There are many misconceptions about menstruation. Beliefs that menstruation is a sickness and that the woman should not exercise during her period are common misconceptions.

Menarche. The first menses, for the average girl, occur between twelve and fourteen years of age; but menstruation may start as early as the ninth year or as late as the seventeenth or eighteenth. Menstruation is only one indication of the onset of puberty. Enlargement of the pelvis, filling out of the breasts, and the appearance of pubic and axillary hair offer physical evidence that the girl is maturing.

The importance of properly preparing a girl for the first menses needs to be understood by all parents. The emotional effect of a first menstrual flow on an uninformed girl can be severe. The possibility of poor adjustment to the menstrual process is reduced by providing sound information before the onset of the menstrual periods.

Dysmenorrhea. Painful menstruation, or dysmenorrhea, is a problem to some women. Much can be done to alleviate this difficulty by developing proper attitudes concerning the normal function of menstruation and by seeking the assistance of a physician to correct remediable defects.

Possible indications of a condition that needs correction are prolonged menstrual flow, irregularity in appearance of the menstrual period, and leukorrhea (a whitish discharge between periods). These symptoms do not always indicate malfunction, but it is advisable to seek the advice of a physician when they occur. They are sometimes caused by infections or malignant growths, and in such a case early treatment is important.

Menopause. Whereas puberty is the beginning of the occurrence of the menstrual cycle, menopause is the period during which the decrease and cessation of menstruation occur. A gradual decrease in the function of the ovaries is the main characteristic of the menopause, or climacteric.

The cessation of ovulation means the conclusion of the childbearing period. Menopause occurs in a majority of women sometime between the ages of forty-five and fifty. Most women have no general disturbance in body function. However, emotional strain is a problem for some during this period of change. Poor attitudes regarding the change and an inadequate understanding of what is taking place are factors that contribute to the difficulties experienced by some women. Assistance by a gynecologist or family physician can be extremely helpful to a woman who experiences bodily disturbances due to endocrine imbalance.

In making and maintaining good adjustments in sexual relations it is important for the woman to understand that the end of the childbearing period does not mean the termination of normal sexual relations.

Unsatisfactory marriages

A most important step that could be taken to reduce unsatisfactory marriages and their end product, divorce, is to improve the selection of marriage partners. The discussion in Chapter 4 concerning choosing a life partner should receive the careful consideration of every person who sincerely desires a happy marriage. Marriages are terminated in the divorce court because husband and wife fail to establish a mutually satisfactory relationship which they deem worth continuing. It is unfortunate that so many couples come to this conclusion. Just as unfortunate, or perhaps even more so in many instances, are the marriages in which individuals fail to attain a mutually desirable relationship and yet continue to remain together under extremely trying conditions over long periods of time.

It is unduly optimistic to expect every married couple to make all the adjustments discussed earlier in this chapter. It is too much to expect every marriage to be a completely happy and satisfying relationship for both partners. However, it is reasonable to expect all individuals who plan to marry to be prepared adequately for such an important undertaking.

Those who seek to escape from an unsatisfactory marriage through a divorce are not necessarily repudiating marriage. The fact that approximately one out of eight married women has been married previously is an indication that these women are not rejecting marriage because of one unsuccessful venture.

HELP FOR THOSE WHO NEED IT

The trend toward establishing more qualified marriage counseling services offers hope in decreasing the problem of unsatisfactory marriages. These services provide help for many marriage partners who are having difficulties. Some couples are unable to work out all their own problems without the aid of trained personnel. They need help in discovering the obstacles to successful marriage and in planning how to surmount them.

The need for qualified personnel to provide the required type of counseling service presents a problem. Many who offer such services are not qualified. Instead of providing assistance, these counselors further complicate the difficulties confronting the marriage partners.

An increase in marriage clinics on college campuses offers to many students a readily available source of qualified assistance.

Following is a partial list of nationally known agencies furnishing information about persons or organizations qualified to provide marriage counseling services:

American Association of Marriage Counselors, Inc., 104 East 40th St., New York 16, New York

American Institute of Family Relations, 5287 Sunset Blvd., Los Angeles 27, California

Family Service Association of America, 215 Fourth Ave., New York 3, New York

National Association for Mental Health, Inc., 10 Columbus Circle, New York 19, New York

Planned Parenthood Federation of America, Inc., 501 Madison Ave., New York 22, New York

DIVORCE

Marriage is not fulfilling its purpose if all possible resources are exhausted and the relationship continues to be unsatisfactory. To desert a mate, to separate informally without dissolving a partnership that really is nonexistent, or to take a new mate without legally ending a former partnership is not a feasible solution if the sanctity of marriage is to be maintained.

Divorce, as a commonly accepted means of terminating unsuccessful marriages, needs to be understood by members of society.

The following statement by Kingsley Davis [3] points out the necessity for understanding all aspects of divorce:

Since divorce is an old institution and is embedded in the social structure in countless ways, there already exist agencies for handling its different aspects. First, divorce is a legal matter, with an elaborate legal machinery and a traditional legal philosophy for handling it. Second, it is a cultural and statistical fact, with fluctuations in time which respond to concurrent economic and social changes. Third, it is an emotional and personal process, with psychologic and psychiatric ramifications. Finally, it is a moral fact, with official and unofficial attitudes toward it that are mutually opposed. All these aspects must be kept in mind if divorce is to be understood.

Divorce is not an easy way out. The individual who assumes that a divorce provides a simple solution to an unsatisfactory marriage can be badly mistaken. Many factors complicate the adjustments required by the termination of a marriage partnership. A few of these factors are considered in the following paragraphs.

Policies regarding divorce vary widely among various religious groups. Some religious codes do not recognize divorce. For some individuals the church position in regard to divorce and remarriage proves to be an insurmountable obstacle.

Alimony payments can constitute a severe handicap to future adjustments by the man. Paying for a past mistake while attempting to make a new adjustment makes the latter extremely difficult.

The task of caring for children, unfortunate victims of an unsatisfactory marriage, presents one of the most difficult aspects of the adjustment following divorce. There is no single solution for the relationship between a divorced couple and their children. Each couple choosing divorce must come to some decision concerning their children. At best this is a difficult decision.

Finally, the individual has to make his personal adjustment to a society in which he has participated previously as a member of a marriage partnership. Examination of our society shows that it is constructed primarily around the activities of married couples and their families. The adjustment to society without the benefit of the marriage partner is more difficult than many persons anticipate. This problem is a distinct handicap to those whose marriage partnership has been characterized by frequent associations with other married couples. The felt need for a partner to satisfy the demands of a couple, or family, society induces some to seek a new mate.

Individuals who do not marry

The importance of planning for marriage has been stressed in the preceding pages. In addition, it is desirable to consider the importance of planning for life as an unmarried person. Some people do not marry and must therefore make adjustments as single individuals in an adult society organized basically around family groups. Some unmarried persons adjust in a completely satisfactory manner. Others are unable to accept their status as unmarried individuals and therefore fail to make desirable adjustments.

The factors that determine why the individual has not married are important in determining his ability to make the adjustment. The most frequently stated reasons for failure to marry are [7, 19]:

Unhappy home experiences during childhood

Failure to achieve emotional independence

³ Kingsley Davis, "Divorce and Its Effects," in Morris Fishbein and Ruby Jo Reeves Kennedy (eds.): *Modern Marriage and Family Living*, Oxford University Press, New York, 1957, p. 101.

Inadequate development of love pattern—homosexuality

Unwillingness to accept obligations involved in marriage

Failure to meet members of the opposite sex

Failure to interest the opposite sex

Failure to take advantage of opportunities to marry

Careers and education delaying marriage too long

Physical or psychological defects

Those who desire marriage but fail to find a mate are most likely to have difficulty in making adjustments as unmarried adults. Persons who desire marriage should recognize some of the obstacles confronting them. It may be necessary to move to another geographical location in order to overcome the uneven distribution of the sexes. The occupation and also activities during leisure time determine the frequency with which eligible members of the opposite sex are encountered. Changing the occupation may be impractical, but planning for new leisure-time activities is advisable. A person who desires a mate should take advantage of every possible opportunity to meet eligible members of the opposite sex (see page 108, Chapter 4).

Those who do not marry have adjustments to make. There are no socially sanctioned sexual outlets for the unmarried in our culture. For this reason, satisfaction of the sex drive poses one of the major adjustment problems. The unmarried may achieve a normal satisfaction of their affectional needs through relationships with other members of their family group or with friends. They can direct their attention toward a successful career and achieve security in this manner. They can make a contribution to society by devoting a portion of their time to service clubs or charitable organizations.

Summary

Marriage is or soon will be a concern of most college students. Each of you expects your marriage to be successful. Successful marriage, however, is more than a matter of expectation. Successful marriage depends upon choosing the right partner and then making adjustments in areas such as getting along with one another, mutual friends, recreation, in-law relationships, family income, religion, children, and sex relations.

One significant aspect of good sexual adjustment in marriage is an understanding of the structure and function of the reproductive systems. In addition, it is essential either to have or to develop wholesome attitudes about sex relations and to appreciate the contribution that a good adjustment in this area can make to a happy marriage.

Persons who are unable to resolve problems that arise in their marriage relationships may need assistance from qualified marriage counselors. They should not hesitate to seek such assistance to save a marriage threatened by adjustment problems too difficult for them to resolve by themselves.

Persons who do not marry are confronted with difficulties because our society is predominantly focused on activities of married persons. The lack of socially sanctioned outlets for the sex drive may also make it difficult for the unmarried. Those who desire to marry should take advantage of opportunities to meet members of the opposite sex in order to improve their chances of finding a marriage partner.

Success in marriage is not automatic. You should prepare yourself for marriage just as extensively as you prepare for your chosen vocation. Tact, intelligence, respect for one's partner, and a sincere desire to succeed in marriage are basic to adjustment in life's most important partnership.

Suggested readings

1. Bee, Lawrence L.: *Marriage and Family Relations: An Interdisciplinary Approach,* Harper & Brothers, New York, 1959.
2. Bernard, Jessie, Helen E. Buchanan, and William M. Smith, Jr.: *Dating, Mating and Marriage,* Howard Allen, Inc., Cleveland, 1958.
3. Blood, Robert O., Jr., and Donald M. Wolfe: *Husbands and Wives: The Dynamics of Married Living,* Free Press, Glencoe, Ill., 1960.
4. Bossard, James H. S., and Eleanor Stoker Boll: *One Marriage, Two Faiths,* The Ronald Press Company, New York, 1957.
5. Bossard, James H. S., and Eleanor Stoker Boll: *Why Marriages Go Wrong,* The Ronald Press Company, New York, 1958.
6. Bossard, James H. S., and Eleanor Stoker Boll: *The Girl That You Marry,* Macrea Smith, Philadelphia, 1960.
7. Bowman, Henry A.: *Marriage for Moderns,* 4th ed., McGraw-Hill Book Company, Inc., 1960.
8. Cavan, Ruth S.: *American Marriage: A Way of Life,* Thomas Y. Crowell Company, New York, 1959.
9. Christopherson, Victor A., Joseph S. Vandiver, and Marie N. Krueger: "The Married College Student," *Marriage and Family Living,* 22:122–128, May, 1960.
10. Duvall, Evelyn M., and Reuben Hill: *Being Married,* Association Press, New York, 1960.
11. Duvall, Sylvanus: *Before You Marry,* new rev. ed., Association Press, New York, 1959.
12. Fishbein, Morris, and Ruby Jo Reeves Kennedy (eds.): *Modern Marriage and Family Living,* Oxford University Press, New York, 1957.
13. Glick, Paul C.: *American Families,* John Wiley & Sons, Inc., New York, 1957.
14. Henry, David: " 'Maturity is the Key' to Successful College Marriages," *U.S. News and World Report,* 48:86–89, June 6, 1960.
15. Hill, Reuben, J. Mayone Stycos, and Kurt W. Black: *The Family and Population Control,* University of North Carolina Press, Chapel Hill, N.C., 1959.
16. Jacobson, Paul H.: *American Marriage and Divorce,* Rinehart and Company, Inc., New York, 1959.
17. Kinsey, Alfred C., and others: *Sexual Behavior in the Human Male,* W. B. Saunders Company, Philadelphia, 1948.
18. Kinsey, Alfred C., and others: *Sexual Behavior in the Human Female,* W. B. Saunders Company, Philadelphia, 1953.
19. Landis, Judson T., and Mary G. Landis: *Building a Successful Marriage,* 3d ed., Prentice-Hall, Inc., Englewood Cliffs, N.J., 1958.
20. McClure, James H.: "Taking the Mystery out of Menopause," *Today's Health,* 38:48–49, November, 1960.
21. Mead, Margaret: "A New Look at Early Marriages," *U.S. News and World Report,* 48:80–86, June 6, 1960.
22. Merrill, Francis E.: *Courtship and Marriage,* rev. ed., Henry Holt and Company, Inc., New York, 1959.
23. National Council on Family Relations: *Marriage and Family Living.* (Quarterly journal)
24. Peterson, James A.: *Education for Marriage,* Charles Scribner's Sons, New York, 1956.
25. Pike, James A.: *If You Marry Outside Your Faith,* Harper & Brothers, New York, 1954.
26. Rutledge, Aaron L.: *Responsible Marriage and Family Living: A Text with Adapted Readings,* Harcourt, Brace and Company, Inc., New York, 1960.
27. Stone, Hannah M., and Abraham Stone: *A Marriage Manual,* rev. ed., Simon and Schuster, Inc., New York, 1952.
28. Whitman, Howard: "Six Ways to Strengthen Your Marriage," *Today's Health,* 37:19–21, March, 1959.
29. "Would You Want Your Daughter . . . ?" Symposium on Mixed Marriage, *U.S. News and World Report,* 49:116–119, May 9, 1960.

SIX

Preparing for responsibilities of parenthood

There is nothing in the life of normal men and women more important to them or to society than the achievement of healthy, happy parenthood. Mothers and fathers are the guardians of our way of life and architects of the future. This was true in the past, and it is true now. Present-day young men and women can and perhaps will do a superior job of being the parents of tomorrow. If traditions are to be maintained and our way of life preserved, they will have to do a superior job.

Most young people marry because they are in love. They wish to establish a happy home. They want children. They hope to rear their families so as to be a credit to themselves, to their community, and to the nation. These noble aspirations can be fulfilled. Understanding children and disciplining them wisely are important, but they are not innate characteristics of parenthood. Such achievements are the result of purposeful and diligent effort.

Facts about readiness for parenthood, human conception, the health aspects of pregnancy, childbirth, the postnatal care of infants, and child behavior should be studied. Such studies need not stop with infancy and childhood. They should continue on through the physical, mental, social, and spiritual growth and development periods, including that interesting and often bewildering state called adolescence.

To stimulate an interest in being an informed parent, and to satisfy the need for such information, professional groups have produced a wealth of pertinent material. Many excellent books, pamphlets, motion pictures, and slides, as well as radio and television programs, are available to parents. Health agencies, state departments of education, colleges, and universities offer guidance in accepted methods of child rearing. There is a need for parent education, and, in a general sense, this need is being met.

An important fact about marriage and parenthood, which sooner or later makes itself known, is that the more insight young men and women have into the status of marriage and parenthood, the happier and more secure their marriage can be made. For those who plan to marry and who want a reasonable assurance of success as parents, a background of facts about the following subjects can be helpful:

What are the personal qualifications for successful parenthood?

What factors indicate a readiness for parenthood?

How does conception take place?

What are the most significant aspects of pregnancy?

How is a baby born?

What care should be provided for infant and mother during the postnatal period?

How should children be reared?

Qualifications for successful parenthood

A factor favorable to effective and successful parenthood, motherhood in particular, is the nutritional status of the mother-to-be. Her physical health augmented by sound nutrition helps to lay the foundation for a healthy baby. Another significant qualification for happy, successful parenthood is emotional maturity on the part of both the husband and the wife. This means that each mate possesses the ability and the experience to meet situations of family life in a way that ensures happiness and increases feelings of love and security for all concerned. At the time of marriage few young persons are fully mature emotionally. This, however, does not mean that they cannot attain such a state. To mature emotionally requires information about growth and development, time for trial and error, patience with one's self and others, and practice in controlling emotions.

Emotional maturity as a requisite to successful parenthood includes such matters as [3]:

ADAPTABILITY. Each mate realizes that his willingness as well as his ability to adapt himself readily to a change of routine or well-laid plans is essential to peace and harmony in the home.

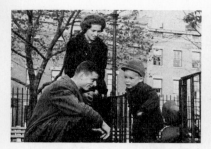

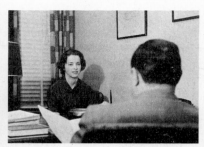

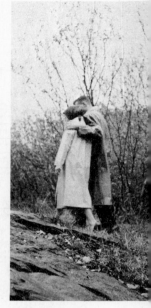

The decision to start a family is one of the most important any young married couple may make . . .

and the choice of a physician to give continuous advice is another serious consideration. Both husband and wife are concerned . . .

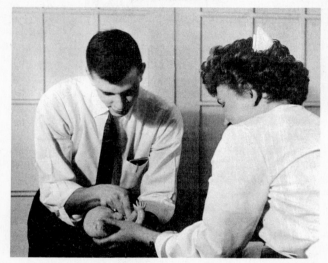

for the prenatal well-being of the prospective mother, for whom walking and other mild exercise is important . . .

and they learn the practical details of parenthood from those with professional experience. Looking forward to the baby's arrival . . .

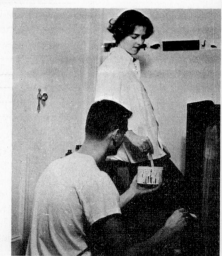

they gradually reorganize the household . . .

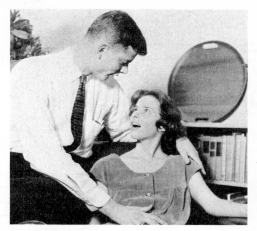

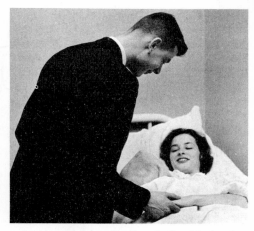

and throughout the pregnancy, in simple, natural ways, they prepare themselves emotionally. Thus with a thoughtful approach to parenthood . . .

a deeply satisfying family relationship begins.

COOPERATIVENESS. Working together as a team by helping to achieve what each partner desires for himself as well as for the children is certain to achieve success in family life.

GOOD JUDGMENT. Sound decisions based on long-range values are quite likely to give feelings of security to all members of the family.

INDEPENDENCE. This means that both mates have a strong desire for independence from parents and others. Such an attitude, however, does not preclude a feeling of interdependence between husband and wife; successful parenthood is a team affair.

KINDNESS. The emotionally mature person realizes that feelings of kindness and gentleness between mates and children are reliable methods of holding a family together.

SENSE OF HUMOR. The ability to see the funny side and to smile at most irritations is a factor basic to happy family living.

SHARING. This means a willingness of mates to enrich one another's lives and the lives of their children by giving cheerfully of their energy, time, love, and talents.

SOUND SEX ADJUSTMENT. Each mate realizes that the highly interpersonal contact of sexual relations should always be on the basis of mutual desire, free from the immature attitude of self-love expressed through the medium of the genitalia.

A harmonious blending of these characteristics is essential to successful parenthood. They are attainable for anyone who consciously works toward achieving them.

Readiness for parenthood

Most young married people want children. This desire is commendable. Marriage counselors agree that children increase the opportunities for establishing a permanent and happy marriage.

There are a number of points of view as to when young married couples should start their family. For example, the feeling among some religious groups that families should start soon after marriage is a strong one. Then there are those who believe that waiting for a year or more while early adjustments are being made will add to the strength and security of the future family. Others adhere to the view that both the wife and the husband should work for a year or more, thus adding greater financial security before starting their family. Still others think that careers are more important and the family function is postponed indefinitely [3].

The problem of when to have the first baby belongs to the husband and to the wife. The decision they make will be influenced by their religious belief, the strength of their desire for children, their income, and their health.

A point that should also be considered is the cost of having a baby. The prenatal care of the mother, the layette, the delivery of the baby, the hospital expenses, the postnatal care of infant and mother, and the services of a pediatrician for a year or more must be carefully estimated. The young couple who early in their marriage learn to budget their income and spend wisely and who discover that inexpensive entertainment can be fun will handle the financial problem of having children with little difficulty.

Conception

Human conception is one of nature's greatest achievements. The physical act resulting in conception reaches a climax when the male deposits between 200 million and 600 million spermatozoa at the entrance of the uterus of the female. Under favorable conditions, these active, microscopic cells begin a fishlike movement which propels them through the cervix and the cavity of the uterus and into the fallopian tubes. The journey is likely to produce many casualties. Sperm that survive keep moving through the oviducts until they meet the ovum. At first the egg appears to resist their advance; however, after repeated attacks, one or more sperm break through the weakened wall of the egg. One sperm reaches the nucleus of the ovum and fertilization, or conception, takes place.

After fertilization, cell division within the egg begins. After several days of continuous dividing, the new combination of cells has moved slowly along the oviduct to a specially prepared lining in the wall of the uterus. Here the embryo comes to rest, to be nourished and protected for approximately nine calendar months.

SEX DETERMINATION

The method nature uses to determine the sex of the fetus has been a subject of specu-
lation for centuries. Before modern science attacked the problem, all sorts of fantastic beliefs prevailed. For example, in France it was accepted that conception before midnight produced a boy and after midnight a girl. The Babylonian Talmud informed parents-to-be that the sex of the child depended upon the parent who could generate the greatest passion. There still persists, in the minds of many people, the idea that diet, the moon, acidity and alkalinity, and hot and cold weather are influences that determine the sex of the child.

It is believed by modern scientists that sex is established at the moment conception occurs and that the male reproductive cell is the determiner. The genes in a special pair of chromosomes are responsible for the sex of the fetus. In the female the chromosomes are always XX; in the male they are always XY. If the ovum, carrying the X factor, is fertilized by an X-bearing sperm, the child will be a girl. If the sperm carries the Y chromosome, the child will be a boy. In other words, the Y chromosome is the determinant.

These data firmly establish the fact that the sex of the child is determined by the father and not by the mother.

Health aspects of pregnancy

Shortly after the embryo becomes implanted in the uterus, nature imparts this fact to the mother by a series of physical and emotional changes. Through the centuries, women have come to accept the following as signs of pregnancy [13]:

EMOTIONAL CHANGES. The mother is easily upset over minor disturbances. This is the earliest indication that she may be pregnant.

CESSATION OF MENSTRUATION. The failure of the menstrual period is accepted universally as an indication of pregnancy. (There are other causes of cessation, which include emotional disturbances, mental illness, exposure to cold, and cysts in the ovary.)

MORNING SICKNESS. This symptom usually occurs about the fifth or sixth week after conception. It is common in more than half of all pregnancies.

CHANGES IN THE BREASTS. Usually by the fifth week the breasts begin to increase in size and firmness. They become tender to the touch and show dark about the nipples.

CHANGES IN SIZE OF ABDOMEN. During the third or fourth month, the abdomen shows an increase in size.

SENSATION OF MOVEMENT. About the fourth or fifth month, movement of the baby can be observed.

FREQUENCY OF URINATION. As the baby grows, pressure on the bladder increases, resulting in an increased desire to urinate.

It is obvious that the first three signs indicate a possible pregnancy and the other four more or less confirm it. However, to leave no doubt, the woman consults her physician. Aided by modern science, a physician can determine with reasonable accuracy whether or not a woman is pregnant. There are at least 40 tests for pregnancy available. The majority of these tests require the injection of a small amount of urine of the patient into a female rat, mouse, rabbit, or frog. If there is a pregnancy, the injection causes swelling, congestion, and hemorrhage of the ovaries and a premature maturation of the ovarian follicles of the animal. There is also a variety of chemical tests, such as Voge's test. In this test urine of the patient is treated with bromine water. If the fluid turns pink, a pregnancy is indicated. An interesting test suggested by Kleitman[1] involves body temperature. Failure of body temperature to drop 0.5 to 0.7°F just before the beginning of the normal cycle of menstruation is an accurate sign of pregnancy.

In late pregnancy the fetal heartbeat can be detected by the use of a stethoscope.

CHOICE OF A PHYSICIAN

The choice of a physician is important. He will guide the mother through the prenatal period. He will deliver the baby. He will probably give postnatal care to both mother and child, and he may be called upon to counsel the parents on rearing their progeny. It is not unusual for the family physician to render these services; however, should serious complications develop during pregnancy or at the time of delivery, the added service of an obstetrician can prove of great importance.

It is possible that the family has no physician or is new in the community. If this is the case, the mother may find helpful counsel at the nearest approved hospital, local health center, or county medical society. For further information relative to choosing a physician, see Chapter 10.

PRENATAL CARE OF THE MOTHER

During the period of pregnancy, each member of the family assumes responsi-

[1] Nathaniel Kleitman, "The Sleep Cycle," *American Journal of Nursing*, 60:677–679, May, 1960.

bilities a bit different from routine family life. The father experiences a stronger protective drive. He usually finds it brings greater happiness to himself and to his wife when he sublimates his sex urges, particularly during the latter part of the pregnancy. The wife, while she may dream about and plan for the baby, does not neglect her husband. She makes him feel that he, too, is important.

As time passes, she finds her weight increasing, her breasts becoming larger and more sensitive, and her walk or gait changing; and she may experience some degree of morning nausea. After these early adjustments have been made, the mother-to-be generally enjoys a high degree of well-being. To ensure maximum health and happiness and to give the fetus its best chances to survive and grow, the prospective mother seeks and follows the advice of her physician in such matters as diet, exercise, travel, sexual intercourse, shoes, wearing apparel, smoking, drinking, the layette, and plans for the delivery. It is common practice for family physicians or obstetricians to provide their patients with a booklet of instructions covering these subjects. The teeth should be inspected frequently. Daily baths are encouraged. The wearing of high-heeled shoes may be dangerous; shoes having low, wide heels should be worn instead. Regular exercise such as light housework, walking, and swimming is encouraged. Automobile trips at high speed, over rough roads, or for long distances are discouraged. Sexual intercourse during the last two or three months of pregnancy usually is forbidden. Alcohol and smoking are usually looked on with disfavor, or their use is reduced or restricted. Apprehensive parents are told that it is impossible to "mark" the baby, and that the sex of the child cannot be accurately determined before birth.

COMPLICATIONS IN PREGNANCY

Most women enjoy normal health during pregnancy, and with proper medical care there is little risk in having a baby. Now and then, complications occur and should have immediate medical attention. A condition that often poses a problem for physician and patient alike is toxemia. This disease is characterized by a sudden increase in weight and rise in blood pressure and the presence of albumin in the urine. Other danger signals are severe persistent or recurring headaches, blurring of vision, spots before the eyes, puffiness of face, hands, and feet, a marked reduction in the amount of urine passed, general depression, and nausea and vomiting. These symptoms are believed to result from the mother's failure to effectively eliminate the waste products of the fetus. If all pregnant women received adequate medical care, the mortality rate for this disease would cease to be serious.

The Rh factor. It was not until 1941 that Levine, Katzin, and Burnham discovered the cause of a circulatory disorder which proved fatal to some infants. This cause is a protein substance in the blood, called the *Rh factor*. This condition is found in man and in the rhesus monkey. It is from the monkey that the symbol Rh was derived. About 85 per cent of the white population and 95 per cent of the Negroes of this country have the Rh factor and are known as Rh-positive. Those who do not have it are called Rh-negative.

As is shown in the accompanying figure, difficulty arises only when the mother is Rh-negative and the father Rh-positive. Even then, it occurs only if the baby has inherited the father's Rh-positive blood. As the end of pregnancy approaches, a few red blood cells of the baby escape into the blood of the mother. If the baby's blood has the Rh protein and the mother's blood does not, the blood of the mother is likely to develop antibodies to counteract the foreign protein introduced by her baby. These antibodies are very small and pass easily from the mother back to her baby. As the antibodies accumulate in the blood stream of the infant, they produce a violent reaction in the child's blood. This

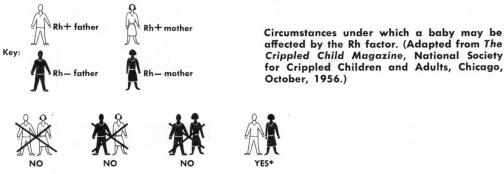

Key:

Rh+ father Rh+ mother
Rh— father Rh— mother

Circumstances under which a baby may be affected by the Rh factor. (Adapted from *The Crippled Child Magazine*, National Society for Crippled Children and Adults, Chicago, October, 1956.)

NO   NO   NO   YES*

*Only one out of 25 babies of Rh+ fathers and Rh— mothers is affected. Of these, one out of twenty suffers brain damage.

condition in the child is called erythroblastosis fetalis. The disease may result in severe brain damage or may be fatal to the infant unless he receives a transfusion of Rh-negative blood shortly after birth. Fortunately it is possible for the physician to test the blood of the mother during the prenatal period in order to determine the extent of the concentration of antibodies and to take steps to counteract any pending danger to the fetus.

A woman who has given birth to a child with erythroblastosis should follow the advice of her physician concerning future pregnancies. He may recommend that pregnancy be avoided for a period of several years. This time interval should be long enough for the antibodies in her blood to disappear. A physician can determine when the antibody-producing cells have ceased to be active.

HOME OR HOSPITAL DELIVERY

If she had her choice, every woman would want her baby to be born in the safest possible place. There is no safer or more convenient place than an approved modern hospital. Most physicians prefer hospital delivery because nurses, technicians, specialists, modern medical equipment, and drugs are immediately available. Not only does the physician benefit, but the mother and baby have greater comfort and security because of these modern facilities. An approved hospital will always have on display a certificate of approval by the American Medical Association or by the American College of Surgeons or American Hospital Association. Such a certificate is issued yearly.

Some women prefer to have their babies born at home. In England and Wales, 45 per cent of babies are delivered in the home; in the United States, 13 per cent. There are things to be said in favor of having the baby born at home. Home deliveries can make the occasion a family affair. The baby is born into the family group and is accepted at once. However, births taking place in the home require special precautions for the protection of both mother and child. Should complications arise, a home delivery can prove unsatisfactory, expensive, and even dangerous to both mother and child.

The birth of the baby

Birth is a natural process. To the baby, it happens but once; therefore, it must go well. To the mother, bearing her first child can be difficult, but, under wise and skillful handling, her preparation, labor, and delivery can be accomplished with a minimum of discomfort. Modern medicine makes the birth of a baby a far cry from childbirth of 50 years ago. Today skillful physicians, the wise use of special drugs, and the modern hospital provide the mother with an assurance that she can deliver her baby with little danger. It may be of interest to note that in the near future hypnosis may offer the possibility of painless childbirth.

To the father, his first child brings mixed emotions of pride and relief. To the physician, there is the great satisfaction of bringing into the world a new personality and at the same time providing maximum protection to both mother and child.

As the date of delivery grows near, the mother's discomfort may heighten. Visits to her physician increase in frequency. She is tired of waiting and looks forward to the birth of her baby. The first indication that the baby is ready to be born may be any one or all of the following:

Abdominal pains, appearing infrequently and at irregular intervals

Rupture of the "water bag," which has surrounded the baby

The "show," a discharge of thick mucus from the vagina

The appearance of any one of these signs is sufficient to warrant calling the physician. In the case of a woman having her first baby, sixteen to twenty hours may pass before the child is born. From the moment the fetus indicates an intent to leave the uterus until it is entirely free from its mother's body, the physician deals with three stages of labor.

The first stage is characterized by contractions in the uterus. These are identified by weak and irregular pains, which usually start in the lower back and move around to the lower part of the abdomen. These pains may occur every fifteen to forty minutes. As this stage progresses, the contractions speed up in frequency and intensity. The first stage of labor comes to an end when the cervix is sufficiently dilated to permit movement of the baby down the birth canal.

The second stage consists in the actual passage of the baby from the body. It is shorter than the first stage, generally lasting from thirty minutes to two hours. The second phase of labor begins when the cervix is fully dilated. If the sac of water in which the baby lived in the uterus has not broken, the physician breaks it. The uterine muscles begin more forceful contraction, and coupled with the strong contraction of the abdominal muscles, labor begins in earnest.

The patient may be assured that her physician will do everything within his understanding and skill to make the experience of giving birth as painless and as safe as possible.

The second stage of labor ends when the baby is free from the body of the mother.

After the baby has been born, the umbilical cord is tied and severed. The physician clears the baby's throat, and, if it has not cried, he administers a gentle pat. As a precaution against possible disease such as gonorrhea, a weak solution of silver nitrate is placed in the child's eyes.

The final stage of labor for the mother consists in expelling the placenta and other membranes from the uterus and birth canal. Its duration is five to thirty minutes. This ends the birth process. The mother is very tired, the father is grateful and relieved, and everyone is happy.

Some fathers register temporary disappointment if the first child is a girl, although it is usually only a short time until they are completely captivated by the new daughter. There is a somewhat greater chance of having a boy than of having a girl: [2]

Although according to the law of chance, there should be 100 boy babies born for every 100 girl babies, nature produces a slight excess of boys, and at birth there are actually about 105 boys for every 100 girls. The sperm

[2] Edith L. Potter, *Fundamentals of Human Reproduction*, McGraw-Hill Book Company, Inc., New York, 1948, p. 49.

cells containing Y chromosomes may be a little more active, or a little more successful in penetrating the wall of an ovum than are those with X chromosomes. No evidence, however, has ever been obtained which satisfactorily explains the preponderance of males over females at birth.

After the baby has been born, the mother is kept in the delivery room for fifteen or twenty minutes to be observed for unfavorable reactions. When her physician is satisfied that she is making a normal recovery, she is returned to her room for a well-earned rest and sleep. It is not uncommon for her to have mild discomfort for a few hours after delivery.

The length of time before the mother may leave her bed and walk varies with her condition. The day following a normal delivery patients are often permitted to sit up and later to walk about the room. Most obstetric patients return to their homes within four or five days after delivery.

Upon returning home, the mother is advised to keep up the convalescent attitude for two or possibly three weeks. This is a temporary health safeguard. Many women become depressed when they must resume household responsibilities immediately after returning home and at the same time assume the entire care of the new baby. For her future health, as well as her baby's, it is important that the mother resume home duties gradually and that she take regular periods of rest each day. The time that must elapse before she returns to social functions, automobile driving, and strenuous exercises varies with the individual. Special exercises are important to her recovery and will be ordered by her physician. Sexual intercourse usually is not resumed until after the physician declares her to be ready for it.

To the mother who cannot breast-feed her baby, menstruation may return as early as six weeks after the birth. If, however, the child is breast-fed, the first menstruation usually begins three to four months after the birth. Breast feeding has a number of advantages over bottle feeding. For example, in breast feeding the infant continues to be closely linked to the nutrition of the mother; an adequate supply of mother's milk usually ensures nutrients needed by the infant; it is also a simple procedure; and there is a satisfying emotional reaction for both infant and mother, which is significant particularly in the growth and development of the baby.

It is also important for the future well-being of both mother and child to establish the practice of having an annual health examination. Such a practice has strong backing from the family physician and the pediatrician. City and county health departments express their approval by providing for frequent child health conferences. All mothers in the community are encouraged to bring their babies for medical examinations and health supervision. Nutritional needs, health practices, mouth health, immunization against diphtheria, tetanus, poliomyelitis, and whooping cough, and vaccination for smallpox are among the major services given children up to five years of age. Many expectant mothers take advantage of the prenatal service offered by public health departments. These conferences are primarily for mothers unable to afford private medical care.

MULTIPLE BIRTH

Twins and triplets are of never-ending interest to most people. What are the chances of multiple birth? Potter[3] says:

In one out of every eighty-five or ninety human pregnancies, more than one baby develops within the uterus. It has been calculated that twins occur about once in every eighty-eight pregnancies, triplets about once in 8,000 and quadruplets about once every 500,000. Prior to 1940, there were approximately forty-five seemingly authentic reports of quintuplet births, the Dionnes being the most famous. According to Professor Horatio

[3] *Ibid.*, p. 50.

Newman, who has spent many years studying multiple birth, sextuplets have been recorded by reliable observers on only four occasions, and none of the children survived. No well substantiated case of septuplets or pregnancy with a greater number of offspring has ever been reported.

At some time during her early pregnancy the mother-to-be is sure to ask her physician, "What are my chances of having twins?" No one can answer this question with accuracy. Authorities agree that out of every eighty-eight human births, two babies are delivered during the same birth period. Although this results in a large number of twins, it gives no assurance that twins will be born in any specific case.

Multiple births consist primarily of fraternal and identical twins. About three-fourths of twins born are the result of the fertilization of two eggs that have been simultaneously discharged from the ovaries, thus producing fraternal twins. They may be of the same or of opposite sex. Fraternal twins are independent individuals, each with his own hereditary traits. Identical twins or triplets occur less frequently. They are the result of a single fertilized egg, which divides to form two or more independent and separate individuals. Identical twins are always of the same sex, with identical hereditary characteristics. Occasionally Siamese twins are born. They are identical twins who have not completely separated.

PREMATURE BIRTH

Despite wishes, calendars, formulas, and science, no one can predict with accuracy the day a baby will be born. If the time of conception is unknown, physicians usually add seven days to the first day of the last normal menstruation and then subtract three months. This will not pinpoint the date, but it will be very close. If the exact date of conception is known, by adding 266 days one can predict with reasonable accuracy the day labor will occur.

Regardless of predictions and precautions, babies are born prematurely. In this country there are about 150,000 such babies born each year. A baby whose birth weight is less than 5½ pounds or who is severely underdeveloped at birth is usually classified as premature.

Premature births have a number of causes. In many cases the cause can be controlled, while in others neither the physician nor the patient can prevent what happens. A woman who wishes to come to a normal term of delivery must exercise extreme care during the last three months of pregnancy. In spite of precautions and good care, premature births occur. Accidents and illnesses may precipitate them. Some of the typical causes of premature births are falls on stairways, on slippery floors, and in bathtubs. Conditions such as an Rh-negative mother and an Rh-positive father, pregnancy toxemia, high blood pressure, heart defects, and kidney diseases can also cause premature births.

A premature birth may take place anywhere. Outside a hospital this can, and usually does, produce great excitement. Until a physician arrives, the most important precautions to remember are:

FIRST. Keep the baby warm. A constant room temperature of 80°F is best. An incubator can be improvised from a bassinet or basket, or even a cardboard carton, lined with a large blanket and heated by hot-water bottles wrapped in towels.

SECOND. Keep the air moist by evaporating water in the room. Handle the baby as little as possible.

THIRD. If it becomes necessary to move a premature baby to a hospital, it is wise to obtain ambulance service. If an ambulance is not available, be sure that the baby is well-wrapped, placed in an improvised incubator, and transported to the hospital in a heat-regulated automobile.

From this it is not difficult to understand why 87 per cent of babies born in this country are delivered in hospitals.

Care of the newborn baby

Once the baby is safely home from the hospital, the new mother and father are usually all "ears and eyes" in their efforts to be good parents. The following selected items are considered to be important in the care of the new baby.

FOOD. In spite of the trend toward bottle-fed babies, breast feeding is still "high priority." Twelve to eighteen hours after birth, the infant is usually offered his first experience in breast feeding. He will not obtain much nourishment, but for his efforts he will receive a yellowish fluid, which is thought to give him protection against disease. This experience also serves to toughen the mother's nipples for the months of breast feeding ahead. While in the hospital, feeding the baby is generally done every three or four hours. At home the feeding schedule should conform to the baby's needs and desires. Some babies are hungry two hours after eating; others may go along for five hours before they want food. Most babies develop a regular schedule of feeding in about a month. During the first three months of life the bottle-fed baby should be held in an upright position while being fed. This tends to prevent middle-ear infection, which may result from getting milk into the nose and hence to the middle ear.

SLEEP. When a newborn baby is not eating, he is probably sleeping. This is normal.

CRYING. Many cartoons have been created depicting exhausted parents walking the floor with "junior" at three o'clock in the morning. This can happen, and it is far from funny. All new babies cry. It is a normal way of expressing certain feelings, and it also gives them exercise. However, crying that persists over ten or fifteen minutes should receive attention. It may be caused by hunger, gas pains, heat or cold, or uncomfortable diapers; sometimes he just needs to be loved.

BATHING. It has been found that daily bathing in clean, warm water, using a soft, warm cloth, keeps the baby clean and fresh. Diaper rash can usually be controlled by promptly changing soiled diapers, washing the body with warm water, and then applying oil or baby lotion to the parts most likely to be irritated. Bathing in a tub or specially prepared bathinet is usually postponed until the baby's umbilical-cord stump falls off. Also, in the case of a baby boy, a general bath is avoided until the circumcision has healed.

When the occasion arises, parents should feel free to consult their physician about the baby on such matters as:

Feeding schedule
Care of the circumcision
Cleaning the nose and ears
Shampooing the baby's hair
Clipping the baby's fingernails
Baby clothes for both day and night
Hygienic care of soiled diapers
When to take the baby out of doors
How to encourage him to exercise
Important things to do when he is ill
How to take a baby's temperature
What to do for convulsions
What supplies are necessary for preparing formula

Being a good parent requires knowledge of the baby's needs, skill in meeting these needs, and at all times letting him feel that he is wanted and is dearly loved [11].

Sterility

Because of inherited or acquired anomalies, it may be impossible for a man or a woman to produce a child. Most authorities agree that one out of nine marriages in this country is infertile. It is estimated that there are 2 million couples of child-

producing age who are without children.
Some of the common causes of sterility in men and women are the following:

Stricture or clogging of the fallopian tubes, which causes one-third of cases of sterility among women

Stricture of the vas deferens (male)

Postinfection state of the testicles or ovaries, which reduces or destroys their efficiency

Defective sperm, the most common defect of the male

Lack of erection—rare

Failure of testes to descend, which is also rare

Emotional factors

Perhaps the best security against a childless marriage is a thorough premarital medical examination. Objective tests and counsel by the physician are available to determine presence or absence of fertility in the male and in the female. It may be of interest to note that sterility is not necessarily permanent. With proper medical care many childless couples have been able to have families of their own.

Adoption of children

Should a couple enter into a marriage and find themselves unable to produce children, there is always the possibility of adoption. The adoption of children is becoming increasingly popular. However, owing to the great interest in adoptions, there is often but one child available for every ten couples who want to adopt a child. This shortage has led to illegal adoption practices. To ensure adequate protection for foster parent and child, many states have enacted adoption legislation. These enactments cover such procedures as permitting children to be legally adopted through independent action, or adoption through licensed agencies or by stepparents. The adoption of an illegitimate child by the natural father is also legal in many states.

Where can one find a child to adopt? The best plan is to go to a responsible licensed adoption or child-placing agency and place a request. State departments of public welfare and local councils of social agencies are prepared to give lists of licensed approved agencies. To avoid legal "headaches," it is best to choose an agency within one's own state.

The growth and development of children

To the average parent, the new baby is a wonderful, bewildering speck of humanity —not well understood, often spoiled, but always loved. It is one thing to marry and produce a child and another to bring that child to his rightful potential. Educators, scientists, and physicians are well aware of this fact, but sometimes parents are not. As a result, there has been no field more carefully studied for the benefit of parents and children than that of the physical, social, mental, and emotional growth and development of boys and girls.

Research studies indicate that parents worry needlessly because their child appears to be slow in growing. Children grow physically because of an innate tendency to do so. Growth is continuous, orderly, and at an individualized rate. It is possible to change the rate and direction of growth, but it is not always wise to do so. When a child's environment fails to provide adequate nutrition, physical activity, sleep, motivation, affection, and discipline, his growth can be markedly changed. Heredity is also a factor in the rate of growth and development of children.

THE THREE FIRSTS

All parents show great interest in the "three firsts" of their babies—the first word, the first tooth, and the first step.

The first word. The first clear verbalizing, such as "bye bye" and "ma ma," occurs by the fortieth week in most babies. At fifteen months, the vocabulary has increased to five or more words, including proper names. "Car car," "all gone," "bye bye," and other expressions are freely used by the year-and-a-half-old youngster. By the time the child is two, three-word sentences are normally achieved. At five he has a vocabulary of about two thousand words and uses them. The six-year-old youngster likes to use big words and enjoys speaking over the telephone. By the time the child reaches ten years, his language has become a tool and is used less to impress himself and others. Verbalization depends largely on temperament and example. The home environment and the speech of the parents tend to set the pattern. If a child is a late talker, he is only expressing his own rate of growth. At no time should he be hurried or placed in competition with other children. He should be given every chance to develop naturally [4].

The first tooth. The appearance of baby's first tooth is cause for great excitement in the average family. It is a lone front tooth that is usually the center of the excitement. It usually erupts by the sixth month. During the following two or three years, all the "baby" teeth (primary; or deciduous, teeth) erupt. From then on until about the sixth year, there is little obvious dental activity. Wise parents make a practice of having routine examinations of their child's mouth beginning as early as two or three years of age. Such procedures serve to acquaint the child with the dentist and the dentist with the oral health of the child. It can be a happy and profitable experience for both. Well-baby clinics conducted by local health departments have been a great boon to the oral health of children. In most communities, such clinics are available to all young children.

When the child is six years old, four significant teeth erupt. They are the first permanent teeth and are referred to as the six-year molars. These teeth are of major importance to the future mouth health of the child. They tend to hold the oral arch in shape while the deciduous teeth are being replaced by permanent teeth. Child, parent, and dentist should form a team to guard these teeth against decay or loss.

From the age of six on through the twelfth year, the child passes through a stage characterized by a mixture of baby and permanent teeth. He has both permanent and deciduous teeth and plenty of vacant spaces. After the twelfth year, he usually possesses all his permanent teeth except the third molars.

The age at which the teeth erupt is not as important as the sequence of eruption. Irregularity in the order of eruption can lead to irregularity in the position of the permanent teeth. A wise parent gives diligent care to the "baby" teeth and so aids nature in providing the child with good occlusion. Some children may show their first tooth as early as three months, and others will keep anxious relatives waiting an entire year. Tooth eruption is basically a matter of individual and family pattern and cannot be hurried [4].

The first step. As in the cases of delayed tooth eruption and delayed speech, there are children who are slow in beginning to walk. Locomotion should not be hurried, nor should the child be placed in competition. A baby will walk when he is ready to walk. By the end of the twelfth month, most children can walk if one hand is held. At fifteen months they are capable of taking a few steps alone. The average year-and-a-half-old child walks freely. By three years he walks erect and is sure of his movements. About the time he enters kindergarten, he walks with ease and has good control over his movements.

HEIGHT AND WEIGHT

Growth in height and weight are subjects of parental interest. Mothers and fathers

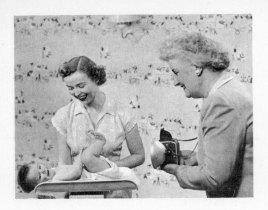

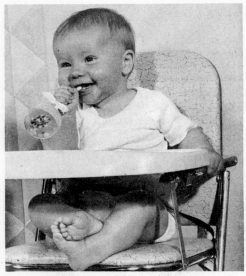

write and speak with great pride about the birth length and weight of their babies. The average newborn baby measures about 21 inches and weighs about 7 pounds. Throughout the period of infancy his growth is very rapid. For example, during the first year the average male child grows nearly 10 inches in height and triples his birth weight. However, nature does not continue as rapid a growth rate as this for any length of time. After two years, the rate of growth slows down and levels off. From then on to the tenth or eleventh year, the child experiences a much slower growth. Starting at about ten years, the growth in weight of the average girl increases in momentum until it reaches maximum acceleration at about the twelfth year. The average boy is slower and does not reach his greatest growth in weight until fourteen. From this time on growth in weight slows and then tends to remain stable in the early twenties. Growth in height reaches its maximum acceleration at about twelve for girls and at fourteen for boys. As with weight, the growth in height finally stops between the sixteenth and twenty-third year [4].

It is a source of pleasure to most children to know that they are growing taller and heavier. It is their business to grow, and they should be able to measure their gains. Unfortunately, there are no 100 per cent accurate height-weight standards.

An unusual system of assessing growth has been advanced by Dr. N. C. Wetzel. He called this appraisal form the "Grid for Evaluating Physical Fitness." By studying the charts of the Grid, it is noted that there are two sets of ruled lines. One set is for height and one for weight. By plotting one's height and weight, a physique channel is determined. The physique channels indicate body build and form the pattern by which one can chart the direction of the child's growth. A youngster who follows a given channel without deviation is following his own growth pattern. Should this growth

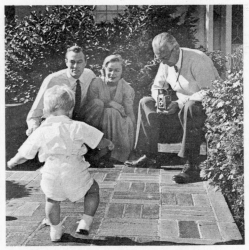

The first word, first tooth, and first step are significant events in the baby's development.

pattern deviate from the channel, it is indicative of an important change and the child should be examined by his physician. This gives the Grid a predictive value. A condition can be detected before it becomes a clinical case. The isodevelopmental lines help to chart the growth progress made by the child each year. They also show the speed of growth achieved. According to Wetzel, direction and speed of growth determine quality of growth.

NUTRITION

A child may be a prize product of heredity, good breeding, culture, and material wealth, but unless he has good nutrition, these factors will profit him little. The nutritional problems of infants and young children are best met by the teamwork of parents, physicians, and nutritionists. Such a team can ensure wholesome physical growth to children by providing a balance of nutrients such as protein, carbohydrates, fats, minerals, vitamins, and water. The daily diet of the growing child should include meat, butter, milk, eggs, citrus fruits or tomatoes, whole-grain cereals, green or yellow vegetables, and raw leafy vegetables in proper proportion. Occasionally, a physician will advise the taking of food supplements to ensure an adequate vitamin supply. Now and then he will withhold certain foods during the transient period of allergies.

Another significant factor in sound nutrition is the emotional climate at the dining table: it can set the pattern for good or poor nutritional practices. Parents who provide wholesome foods, a happy social experience, and good fellowship, well mixed with a leisurely attitude while dining, are providing the child with the best possible opportunity for establishing wholesome eating practices. Other factors that influence nutrition are adequate sleep and rest, wholesome physical activity, avoidance of overfatigue, and good elimination.

POSTURE

A happy, healthy, well-adjusted child has an enthusiasm for living and expresses this through a variety of body movements. When the control of his body is good, he grows in physical efficiency; when he is awkward or his muscles are weak, his physical efficiency is impaired. So-called "good" and "poor" postures have been fairly well established. For example, a good standing posture can be determined by using the plumb-line test. This test is conducted from a side view. The body is in good alignment if a straight line can be drawn from the ear through the shoulder, elbow, hip, and knee joints and to a point just in front of the ankle bone.

The posture of a baby is usually of little concern to the parent. However, babies do have bowed legs and knock knees. Fortunately, these conditions tend to correct themselves as the child begins to walk. By the time he is six years of age, his legs are usually straight. Sometimes parents become concerned because their child has a hollow back and a protruding abdomen. This condition is also transient. Because the preadolescent has a great desire for activity, he reduces this protruding abdomen in a natural way. By the age of ten, the average youngster carries his head, neck, and shoulders in good balance [2].

It is the posture of the adolescent that usually gives parents and teachers concern. Between the ages of twelve and seventeen, the boy and girl undergo a variety of changes. Their growth is rapid; their muscles range from weak to strong. They have feelings of security and insecurity, happiness and unhappiness. They make satisfactory and unsatisfactory social-emotional adjustments, and their personal regimen is good and again it is poor. These factors have much to do with posture, and good posture can favorably influence a youth's physical and social well-being.

SOCIAL-EMOTIONAL ADJUSTMENTS

Of great significance to the immediate as well as the future happiness of both child and parent are the ways by which the emotional needs of children are met. It is believed by many psychiatrists that all children must have a feeling of belonging or security; they must adjust to the world as it is; they must discover that they are like other people; they must have opportunities for creative expression and status within their own group. How successfully parents meet these needs may make the difference between an efficient, well-adjusted personality and one who is unhappy and a source of trouble to himself and his fellows (see also the discussion of adjustment, Chapter 3).

There comes to every parent moments when he wonders just how successful he has been as a parent. These are natural feelings and can be dispelled if in early parenthood a few simple rules on child care are developed. These rules should be mutually agreed upon, they should be functional, and they should be followed consistently. These rules should cover such matters as [3]:

Showing your children that you love them

Cooperating with them, their associates, and their friends

Teaching them to be friendly

Helping them to develop self-confidence by showing confidence in them

Encouraging them to recognize their problems and teaching them to seek their own solutions

Teaching them to recognize the sex function in life and helping them develop wholesome attitudes toward it

Teaching them very early a respect for law and authority

Helping them establish worthwhile values

Experience and observation

Up to this point the discussion has centered largely on preparation for parenthood through readings and by attending lectures on child growth and development, family living, personal adjustments, and health education. One can supplement these readings and courses by the following means:

Observe closely how parents meet, either successfully or unsuccessfully, the problems inherent in rearing children.

Become a baby sitter. Both college men and women are proving that baby-sitting not only is financially profitable but provides experience in how to play with children, what to read to children, how to stop babies from crying, how to feed them correctly, and the like.

Observe young brothers or sisters or other children. It is helpful to note the best ways of motivating their interest in doing things they like as well as things they dislike.

Volunteer in youth services programs. Time spent as a camp counselor or leader in YMCA clubs, Boy or Girl Scouts, Campfire Girls, children's clinics, and child-care centers can be both interesting and constructive.

In short, you as a college student have a laboratory rich in opportunities for learning how to deal with children before having to care for your own.

Summary

There is nothing in the life of normal men and women more important to them or to society than achieving healthy, happy parenthood. Two factors favorable to effective parenthood are the sound nutritional status of the mother-to-be and emotional maturity of husband and wife.

Parents need to be assured that intelligent planning can make their responsibilities both stimulating and satisfying. Wise parenthood is concerned not only with aspects of reproduction but also with the place in which the baby is to be born, the prenatal, natal, and postnatal care of the mother and child, and the growth and development patterns of children. Continuous guidance and supervision by the family physician and other qualified persons assists parents in successfully carrying out their responsibilities.

Parenthood—a biological gift, a modifier of personality, a happy adventure, and a worthy challenge to the energies of normal men and women—is a highly satisfying experience.

Suggested readings

1. Chenoweth, Alice: "Postnatal Period—General Scope," *Journal of the American Medical Association,* 172:419–422, Jan. 30, 1960.
2. Cleveland, Anne: *The Parent from Zero to Ten,* Simon and Schuster, Inc., New York, 1957.
3. Eckert, Ralph: *What You Should Know about Parenthood,* Science Research Associates, Inc., Chicago, 1953.
4. Gesell, Arnold, and Frances L. Ilg: *The Child from Five to Ten,* Harper & Brothers, New York, 1946.
5. Green, Margaret C. L.: *Learning to Talk,* Harper & Brothers, New York, 1960.
6. Heider, Grace M.: "What Makes a Good Parent?" *Children,* Children's Bureau, U.S. Department of Health, Education, and Welfare, 7:207–212, November-December, 1960.
7. Jenkins, Gladys G.: *A Guide for Family Living,* Science Research Associates, Inc., Chicago, 1956.
8. Kreig, Margaret B.: "Blotting Out Pain through Hypnosis," *Parents' Magazine,* 25:73, October, 1960.
9. Lundeen, Evelyn C., and Ralph H. Kunstadter: *Care of the Premature Infant,* J. B. Lippincott Company, Philadelphia, 1958.
10. Lynch, Harold D.: *Your Child Is What He Eats,* Henry Regnery Company, Chicago, 1958.
11. Riker, Audrey P., and John T. Burns: "New Baby in the House," *Parents' Magazine,* 35:40–41, 107–109, December, 1960.
12. Shepard, Kenneth S.: *Care of the Well Baby,* J. B. Lippincott Company, Philadelphia, 1960.
13. Williams, Jennie: *Family Health,* J. B. Lippincott Company, Philadelphia, 1959.

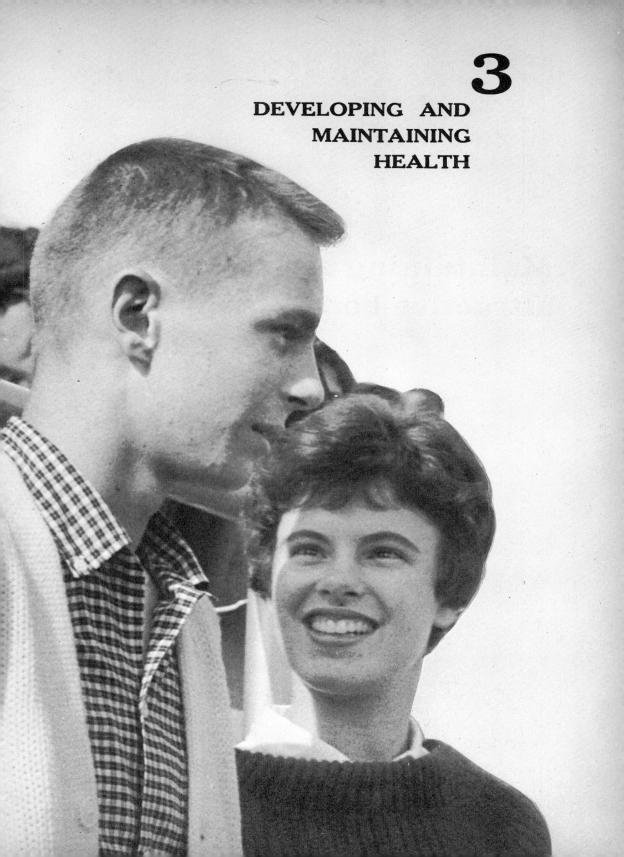

SEVEN

Maintaining a healthy and attractive body

The physically fit, well-developed human body is one of man's supreme achievements. Of all the qualities and characteristics that make up the integrated personality, and there are many, having a fit body is one of the most desirable. This wonderful human body has its beginning when the sperm and ovum unite. It grows, develops, and finally becomes a compact, coordinated organism composed of trillions of active cells. It is capable of reproducing itself; of giving protection to its vital organs; of repairing much of its damaged tissue; of maintaining a constant temperature; of neutralizing and destroying disease germs and their by-products; of converting food into energy and tissue; of expelling waste products—in short, of an amazing number of biological and psychic phenomena.

Maintaining our bodies in a healthy and attractive condition requires disciplined living—living that makes much of good nutrition, sound emotional and social controls, freedom from diseases, vigorous physical exercise, proper care of eyes and ears, sound care of teeth and gums, intelligent attention to organs of elimination, good posture and grooming, and rational controls of beverage alcohol and tobacco. Such a regimen is basic to total fitness.

Physical fitness

Just how fit are you? It has been said by scientists that scarcely 25 per cent of the adult male population in this country would be able to survive a natural test of their physical fitness [10]. Our modern pattern of bringing up children might give one clue to the reason for this situation. For example, in urban living a baby gets his exercise in a small playpen. After he learns to walk, he is placed in a stroller and his mother gets the exercise. When it is time for him to start to school, a bus or the family automobile saves him the much-needed exercise of walking. At the end of the school day he all too often finds a comfortable spot in front of a television set to be entertained for an hour or more. As he grows older, preparing homework assignments tends to supplant physical activity. By this time he has developed a well-established attitude and a pattern of behavior that expresses itself through a reduction of physical activity rather than a program of vigorous physical exercise. This, unfortunately, is the pattern that leads to softness. Individual and national softness—physical, mental, and even moral—is becoming so pronounced that early in his administration President Kennedy issued an appeal to the nation to upgrade its national fitness through vigorous physical activities. He stated: [1]

[1] John F. Kennedy, "The Soft American," *Sports Illustrated*, 13:15–23, Dec. 26, 1960.

For physical fitness is not only one of the most important keys to a healthy body; it is the basis of dynamic and creative intellectual activity. The relationship between the soundness of the body and the activity of the mind is subtle and complex. Much is not yet understood. But we do know what the Greeks knew: that intelligence and skill can only function at the peak of their capacity when the body is healthy and strong; that hardy spirits and tough minds usually inhabit sound bodies. In this sense, physical fitness is the basis of all activities of our society. And if our bodies grow soft and inactive, if we fail to encourage physical development and prowess, we will undermine our capacity for thought, for work and for the use of those skills vital to an expanding and complex America.

How fit are you? Before answering this question, let us identify some of the components of fitness. In a broad sense fitness is a combination of physical, mental, emotional, social, and spiritual components. The ability of the individual to function effectively in his environment depends on how smoothly these components function as a whole. In other words, if you would satisfy your own needs and at the same time contribute your share to the welfare of society, you should possess:

Optimum organic health consistent with heredity and the application of present health knowledge

Sufficient coordination, strength, and vitality to meet emergencies as well as the requirements of daily living

DEVELOPING AND MAINTAINING HEALTH

Emotional stability to meet the stresses and strains of modern life

Social consciousness and adaptability to the requirements of group living

Sufficient knowledge and insight to make suitable decisions and arrive at feasible solutions to problems

Attitudes, values, and skills that stimulate satisfactory participation in a full range of daily activities

Spiritual and moral qualities that contribute the fullest measure of living in a democratic society

Fitness of this quality not only makes possible a desirable kind of citizenship, it is also a strong factor in keeping democracy a potent force in the world today.

When people talk about physical fitness, someone usually wants to know, "Physically fit for what?" Fitness can mean different things to different people. For example, the vitality, strength, and endurance necessary for success as a coal miner are not necessary in the same proportions for success as a bookkeeper. Yet both the miner and the bookkeeper can be physically fit; that is, both can do a satisfactory day's work and still have enough strength and energy for emergencies, for off-the-job responsibilities, and for recreation after the working day has ended. This concept, with its implications, also holds true for the college student. Success, whether on or off the campus, means not only academic achievement but productive participation in home and community affairs and in leisure-time activities as well.

A study of the three questions that

follow may help the student gain a better understanding and appreciation of his body and develop insights into ways of keeping it physically fit:

What are the significant relationships between body types and their adaptability to physical activities?

How can a person determine his present state of physical fitness?

What are some of the activities which help develop and maintain a strong, healthy body?

BODY TYPES

Almost everyone would like to have an attractive figure. For women this means being truly feminine; for men, being muscular and athletic; for both, a body well-conditioned by participation in vigorous physical activities. Contrary to common belief, participation in vigorous games and sports by women does not result in a "masculine build." In fact, muscular strength and endurance are of greater significance to skill in physical activity for women than is body build.

Studies of body builds show a variety of constitutional types—types that are not only different in appearance but in adaptability to physical exercise as well. To achieve maximum pleasure from physical activities and to improve one's quality of well-being, it is important to select games, sports, gymnastics, etc., appropriate to one's physical endowment.

After a comparative study of the physiques of 4,000 college students, Sheldon discovered that body types could be classified in terms of three compo-

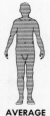 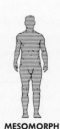 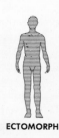

Sheldon's classification of body types. (Adapted from Laurence Morehouse and Augustus Miller, Jr., *Physiology of Exercise*, The C. V. Mosby Company, St. Louis, 1953.)

AVERAGE   ENDOMORPH   MESOMORPH   ECTOMORPH

nents, based on the three layers of the human embryo: [2]

1. The *endoderm,* an inner layer of cells from which develop the organs of digestion, the bladder, and the urethra. The component based on this layer is termed *endomorphy,* and individuals in whom that component is dominant are *endomorphs.*

2. The *mesoderm,* a middle layer which produces the skeleton, musculature, and circulatory system. The component based on this layer is termed *mesomorphy,* and individuals in whom that component is dominant are *mesomorphs.*

3. The *ectoderm,* the outermost layer predominating in the production of the skin, hair, nails, and nervous system. The component based on this layer is termed *ectomorphy,* and individuals in whom that component is dominant are *ectomorphs.*

This brief description should not be considered a rigid classification of body types, since allowances must be made for individual body structure, and each component is found in everyone in varying proportions. This can be denoted numerically. Thus, for the somatotype individual classified as 731, the figure 7 indicates a predominance of the inner layer of the endomorph, the 3 indicates some degree of the mesomorph, and the 1 shows a small proportion of the ectomorph.

What meaning has this for a student attempting to find games and sports appropriate to his physical endowments? In general, it means that, although these three components are found in everyone, the extremes of dominating characteristics become the differential in individual reaction to games and sport competition. For example, the extreme endomorphs, or viscerotonic persons, are

generally fat and relaxed and love comfort and sociability. They have large digestive organs and poorly developed muscular tissue. They are fond of food and need companionship. They are usually uncomfortable in the gymnasium but often enjoy the swimming pool. Their strongest forte is in recreational activities such as fly and bait casting, card games, skating, table tennis, horseshoes, shuffleboard, boating, photography, and informal group games.

The mesomorphs, or somatotonic individuals, are the athletic type with hard, firm muscles. They are energetic and muscularly active, with vigor and push. In personality traits they are adventurous, competitive, and aggressive. The mesomorphs have a direct approach to all problems and show a need for and enjoyment of physical exercise. They love competition and excel in most athletic activities, whether they are team games or single or dual activities [15].

The extreme ectomorphs, or cerebrotonic persons, are characterized by restraint and tightness in posture and movement. They are quick to act, mentally overtense, and self-conscious; they love privacy, fear people, and seek solitude when troubled. In build they are tall and slender, with fragile bones and stooped, hesitant posture. They prefer to watch physical activities rather than take part in them. However, should their mesomorphy component be above 3 or 4, they welcome active participation in athletic games and sports. They will achieve success in fencing, archery, golf, tennis, squash, track and field events, and other nonteam activities.

INDEXES OF PHYSICAL FITNESS

Total fitness has been identified as a state of well-being marking the high degree of efficiency with which a person is able to perform his daily tasks. Further, it implies that one has ability to function skillfully and that this ability is heavily influenced by the smoothness

[2] W. H. Sheldon, "Constitutional Factors in Personality," in J. McV. Hunt (ed.), *Personality and the Behavior Disorders,* The Ronald Press Company, New York, 1944, vol. 1, pp. 526–545.

Table 7.1 Body types and physical fitness

Mesomorphic endomorphs (S-types: 631, 532, 541, 542, 543)	Endomorphic mesomorphs (S-types: 452, 361, 462, 451, 453)	Extreme mesomorphs (S-types: 171, 162, 262, 172, 252)	Ectomorphic mesomorphs (S-types: 253, 254, 163, 164, 265)	Mesomorphic ectomorphs (S-types: 235, 126, 136, 145, 146)
Table tennis	Baseball	Sprints	Lightweight wrestling	Bicycling
Floating (swimming)	Football (lineman)	Basketball	Long-distance running	Cross-country
Croquet	Heavyweight boxing	Middleweight boxing	Tennis	Table tennis
Fly and bait casting	Heavyweight wrestling	Middleweight wrestling	Gymnastics	Basketball center (short periods)
Bowling	Swimming	Quarterbacks	Weight lifting	Archery
	Soccer (backs)	Football (backs)	Javelin	Also many athletic games, except those requiring weight and sheer strength
	Ice hockey (backs)	Divers	Pole vault	
	Weight tossing	Tumbling	High jump	
		Lacrosse	Fencing	
		Soccer (forward)	Badminton	
		Ice hockey (forward)	Skiing	
		Handball	Jockey	

Source: Carl E. Willgoose, "Body Types and Physical Fitness," *Journal of Health, Physical Education and Recreation,* 27:27, September, 1956.

with which the physical, mental, social, emotional, and spiritual components operate. In fact, if one is to satisfy needs and desires and make a worthy contribution to the present-day social order, these components must function as a whole and to the mutual advantage of each other.

As indicated previously, being physically fit can mean different things to different people. There are also a variety of expressions by which health authorities have identified or defined physical fitness. For example, Keeney suggests that we think of physical fitness as a person's capacity to do work. This capacity, of course, will depend upon his strength, endurance, and coordination and on the length of time and degree these components have worked together [11].

The United States Naval Institute uses the Harvard Fatigue Laboratory Test to determine physical fitness. This consists of stepping up to and down from a raised platform in marching rhythm for a period of five minutes. The purpose of the test is to determine an individual's ability to withstand vigorous sustained physical exercise. His capacity is measured by his circulatory adjustment at the conclusion of the five-minute period [18].

Balke believes that the best test of physical fitness is man's ability to survive under extreme biological demands. For example, he found that the physically well-trained person can mobilize and use nutrients within his body more effectively than the person with less training. He also noted that when the untrained person reaches a condition of metabolic exhaustion, that is, with little energy remaining, he stops and can go no further, whereas the physically fit individual seldom reaches this state of complete exhaustion. He seems to have reserve energy that permits him to continue the activity on a reduced scale [10].

Steinhaus lists four tests to determine physical fitness:

Burpee Test for Agility and Heart Response

The curl, a test to determine abdominal strength

The pull-up, a test to determine arm and shoulder strength

The Sargent Chalk Jump, a test to determine leaping strength

These tests and scoring tables are described in a booklet by Steinhaus called *How to Keep Fit and Like It* [24].

McCloy, in an article on physical fitness, says: [3]

To be physically fit in the sense of the functioning of the neuro-muscular system, one needs an adequate amount of strength and endurance. . . . The amount of strength and of endurance should be more than completely adequate for that person's emergency needs, for off-the-job work, and for recreation.

Morehouse and Miller classify the components of physical fitness into anatomical, physiological, and psychological fitness. They believe that when a person is anatomically fit, he has intact all parts and all organs of his body necessary for doing the job at hand. When he possesses muscular strength, endurance, and motor skill to perform skillfully and to recover from fatigue quickly, he is physiologically fit. Psychological fitness means that the individual combines effectively intelligence, drive, educability, and emotional stability in doing a task. Further, they indicate that the difference between a person who is fit and one who is not,

when both individuals are of the same height and weight and are committed to performing the same piece of moderate work, is as follows:

In the physically fit person there is [15]:

A slower pulse rate during the working period and a faster recovery to normal at the conclusion of the task.

A slower rise in blood pressure during the physical exercise and a quicker return to normal.

A lower intake of oxygen during the exercise. This is the result of a better-conditioned oxygen transportation mechanism.

A larger stroke volume of the heart. This means that the heart is in good condition and that there is a larger amount of blood sent out from each ventricle during exercise than in the less well-conditioned heart.

A lower blood lactate level during the period of exercise. This indicates that the individual in good physical condition has fewer fatigue products in the blood and will not tire as rapidly as the less fit person doing the same amount of moderate work.

From the foregoing, it can be concluded that being physically fit not only is a highly desirable quality but is essential for effective living. Physical fitness is never a gift, nor is it static. It is dynamic and changes with environment and with need. It is the result of disciplined living.

In summary, you as a college student may be said to be physically fit for your job if you:

Function as a total personality with efficiency and without discomfort.

Possess sufficient muscular strength and endurance to maintain an effective posture, successfully carry on the duties imposed by the academic environment, and meet emergencies satisfactorily and also have enough energy both for recreation and for social obli-

[3] C. H. McCloy, "What Is Physical Fitness?" *Journal of Health, Physical Education and Recreation*, 27:15, September, 1956.

gations after the "work day" has ended. Meet the requirements of your environment through efficient functioning of your sense organs. Possess the resilience to recover rapidly

from fatigue and tension without aid of stimulants.

Enjoy natural sleep at night and feel fit and alert in the morning for the job ahead.

Developing and maintaining a strong and healthy body

The wonderful human body is truly a precision instrument, capable of great achievements. It is delicately adjusted and easily put out of order, yet it is exceedingly tough and resilient. If given the right care, it is capable of high accomplishments; if allowed to become ill or to degenerate, it can be the source of inefficiency and unhappiness. Few persons have a perfect body. Almost everyone has one or more physical imperfections. The important point is to accept these imperfections, to make the most of what one has, and to strive constantly for improvement.

Keeping such a precision instrument as the body fit and functional is no job for the uninformed or careless person. It requires an understanding of the body, sound health practices, and disciplined living. The result of such a regimen can be measured in happiness and high achievement. The discussion that follows on physical exercise, dental health, vision and hearing, elimination, grooming, and posture can be helpful to the student in achieving these goals.

PHYSICAL EXERCISE

Science has established the fact that the functional efficiency of the body will improve when it is used and will regress when it is not used. This means that all normal organs of the body perform more effectively and efficiently when they are given frequent opportunities to act. Conversely, when muscles, nerves, heart, lungs, and other organs are subject to extended periods of little activity, they lose tonus, become flabby, and, if forced into

sudden action, render limited service.

The body is built to be active. It thrives on exercise. In fact, vigorous physical exercise comes close to being a necessity if the body is to maintain a healthy state. A regimen of games, sports, dancing, and conditioning exercises, engaged in faithfully, builds up the endurance of the heart, lungs, and muscles; stimulates the liver and kidneys; reduces nervous tension; and creates a satisfying feeling of emotional and social well-being. By way of illustration, conditioning exercises, which are growing rapidly in popularity, can be fun; they are healthful and they can be performed almost anywhere: in plush commercial settings, in school gymnasiums, or at home. All that one needs is an honest desire to get into condition, a series of appropriate exercises, and a convenient place to perform them.

Most college students make a serious effort to engage regularly in some kind of physical exercise. There are days, however, when an overcrowded schedule precludes physical activity. It is then that the practice of conditioning exercises can prove their value. The normal student performing the following exercises each morning for five or ten minutes finds that, after getting used to the routine, he will be able to start his day with added zest and with an increased feeling of well-being:

1. From a standing position, begin the exercise by running in place. Swing the arms vigorously. Keep the head up. Do this for one to two minutes.
2. Stand with the feet wide apart. Bend

forward from the trunk and touch the floor with your hands. If it is more comfortable, bend the knees. Repeat this 5 to 10 times with increasing cadence.

3. Stand with the feet a few inches apart. Bend the knees so that the body is in a half-squat position. Return to a standing position. Repeat this 5 to 10 times.

4. Lie on your back with hands at the sides. Slowly raise the head and shoulders so that you can touch the knees with your fingers. Return to the lying position. Repeat this 5 to 10 times. You may find it necessary to hook your feet under a dresser, table, or bed in order to help raise the body to a sitting position.

5. Now lie face down with arms at the sides. Slowly lift only the head and shoulders. Return to starting position. Repeat this 5 to 10 times.

6. Take a standing position. Keep the feet well apart. Hold the left hand high over the head, with arm straight. Hold the right arm close to the body. Now bend the trunk sideward to the right. Alternate with the right arm over the head and bend the trunk to the left. Repeat this exercise 5 to 10 times, alternating first to the right, then to the left.

7. Finish the series of exercises by running in place for one to two minutes.

If you follow this series of exercises with a shower and a brisk rub with a bath towel, you should feel ready for the day's activities. If you desire additional exercises of a more strenuous nature, note the exercises described in Suggested readings Nos. 18 and 24.

The problem of physical exercise and its relation to fitness has been studied with great diligence by scientists both in this country and abroad. For example, during the 1960 Olympic Games 10 scientific sessions were held, bringing together sports physicians, scientists, and physical educators from 15 countries. The Athletic Institute of this country brought together a similar group of distinguished physicians, physiologists, psychologists, and physical educators to discuss the subject "Exercise and Fitness." Selected statements from the findings of these two groups and others [10, 23] indicated some significant facts about the physiology of exercise. In relation to *food and physical condition,* they noted that:

Physical exercise has a favorable influence on metabolic functions.

Fatty deposits in the liver can be reduced by physical exercise.

A lack of physical exercise is a factor in raising blood cholesterol.

The well-conditioned athlete appears to suppress the blood cholesterol level, making it less likely that he will develop a cardiovascular disease because of the presence of unneeded fats.

The nutritional requirements of the athlete are essentially the same as those of the nonathlete except in the amount of food consumed. The most satisfactory diet for the athlete is one that he enjoys and that at the same time provides him with a variety of needed nutrients.

"Crash diets," combined with a low fluid intake, which enables an overweight athlete to qualify for a lower weight classification, are too drastic and can be dangerous to his well-being.

Vigorous physical exercise depresses action in the stomach. If vigorous exercise should follow a meal, the subject is likely to have distress with nausea and vomiting. Light physical exercise before or after a meal usually does not interfere with the digestion of food.

In relation to the *heart and physical exercise,* they noted that:

The better the physical condition, the less work is required of the heart.

There is sufficient evidence to support the hypothesis that individuals engaged in occupations requiring physical activity are less likely to develop arteriosclerotic heart disease than those whose jobs require little or no physical exercise.

In relation to *muscles and physical exercise,* they noted that:

Physical exercise improves muscle strength, and strength is basic to physical fitness.

Increase in muscular strength during emotional excitement is caused chiefly by secretions from the adrenal glands acting on striated muscle tissue.

The following additional points brought out by these groups indicate that a variety of factors influence the body during physical exercise:

Athletes performing at high altitudes will take longer to recover from fatigue incurred during exercise but will usually have little difficulty performing in speed or in strength events.

Blood viscosity and clotting time are unfavorably influenced by stress and tension of everyday living.

Regular physical exercise, rest, and relaxation favorably influence all body functions.

Excellence in athletic performance involves long periods of both physical and mental conditioning. This means that through proper physical exercise and dogged determination, the athlete conditions his nervous system to act in a manner conducive to maximum coordination of all body organs.

There is no accepted research to show that the athlete ingesting drugs prior to a contest can improve his performance.

A system of regular physical exercise can make a fifteen- to twenty-year difference in maintaining fitness in the adult (resistance to physical deterioration).

Physical exercise is nature's remedy for tenseness and stress so common to modern living.

Exercising when the temperature is high places a large burden upon the cardiovascular system. This is caused by an increased blood flow to the dilated skin blood vessels, to the muscles, and to the brain. As a result, activity becomes difficult because of the inability of the heart to increase its output. When this occurs, symptoms of heat exhaustion develop and athletic performance is greatly impaired.

These are but a few excerpts from a long list of research reports given by the groups previously mentioned.

Games and sports are also excellent conditioners. They contribute not only to physical vigor but to mental, social, and emotional health as well.

The late Ralph LaPorte [4] and a national committee compiled a comprehensive list of popular physical activities— games and sports—in order of their contribution to well-being. A summary of the report follows:

PHYSICAL AND ORGANIC HEALTH. Swimming and diving, boxing, wrestling, basketball, football, soccer, speedball, handball, tennis

SOCIAL HEALTH. Football, softball, soccer, speedball, touch football, volleyball, water polo, baseball, lifesaving

EMOTIONAL HEALTH. Football, lifesaving, basketball, softball, soccer, speedball, tennis, water polo, track and field

SAFETY SKILLS. Lifesaving, swimming and diving, boxing, wrestling, tumbling

RECREATIONAL SKILLS. Swimming and diving, baseball, softball, soccer, volleyball, archery, golf, handball, horseshoes, squash, tennis, folk dancing

ALL-ROUND CONTRIBUTION TO WELL-BEING. Swimming and diving, football, soccer, basketball, softball, lifesaving, tennis, baseball, speedball, volleyball, boxing, wrestling

The student making a serious effort to keep in good all-round condition will find that active participation in aquatics, conditioning exercises, individual sports, team games, gymnastics, combative sports, dancing, or a combination of these activities will give him good variety and a medium for maintaining a strong, healthy, and attractive body.

[4] Ralph LaPorte, *The Physical Education Curriculum,* University of Southern California Press, Los Angeles, 1953, p. 13.

Dental health

Perhaps no single part of the human body has been studied with more intensity or treated and repaired with more frequency than have the teeth and the gums and bone supporting them. An entire profession of over 90,000 dentists and thousands of allied workers are dedicated to the welfare of these organs. However, in spite of this great effort, dental caries and periodontal diseases continue to increase at a rate faster than either programs of repair or dental health education.

Advanced as we are in health services, there is still a serious dental problem among the American people. For example, by sixty years of age the average adult has only 10 of his original 32 teeth; 22 teeth have been lost because of disease and accident, mostly due to ignorance and carelessness. Approximately 60 per cent of all patients twenty to thirty years of age seeking dental care have one or more missing teeth. Extractions occur five times as often among patients who visit their dentists during a three-year interval as those who have had dental attention in a six- to twelve-month period. Dental decay among school children is exceedingly high. By sixteen years of age the average youth has seven decayed, missing, or filled teeth. These facts are revealing. They amplify the plea of the dental profession for more functional dental health education, application of known preventive and control methods against decay and other diseases, and continued research to discover acceptable means of ensuring better dental health for all [1].

STRUCTURE AND FUNCTION OF TEETH

An understanding of dental health and proper care of teeth and gums can have no more ardent supporter than the person who loses his teeth and discovers too late how vital they were to the enjoyment of a delicious meal, the complete mastication of food, the art of good speech, and a pleasing personal appearance.

Fortunately the enamel of our teeth is the hardest substance in the body and, if given proper daily attention, will last a lifetime. Each tooth has two important parts: the *roots,* which anchor it to the jawbone; and the *crown.* To make sure they last for life, nature builds each tooth from four highly efficient tissues: the *enamel,* which is very hard and cov-

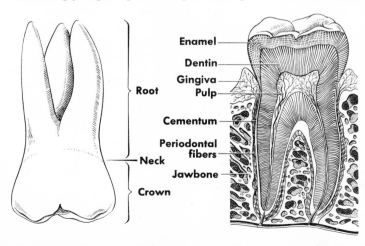

Enamel
Dentin
Gingiva
Pulp
Cementum
Periodontal fibers
Jawbone
Root
Neck
Crown

The structure of the teeth. (Adapted from *Dental Health Facts,* American Dental Association, Chicago, 1956.)

ers the crown; the *dentin,* again a very hard tissue, which makes up the main portion of the tooth; the *cementum,* which covers the roots; and the *dental pulp,* the "heart" of the tooth, which contains the blood vessels, nerves, and lymphatics. Nature went one step further to secure maximum service and protection by providing a thin tissue called *periodontal membrane,* which attaches the root to the jawbone and which acts as a cushion to lessen shock when the teeth come together in the act of chewing (see the figure on page 183).

Fortunately everyone is provided with two sets of teeth. The first set, called *primary,* or *deciduous teeth,* begins to form at about the sixth week of prenatal life. By the time a child is two and one-half years of age, he should have a full complement of 20 primary teeth. About 15 per cent of our population has congenitally missing or supernumerary teeth. Only X-ray examination can disclose these conditions, which are hereditary. In keeping with the size of the jaws, primary teeth are smaller than the permanent set. They also serve as training media in the proper care of teeth before the lifetime set makes its appearance [1].

The permanent teeth begin to calcify shortly after birth, and the first four erupt at about six years of age. These first four permanent teeth are popularly called the six-year molars. They are of great help in determining the shape of the lower part of the face. They hold the line while the deciduous teeth are shedding and the permanent teeth are erupting. When all the permanent teeth have erupted, there will be 16 in each jaw, for a total of 32 teeth. Between the ages of seventeen and twenty-one years, the last four molars, or wisdom teeth, erupt. Usually they come through without difficulty, but now and then they have an annoying way of becoming impacted below the gum line. Only by regular examination, including X ray, can the dentist discover this tendency in time to prevent serious problems.

DENTAL CARIES

The cause of dental decay (caries) has been the subject of intensive study by scientists for many years. Researchers at the National Institute of Dental Research, in Bethesda, Md., indicate that a specific strain of *Streptococcus* bacteria may be an important cause of dental decay.

The American Dental Association stresses the following as significant factors in producing caries [22]:

A translucent gelatinlike film adheres to the teeth and to surrounding mucous membranes. It is called *dental plaque,* or *zooglea.* It can be removed temporarily by cleaning the teeth. The zooglea provides a protective medium for bacteria including *Lactobacillus acidophilus* and *Streptococcus.* Working with trapped food, these bacteria produce an acid that destroys the enamel of the teeth. Certain fermentable foods, such as sugar and refined starches, easily penetrate into this bacterial mass, and within minutes destructive acids are produced.

The strength of these destructive acids and the power of the saliva in the mouth to neutralize them are important

Progress of decay. Left to right: (1) Early stage of dental decay. The enamel has been penetrated. (2) The softer dentine has been attacked. (3) The pulp has been killed and an abscess formed. (4) The molar is extracted; the bicuspid is abscessed. (Adapted from *Dental Health Facts,* American Dental Association, Chicago, 1956.)

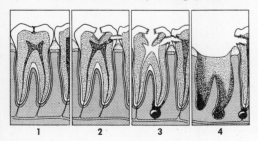

1   2   3   4

factors in determining the amount and rate of tooth decay.

A third and vital factor in tooth decay is the length of time the teeth are exposed to the destructive acids, as well as the frequency of exposure. For example, sucking hard candies for 20 to 30 minutes or eating fermentable foods such as sugars and starches at bedtime without cleaning the teeth afterward can be highly damaging to tooth enamel.

Finally, there is always the possibility that one may have inherited a tendency to dental decay.

Dental decay affects a high percentage of the population of this country. In some communities almost everyone has decayed teeth, whereas in others, where good dental health practices are followed or where natural fluorides in optimum amounts are found in the drinking water, the percentage is much less. It is doubtful that all dental decay can be prevented, but much of it can be avoided. As previously indicated, a major cause of tooth decay is an excessive use of sugar and other refined carbohydrates.

It takes approximately three minutes after eating "sweets" for destructive acids to be formed and start attacking the surfaces of the teeth. The greatest amount of damage occurs within the first fifteen to thirty minutes. Brushing the teeth would be best, but rinsing the mouth with water immediately after eating helps prevent dental decay.

The belief that women have an increased number of carious teeth during pregnancy is without clinical proof. Should such an increase occur, it is probably caused by faulty diet or improper oral health; there is also the possibility of regurgitation of stomach acids.

Controlling dental caries is a matter of frequent dental examinations, including the use of X ray; proper brushing of the teeth; restricted use of sugar and other refined carbohydrates; and the use of fluoride, either by its inclusion in the drinking water or by topical application to the teeth.

PERIODONTAL DISEASES

After thirty-five years of age, the chief single cause of loss of teeth appears to be periodontal diseases. The tissues within the mouth usually affected are the gums (gingiva); the periodontal fibers (this includes the tissue that holds the teeth to the jawbone); the cementum; and bone. The dental profession estimates that one-tenth of the adults in this country need treatment for gum disorders. Over 30 per cent more men than women lose their teeth because of periodontal diseases. By forty-five years of age, one out of every two men in the United States either has lost all his teeth because of periodontal diseases or is suffering from this disorder [1]. It has been noted that chronic mouth breathing in children may lead to inflammation of the gums. If this condition remains uncorrected, it can contribute toward periodontal disorders and loss of teeth.

Gingivitis. This is a typical gum disease and, if left untreated, may lead to pyorrhea. It is characterized by swollen, inflamed gums. Any of the following conditions may lead to gingivitis [1]:

An accumulation of tartar on the teeth
Food lodged between the teeth
Irregular edges of filled teeth
Injury to the gums or to the teeth
Incorrect brushing
Glandular changes during periods of adolescence or pregnancy
Infectious bacteria
Allergies
Crowded or separated teeth
Some drugs

Gingivitis can be successfully treated by a dentist. Further recurrence usually can be prevented by brushing the teeth and gums correctly and at appropriate times, by having the teeth cleaned regularly, and by eating well-balanced meals.

Periodontitis (pyorrhea). A second variety of periodontal disease results when gingivitis remains untreated. For example, unremoved tartar will cause the gums to recede from the teeth, leaving small crevices; inflammation develops and spreads; pockets are formed and fill with pus; the supporting structures of the teeth become weakened; and, unless treatment begins at once, the teeth may be lost.

Vincent's infection. If this third type of periodontal disease is not treated promptly, it is likely to lead to serious illness. Factors predisposing to Vincent's infection include untreated gingivitis; loss of sleep; allergies; blood diseases; and excesses in food, tobacco, and alcohol, as well as poor mouth health. During the acute stage of the infection, the gums are inflamed, sore, and ulcerated; they have a foul odor and bleed easily; and there is excessive salivation. Without proper treatment the disease becomes chronic, and the gums are destroyed. In severe infection, glands in the neck and the area about the chest may become involved, and the results can be serious. The patient should be under competent dental and medical care [1].

Progress of pyorrhea. Left to right: (1) Irritations cause gums to withdraw from teeth. (2) Further destruction. (3) Pyorrhea has destroyed most of the tissues. (4) One tooth is lost, the other weakened. (Adapted from *Dental Health Facts*, American Dental Association, Chicago, 1956.)

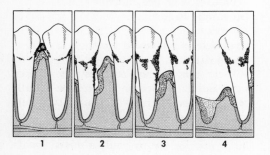

1   2   3   4

DIET AND DENTAL HEALTH

Like all growing tissue, growing teeth need adequate amounts of protein, minerals, fats, and other food elements. These are obtained through the blood that supplies the pulp area of the tooth. If there is a limited or poor supply of food, the blood will take the necessary elements from other body tissues. It is therefore imperative that a balanced diet be provided for proper growth of teeth. This is especially true of children.

Once all the permanent teeth are completely formed, calcified, and erupted, their need for nutrients such as calcium decreases. This, of course, does not mean one should stop the intake of high-calcium foods. Adult teeth no longer need calcium, but the bone tissue that keeps the teeth in place must be supplied.

The concept that excessive amounts of sugar and refined starches are the chief offenders in dental health is not a new one. Research as early as 1867 indicated there was a relationship between the ingestion of sugar and tooth decay. Fortunately, the saliva of most individuals has a tendency to neutralize harmful acids produced by bacteria on foods, confections, and beverages consumed. The more rapidly the saliva flows about the mouth, the less opportunity there is for destructive acids to work. If the saliva has a high alkaline content, it offers greater protection. Fibrous foods, such as fruits and vegetables, are also helpful in keeping the mouth clean and free from acid-producing factors [21].

Sugar in its many forms is consumed by the American public at a rate 10 times greater than that of our ancestors of 100 years ago. It is estimated that the average person consumes over 120 pounds of sugar each year. A person scarcely realizes how much sugar he consumes until he takes stock of the amount of candy, cake, pie, puddings, and sweet drinks he eats and drinks each day. Add to this the ½ teaspoon of sugar in each stick of gum he chews, and he has a sizable amount of sugar and a formidable threat to the security of his teeth. Remember, however, that it is not always the amount of sugar that is harmful. It is the continual exposure that keeps the teeth in a constant state of attack by harmful acids.

In September, 1953, the House of Delegates of the American Dental Association in their *Transactions* stated: [5]

Whereas, convincing evidence has been accumulated over many years concerning the hazards to dental health resulting from the consumption of sugar, and

Whereas, dentists have been bringing this evidence to the attention of their patients and the general public, and

Whereas, The Council on Foods and Nutrition of the American Medical Association has reported that sugar in the diet too frequently becomes a substitute for foods of higher nutritive value, and

Whereas, it is the responsibility of the health professions to recommend desirable dietary habits, and

Whereas, these recommendations have been challenged in the advertising of products, such as sweetened drinks and confections, that contain large amounts of sugar, and

Whereas, a recent report adopted by the Council on Dental Health and the Council on Dental Therapeutics provides a comprehensive review of the published evidence of the dental hazards of high levels of sugar consumption, therefore, in the interest of public health, be it

Resolved, that the Association recommend voluntary restriction in the consumption of sweetened beverages and confections, and be it further

Resolved, that the Association recommend that dental societies call to the attention of school administrators the need for eliminating from the schools the sale of sweetened beverages and confections, and be it further

Resolved, that the Association emphasize the responsibility of the manufacturers of sweetened beverages and confection for devising suitable methods to eliminate the dental health hazards associated with the consumption of their products, and be it further

Resolved, that the statement adopted by the Council on Dental Health and the Council on Dental Therapeutics entitled, "Sugar

[5] American Dental Association, *Handbook for Dentists,* Chicago, 1956, p. 18.

and Dental Caries," be referred to the Editor of *The Journal of the American Dental Association* to be used as a criterion in administering the standards for advertising.

DENTIFRICES

Brushing the teeth after eating pays off in money saved, time, energy, and appearance of the teeth. Each person should have his own toothbrush, preferably two brushes for alternate use. They should be kept clean and permitted to dry between brushings. A satisfactory brush has a flat surface for brushing, firm bristles, and a head small enough to permit easy access to all surfaces of the teeth and gums.

The commercial dentifrices (tooth powders and pastes) are pleasant to use, and there is increasing evidence that some dentifrices containing stannous fluoride prevent dental caries [6]. For an inexpensive dentifrice the dental profession suggests ordinary baking soda (bicarbonate of soda) and powdered table salt as satisfactory. The formula is 3 parts of bicarbonate of soda mixed with 1 part of salt.

Ammonium compound, chlorophyll, and antienzyme found in many commercial dentifrices are not miracle products. One should be wary of claims for these products. To keep the teeth and gums in a healthy state, it is important to brush them properly immediately after eating; consume a balanced diet low in sugar; and have the teeth examined and cleaned regularly by a dentist.

Mouthwashes. The unsupervised and indiscriminate use of mouthwashes by the public does not have the support of the Council on Dental Therapeutics of the American Dental Association. There is little or no therapeutic value in mouthwashes. The normal healthy mouth does not require medication. One who suffers from persistent mouth odors or other mouth disorders should consult his dentist and physician. It is unwise to mask abnormalities of the oral cavity with medicated mouthwashes or scented "sweets."

FLUORIDATION

One significant answer to the great rise of dental decay in the mouths of American children and youth is protection by fluoridation. Although there is no 100 per cent protection against dental caries, the fluoridation of drinking water in more than 1,800 American communities with a population of over 37 million is making a sizable reduction in the number of decayed teeth among the children [26]. Over 4 million people in the United States are using water that contains natural fluorides. Although health authorities recommend only 1 part of fluoride to each million parts of water, thousands of people in this country are drinking water containing three to seven times this amount in a natural form. As yet there have been no adverse effects on these people, with one exception: where the fluoride concentration is excessively high, there are instances of mottled enamel on the teeth [1, 3].

As early as 1892 Sir James Crichton-Browne indicated that there might be a relationship between the high rate of dental decay in England and a lack of fluorides in the diet. In 1902 Dr. J. M. Eager, a U.S. Marine Hospital medical officer, first described dental fluorosis (mottled teeth). In 1908 investigation of the "Colorado brown stain" by Black and McKay laid the foundation for the studies which led to the discovery of the caries-preventing value of fluorides in drinking water. The actual identification of fluoridation as the causative agent of mottled enamel occurred in 1931. The tendency of fluoride waters to prevent the development of dental caries was established in 1942 [1].

Comparative studies of tooth decay and loss of teeth in the cities of Boulder, Colorado, which uses fluoride-free drinking water, and Colorado Springs, where the water contains 2.5 parts of fluoride per million of water, are revealing. Among 40 forty-four-year-old persons in Boulder, there were, on an average, 22 decayed teeth, whereas the same age group

Proper technique for brushing the teeth. (Adapted from *Dental Health Facts*, American Dental Association, Chicago, 1956.)

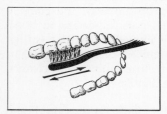

Brush the chewing surfaces of your upper and lower teeth,

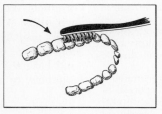

the outside surfaces of your upper teeth,

the inside surfaces of your upper teeth,

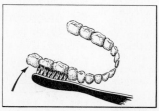

the outside surfaces of your lower teeth,

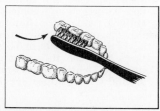

and the inside surfaces of your lower teeth.

in Colorado Springs had only 10 carious teeth. Both groups had been exposed to the drinking water of their respective communities since childhood.

In Grand Rapids, Michigan, a cooperative study conducted by the U.S. Public Health Service, the University of Michigan, and the state public health department disclosed similar findings. Fluoride was added to the normally fluoride-free lake water used by the people of Grand Rapids. The ratio of concentration was 1 part of fluoride to 1 million parts of water. The study began in 1945. Children born in Grand Rapids and raised on fluoride water showed *65 per cent less tooth decay than children of the same age group prior to fluoridation in 1945.*

In Newburgh, New York, after ten years of using fluoridated water, children drinking that water since birth showed 60 per cent lower incidence of tooth decay than children drinking fluoride-free water in the nearby city of Kingston. Extensive medical examination of the Newburgh children, including X rays of the extremities, disclosed no harmful results. As an aftermath of this ten-year study, Kingston requested that its water supply be fluoridated.

A detailed medical examination of people born and reared in Cameron, Texas, where the water supply has a natural amount of fluoride (0.4 parts per million), and Bartlett, Texas, which has twenty times that amount, or 8.0 per million, revealed no significant physiological or functional effects from drinking either water.

The question has been raised whether adding fluorides to the drinking water of the community is an economical way to reduce dental caries. The cost varies from city to city, but in the majority of communities it is about 10 cents per person per year. Information released by the U.S. Public Health Service indicates sources of fluorides that will be much lower in cost. This means that if an individual lives for 70 years in a community where fluorides are placed in the drinking water, it will cost the community on the average about $7 or less for his protection. In Madison, Wisconsin, before fluoridation began it is estimated that by the time a child reached the age of sixteen, the average family had spent $180 for his dental care [1].

Every major health organization in this country has approved the program of water fluoridation. Following is but a partial list of organizations that have endorsed the program after careful and detailed study:

The American Dental Association
The American Medical Association

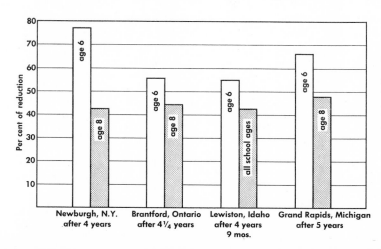

Reduction of dental caries in permanent teeth as a result of fluoridation of water supplies in four areas. (Adapted from *Dental Health Facts*, American Dental Association, Chicago, 1956.)

Per cent of reduction

| Newburgh, N.Y. after 4 years | Brantford, Ontario after 4¼ years | Lewiston, Idaho after 4 years 9 mos. | Grand Rapids, Michigan after 5 years |

The National Research Council
The U.S. Public Health Service
The American Hospital Association
The Association of State and Territorial Health Officers
Most state and local medical and dental societies

Frank E. Law, Chief, Operational Research Branch, Division of Dental Public Health, Public Health Services, U.S. Department of Health, Education, and Welfare, in an address before the National Congress of Parents and Teachers, in San Francisco, summarized the arguments in favor of fluoridation as follows:

The dental health problem in this country is so tremendous that prevention through fluoridation is the only solution.

Water fluoridation is effective—a 65 per cent reduction in tooth decay results.

Water fluoridation is safe—extensive laboratory, animal, and human studies prove there is no hazard to health at the recommended level.

Water fluoridation is economical—for an average of 10 cents per person per year, a community can benefit from this public health measure.

It is readily applied and controlled—no problems of operation or maintenance of the desired fluoride level have been reported.

The method is legal. The courts of 13 states where fluoridation was contested have upheld it as a valid community activity involving no infringement on personal liberty.

It has the overwhelming support of qualified professional health workers and of other groups that are interested in the health and the welfare of our people.

Authorities indicate that it is practical to fluoridate the water supply of 90 per cent of our country's urban population. When this occurs, more than 39 million children under sixteen years of age will receive effective protection from dental decay.[6]

Vision

Of all the senses that make us aware of the world about us, none gives more opportunity for learning and for pleasure than does vision. People live by their eyes; they work, talk, play, and love with them. More than four-fifths of their awareness of things in their environment comes through the eyes. Because life in our society is visually oriented, the ability to see and to see accurately is closely related to progress and success. By the time a person reaches college he is usually aware of this fact; aware that his past achievements have been closely related to the quality of his power of sight; aware that during the next four or five years of college living his success depends to a large degree on how well he protects and maintains this power of vision. All too frequently, however, he is unaware of the facts and techniques comprising sight conservation. The discussion that follows may be helpful as a guide to effective care of the eyes and the function of vision.

The act of seeing is highly complicated. Light rays reflected from a viewed object pass through the cornea, pupil, aqueous humor, lens, and vitreous humor to the retina. Here the nerve endings, cones, and rods are stimulated by the light image, and energy is carried along the optic nerve to the occipital lobe of the brain, where we see. Acting with the eyeball, the optic nerve, and the visual center in the brain are a number of accessories to the visual function—accessories that provide both protection and

[6] U.S.Public Health Service, "Control of Dental Caries through Fluoridation of Central Water Supplies," *Social Legislation Information Service*, No. 73, Oct. 24, 1960.

ease of operation of the eye. These organs include [7]:

EYEBROWS. They give protection from light, sweat, blows, etc.

EYELIDS. They aid sleep and protect against excessive light and foreign bodies. The glands in the lids lubricate surfaces of the eyeball.

LACRIMAL APPARATUS. These glands keep the eye moist and free from foreign bodies.

MUSCLES OF THE EYEBALL. The ciliary muscle and a ligament help to control the position of the lens and the contraction and dilation of the pupils. The extrinsic muscles hold the eyeball in place and control its movements.

FASCIA BULBI. This is the capsule in which the eyeball rotates.

The actual mechanism for sight consists of:

EYEBALL. It is usually uniform in size, but is slightly larger in the male. It has three tunics or coats. The outer coat or fibrous tunic, called *sclera,* gives protection. The choroid or vascular coat containing the blood vessels, pigment, and muscles gives color to the eye and regulates the amount of light entering

it. The retina or nervous coat contains neurons (rods and cones). It is highly sensitive to light rays and through a physical or a chemical process (as yet unknown) develops a nerve impulse which travels to the visual center of the brain.

VISUAL CENTER. When light rays reach the retina, they have been refracted, that is, bent. This happens as light passes through the cornea, the aqueous humor, the lens, and the vitreous body. Bending of the rays occurs because light rays travel at a different speed as they pass through the varying density of these tissues. When the image is cast upon the delicate membranes of the retina it has been refracted to the extent that it is upside down; that is, as light comes to focus on the retina, the rays from the top of the object are projected to the bottom of the image and the bottom rays are now at the top. The portion of this inverted image on the inner halves of the retina travels over the optic nerve to a crossover point (optic chiasma). Here they cross and move on to opposite sides of the visual center of the brain. The inverted

Section of the right eyeball. (Adapted from *The Most Wonderful Eyes in the World,* Society for the Prevention of Blindness, New York, 1956.)

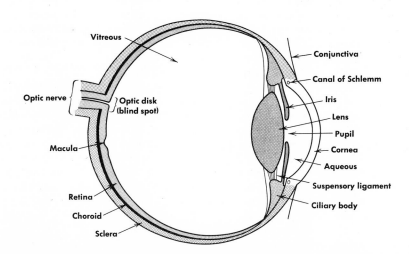

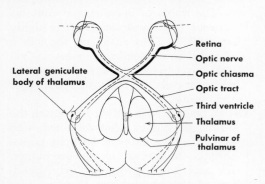

Lateral geniculate body of thalamus

Retina
Optic nerve
Optic chiasma
Optic tract
Third ventricle
Thalamus
Pulvinar of thalamus

Optic chiasma. (Adapted from Russell M. DeCoursey, *The Human Organism,* McGraw-Hill Book Company, Inc., New York, 1955.)

impulses coming from the outer side of the retina are transmitted to the brain without crossing.

The crossing of the nerve fibers is believed to help toward the correlation of eye movements and visual perception. And so this inverted image on the retina is transmitted to the brain. From the visual center these impulses are relayed to associated areas of the brain, the object is recognized, and action predicated on past experience results.

REFRACTIVE ERRORS

Conditions in which the images are focused improperly on the retina are called refractive errors. The most common of these are myopia (nearsightedness), hyperopia (farsightedness), presbyopia (poor accommodation), and astigmatism (defect of curvature of refracting surfaces).

Myopia. When one has myopic vision, near objects are usually clear and those in the distance are blurred. Nearsightedness is classified as primary (physiologic) and secondary (pathologic). The great majority of cases are primary. They are corrected with concave (minus) lenses. These lenses are ground so as to be thin in the center and thick at the edges. This shape permits the light rays that are focusing in front of the retina (too soon)

to diverge and converge on the retina, giving a clear image. Secondary myopia results from disease of the various tunics of the eye. The cause is largely unknown.

Hyperopia. Hyperopia, or farsightedness, happens when the eyeball is too short or the lens or the cornea is flattened. This causes light rays to converge too late or behind the retina. A convex lens is used to correct this condition. It should be understood that glasses do not cure refractive errors; they only compensate for them.

Presbyopia. This is a loss of elasticity of the lenses and a lowered tone of the ciliary muscle. It creates a condition where objects in the distance can be seen clearly but objects close to the eye are indistinct. It is often referred to as the "farsightedness of the aged." The correction is properly fitted convex lenses.

Astigmatism. An imperfect curvature of the refracting surface of the cornea prevents a single focus on the retina. When looking at a bright light, a person with astigmatism sees shafts of light extend outward from the center of light like a star. To correct the imperfect refractory surface of the cornea, cylindrical lenses are ground, which, when worn as glasses, equalize the vertical and horizontal refractive surfaces of the cornea.

SYMPTOMS OF FAULTY VISION

Evidences of faulty vision are not difficult to recognize. The National Society for the Prevention of Blindness [7] believes the following symptoms indicate a need for an eye examination:

BEHAVIOR

Walks with extreme caution looking closely or feeling with the foot for a step up or a step down or for small

[7] Winifred Hathaway, *Education and Health of the Partially Seeing Child,* National Society for the Prevention of Blindness, Inc., Columbia University Press, New York, 1954, p. 19.

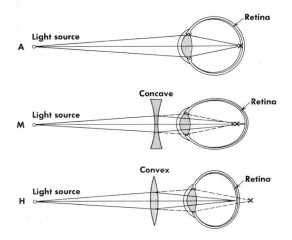

Normal eye (A): light rays focus on retina for accurate vision. Myopia (M): light is focused in front of the retina; the concave lens corrects this error. Hyperopia (H): light is focused behind the retina; the convex lens corrects this error.

obstructions; trips or stumbles frequently.

Holds reading materials or other types of fine visual work close to eyes or at a greater distance from the eyes than is normal.

Attempts to brush away blur; rubs eyes frequently; frowns; distorts face when using eyes for either distance work or close work; shuts or covers one eye; tilts head to one side or thrusts it forward.

Fails to see distant objects readily visible to others.

Is unduly sensitive to light.

Is unable to distinguish colors.

Is unable to estimate accurately locations of objects, hence frequently runs into them or fails to place objects properly.

Fails to see objects, not directly within the line of vision, which are clearly visible to the average person, while the eyes are fixed looking straight ahead.

APPEARANCE OF EYES

Red-rimmed, crusted, or swollen eyelids

Frequent sties

Watery or red

Crossed or not functioning together

Discharge of pus

Bloodshot

COMPLAINTS DUE TO USE OF EYES

Dizziness

Headache

Nausea

Pain in the eyes

Blurring of letters or objects

TESTS FOR VISUAL ACUITY

Symptoms such as the ones just listed indicate a need for an examination. Simple screening tests for visual acuity by qualified personnel (nurses, teachers, etc.) often reveal visual difficulties that have been previously undiscovered. These tests are for screening purposes only and are not intended to take the place of an examination by competent specialists.

The Snellen test. The Snellen visual acuity charts are familiar to all. They are used in most college health examinations and are the mainstays in vision screening in elementary and secondary school testing programs. The test requires the reading of letters or figures on a well-lighted chart at a distance of 20 feet. The letters are graduated in size according to optical principles established by research. Each line of letters is numbered to indicate the standard distance at which an individual with normal sight should be able to read.

For example, if a person can identify the letters on the 20-foot line at 20 feet from the chart, he is listed as having normal central visual acuity. This is expressed in fractions such as $^{20}\!/_{20}$, indicating that the 20-foot line was successfully read at 20 feet. The fraction $^{20}\!/_{30}$ means that the 30-foot line was read at 20 feet. For many people, $^{20}\!/_{15}$ vision represents an extraordinary ability to see. It may also indicate a minor hyperopia. At 20 feet the individual reads accurately the 15-foot line. In each reading, the top figure of the fraction indicates the distance from the chart, and the bottom figure shows the line the individual was able to read.

TESTS FOR COLOR VISION

Most people can recognize color. There are many who are color-weak, and a few are totally color-blind—that is, they see black and white only. The most common type of color blindness is red-green blindness. These people see the entire color spectrum in yellow and blue tones. Apparently this condition is inherited as a sex-linked trait. It is more common in men than in women, affecting between 5 and 8 per cent of the male population. Color vision can be determined by many pseudoisochromatic tests. One of the simplest is the Dvorine color-perception test. The person being tested reads the numbers on a series of pages, which is a matter of identifying patterns of colored dots on a background of similar dots of a different color.

Before a student does much in planning his vocation, he should first determine his color perception. For example, if he is color-blind, he should not plan on a career in the Navy, the Air Force (as a pilot), interior decorating, chemistry, electronics (where electrical components are color-coded), repairing color television sets, or fashion designing. In each of these occupations accurate color perception is essential.

TELEVISION

The eyes, like other organs of the body, are subject to fatigue. Eye fatigue can be avoided while watching television if the picture is clear, if the viewer is sitting at a distance commensurate with visual comfort, and if there is no sharp contrast between the bright screen and the surrounding light in the room. The eyes should be given periodic rest while a program is in progress. It is also important to place the set directly in front of the audience and make sure that the screen is at eye level. A large screen permits more comfortable viewing than a small one and gives a clearer picture at a greater distance. If all rules for good viewing are met, color television should not cause undue eye fatigue. If one's eyes are uncomfortable in spite of the fact that the picture is adjusted correctly and the room is properly lighted, an eye examination is indicated.

SUNGLASSES

The wearing of sunglasses has become a popular practice in this country. The need for sunglasses varies with individuals. If they provide comfort from constricted eyelids and from squinting while exposed to sunlight, then they should be worn. They may also be needed for special environments such as the beach, for skiing in bright sunshine, driving on desert highways, fishing in the ocean or lake, or under any situation when the eyes are exposed to glare. Colored glasses can add to the enjoyment of such out-of-door experiences. Sunglasses not only provide relief from glare from the sun but also help keep dust out of the eyes, protect against windburn of the conjunctiva, and provide a certain amount of confidence to some people by permitting a psychic withdrawal from personal contacts with the world about them. Sunglasses should be properly fitted and approved by an eye specialist.

DISEASES OF THE EYE

Glaucoma. The chief cause of blindness in the United States is glaucoma. There are over 800,000 men and women in this country who are slowly losing their sight because of this disease. The National Society for the Prevention of Blindness suggests three points to remember about glaucoma:

It occurs most frequently after forty years of age.

It is not easy to recognize in its early stages.

The progress of the disease can be stopped if there is an early diagnosis.

The symptoms of glaucoma are of two types—acute and chronic. The acute type comes on suddenly. The vision becomes cloudy and may be accompanied by severe pain around the eyes. The chronic type comes on slowly and painlessly. Anyone who needs a frequent change of glasses with little or no improvement in vision, who fails to adjust to darkened areas, who has loss of side vision or blurred vision, and who sees colored rings around lights should contact his physician at once.

Cataracts. There is no known cause of cataracts. Some authorities believe vitamin deficiencies (riboflavin) and the parathyroid hormone may be involved. In cataract the crystalline lens of the eye or its capsule or both become less transparent, which results in a loss of visual acuity. Surgery may help restore partial vision.

SAFETY GLASSES

A plastic lens first introduced in the United States in 1937 has largely solved the problem of lightweight and safety glasses. The new hard-resin lenses rest lightly on the nose, reduce fogging of lenses by about 75 per cent, and give greater protection to men engaged in eye-hazardous employment as well as to athletes and children who are required to wear glasses.

CONTACT LENSES

Contact lenses have stimulated interest on the part of many persons. Those who are wearing glasses or who are about to be examined and fitted for a visual problem are particularly interested. The physical contour of some persons' eyes is suited to this type of fitting more than others. Many persons employed in sports or in some of the creative arts use such lenses. The decision about fitting contact lenses rests with the professional examiner selected.

CARE OF THE EYES

The student who wants maximum use of his eyes now and the assurance of satisfactory vision later on in life will take these precautions:

Have a periodic examination of the eyes and visual acuity.

Obtain the approval of qualified specialists before wearing colored glasses continuously.

Wear safety glasses where there is danger to the eyes.

Provide adequate nonglare illumination for study and work areas.

Rest the eyes frequently when doing close work or watching motion pictures.

Consult a specialist about any unusual symptom in seeing or in the appearance of the eye.

Hearing

The ability to hear and to see accurately is fundamental to the learning process. Fortunately the great majority of students in our colleges see and hear with little difficulty. It is interesting to note that those with a slight hearing loss have overcome this by "learning to listen"; that is, they listen to one person at a time, they concentrate on consonants, and they learn to read lips.

To protect the ear and to promote accurate hearing, the following steps are important:

Have a complete medical examination periodically, including a hearing test.

Consult a physician upon the first indication of discharge from the ear, or if there is a tendency to move closer to a speaker or cup the ear to hear better, or if there are earaches or irritating noises in the head.

Avoid an environment where high, shrill noises or sharp explosions occur.

Avoid using matches, hairpins, toothbrushes, etc., to clean the ears.

Lower the head, face down, to blow the nose—sometimes it is better to tilt the head back and snuff backward until the nose and throat are clear.

Clear up excessive pressure within the ear by chewing or swallowing.

Practice sound nutrition, cultivate good mental health, and avoid excessive use of tobacco.

Elimination of body wastes

Each time food and liquids are taken into the body and have been digested, residue in the form of waste material has to be removed. This is the job of the large intestine, the kidneys, the lungs, and the skin. When these organs perform normally, they add substantially to the comfort and health of the body; when they fail, the body undergoes discomfort and illness. To keep these organs in good condition and working naturally one ought to know how they function and establish practices that keep them healthy and efficient.

Temporary storage of undigested food residue from the small intestine is the function of the *large intestine*. As the feces move through the colon, changing from a liquid to a more solid consistency, bacterial decomposition takes place. This chemical action results in the unpleasant odor associated with fecal matter. As the feces enter the rectum, sensory stimulation brings about an awareness of the impending act of elimination. To maintain regularity of bowel evacuation one should always heed this warning. The most common cause of constipation is the failure to empty the lower colon and the rectum when there is a desire to do so.

The use of a laxative to relieve pain in the abdomen is not wise; such a practice could result in a ruptured appendix.

The *kidneys* have a threefold function in keeping the body healthy:

They extract excessive amounts of acid and alkaline substances from the blood.

They conserve or excrete water as the situation arises.

They control the excretion of salts such as calcium, potassium, magnesium, and sodium.

The primary responsibility for doing this job lies with thousands of tiny ball-like tissues of the cortex of the kidney. They are called *glomeruli.* (For details on the function of the kidneys, see Chapter 12.)

The *lungs* and *skin* are also excretory organs. The lungs excrete carbon dioxide and at the same time permit water and heat to escape. The skin has a variety of functions. Its primary excretory job is to eliminate water and salts in the form of perspiration. A more complete coverage of the skin will be found under the discussion on grooming.

To aid the body in eliminating wastes one should:

Establish a regular time for bowel evacuation (an occasional change in timing is no cause for concern)

Include in the diet adequate amounts of fruits and vegetables

Drink enough water to meet daily needs

Engage in vigorous physical exercise (adapted to one's need)

Avoid habitual use of laxatives

Have an annual health examination, which includes a stool specimen and urinalysis.

Grooming

Good grooming is an asset to success both socially and in the world of business. As an effective adjunct to personality, it has no peer. Good grooming combines the quality of good taste with good personal health practices.

Good taste per se is not easy to define, yet its presence or absence is readily discernible to even the casual observer. One cannot purchase good taste, but it can be developed. For example, a person can study his body build and choose a wardrobe consistent with his figure. Good taste in clothes and accessories means knowing what to wear, when to wear it, and how to accent favorable points of personality.

In the use of cosmetics, good taste has one important rule—a light touch goes a long way in assisting nature. The key to being attractive is to be natural.

Well-groomed men and women are meticulous about their *personal health practices*. With them, the care of the hair, the skin, and the nails is never left to chance.

CARE OF HAIR

For men, hair grooming is not quite the problem it is for women. Having his hair cut and combed according to the dictates of his social or business group, regularity in shampooing, and the control of dandruff seem to meet most of a man's needs. Of course, there is the matter of baldness. How can one stop falling hair? This question has been asked since the earliest times. One of the first prescriptions known to medicine was used by the ancient Egyptians in an effort to grow new hair. The prescription was made up from fats of snakes, geese, lions, the hippopotamus, and the crocodile. But up to the present time, hundreds of remedies have been tried to restore hair—none of which has been effective. A complete medical examination by the family or college physician is the first step to take when one discovers he is losing his hair. Beginning cases of baldness have been stopped by prompt treatment of infections and glandular disturbances.

For the well-groomed woman, care of the hair usually involves an investment of time, energy, patience, and money. Added to the possible problems of dandruff and dry or oily scalp are those of shampooing, waving, permanent, cutting, styling, dyeing, bleaching, and superfluous hair. One solution is to seek the services of a cosmetologist. However, one should never underrate what a systematic home program of correct massage of the scalp, of brushing the hair, of shampooing, and of proper food can do to maintain healthy, attractive hair.

Massaging. Scalp massage is essential to attractive hair. To stimulate the oil glands located near the hair roots, place the pads of the fingers at the base of the neck and, with a firm, rotary motion, work the fingers slowly up the head, covering every portion of the scalp. This exercise should be practiced both morning and evening. It is equally effective for dry or oily scalps.

Brushing. Brushing the hair should always follow the scalp massage. Use only the best brushes. The bristles of a good brush are strong and moderately stiff. Hair should be brushed starting at the hairline and working in from the edges, always with long, smooth strokes in an upward sweep. Most authorities suggest lowering the head when brushing the hair, to increase the flow of blood to the hair follicles.

Shampooing. Frequency of shampooing is relative. For example, persons ex-

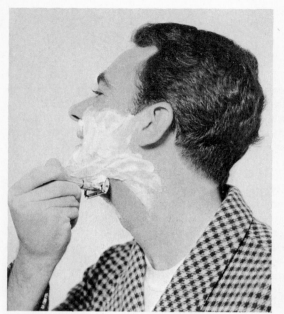

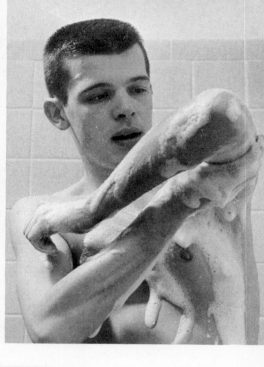

A clean shave indicates to the world that a man is interested in looking his best.

A warm shower with soap followed by a brisk rub is refreshing to both mind and body.

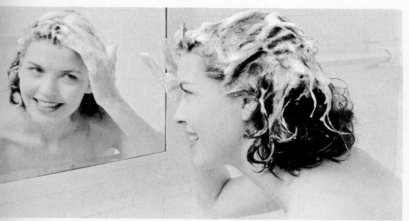

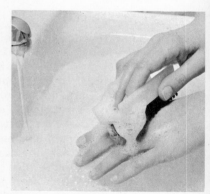

Massaging the scalp while shampooing relaxes it, deep-cleans it, and works wonders for the sheen and texture of your hair.

A thorough scrubbing of the hands with a nail brush and rich soap suds is essential to good grooming.

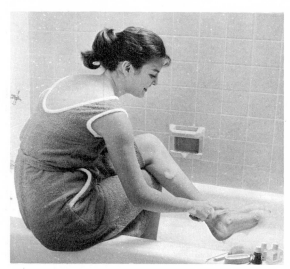

Good grooming includes a thorough scrubbing of the feet daily.

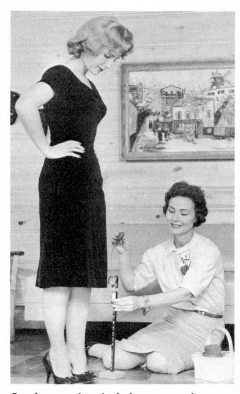

Good grooming includes appropriate length of dress and perfect hem line.

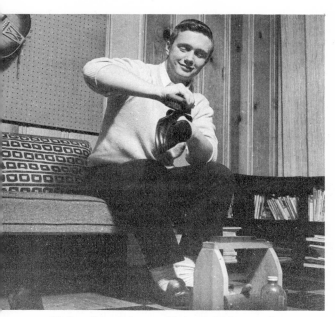

Well-polished shoes add the finishing touch to the well-groomed person.

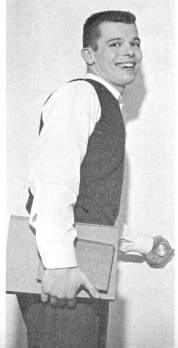

A well-groomed student can start his day with confidence—and a smile.

posed to dust, those with oily scalps, or women who wear their hair loose and flowing may find it necessary to shampoo frequently. On the average, the normal scalp needs to be washed every ten to fourteen days. Care should be used in choosing the shampoo. A good course to follow is to seek the advice of a cosmetologist.

Proper food. A well-nourished body usually means well-nourished hair. A properly balanced diet for healthy skin and hair includes food selected from *A Daily Food Guide* (see Chapter 9). The diet should also include adequate amounts of water daily.

CARE OF THE SKIN

Attractive women and men have healthy skin. A healthy skin is dependent on a well-nourished body, vigorous physical exercise to stimulate circulation, and cleanliness (the face should be washed with a mild soap and warm water each day—in case of a dry skin, application of face cream can be helpful). Pure preparations of rouge, lipstick, face creams, and powder are harmless and can be beneficial in complementing beauty. At no time should cosmetics be employed to disguise skin disorders.

Acne. This skin disorder, which is common to young people, is an infection involving the sebaceous glands and the pores of the skin. These glands are subject to enlargement and the accumulation of sebum. If sebum is retained, it tends to become discolored and gives rise to blackheads. Blackheads in themselves are harmless. However, if they are carelessly handled by incorrect squeezing, pus-forming organisms invade the area and infection results. Emotional disturbances, greasy foods, chocolate, sluggish intestinal tract, menstrual disorders, inadequate sleep, poorly balanced diet, lack of exercise, lack of fresh air and sun-

shine, unclean skin and scalp, and overuse of creams and grease on the face tend to contribute to the development and spread of acne. Mild or severe cases of acne or other skin blemishes should be treated by a dermatologist. Modern techniques employed by competent physicians can control and, in many cases, eliminate skin disorders [4, 20].

BODY ODORS

A person should never wait to be told he has body odors. Anyone who perspires is subject to them. They are caused by the accumulation of decomposed perspiration. When perspiration is absorbed into the clothing, the garment will also give off an unpleasant aroma. Good grooming prevents objectionable odors by regular bathing, by the use of a deodorant by men as well as women, and by the wearing of freshly laundered or clean apparel.

CARE OF THE NAILS

The nails and the hair have much in common. The hair grows from its follicle; the nail, from a funnel-like fold of soft cells. Both are outgrowths of the skin, and a diet that nourishes the skin nourishes them. In prehistoric times, when fingernails were used as weapons for fighting, they were permitted to grow long and assume a clawlike appearance. Today, together with their natural function of protecting the fingers and toes, nails are important adjuncts to grooming.

The well-cared-for nails are polished, trimmed, cleaned, and, in the case of women, colored in good taste. To avoid ingrown toenails, particularly of the big toe, the nail should be cut straight across. When fingernails or toenails have been cut to the desired length, they should be smoothed with a file. It is unwise to trim the cuticle; it should be pushed back gently.

A common complaint about fingernails

is their extreme dryness. Too frequent application of nail-polish remover and harsh detergents in water have a tendency to dry the nails. There is no internal treatment to correct this condition. Avoidance of detergents for a while and a less frequent use of polish remover will restore the natural oil to the nail.

Posture

There is no one good posture for every one or for every occasion. Posture varies with individuals and their needs. The most effective posture is the one that is best adapted to the task at hand and that requires the smallest expenditure of energy. Any posture that permits freedom of body movement with a minimal use of energy and is adaptive to the individual and his environment can be considered a normal posture.

TYPES OF POSTURE

In the discussion that follows, emphasis is placed first on the *static* forms of posture and then on the *dynamic* forms [5, 14].

Attention or military posture. In this alignment the head is held erect with the chin in, the chest high, the hands stiffly at the sides, and the feet together. This is an unnatural posture, and if it is held for a long time, it will adversely affect blood circulation and produce fatigue.

Standing posture. Dentists, barbers, clerks, machine operators, laboratory workers, etc., who stand for long periods, find it desirable to move as much as possible for the sake of circulation. They will also find it less fatiguing if they wear shoes that fit loosely, stand on a soft or elastic surface, keep the weight evenly distributed on the feet, and hold the head as erect as possible.

Sitting posture. For those who sit while working, it is important to keep the head erect and well-balanced, the hollow of the back or lumbar curve well supported, the height of the chair, bench, or stool adjusted so that the hip, the knee, and the feet are at right angles to the trunk of the body, and the feet placed firmly on the floor. The height of the writing desk or table should be adjusted so that the arms are parallel with the hips and the knees. Short individuals may find it necessary to have a platform for their feet. It will add to comfort when

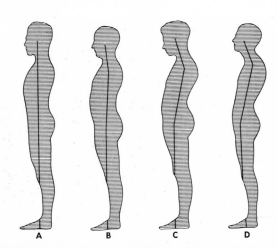

A   B   C   D

Posture silhouettes. **(A) Good:** head, trunk, and thigh in straight line; chest high and forward; abdomen flat; back curves normal. **(B) Fair:** head forward; abdomen prominent; exaggerated curve in upper back; slightly hollow back. **(C) Poor:** relaxed (fatigue) posture; head forward; abdomen relaxed; shoulder blades prominent; hollow back. **(D) Very poor:** head forward badly; very exaggerated curve in upper back; abdomen relaxed; chest flat-sloping; hollow back. (Adapted from Posture Silhouette Photographs, University of Southern California, Department of Physical Education.)

sitting in a favorite reading chair if a person tilts slightly backward and gives support to his hips, lower back, and head.

Reclining posture. Regardless of the position one assumes for sleeping, it will change many times during the night. This is nature's way of keeping blood properly circulated. The position of the pillow is important to sleep. There are those who disdain its use; others like one to three pillows under their head and shoulders. If a pillow is used, it should help to keep the head and neck straight without tension. Usually the pillow is bunched for those who sleep on their side and flat for those in a supine (on the back) or a prone (face down) position. It is important that the mattress and bedsprings should support the body and not permit sagging.

Walking posture. The old proverb that one picture is worth a thousand words has ready application when motivating a person to make changes in his walking posture. By studying motion pictures of your walking posture, you observe faults that might otherwise pass unnoticed.

Most persons can develop a graceful and easy stride. When attempting to correct walking posture, make a point consciously to follow each of these suggestions:

Keep the head and shoulders squarely balanced on the trunk.

Swing the leading leg forward from the hips.

Transfer the body weight forward so that it rests on the outside of the forward foot.

The back leg, which is ready to push off, should form a straight line with the head and trunk.

Swing the back leg forward; at the same time, shift the weight from the outside of the foot of the lead leg to the toes; now push off, transferring the weight to the foot of the forward leg.

By keeping the head balanced, with the toes pointed straight ahead, and shifting the body weight as the legs alternate in their forward swing, one can develop an acceptable walking posture.

Working posture. When lifting a heavy object, it is wise to keep the trunk erect, pull in the abdominal area, stand close to the object to be lifted, adjust the feet to give good balance, and bend the hips, the knees, and the ankles. Actual lifting is accomplished by straightening these joints and assuming a standing posture. To lower an object, reverse the lifting procedure. When carrying a heavy object, keep it close to the body. When carrying a heavy suitcase or similar object, tilt the body to the opposite side to compensate for the weight of the object.

POSTURE AND ORGANIC FUNCTION

The function of the major organs of the body depends significantly on the support they receive from body postures. For example, faulty postures are likely to cause a variety of harmful pressures and malfunctions of organs such as the liver, pancreas, stomach, intestines, and kidneys. The liver, normally held in place by its suspensory ligament, may be pressed downward and forward by faulty body mechanics, thus creating a congestion in both the liver and the gallbladder.

The pancreas is in a fixed position and is not easily displaced. However, it too is subject to pressure by unfavorable postures. This can interfere with its function and may impede the secretions from the islets of Langerhans in this organ.

The stomach in the slender-body type of individual is long and has a fishhook shape. A sagging posture in this person is quite likely to result in further lowering of the stomach, increasing its sag and producing many functional disturbances (gastritis, ulcers, etc.) In the stockily built individual the stomach is less likely to be displaced downward by poor posture. However, it too is subject to pressures, which accounts for some of the abdominal distress encountered by these people [8].

The small intestine in the slender-body type is much longer than in the stockily built person. Faulty posture in the slender person can cause downward displacement of the intestines and result in a failure of this organ to do a good job of absorbing necessary food elements.

The kidneys, which are held in position by heavy fat deposits, are also affected by faulty body mechanics. In a person with sagging posture the diaphragm relaxes, the liver is forced onto the kidney, the fat protection is lost, and ptosis, or loss of muscle tone, results [8].

It is obvious from these brief illustrations that uncorrected faulty postures can lead to a variety of physical disorders and illness. On the other hand, good posture—correct body mechanics and dynamics—pays off in effective organic functioning and sound health.

Summary

In a broad sense, *fitness* is a combination of physical, mental, emotional, social, and spiritual components. The ability of the individual to function effectively in his environment depends on how smoothly these components function as a whole. Of all the qualities that comprise an integrated personality, a well-developed, physically fit body is one of the most desirable.

A person may be said to be physically fit if he functions as a total personality with efficiency and without discomfort, possesses sufficient muscular strength and endurance to maintain an effective posture, successfully carries on the duties imposed by the environment, meets emergencies satisfactorily and has enough energy for recreation and social obligations after the "work day" has ended, meets the requirements of his environment through efficient functioning of his sense organs, possesses the resilience to recover rapidly from fatigue and tension

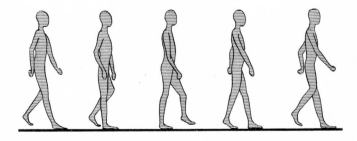

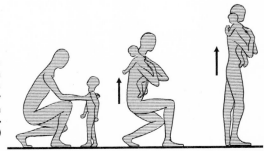

Walking posture (above). Always prepare a new base before leaving the old. Lifting a weight (below). The weight of the baby is held close to the center of gravity directly above the pushing force. (Adapted from Eleanor Metheny, *Body Dynamics*, McGraw-Hill Book Company, Inc., New York, 1952.)

without the aid of stimulants, and enjoys natural sleep at night and feels fit and alert in the morning for the job ahead.

Keeping the body fit and functional is no job for the uninformed or the careless person. It requires an understanding of the body, sound health practices, and disciplined living. The results of such a regimen can be measured in happiness, health, and high achievement.

Suggested readings

1. American Dental Association: *Dental Health Facts,* The Association, 1956.
2. Anderson, Odin W., and George Rosin: *An Examination of the Concept of Preventive Medicine,* Health Information Foundation, New York, 1960.
3. Changing Times: "What's Holding Up Fluoridation?" *The Kiplinger Magazine,* 15:15–18, August, 1961.
4. Cohn, Milton M.: "The Skin from Infancy to Old Age," *American Journal of Nursing,* 60:993–996, July, 1960.
5. Cooper, John, and Ruth Glassow: *Kinesiology,* The C. V. Mosby Company, St. Louis, 1962.
6. Council on Dental Therapeutics: "Evaluation of Crest Tooth Paste," *Journal of the American Dental Association,* 61:273, August, 1960.
7. DeCoursey, Russell M.: *The Human Organism,* 2d ed., McGraw-Hill Book Company, Inc., New York, 1961.
8. Goldthwait, Joel, Lloyd Brown, and John Kuhns: *Essentials of Body Mechanics,* 4th ed., J. B. Lippincott Company, Philadelphia, 1945.
9. Jahr, Herman M.: *As Others See Us,* American Medical Association, Chicago, 1959.
10. Johnson, Warren, and others: *Science and Medicine of Exercise and Sports,* Athletic Institute, Chicago, 1960.
11. Keeney, Clifford E.: "Working Capacity," *Journal of Health, Physical Education and Recreation,* 31:29–30, September, 1960.
12. Kennedy, John F.: "The Soft American," *Sports Illustrated,* 13:15–23, Dec. 26, 1960.
13. Lowman, C. L., and Carl H. Young: *Postural Fitness Significance and Variance,* Lea & Febiger, Philadelphia, 1960.
14. Metheny, Eleanor: *Body Dynamics,* McGraw-Hill Book Company, Inc., New York, 1952.
15. Morehouse, Laurence E., and Augustus T. Miller, Jr.: *Physiology of Exercise,* The C. V. Mosby Company, St. Louis, 1959.
16. Morehouse, Laurence E., and Philip J. Rasch: *Scientific Basis of Athletic Training,* W. B. Saunders Company, Philadelphia, 1958.
17. Nagle, Francis: "How Much Fitness?" *Journal of Health, Physical Education and Recreation,* 31:28, September, 1960.
18. Oerman, Karl C. H., Carl H. Young, and Mitchell J. Gary: *Conditioning Exercises, Games, Tests,* The United States Naval Institute, Annapolis, Md., 1960.
19. Rash, J. Keogh: "Fourfold Fitness," *Physical Educator,* 17:92–94, October, 1960.
20. Rattner, Herbert, and Paul Lazar: "Dermabrasion for the Improvement of Acne Scars," *Journal of the American Medical Association,* 171:2326–2331, Dec. 26, 1959.
21. Sandel, Perry J., and Sumter S. Armin: "How to Educate High School Students in Oral Hygiene," *Journal of Health, Physical Education and Recreation,* 31:33–40, October, 1960.
22. Staff of the American Dental Association: "Your Teeth and How to Keep Them," *Today's Health,* 39:59–62, January, 1961.
23. Staley, Seward C., and others: *Exercise and Fitness,* Athletic Institute, Chicago, 1960.
24. Steinhaus, Arthur H.: *How to Keep Fit and Like It,* The Cartnell Corp., Chicago, 1957.
25. Tucker, W. E.: *Active Alert Posture,* The Williams & Wilkins Company, Baltimore, 1960.
26. U.S. Public Health Service: "Control of Dental Caries through Fluoridation of Central Water Supplies," *Social Legislation Information Service,* No. 73, Oct. 24, 1960.
27. Van Huss, Wayne, and others: *Physical Activity in Modern Living,* Prentice-Hall, Inc., Englewood Cliffs, N.J., 1960.

EIGHT

Utilizing opportunities for rest and recreation

CONSTRUCTING A DAILY SCHEDULE

CONTROLLING FATIGUE

REST, RELAXATION, AND RECREATION

SLEEP

How many students have stopped long enough in their drive for achievement to sit down and attempt to relax, only to find to their surprise that this is more difficult than they thought? What they discover is that, in meeting the demands of the college program and possibly in spending some hours earning a few dollars, they have developed tensions that do not subside automatically. Is this condition undesirable? To the normally active student, with reasonably good resilience, a temporary state of tension probably does little harm. In fact, it often helps accomplish considerable work. However, excess tension accompanied by fatigue that persists day after day is not desirable and can lead to serious conditions.

Throughout life the individual moves in a pattern which is

fundamentally rhythmic. He experiences the flow of seasons, day and night, hunger and food, fatigue and recovery, cardiac and respiratory regularity, and muscle-nerve coordination, all of which give balance, understanding, and beauty to his utilitarian, cultural, and creative efforts.

Such a rhythmic pattern exists for all the dynamics of life. Whether one is a day laborer or a student in an institution of higher learning, the sooner he makes a conscious effort to integrate a pattern of balance into his daily living, the more tranquil, harmonious, and constructive will be his periods of work, exercise, rest, sleep, and recreation.

The principle of balance among work, rest, relaxation, and recreation is not new; it has been employed in all successful business and industrial institutions for many years. This principle is also applicable to the life of the college student. It is important for him during his time of preparation in college to put into practice a schedule or plan which will assure him a smooth transition into the business and professional world. Such a plan starts with a well-balanced program of daily activities.

The discussion that follows is organized to help you answer such questions as these:

How should I plan my daily schedule so as to make the most effective use of my time?

How can I guard against fatigue?

Where are the opportunities in the daily schedule for rest, relaxation, and recreation?

How significant is sleep to my well-being?

Constructing a daily schedule

All students need to construct a daily program early in their college careers and then evaluate the time allotted for work, rest, relaxation, recreation, and sleep.

Because students can be sure of some kind of a daily program, the question is, What kind shall it be? Experience has shown that a schedule can become a taskmaster, a producer of fatigue, discouragement, illness, and inefficiency; or it can be an orderly disciplinarian, holding a balance among work, relaxation, recreation, rest, and sleep. At best it is demanding and can be fatiguing; however, schedules are a combination of faculty and student planning and can be constructed in keeping with student needs and interests. Table 8.1 illustrates a sample daily program of a freshman majoring in business administration. It is not a perfect schedule, but it is functional and illustrates a broad pattern of work, then rest; work, then recreation; work, then rest and sleep. To the healthy student this 24-hour schedule, consistently employed, provides a means of achieving scholastic excellence, with no neglect of social and physical activities and with a minimal drain on his energies.

It would be naïve to believe that such a schedule is inviolate. Unforeseen happenings and just plain desire to change the pace are to be expected. In fact, once in a while it is good to break with routine. Such a break can be stimulating, and it does not defeat the rhythm principle; but a basic routine is still desirable. Some people are temperamentally unsuited to a regular routine and find it difficult to follow. However, dangerous wear and tear occur when there is little opportunity for repair of body tissues and when the pace or rhythm of daily living is irregular, with constant fluctua-

Table 8.1   Sample daily program (major: business administration; freshman, or 13th, year)

Activity	Time	Monday	Tuesday	Wednesday	Thursday	Friday
Classwork	8	Business math		Business math		Business math
	9	English	Physical education	English	Physical education	English
	10	Economics		Economics		Economics
Free time	11					
Lunch	12	Lunch	Lunch	Lunch	Lunch	Lunch
Classwork	1	Psychology	Orientation	Psychology		Psychology
	2	Health education		Health education		Health education
Free time	3					
	4					
	5					
Dinner	6					
	7					
Study	8					Social activities
	9					
	10					
Sleep	11 to 7	Retiring at 11 and arising at 7 provides 8 hours of sleep				

tion. For example, a student may follow the suggested schedule on Monday, but on Tuesday he may miss classes, take lunch on the run, disregard rest and recreation, and gulp his dinner—all for the sake of concentrated study. On Wednesday, being tired, he sleeps in classes, cuts out recreation, and in the evening turns completely to social activities. Thursday, he makes a desperate effort to return to the schedule, with some success. Friday, the desire to get away from it all results in cutting classes and much play, followed by a great desire to sleep. It is this kind of irregularity repeated often which produces physical and emotional disharmonies, tensions, chronic fatigue, irritability, lack of interest in schoolwork, and, eventually, scholastic failure.

Controlling fatigue

Although the irregular kind of living just described is not typical of college students, neither is it a rare occurrence. When it does occur, fatigue in some form and degree results. In fact, college health service records of physical examinations indicate that the so-called tired feeling is one of the most common complaints among college students.

It should be understood that fatigue is not all bad. In fact, metabolic products that include fatigue elements resulting from proper warm-up practices appear to be necessary for good mental and physical performance. Chemical changes and temperature elevation within the tissues lower their viscosity so that contraction and relaxation occur with greater speed and efficiency. Fatigue is also nature's way of forcing the body to slow down and rest.

The specific causes of muscular fatigue, which eventually results in lower efficiency, are not fully understood. One cause is believed to be the inability of the synapses of the nervous system and the motor end-plates (between muscle and nerve fibers) to transmit impulses to the muscles. This inability is probably due to an inadequate amount of a chemical called *acetylcholine*. When the body is fatigued, there is a decreased amount of acetylcholine; when the body has recovered from fatigue, acetylcholine is present in the synapses and the motor end-plates and a normal transmission of impulses results [17].

Fatigue of the body takes many forms: *muscular* fatigue, in which the capacity of the muscle is diminished; *cardiac* fatigue, which results in a lower stroke volume and a progessively lessened amount of blood leaving the ventricles of the heart; *postural* fatigue, resulting from long standing, in which the brain receives less blood and the feet and legs too much; *visual* fatigue, shown by ex-

cessive secretion of tears and blocking of movements of the eye; and *auditory* fatigue, which results from exposure to noise [17].

Fatigue may be general, or it may be chronic. In general fatigue the whole body is affected to a slight degree.

The onset of general fatigue in a person doing light work is seldom noticed by the subject. He is unaware that his standards of performance are deteriorating and he may even believe that his efficiency is steadily increasing. His sense of timing is the first to fail and errors and accidents begin to appear. As fatigue advances the worker's grasp of the over-all plan of the operation begins to fade so that eventually only the most prominent features of the task are performed and the rest are ignored. Attention is finally shifted from the performance of the task to the discomfort of the body. Deterioration in skill now proceeds rapidly.[1]

Usually a night's sleep is enough for full recovery.

Chronic fatigue is much more profound. It is usually the end result of worry, an excessive amount of work, inadequate nutrition, and insufficient sleep over a long period of time. The symptoms are easily observed; some of the most typical are the following:

Lack of interest in almost everything, even food

Loss of weight

A feeling of exhaustion at the end of the day

Constipation

An increased feeling of irritability

Lowered resistance to infection

A desire to be alone

Restlessness

Paleness

Loss of interest in studies and social events

Shortness of breath on exertion

[1] Laurence E. Morehouse, and Augustus T. Miller, Jr., *Physiology of Exercise*, The C. V. Mosby Company, St. Louis, 1959.

Disturbance of sleep by dreams, a tendency to awaken early in the morning
Increasing desire to adjust through excessive use of coffee, tobacco, or beverage alcohol [17].

With a combination of causes such as worry, excessive work, irregular hours, insufficient sleep, and inadequate nutrition producing this kind of continuous fatigue and its symptoms, one finds that a complete recovery not only takes time but requires the establishment of a new daily schedule as well, a schedule that has adequate provision for work, rest, relaxation, recreation, sleep, and sound nutrition.

Rest, relaxation, and recreation

The daily program previously discussed suggests time for work, rest, relaxation, recreation, and sleep. Authorities believe such a schedule is beneficial. In present-day society, the pace at which people live is rapid and sustained. Competition is part of every waking hour. And when a job depends equally upon personality and skill, extreme pressure can be inflicted and severe tension develop. Without some planned form of release, rest, relaxation, and recreation, ill health and inefficiency may result.

The modern college campus can also be a tension-producing environment. Unless the student is on guard, he can find much to harass him and build up fatigue. Long and late hours of study, problems about finances and grades, lack of sleep, illness, and conflicts are tension-producing factors. However, it must be pointed out again that tensions are not all bad. In fact, to reach top performance in almost any physical or mental pursuit, it is necessary to develop a certain amount of neuromuscular tension. But such tensions cannot be maintained indefinitely; there must be a letdown, a release, or ultimately there results a profound accumulation of fatigue, irritability, and loss of efficiency that can culminate in illness. The letdown, or period of rest, is a specific antidote to excessive tension and chronic fatigue.

REST

If tensions are by-products of curricular pursuits, and they probably are, rest is both a healer and a deterrent and can help to balance a strenuous schedule.

In rest there is a diminishing or cutting down of sensory and motor stimulation. There is no activity. The chief purpose of rest is to reduce tension—to recover from fatigue. The length of the rest period should be in proportion to the length and type of exertion. A tennis, handball, or basketball player, who is participating for fun, rests frequently. As the game progresses, he takes more time-out periods. He finishes the game tired, but never exhausted. A student studying for two to three hours without interruption builds up a substantial amount of fatigue. It is better to employ rest periods at regular intervals.

A busy day on the campus does not afford many opportunities for rest. However, there are times when rest can be taken, and with profit. The time between classes offers a few minutes' letdown. Some colleges provide rooms where students can pause for quiet and meditation. The time prior to and immediately after lunch or dinner may be used for rest and quiet.

Rest is necessary to all forms of animal life. Even plants and trees have periods in which they are dormant. A wise student understands and recognizes his need for rest and consciously employs techniques to enjoy it each day.

RELAXATION

Relaxation differs from rest. In rest there is no obvious activity, whereas in relaxa-

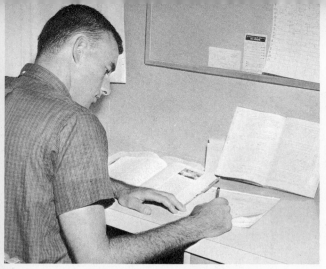

Too long periods of study tend to build up a substantial amount of fatigue and tension.

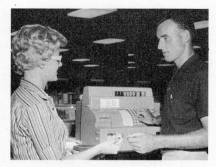

Long periods of time spent on outside jobs or activities also build tensions.

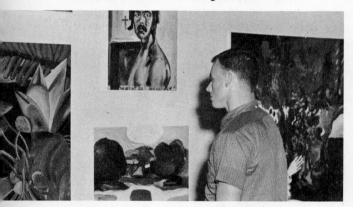

Relaxation and recreation are perhaps the most positive factors in reducing tensions. You may find that regular visits to art galleries, concerts, and the like remove tensions or that . . .

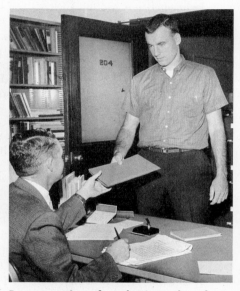

Proper spacing of academic work and handing in assignments on time tend to relieve tensions.

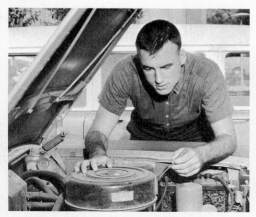

tinkering with your automobile is a pleasant and rewarding diversion.

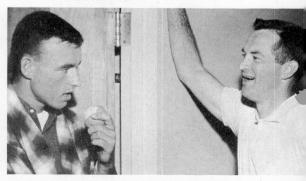

An informal chat with a roommate or friend may help greatly to clear the atmosphere.

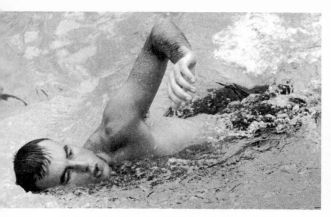

Swimming is a healthful exercise which can give you a delightful feeling of relaxation.

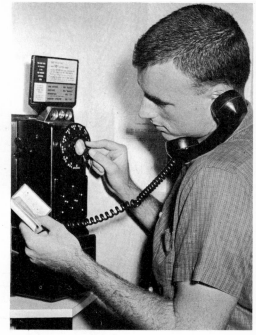

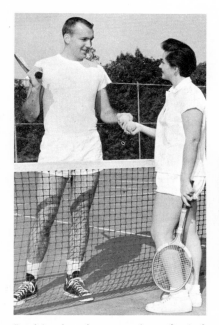

Planning, organizing, and participation in social activities can provide relaxation if not carried to excess.

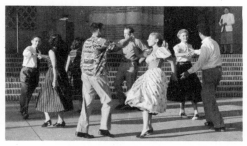

Dancing is a highly satisfying way of relaxing.

Participation in recreative physical activities goes a long way in reducing tensions. Tennis, for example, offers not only desirable physical exercise, but is also a fine opportunity for dating.

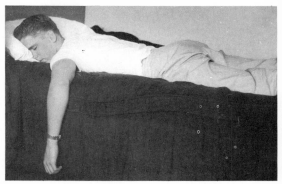

If tensions are by-products of college living, rest and sleep are natural healers and offer a sound way of restoring energies.

tion the individual may reduce action without abolishing the tension necessary for a good performance. This holds true for the performer and the spectator alike. The relaxed person usually finds more satisfaction in recreational activities than the person who holds on to his tensions. However, although relaxation and recreation are not the same, they do complement each other.

Relaxation, which is so important to a satisfying regimen of recreational activities, is not always the same for all people or for all occasions. A well-known surgeon found it important to leave his office at lunch time to seek the seclusion of a darkened motion-picture theater, where he could either rest or relax. A business executive found that driving slowly along a highway adjacent to the ocean relaxed and refreshed him. Rathbone believes that simply changing the pace is only part of the answer. Along with the change of pace, she believes that rhythmic exercise, constructed specifically for tension reduction, should be employed. In her book *Relaxation,* she suggests techniques for accomplishing this. She describes a series of rhythmic exercises which permit the arms and the legs to swing freely; the spine to "sway," to twist, and to move backward and forward; the tissues of the joints to be fully stretched; and restrictions on normal breathing to be released. These exercises are worth the attention of the student [18].

Jacobson believes that by lying quietly and comfortably, then tensing muscle groups, tension can be reduced—for example, tensing muscles in the hand, then relaxing them. This is then repeated for muscles of the neck and of the abdomen. He also illustrates methods of relaxing while active. In fact, he states that one can relax most of the muscles of the body while reading or writing. Relaxation is a matter of training [8].

Relaxing the skeletal muscles at will is difficult at first. It requires many hours of work under the direction of well-qualified personnel. Most college physical education departments provide this kind of instruction. Students lie on mats or firm cots in a comfortable position. The room is quiet. Instructions are given slowly, rhythmically, in a low, pleasant voice, often accompanied with soft music.

The supine position can be very comfortable and should encourage total relaxation. A small support to the neck and one to the lower back can add to one's comfort. The knees should be raised slightly, supported by rolls if necessary. The thighs should be permitted to rotate outward. The arms lie parallel to the body. Instruction in relaxing isolated muscles may then follow.

Characteristics of a relaxed person. Skill in relaxing mind and body helps sustain efficiency. A person in good health who is relaxed [18]:

Moves with ease and with freedom of all parts of the body.

Shows no extra motility; that is, has no nervous mannerisms.

Maintains body postures that permit him to function effectively.

Has good mobility in the joints, especially in the spine.

Has no difficulties with the respiratory system (asthma, irregular breathing, etc.).

Has normal blood circulation (extremities not cold, no excessive sweating, cramps, or flushing of skin).

Has no discomfort from the visceral organs (no constipation, diarrhea, or indigestion).

Has no exceptional or unusual urinary action.

Has a normal menstrual period (women).

Has skeletal muscles which function easily without discomfort.

Makes wholesome adjustments to irritating factors in his environment (people, noise, criticism).

Enjoys periods of rest, and finds it easy to reduce his tensions.

Has no difficulty in going to sleep, and sleeps well.

Has a feeling of security.

Adjusts quickly to the demands of his job.

Avoids the stamp of perfectionism and is satisfied with reasonable accomplishments.

Creates time for recreation and hobbies.

Finds happiness in things of beauty.

Finds satisfaction in spiritual things.

The well-adjusted student will approximate these characteristics. For the student whose score is low, however, it may be time to readjust his goals as well as his daily program. Perhaps it will be necessary to increase the opportunities for rest, relaxation, and recreation. Once these periods are firmly established and a rhythmized program is functioning, excessive tension and fatigue are less likely to occur.

RECREATION

Whereas rest precludes activity and relaxation involves action on a sliding scale, recreation is activity. It is activity motivated by freedom and joy and expressed through mind and body, with revitalizing effects.

Recreation can be many things to many people. It can stimulate the imagination for creative expressions; encourage the use and expansion of artistic and physical skills; serve to develop insights, understandings, and appreciation of the beauty in nature; provide opportunities for social recognition and acceptance; and help to reduce the tension and fatigue of modern living. Recreation varies with individual needs and interests. That which brings joy and satisfaction to one may be hard work and a backache to another. Gardening can be fun or just plain drudgery. Fishing is often acclaimed as the king of recreational sports, but those who think of a stream, lake, or ocean as something to swim in, go boating on, or photograph are left cold by thoughts of a fishing trip. An art gallery or a modern dance concert can bring release, happiness, and spiritual uplift, or it can bore, fatigue, and induce a spirit of derision. Evenings of social, square, and folk dancing, satisfying and popular as they are to some, are times of torture and embarrassment for others. Carpentry and home hobbies of the craft type give hours of satisfaction and pleasure to the skilled or to those with an aptitude for them but produce feelings of frustration in the unskilled. Watching games and sports either at the scene or on television passes many interesting hours and provides conversational topics at business or social gatherings to most men. To some women they offer little that is revitalizing.

Reading, running the scale from comic books to classics, and watching television appear to hold priority over most indoor pastimes. Singing, playing a musical instrument, or listening to music can afford experiences of great spiritual depth.

In short, any force that helps to expand and enrich human personality by developing potentialities and giving them quality and direction is a major factor in the ultimate success and happiness of the individual [16]. This is recreation. The college student is in a strategic place to take full advantage of such forces. Recreational skills learned during student days not only give satisfaction then but tend to ensure the future for effective living.

Hobbies. A highly important part of recreation and one that will become increasingly significant in the future is the broad field of hobbies. Probably no area of living can contribute so richly to man's leisure time as a hobby. Menninger[2] expresses it this way:

Some hobbies are for the solitary; some are for the gregarious; some, like sports, are active; and others, like reading, are passive. Writing is creative and bridge is competi-

[2] William C. Menninger, *Enjoying Leisure Time,* Science Research Associates, Inc., Chicago, 1950, p. 31.

tive. But the nature of each of these activities can be changed according to the desires and goals of the individual. You can study the lives of great writers, as well as plot your own stories, and thereby combine creative activity and educational activity. You can read about sports, participate in them, or collect facts, autographs, and statistics. In other words, the way you carry out your hobby, the kind of activity you want to find in it is largely up to you.

It is never too late to start a hobby. If you have one, you possess a powerful deterrent to boredom. If you are still undecided about a hobby it is time to look over the following list and start one now. In the *creative* field one can find profitable fun in such things as carpentry, ceramics, composing, flower arrangement, hat design, leatherwork, photography, shipbuilding, woodwork, and writing. The field of *collecting* offers much in antiques, autographs, china, coins, glass, guns, paintings, recipes, records, stamps, etc. In *educational* activities one may find enjoyment in studying animals or bees, conducting experiments in physics and chemistry, or just traveling. *Competitive games and sports* offer a rich variety of physical activities. *Noncompetitive physical activities* include such things as bicycling, camping, dancing, fishing, hiking, riding, hunting, skating, skiing, and swimming. The range of *spectator activities* is unlimited. *Social group activities,* including membership in recreational groups, glee clubs, orchestras, dance clubs, and choirs, are highly rewarding [16]. The important point is, if you are wondering what to do with your leisure hours, adopt a hobby.

One of the great tragedies of life occurs when an individual reaches the age of sixty-five, is retired, and finds himself with leisure time but with no skills or interests beyond the scope of his former job. William P. Shepard, of the Metropolitan Life Insurance Company, addressing a National Industrial Health Conference, said: "A fellow who never has had any other interests but his job suddenly dries up and blows away when he is retired. But people who have a number of outside interests live to a ripe old age."

During the past few years, colleges and universities in this country have made time, space, equipment, and recreational leadership available so that their students can develop these outside interests. Campus recreation associations are now integral parts of the college program. Students are encouraged by faculty and fellow students to become participating members of recreation clubs devoted to such interests as badminton, boxing, bridge, bowling, ceramics and other crafts, cycling, dancing, fencing, fiction, flying, fishing, golf, gardening, hiking, polo, painting and allied art work, photography, rod and gun, riding, skating, singing, swimming, sailing, tennis, and wrestling. Experience has shown that, where these clubs are cooperatively controlled, students find unexcelled opportunities for improving their recreational skills under expert instruction, for developing friendships, and for establishing status—a feeling of belonging.

The scope of activities is so impressive and broad that there may be a problem in selecting recreational activities for the first time. In choosing your recreational activities, you should consider the following points:

What is the initial cost of the equipment?

Is the activity primarily group or individual?

Does it require active or passive participation or both?

Is it convenient for me in relation to the rest of my program?

A brief consideration of these questions may be helpful in making wise selections.

THE INITIAL COST OF THE EQUIPMENT. Most equipment for recreation of the active type is expensive. However, it is not necessary to purchase the most expensive or the newest equipment, and it is possible that the college may furnish part of it. Good equipment is essential to efficient performance. If an activity is worth participating in, it is wise to purchase the best equipment within one's means.

INDIVIDUAL OR GROUP ACTIVITY. The choice between joining a club which emphasizes group or individual activity is made on the basis of interest, friendships, and the desire to acquire a new skill. During the four or five years in college it is a good practice to have experiences in both group and individual activity.

ACTIVE OR PASSIVE PARTICIPATION. There are times in life when participation in vigorous recreational games and sports is impossible. It is then that skills in the passive or less active form pay dividends. Before graduation the student should have participated in both types of recreation.

APPLICATION TO ONE'S PROGRAM. Earlier in the chapter, emphasis was placed on the importance of balance so that the student's daily program may conform to some type of broad, harmonious rhythmic pattern. The advantages of such a pattern, including time for work, recreation, rest, relaxation, and sleep, previously have been emphasized. In constructing the first program of the year, it will pay to make sure that there is an adequate place the three R's—rest, relaxation, and recreation.

Sleep

During the summer months, in the temperate zone, there occurs a cycle of about fifteen hours of daylight and nine hours of darkness. In the winter, the ratio is reversed, with fifteen hours of darkness and nine hours of daylight. Early man established his living schedule by this natural arrangement of light and dark. The behavior pattern of people up to modern times was influenced by it. Today, however, by the flip of a switch or the pressure of a finger, there is no darkness. Modern man has broken the cycle. He turns night into day. He changes the work and play patterns of his fellow man. He is in full control of what was once nature's business. However, man still needs, at regular intervals, opportunities to withdraw from activity and seek the quiet seclusion of darkness, to rest and sleep.

Scientists agree that natural sleep is the most satisfying form of recuperation from fatigue. During sleep all vital functions of the body are reduced. Body cells that have been used during activity are repaired. The metabolic rate is lowered, and energy is restored.

Students often ask questions about sleep, such as, What is sleep? What is the purpose of sleep? How much sleep should I get? Would it hurt me to study all night? Will my efficiency be impaired if I go without much sleep? Is it normal to twist and turn during sleep? Only partial answers can be given to some of these queries.

Sleep is a natural phenomenon common to all animal life. It is a position on the scale of consciousness—a periodic interruption of wakeful hours. As yet there has been no fully accepted scientific explanation of this phenomenon. The ancient theory that blood leaving the brain produces sleep is still a popular one, but it is not accepted by modern scientists. The belief that an accumulation of fatigue products influences a "sleep center" in the thalamus of the brain has some support, but again this is not an accepted explanation. Whereas there is no widely accepted theory of the cause of sleep, many interesting observations about sleep have been made. For example, everyone accepts the fact that sleep is necessary for life. It is also the main factor in recovery from fatigue. If left to his own choosing, the healthy human adult under normal conditions will sleep between seven and eight hours each night. When he has had all the sleep necessary for a refreshed body he will awaken slowly and naturally without mechanical aids.

Apparently there are several levels of intensity of sleep. As one lies quietly in his bed anticipating sleep, he drifts slowly from a stage of drowsiness to a light stage of sleep and then to a very deep sleep. When the body has reached this deep level, certain changes occur [12, 13, 14]:

There is total unconsciousness.

The blood concentrates in the large organs of the viscera.

The systolic blood pressure falls.

The blood supply to the skin increases.

There is less oxygen in the blood.

The chemical composition of the blood changes (less calcium in the blood and more at the base of the brain).

The body temperature falls slightly.

Ventilation of the lungs slows down.

Skeletal muscles relax.

The sense of smell is diminished.

The average normal adult sleeps best in a comfortable bed to which he is accustomed. It must be out of drafts and in a room that is cool and dark. Natural sleep is more apt to come to one whose mind is free from worry and whose body is free from pain or irritation. During a normal night's sleep, the average person changes his sleeping position every eleven to twelve minutes [12, 13, 14].

An occasional loss of sleep happens to everyone and is nothing to fear. Research indicates that normal adults suffer no major physiologic change after as much as 200 hours of induced insomnia. Veterans of both world wars recall many instances of men and women forced to go without sleep from forty-eight to seventy-two hours who made normal physical recoveries after twelve to fourteen hours of sleep. It appears that the significant change after prolonged insomnia or loss of sleep is in the central nervous system [12]. Edwards observed that after 100 hours of wakefulness his subjects were irritable and restless and suffered from headaches. It took seven days of normal living and sleeping for them to return to the pretest status. Kleitman found that in his subjects, the feeling of drowsiness came in waves, the most difficult periods occurring at 3 A.M. and 6 P.M. [12].

Studies have been made as to the influence of the seasons of the year on sleep. Laird reports that one is likely to sleep less well in spring than in autumn. He believes that this change varies with calcium metabolism, which appears to be at its lowest during the spring months. Kleitman, on the contrary, believes that in the spring of the year one falls asleep with greater ease and has less motility (movement) [12].

Nevertheless, these findings do have a significant fact in common: that normal sleep provides a great margin of safety not only during the experiments but in actual emergency situations as well.

In view of the research that has been done on sleep, the physically well student can take comfort in the fact that occasional loss of sleep is not necessarily harmful to his health or to his efficiency. It is the continuous loss that produces chronic fatigue and can be harmful to health.

There are times when it is difficult to reduce body tension enough to go to sleep. Such a state is not uncommon and is no cause for alarm. A restful night's sleep can be induced by the use of drugs or by following a planned routine for relaxing the body naturally. The practice of using sleeping pills can be harmful to effective living. Health authorities condemn their unrestricted use (see Chapter 13, Understanding Depressants and Stimulants). Any drug taken internally to induce sleep should be used only in an emergency and upon the advice of a reputable physician.

Getting enough sleep can be a problem for some people, but difficulty in getting *to* sleep is all too often a source of annoyance to many. Tensions built up during the day and evening become deterrents to sleep. The following suggestions may be helpful in reducing these tensions before retiring:

Begin a conscious relaxing of the body muscles while sitting in a comfortable chair.

Make all body movements slow and deliberate.

Read, listen to the radio, or watch TV, whichever is the most relaxing.

Sip a warm or cool drink (let experience dictate which temperature).

When the desire to sleep comes, move very slowly through the routine of preparation for retiring.

Keep the mind set on total relaxation.

Move slowly into bed, stretch, concentrate on how good the softness feels; banish all worries, plannings, or recapitulations; and go to sleep [15].

A restful sleep is a satisfying experience. It is nature's insurance against a complete nervous breakdown of the human race. Of all the pleasures man enjoys, sleep is one of the most rewarding, and, interestingly enough, it can be appreciated and enjoyed only afterward.

Summary

Opportunities for work, rest, relaxation, recreation, and sleep during a twenty-four-hour period can be planned so that you will have ample time to meet your obligations. This principle of balance among work, sleep, rest, relaxation, and recreation is not new; it has been employed in business and industrial organizations for many years.

Perhaps the first essential in achieving this objective is to construct a balanced daily schedule. Such a schedule, consistently employed, can help you provide an effective means for achieving scholastic excellence, with no neglect of your social and physical activities and with a minimal drain on your energies.

One pronounced result of employing a balanced daily schedule is that it helps to control fatigue. An active body becomes fatigued. This is a normal physiologic reaction. Body fatigue may be general or chronic. General fatigue is an experience common to all of us. Usually a night's sleep is enough for a full recovery. Chronic fatigue is more profound. It may occur as the result of worry, excessive work, inadequate nutrition, and insufficient sleep over a long period of time. Recovery from this condition involves the establishment of a more healthful daily schedule.

It is generally agreed that natural sleep is one of the most satisfying forms of recovery from fatigue. The healthy adult under normal conditions will sleep between seven and eight hours each night. When he has had all the sleep necessary for a refreshed body, he awakens slowly and naturally without mechanical aids.

Work, rest, relaxation, and recreation, which includes hobbies, are also effective and essential components of a balanced daily schedule.

Suggested readings

1. Brauchi, John T., and Louis J. West: "Sleep Deprivation," *The Journal of the American Medical Association,* 171:11–14, Sept. 5, 1959.

2. Brown, Pete: "A Woodland Refuge on Campus," *Recreation,* 54:66–67, February, 1961.

3. Carter, Joel: *How to Make Athletic*

Equipment, The Ronald Press Company, New York, 1960.

4. Collin, Lore: *Stampcraft,* Charles E. Tuttle, Rutland, Vt., 1959.

5. Gabrielsen, M. Alexander, Betty Spears, and B. W. Gabrielsen: *Aquatics Handbook,* Prentice-Hall, Inc., Englewood Cliffs, N.J., 1959.

6. Hooley, Agnes M.: "Leisure-time Pursuits in College," *Recreation,* 53:83–84, February, 1960.

7. Hunt, Valerie V.: *Recreation for the Handicapped,* Prentice-Hall, Inc., Englewood Cliffs, N.J., 1955.

8. Jacobson, Edmund: *You Must Relax,* 4th ed., McGraw-Hill Book Company, Inc., New York, 1957.

9. Kamiya, Joe: "How Much Sleep Do You Really Need?" *U.S. News and World Report,* 60:68–74, Feb. 6, 1959.

10. Kaplan, Max: *Leisure in America,* John Wiley & Sons, Inc., New York, 1960.

11. Kearney, Paul W.: "A Heart Stops Beating," *Skin Diver Magazine,* 10:42, April, 1961.

12. Kleitman, Nathaniel: *Sleep and Wakefulness,* University of Chicago Press, Chicago, 1950.

13. Kleitman, Nathaniel: "The Sleep Cycle," *American Journal of Nursing,* 60:677–679, May, 1960.

14. McBrooks, Chandler: "The Mysterious State of Sleep," *Yale Scientific Magazine,* 31:31–35, January, 1957.

15. Metheny, Eleanor: *Body Dynamics,* McGraw-Hill Book Company, Inc., New York, 1952.

16. Menninger, William C.: *Enjoying Leisure Time,* Science Research Associates, Inc., Chicago, 1950.

17. Morehouse, Laurence E., and Augustus T. Miller, Jr.: *Physiology of Exercise,* The C. V. Mosby Company, St. Louis, 1959.

18. Rathbone, Josephine: *Relaxation,* Bureau of Publications, Teachers College, Columbia University, New York, 1950.

19. Stocker, Stanley W.: "Winter Camping," *Recreation,* 53:68–69, February, 1960.

NINE

Selecting and eating wholesome foods

NUTRITIONAL STATUS OF THE AMERICAN PEOPLE

MISCONCEPTIONS ABOUT FOODS

OVERWEIGHT AND UNDERWEIGHT

BASIS FOR PLANNING THE DIET

FUNCTIONS OF FOOD IN THE BODY

ESSENTIAL BODY NUTRIENTS

PREPARATION OF FOODS TO CONSERVE NUTRIENT VALUE

CONVERTING FOOD FOR BODY FUNCTIONS

DISORDERS OF THE DIGESTIVE SYSTEM

Nutritional practices of many Americans are difficult to understand. In a land of nutritional plenty many individuals are undernourished—and not all because of lack of money. Individuals spend excessive amounts of money to purchase foods that do little but add pounds; then the same persons spend more money for products and services to help them lose pounds. We generally find eating to be a pleasurable activity, yet some persons replace a daily meal or meals with a complete formula food or they use the mealtime to upset family members with discipline activities or discussion of unpleasant problems.

Individuals pass up the fruit and vegetables, whole grain foods, and milk and buy their vitamins and minerals in drugstores. Parents attempt to force their children to eat certain foods which they themselves refuse. It is generally agreed that a nutritious breakfast is an important part of sound nutrition, yet parents fail to prepare such a breakfast for their children and many persons fail to get up in time to have breakfast.

Many persons are unhappy because they lack money to buy materials they want, yet they support both faddists and reputable pharmaceutical firms by spending money for special foods and supplements that a balanced diet would provide. We spend millions annually for laxatives, when proper diet would, in most cases, promote proper elimination of waste material from the digestive tract.

College students reflect many influences, including those of their family, their friends, and their own personal feelings, in their selection of foods. Poor nutritional habits may be difficult to change, but *they can be changed*. Selecting an adequate diet and establishing good eating habits are challenges that you should be sufficiently mature to accept.

Understanding and applying information elicited by the following questions provide a basis for improved nutritional practices:

What are the common weaknesses in the diet of American people?

What are common food fads and fallacies that you should understand in order to avoid?

What is the significance of overweight and underweight to the health status of individuals?

What essential nutrients are required to satisfy the functions of food in your body?

How can you plan effectively to meet the nutritional needs of your body?

Nutritional status of the American people

Studies provide evidence that the nutritional status of Americans, on the whole, is probably superior to that reported for any similar population group [21]. Studies also provide evidence, however, that a substantial number of individuals have dietary deficiencies. In addition, there is evidence that certain deficiencies are common among certain groups in our society. An understanding of the more common deficiencies is helpful to those interested in providing for their body's nutritional needs.

College students, as well as other adults in the population, can profit from the findings of an extensive nutritional-status study in the United States [21]. Included in the sample of the population

in this study were students in the 13–20 age group. The diets of boys were adequate or more than adequate in amount for all nutrients except vitamin C. The girls, on the other hand, were high in only three nutrients: vitamin A, riboflavin, and niacin. Their average intake of calcium, iron, thiamine, and vitamin C was seriously low and for calories and proteins was borderline low. Girls in the 13–20 age group demonstrated the least favorable nutritional status of all the individuals examined.

A report on the eating habits of college students indicates that this group does not exhibit improvement over other groups in the population [12]. This same report shows that in a series of studies a number of students, from a low of 9 per cent to a high of 25 per cent, missed having breakfast at least two days each week. In addition, it was found that many other students did not include recommended foods in their morning meals.

Some of the reasons commonly given for failure to include recommended amounts of nutrients in the diet are:

Lack of income

Size of family

Lack of knowledge

Failure to apply knowledge

Failure of the homemaker to take sufficient time for meal planning

Continuation of faulty family eating patterns from generation to generation

Personal likes and dislikes for specific foods

It is significant to note that the findings of one study show that the extent of the formal education of the homemaker seemed to be the most important single factor in her knowledge of nutrition [35].

High income makes it possible to provide the recommended amounts of nutrients, but it does not ensure that these nutrients are provided. One study shows that families failed to meet the nutritional recommendations of the Food and Nutrition Board of the National Research Council with meals that averaged 40 cents, whereas other families more than met the recommendations with meals averaging 25 cents [18]. Another study shows that certain nutrients are more likely to be related to income than are others [33]. Vitamin C is the nutrient most closely related to income and thiamine the least related. Higher income is closely related to the purchase of good food sources of vitamin C, the citrus fruits in particular. High-income families fail to include adequate amounts of thiamine as frequently as do low-income families. High-income families tend to reduce the amount of grains and pork, two of the best sources of thiamine.

One unsatisfactory eating habit of many Americans is their failure to start the day with an adequate breakfast. The data in Table 9.1 show a variety of breakfasts served to a group of adults and the percentage of individuals who had each of these breakfasts. As can be seen by checking the table, only slightly over 60 per cent of the homes served breakfasts containing fruit, carbohydrate foods, and protein foods. In another study the breakfasts reported for adolescents were found to contribute approximately one-fifth instead of the recommended one-third to one-fourth of the daily allowances of nutrients [21]. The breakfasts, especially for girls, were most frequently deficient in calories, protein, iron, vitamin A, and niacin.

Despite evidence to show that Americans, on the whole, are extremely well-nourished in comparison with other population groups, there is a need for more widespread understanding and application of sound nutritional information. The frequency of deficiencies reported in

Table 9.1 Types of breakfasts served adults

Type of breakfast	Percentage of homes	
	Rochester	Syracuse
None	1	2
Coffee or juice and coffee	2	2
Carbohydrate and coffee	8	4
Carbohydrate and milk†	9	9
Fruit, carbohydrate†	7	8
Fruit, carbohydrate, milk†	26	27
Fruit, egg, carbohydrate†	14	15
Fruit, egg, carbohydrate, milk†	22	21
Egg, carbohydrate†	5	6
Egg, carbohydrate, milk†	5	5
Fruit, egg	1	1

† Might or might not include coffee.
Source: Charlotte M. Young and others, "What the Homemaker Knows about Nutrition: IV. Her Food Problems, Shopping Habits, and Sources of Information," *Journal of the American Dietetic Association*, 32:433, May, 1956.

the diets of individuals and the widespread acceptance of the recommendations of food faddists are an indication that a concentrated effort is needed to raise the nutritional status of Americans to a higher level. We need to be aware of some of the reasons why we fail to apply sound nutritional practices in daily living. We should approach meal planning and food selection with the idea of increasing our pleasure from eating; at the same time we should eat foods that supply nutritional needs.

Misconceptions about foods

Extravagant claims for any single food should arouse suspicions about either the value of the food or the purpose of the person making the claim. With the exception milk, which serves as the only source of nourishment in the very early period of life, no single food has extraordinary qualities of the kind that quacks or faddists claim for their favorite products. Milk has sometimes been referred to as "the most nearly perfect food," but milk alone provides an inadequate diet for anyone except the very young infant. Following the recommendations included in *Food for Fitness: A Daily Food Guide* (see page 230) is much more likely to provide your body with the required nutrients than following the suggestions of some person who is either misinformed or interested primarily in making money at your expense.

WHY FOOD FADDISTS?

Food faddists make their claims for a variety of reasons. Some are firmly convinced that they have an idea that will benefit mankind; unfortunately, though they have little scientific evidence to support their claims, they do have sufficient persuasive power to convince many gullible persons to take their advice. Others undertake the promotion of a particular product for personal gain. The persuasive power they exert is no less effective than that of the rightful crusaders.

Characteristics of individuals who are most often persuaded by the faddist are not always clear-cut and easily defined. There are, however, some types of individuals who are more likely to fall victim to the exaggerated claims of the faddist. There are persons who are swayed easily and who tend to follow the advice of anyone who sounds plausible. This type is likely to switch allegiance from one faddist to another. There are persons with health problems, real or imaginary, who seek constantly a new way to resolve their problems with or without the advice of a qualified medical adviser. This group, which includes the hypochondriacs, is made up of individuals grasping at one straw and then at another in hope of finding a solution to the health problem. There are other persons who follow blindly ideas that have persisted in their family from one generation to another. There are still others too poorly informed about nutrition to make intelligent choices concerning foods. These persons find it difficult to detect the half-truths and misleading statements included in faddist propaganda. Individuals in most of the above categories can be helped to make more intelligent choices through a sound educational program (see Chapter 10 for information on consumer health).

COMMON FOOD FADS

Food fads change with the times, but the problems associated with them are much the same. In some instances the recommended product is harmful to the user. Frequently the danger is not directly from the product itself but results from the failure of the user to eat foods needed to provide nutrients for normal body functioning. Because of false security developed as a result of claims made by the faddist, some serious consequences may result from the failure to seek qualified medical assistance. Still another problem is the expense of purchasing the product recommended by the faddist, which is usually considerably more than the cost of equivalent nutrients in regular foods. Consideration of some past fads may help demonstrate the nature of claims commonly made.

Exaggerated claims for specific foods. Various claims have been made for specific foods at different times. The stress on fish as a brain food, celery as a nerve tonic, and onions as a cure for a cold are examples of such exaggerated claims. More recently, some faddists have extolled the virtues of yoghurt, honey, vinegar, and royal jelly as super foods. Yoghurt is made from milk and has whatever values milk contributes to the diet. Because it consists of milk alone, it provides only those substances found in milk. It is a good food, but the price of yoghurt makes it a rather expensive source of nutrients found in more reasonably priced milk or milk products.

Honey and vinegar have received particular emphasis as a result of a book on folk medicine. Nutritionists are appalled at the claims made by the author and at the popular reception of the publication. The claim that apple-cider vinegar has a high potassium content—a statement disproved by food composition tables—and that two teaspoons of vinegar in a glass of water at mealtime will make it possible for the body to burn fat instead of storing it are examples of the farfetched statements made [31].

Royal jelly, the food of the queen bee, is another example of a food product for which unreasonable claims have been made. Nutritionists suggest that the jelly may be excellent for the queen bee but that for humans it is of no practical benefit as a food or as a drug or cosmetic, two other uses suggested by its proponents [31].

Considerable caution should be exer-

cised in accepting sweeping claims about specific food products. Sound, scientific information should be available on products before one decides to use them to the exclusion of other foods.

Myth of overprocessing. This faddist claim is developed around the idea that the only food which is good is "natural" food. It is claimed that foods that have been processed are lacking in essential nutrients. This concept is an exaggeration of the fact that there is a loss of nutrient value as a result of some processing and cooking of foods. The fact that processing of foods is based on preserving nutritional values or in restoring them to foods is overlooked by the faddist.

This type of faddist usually has a specific product that he is selling, and he generally demands a premium price. If we were to eat only the so-called natural foods, we would have to exclude a large portion of the food commonly included in the American diet.

Fortunately, the answer to the question of raw foods as opposed to cooked foods is not one or the other, but a combination. Some foods are more readily digested when cooked properly. Some foods tend to lose part of their nutrient value when cooked, especially when improperly cooked. The superiority of raw foods as the primary constituent of meals in this country at the present time cannot be substantiated. The general opinion of authorities is that the diet of most individuals can profitably include some cooked and some raw fruits and vegetables.

Myth of soil depletion. This claim is based on the idea that repeated farming of land has so depleted the soil that all foods grown on it are nutritionally inferior. Many faddists claim that the depleted soil can be restored to normal only by the use of organic fertilizers and that chemical fertilizers are not only worthless but also dangerous. The U.S. Department

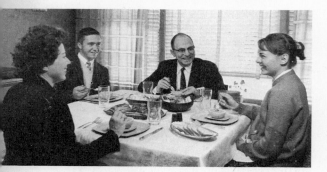

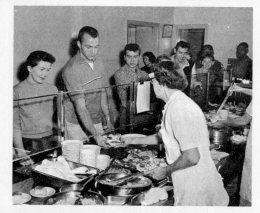

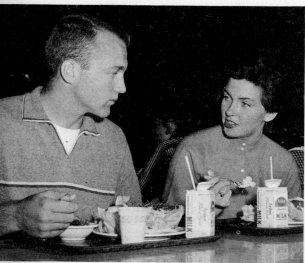

Mealtime can be enjoyable and nutritious in a pleasant family atmosphere or in the college cafeteria with a wise choice of food and a friendly companion.

of Agriculture, on the basis of scientific tests, concludes that there is no evidence to support the claim that foods are nutritionally inferior due to soil depletion. Poor soil will give a smaller yield, but there will not be less nutrients in the food produced. If it were true that the amount of nutrients in a given food was related to the quality of the soil, it would be useless to prepare tables showing the composition of foods. The only known essential deficiency in soil that results in a deficiency in foods grown in it is iodine. Deficiency of iodine in foods grown in some areas is made up by adding iodine to common table salt for use in seasoning food [33].

Claims associated with subclinical deficiencies. Faddists who use this subterfuge claim that persons who feel fatigue or have aches and pains probably feel this way because of subclinical deficiency; therefore, they should be supplementing their diet with some particular product— one sold by the faddist, of course. Proponents of this approach indicate that a subclinical vitamin deficiency does not produce observable evidence of the deficiency but merely that the general symptoms indicated above suggest the suspected deficiency.

It would be a rare individual who did not exhibit such symptoms occasionally, but there is no sound basis for assuming that the symptoms are due to subclinical deficiencies, as claimed. Even if the claims were true, it could not be safely assumed that the advertised products would be of value. Components of products sold by one company included alfalfa, ground bones, juices from cereal plants, garlic, lecithin, wheat germ, volcanic ashes, and water. The producer in this case was convicted of false claims in labeling [31].

The food-supplement story is best illustrated by a product composed of a concentrated extract of alfalfa, water cress, and parsley and some 30 vitamins and minerals, among other ingredients. This product has been purchased by an estimated 3 million persons, who spent more than $200 million. Despite numerous court appearances and convictions, the vendors of this product have continued to reap a monetary harvest from the public [30, 31].

The possible harm through needless expenditure of money and development of false feelings of security from such products is difficult to assess. The readiness with which individuals accept an easy way of meeting nutritional needs substantiates the importance of an improved understanding of nutrition by the general public.

Vitamin preparations. Even the vitamin salesmen admit that most persons can obtain all the vitamins they need from a well-balanced diet. They suggest, however, that, in order to be sure that vitamin needs are met, the individual should take a vitamin preparation. Some persons respond to this suggestion by deciding that if a given amount of vitamin is good, then more of the vitamin will be better. They do not realize, unfortunately, that too much of certain vitamins can be harmful or that the excess amounts of others are simply excreted by the body. On the one hand, there is a danger from an excess, and on the other, a waste of money for extra amounts that the body is unable to use.

Some individuals, among them Norman Jolliffe, Chief of the Nutrition Division, New York City Health Department, take the viewpoint that many persons should supplement their diet regularly with vitamin preparations. In general, this belief is based upon the premise that these persons cannot or will not eat a balanced diet and that supplementing is the only logical answer. A better answer would be to have these persons improve their dietary practices to the extent that the nutrients required for normal body functioning are included in the daily diet.

The position of the Council on Foods and Nutrition, American Medical Association, is: [1]

Healthy persons whose diets are normally considered adequate may benefit from supplementary vitamins at certain special periods of life, such as during pregnancy and lactation. Vitamin supplementation is useful during periods of illness or deranged mode of life, which may result in impairment of absorption of nutrients or deterioration of dietary quality. Supplementation may also be of value to the individual who, through ignorance, poor eating habits, or emotional or physical illness, does not eat an adequate diet. The physician's primary responsibility for these patients is to remove these disturbing factors rather than merely to alleviate their results. Nevertheless, until the disturbing factors have been discovered and, when possible, removed, supplementary vitamins are valuable in assuring adequate intake.

The Council also recommends that when multivitamins are used for ordinary diet supplementation, the preparations should supply about one-half the recommended daily dietary allowances. Preparations containing more than one-half the daily recommendations should be used only for therapeutic purposes as prescribed by the physician.

Complete formula foods. Considering the pleasure and satisfaction that most people derive from eating, it would seem that complete formula foods to replace meals would have little appeal. The early success of such products, from the producer's standpoint, indicates that the appeal was great. Apparently there are many persons who prefer to overeat at some meals or for periods of time and then put up with the crash dieting program suggested by producers of the complete formula foods. There seems to be little disagreement among nutritionists with the claim that the better complete formula foods do seem to be nutritionally

[1] Council on Foods and Nutrition, American Medical Association, "Vitamin Preparations as Dietary Supplements and as Therapeutic Agents," *Journal of the American Medical Association*, 169:42, Jan. 3, 1959.

complete except for the shortage of calories. The primary concern with use of complete formula foods is the danger of self-imposed crash dieting and the over-all efficacy of most forms of "popular" dieting.

It is apparent that diet planned around complete formula foods can cause weight loss and can be safe if supervised by a physician. The history of dieting over the years has indicated, however, that most individuals gain only temporary benefit from dieting that is not related to establishing sound eating habits, which can be followed when the immediate purpose of the diet is accomplished. From a health standpoint, little can be said in favor of alternating gains in weight and dieting to lose weight.

A college student would do well to plan meals so that he meets his needs through a variety of foods and enjoys both eating and the consequences of eating. There is little need for complete formula foods when an ample supply of a variety of good foods is available and within our means.

Fads emphasizing weight control. Faddists have responded to the emphasis placed on the dangers of overweight. Overweight persons are literally bombarded with a variety of diets and special products guaranteed to help them lose pounds without suffering from hunger. Some of these diets, which are lacking in sufficient amounts of protein or are deficient in other ways, can be dangerous if followed for any prolonged period of time. It should be emphasized that there is no ideal reducing diet that fits all persons. Drugs that are suggested as an aid to reducing may be potentially dangerous to some users. This highly exploited nutritional problem should be combated in a logical and sensible way and not by the use of products, diets, and devices suggested by some promoter, whose primary concern is to make money at the expense of the overweight person.

Overweight and underweight

Underweight persons are malnourished, at least to the extent that they are providing too few calories to maintain normal weight. It is a fallacy to assume, however, that all malnourished persons are underweight. It is possible to be overweight and, at the same time, deficient in vitamins, minerals, or proteins. The individual who permits himself to become either excessively overweight or excessively underweight is placing a burden upon his body functions. For a longer life and for better health he should attempt to maintain his weight at a normal level.

OVERWEIGHT

Although it has been stated that the best way to determine obesity is to view one's self in the mirror, it is difficult to determine normal weight. The wide variation in body build reduces the value of height-weight tables in assessing normal weight.

However, the revised tables of desirable weights prepared by the Metropolitan Life Insurance Company are helpful in appraising weight status (Table 9.2). An individual is considered to be overweight if he is 10 per cent above his ideal weight and obese if he is 20 per cent or more above his ideal weight.

An observant individual sees many obese and overweight persons around him. Studies confirm the prevalence of overweight persons. In one nationwide study it was found that from one-fourth to one-half the women examined in different geographical areas of the country were 10 per cent or more overweight; more than half of them were more than 20 per cent overweight. The number of men examined was considerably smaller, but the percentage of overweight persons was about the same as for women [21].

It is accepted generally by authorities

Table 9.2 Desirable weights for men and women according to height and frame (ages twenty-five and over)

Height in shoes	Weight in indoor clothing, pounds		
	Small frame	Medium frame	Large frame
Men			
5' 2"	112–120	118–129	126–141
3"	115–123	121–133	129–144
4"	118–126	124–136	132–148
5"	121–129	127–139	135–152
6"	124–133	130–143	138–156
7"	128–137	134–147	142–161
8"	132–141	138–152	147–166
9"	136–145	142–156	151–170
10"	140–150	146–160	155–174
11"	144–154	150–165	159–179
6' 0"	148–158	154–170	164–184
1"	152–162	158–175	168–189
2"	156–167	162–180	173–194
3"	160–171	167–185	178–199
4"	164–175	172–190	182–204
Women			
4'10"	92–98	96–107	104–119
11"	94–101	98–110	106–122
5' 0"	96–104	101–113	109–125
1"	99–107	104–116	112–128
2"	102–110	107–119	115–131
3"	105–113	110–122	118–134
4"	108–116	113–126	121–138
5"	111–119	116–130	125–142
6"	114–123	120–135	129–146
7"	118–127	124–139	133–150
8"	122–131	128–143	137–154
9"	126–135	132–147	141–158
10"	130–140	136–151	145–163
11"	134–144	140–155	149–168
6' 0"	138–148	144–159	153–173

Note: Prepared by the Metropolitan Life Insurance Company. Derived primarily from data of the *Build and Blood Pressure Study*, 1959, Society of Actuaries.
Source: Metropolitan Life Insurance Company, *Statistical Bulletin*, 40:3, November-December, 1959. By permission.

that the mortality rates for overweight persons exceed those for standard-weight persons. Implications of overweight in the occurrence of degenerative disorders are considered in Chapter 12.

Causes. Except for a relatively few cases due to glandular malfunction, probably no more than 1 per cent of all cases, people are overweight because they overeat. Overeating is strictly an individual matter; what would be a normal diet for one person may mean added pounds to another. The factors discussed in the consideration of metabolism (see pages 231–232) determine whether the amount eaten causes weight gain, loss, or maintenance. The factors that determine the amount eaten are varied and are not as well understood as those which influence metabolism.

Some of the reasons for overeating are:

Following a family pattern of eating

Overeating during convalescence from an illness and continuing after recovery

Eating to meet demands for heavy activity and then reducing activity without changing eating habits

Eating due to boredom, loneliness, or discontent

Poor eating practices such as eating between meals and excessive use of calorie-rich foods

Parents play an important role in establishing eating practices for weight control as well as for supplying needed nutrients. Parents should not be blamed indefinitely, however, for practices that a mature individual should be able to improve over a period of time. Whatever the reason for overeating, the end result, if the practice is continued, is an overweight person.

Reducing safely. Obesity is a major health problem. It is advisable for the obese individual to consult his physician and to follow his suggestions for protecting health while reducing weight. He should beware of the glittering promises made in advertising simple, safe methods of losing weight without changing eating habits. Reducing compounds can injure the health. The Council on Foods and Nutrition, American Medical Association, has issued a warning against indiscriminate use of formula diets, which have received widespread publicity during the early 1960s. Rapid weight loss, which may occur as a result of using formula diets, can be dangerous to health [9].

The way to lose weight is to take in fewer calories than the body requires. Body fat is then used to supply the extra calories, and weight is decreased. However, a safe diet does not omit all car-

bohydrates or all fats or all of anything. The individual should be certain that nutrients are supplied in required amounts. He should choose his calories by the company they keep; that is, calorie sources should also provide minerals and vitamins.

Moderate, consistent exercise suited to the individual plays an important role in the control of body weight. It is a fallacy to assume that it is a simple matter to exercise away quickly the many pounds accumulated over a period of time. It is likewise a fallacy to assume that exercise is of little value because of the relatively prolonged period of activity required to burn up 1 pound of body fat. The value of exercise is indicated by the following example. Table 9.4 shows that an individual uses 0.7 calories per pound per hour while sitting at rest and 1.4 calories per pound per hour while walking at moderate speed. A man weighing 160 pounds would use approximately 112 calories while sitting at rest for one hour and approximately 224 calories while walking for the same period of time. The difference of approximately 112 calories, if allowed to accumulate as fat each day, would at the end of a year total 11 to 12 pounds of body fat. Among the many benefits that exercise can offer is that of aiding in normal weight maintenance.

It is easier to keep pounds off than to take them off. The ideal weight-control program begins while weight is normal. Eating to satisfy the energy needs of the body and to maintain weight sets a pattern that can be maintained with minor changes as one grows older and/or changes his activity program. Eating to lose weight rapidly frequently leaves an individual dissatisfied and sets a pattern he is not likely to follow when he has returned to normal weight. A weakness of most reducing diets is that they are temporary; they do not represent an effort to establish a dietary pattern that the individual can or will continue. See

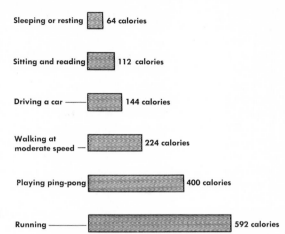

Sleeping or resting — 64 calories

Sitting and reading — 112 calories

Driving a car — 144 calories

Walking at moderate speed — 224 calories

Playing ping-pong — 400 calories

Running — 592 calories

Caloric expenditure by a 160-pound man for one hour of selected activities.

Table 9.5 for information on the nutrient value of selected foods.

UNDERWEIGHT

The individual more than 10 per cent under his ideal weight is likely to be functioning at a level somewhat below optimum. The reduced vitality and stamina consequent to such a condition may be dangerous to his health.

Some disadvantages of being underweight include a scrawny appearance, a tendency to chill easily as a result of inadequate subcutaneous fat, irritability, lack of ambition, inability to concentrate, a tendency to tire easily, a tendency to digestive disorders, and lowered resistance to disease germs [4]. The under-

weight individual needs the advice of his physician in order to determine whether or not the condition is due to an organic cause. If the condition is simply a matter of an insufficient supply of nutrients to meet the needs of the body, he can add more of these nutrients to the daily intake of food. High calorie content is a primary objective of a diet to increase the weight, but added amounts of protein, minerals, and vitamins are equally important.

One of the basic objectives of meal planning is to provide a diet that enables ideal weight to be maintained and at the same time includes adequate amounts of all of the nutrients that are necessary.

Basis for planning the diet

A sound basis for planning your diet is to understand what influences the kind and amount of food that an individual eats and to have a sound guide to use as a basis for meal planning. A sound guide as a basis for planning is readily available and is discussed in detail in the following paragraphs. The factors that influence the kind and amount of food eaten are not as clearly understood.

It is apparent that each individual, by

the time he has reached college age, has established eating practices and patterns that may be difficult, but not impossible, to change. He is a product of his home environment and other influences in the types of food to which he is accustomed, mealtime atmosphere, specific likes and dislikes, use of foods for satisfaction lacking from other sources, peer pressures to eat a variety of snack foods, fashion demands for body build, and the pure pleasure of eating good food. He is under a constant barrage from advertising men, who push foods guaranteed to do such things as add weight, take off weight, simplify eating, increase pleasure, and save money. He is aware that a good breakfast is desirable, but he may have been brought up on the basis of a few minutes' extra sleep and a breakfast on the run.

College students with poor nutritional practices can make some improvements, if they are willing to face up to the reasons why their practices are poor and establish a plan of action to make changes. As indicated in Chapter 5, many college students are married and most of them will eventually marry. When children are added to the family, the eating habits of the parents will in turn influence those of the children. It behooves parents to give careful consideration to the ultimate effect of poor eating practices on the health of their children.

During World War II, when the Ameri-

can people were being prepared for any eventuality, considerable emphasis was placed on the problem of conserving food and, at the same time, being certain that the diet was meeting nutritional needs. As a result of the research carried on, the Basic Seven food groups became widely publicized as a sound basis for meal planning. More recently these same food groups have been reorganized into four groups as presented in *Food for Fitness: A Daily Food Guide* [32].

A DAILY FOOD GUIDE

The food groups in *A Daily Food Guide* provide a sound basis for planning the variety of food that should be included in the daily diet. In addition, foods such as butter, margarine, other fats, oils, sugars, or unenriched refined grain products are used to some extent to satisfy the appetite. (See Table 9.3.)

Many persons who speak glibly about vitamins and minerals actually understand little about these nutrients or about

Table 9.3   Food for fitness: A daily food guide

Food group	Contribution to diet	Amount
Meat	Foods in this group are valued for their protein, which is needed for growth and repair of body tissues—muscle, organs, blood, skin, and hair. These foods also provide iron, thiamine, riboflavin, and niacin.	2 or more servings Beef, veal, pork, lamb, poultry, fish, eggs As alternates: dry beans, dry peas, nuts
Milk	Milk is our leading source of calcium, which is needed for bones and teeth. It also provides high-quality protein, riboflavin, vitamin A, and many other nutrients.	Children: 3 to 4 cups Teen-agers: 4 or more cups Adults: 2 or more cups
Bread and cereal	Foods in this group furnish worthwhile amounts of protein, iron, several of the B vitamins, and food energy.	4 or more servings Whole grain, enriched, or restored
Vegetable and fruit	Fruits and vegetables are valuable chiefly because of the vitamins and minerals they contain. In this plan, this group is counted on to supply nearly all the vitamin C needed and over half of the vitamin A. Vitamin C is needed for healthy gums and body tissues. Vitamin A is needed for growth, normal vision, and healthy condition of skin and other body surfaces.	4 or more servings A citrus fruit or other fruit or vegetable important for vitamin C A dark-green or deep-yellow vegetable for vitamin A—at least every other day Other vegetables and fruits, including potatoes

Source: *Food for Fitness: A Daily Food Guide.* U.S. Department of Agriculture, leaflet No. 424, 1958.

the best food sources for obtaining them. Fortunately, it is not necessary to be an authority on minerals and vitamins, but the informed student is more likely to recognize the need for using some guide to ensure the inclusion of all the essential nutrients in his daily diet.

Unlike the rigid diet prescribed by a physician for a patient with some specific ailment, *A Daily Food Guide* provides a wide range of choices within the food groups. One should not assume, however, that all the foods in each group are equivalent in value. It is recommended that an individual plan for variety within each group as an additional guarantee of supplying all the nutrients in ample amounts.

Functions of food in the body

The food we eat fulfills certain essential functions within the human body. *A Daily Food Guide* provides for foods to serve each of the functions essential to optimum efficiency of the body. The three general purposes for which food must be provided in adequate amounts are:

Fuel for energy and warmth

Materials for building new tissues and repairing old tissues

Regulating substances to control the complex functioning of the body

Foods, wisely selected, supply raw materials, which can be converted by the body into substances that satisfy these requirements.

FUEL

Fuel must be oxidized by the body to produce energy, which in turn results in motion. Motion is not limited, however, to external movements such as walking, writing, or talking. Activity is going on continuously within the body as long as a spark of life remains.

Basal metabolism. Internal activities that require energy include the beating of the heart, the communication functions of the nervous system, the contraction and relaxation of the breathing muscles, the peristaltic movements of the digestive tract, the filtering activities of the kidneys, the hormone-producing activities of the endocrine glands, and maintaining of muscle tone in the skeletal muscles of the body. The energy demands of the activities that go on continuously, whether the individual is asleep or awake, are referred to as *basal metabolism.* These energy demands are the minimal, or basal, requirements to maintain life processes.

The basal metabolic rate (BMR) is determined by measuring the amount of oxygen consumed during a given period of time and calculating the amount of heat resulting from the oxidation. This measurement is accomplished by having the subject breathe through a respiration apparatus, which controls and measures the amount of oxygen used. The measurement is made when a person is relaxed and lying at complete rest and has not had food for at least twelve hours. The BMR is expressed in calories per square meter of body surface per hour.

The basal metabolic rate is influenced by several factors. The rate is highest during the first two years of life and declines from that point on until adolescence, when there may be a slight rise followed by a slow progressive decrease for the remainder of life. Women have a slightly lower rate than men. Secretions of the thyroid and adrenal glands have a pronounced effect upon metabolic rate [4, 8].

An individual's basal metabolism is lower during sleep because of the relaxation of muscle tension. The degree of muscle tension when one is awake likewise affects the energy demands for internal activities: the more tense the individual, the greater the energy demand. Emotions are still another influence, to a degree, through their effect upon the endocrine glands and upon muscle tension. The aftereffects of exercise influence the basal metabolic rate for a period of time following a day when the activity rate has been high. The aftereffects of food also carry over to some extent into the resting stage, as does exercise, with a higher protein intake resulting in a higher metabolic rate during the follow-up period. Prolonged fasting, on the other hand, results in a lowered metabolic rate [4, 8].

The basal metabolic rate at any given time is significant in that it influences the body's demands for calories and provides the physician with clues about normal body functioning. A high metabolic rate, for example, may indicate to the physician that the thyroid gland is overproducing the hormone thyroxin (hyperthyroidism). A low metabolic rate may indicate an underproduction of thyroxin (hypothyroidism). A person with a higher basal metabolic rate can eat more food proportionally without adding weight than can a person with a low metabolic rate. Basal metabolic rate plus other activities determines total energy requirement.

Individual energy requirement. In addition to energy requirements indicated by the basal metabolic rate, each individual requires energy to participate in voluntary activities, to digest the food he eats, and to adjust to external heat or cold to which he is exposed. A large individual has a greater energy requirement for basal metabolic needs. An active person, likewise, needs a greater amount of energy. Table 9.4 provides for a comparison of the difference in energy requirement for different degrees of activity (see page 228 for an example of energy demands and weight control).

Calories. A calorie (large calorie) is the amount of heat (energy) required to raise one kilogram of water one degree Centigrade. The caloric value of different foods has been determined and is shown in Table 9.5. When an individual supplies his body with food to meet his caloric needs, he maintains his weight. Too many calories result in added weight and too few calories result in loss of weight.

BUILDING AND REPAIR OF TISSUES

In addition to supplying energy, food also must provide material for building and repairing tissues of the body. The greatest demand for building material occurs during periods of rapid growth.

Table 9.4 Energy expenditures for everyday activities

Activity	Calories per pound per hour
Dressing and undressing	0.8
Driving a car	0.9
Exercise:	
Light	1.0
Active	1.9
Severe	2.8
Very severe	3.8
Household tasks (cleaning, dusting, sweeping, etc.)	1.2
Knitting	0.8
Playing piano	0.9
Playing Ping-pong	2.5
Running	3.7
Sitting, eating, hand sewing, reading, sitting in bus or subway, smoking	0.7
Standing, cooking, dishwashing, ironing, paring potatoes	0.9
Sleeping or resting	0.4
Swimming	4.1
Typing	1.0
Walking slowly	1.1
Walking, moderate speed (3 miles per hour)	1.4
Walking down stairs (no. of flights * ___)	0.01
Walking up stairs (no. of flights * ___)	0.02

* Disregard time and multiply the number of flights (15 steps to one flight) by calories per pound per hour.
Source: Clara Mae Taylor, *Food Values in Shares and Weights*, 2d ed., The Macmillan Company, New York, 1959, p. 12.

Building and repair, however, continue throughout life. The function of the different nutrients in growth and repair are discussed in detail later in the chapter.

REGULATING BODY ACTIVITIES

Control of the complex activities of the human body requires an extremely fine balance of regulating substances. Minute amounts of a substance can upset the balance and result in either minor or extreme divergences in the normal growth or activity pattern of the organism.

The effect of too much or too little thyroxin has been discussed in relation to basal metabolism. Hormones, such as thyroxin, exert their influence on various body activities. Excessive production of a growth hormone by the pituitary gland before puberty results in gigantism. An insufficient production of insulin by the islets of Langerhans in the pancreas makes it impossible for the body to oxidize sugar properly, and diabetes mellitus results. The menstrual cycle in the female is largely controlled by hormones secreted by the pituitary gland and the ovaries. See Table 2.1, on pages 52 and 53, for additional information on hormones.

It is amazing indeed that such infinitesimal amounts of these regulating substances are able to exert such a profound influence upon the body activities. It is even more amazing that the body remains in a normal state of balance to the extent that it does. It is essential that ingested foods contain the raw materials from which the body tissues can secure the components to make up the various regulating substances that can be manufactured by the tissues. Other substances, such as vitamins, minerals, and certain amino acids, must be obtained from food sources because the body is unable to synthesize them satisfactorily.

Essential body nutrients

The food groupings in *A Daily Food Guide* are organized according to the primary contributions that foods make to the body for use as fuel, in building and repair, or in regulating functions. The specific nutrients included in foods are 35 or more in number, but they are classified conveniently into six groupings: carbohydrates, fats, proteins, minerals, vitamins, and water. Although it has no nutrient value as such, roughage sometimes is considered under a separate heading because of its regulating effect in the elimination of waste from the alimentary canal. The following discussion considers the nutrients in relation to functions they serve in the body and foods from which they are derived.

CARBOHYDRATES

Carbohydrates are composed of carbon, hydrogen, and oxygen. The combination of these three elements to form either sugars or starches provides a primary source of fuel for the body. Carbohydrates are chiefly of plant origin. Milk sugar, or lactose, is an exception, being an animal product.

The carbohydrates are classified under three headings:
Monosaccharides (simple sugars): glucose, fructose, galactose
Disaccharides (double sugars): sucrose, maltose, lactose
Polysaccharides (many sugar groups per molecule): starch, dextrins, glycogen, cellulose, hemicellulose

The body is able to absorb the simple sugars directly through the wall of the intestinal tract. The disaccharides and polysaccharides must be broken down by the digestive process and converted to simple sugars in order for absorption to take place. All the simple sugars are then converted to glucose, primarily in the liver, and made available for use by the

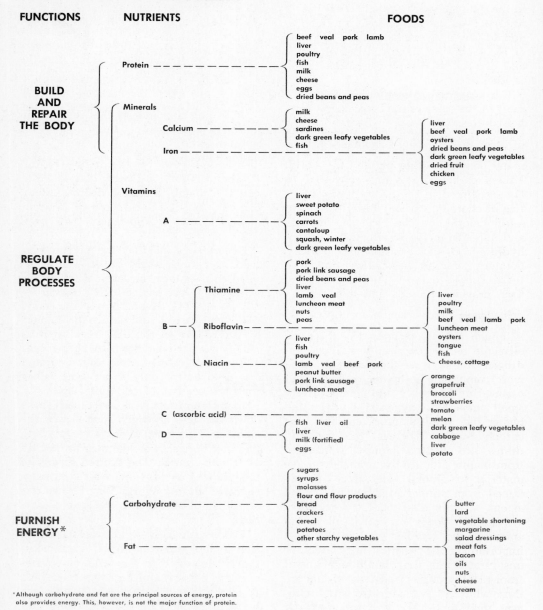

FUNCTIONS   NUTRIENTS   FOODS

BUILD AND REPAIR THE BODY

Protein —
- beef veal pork lamb
- liver
- poultry
- fish
- milk
- cheese
- eggs
- dried beans and peas

Minerals

Calcium —
- milk
- cheese
- sardines
- dark green leafy vegetables
- fish

Iron —
- liver
- beef veal pork lamb
- oysters
- dried beans and peas
- dark green leafy vegetables
- dried fruit
- chicken
- eggs

REGULATE BODY PROCESSES

Vitamins

A —
- liver
- sweet potato
- spinach
- carrots
- cantaloup
- squash, winter
- dark green leafy vegetables

B —

Thiamine —
- pork
- pork link sausage
- dried beans and peas
- liver
- lamb veal
- luncheon meat
- nuts
- peas

Riboflavin —
- liver
- poultry
- milk
- beef veal lamb pork
- luncheon meat
- oysters
- tongue
- fish
- cheese, cottage

Niacin —
- liver
- fish
- poultry
- lamb veal beef pork
- peanut butter
- pork link sausage
- luncheon meat

C (ascorbic acid) —
- orange
- grapefruit
- broccoli
- strawberries
- tomato
- melon
- dark green leafy vegetables
- cabbage
- liver
- potato

D —
- fish liver oil
- liver
- milk (fortified)
- eggs

FURNISH ENERGY*

Carbohydrate —
- sugars
- syrups
- molasses
- flour and flour products
- bread
- crackers
- cereal
- potatoes
- other starchy vegetables

Fat —
- butter
- lard
- vegetable shortening
- margarine
- salad dressings
- meat fats
- bacon
- oils
- nuts
- cheese
- cream

*Although carbohydrate and fat are the principal sources of energy, protein also provides energy. This, however, is not the major function of protein.

The functions of food in nutrition. (National Live Stock and Meat Board.)

body tissues. Excess amounts of glucose in the liver are converted to glycogen, a storage form of animal starch.

In *A Daily Food Guide* the food groups that supply carbohydrates include the vegetable and fruit group and the cereal and bread group. In addition, the average person obtains more carbohydrates from sirups, preserves, and white and brown sugar, which constitute regular "extras" in the typical American diet. These extras are not essential in the diet, but they do add to the enjoyment of meals. Because of the danger of increased dental caries and obesity, moderate use of the extras is advisable.

Carbohydrates, along with fats, supply most of the calories the body needs. Carbohydrates supply approximately 50 per cent of the calories in the American diet and considerably more in the diet of many people in other parts of the world. Excess carbohydrates are converted to fat and stored in the body. A wise practice in choosing carbohydrate foods is to select calories on the basis of vitamins and minerals included with them. Carbohydrate foods such as whole-grain cereals, potatoes, starchy vegetables, and ripe fruits supply calories and at the same time provide vitamins and minerals.

FATS

Although fats are composed of the same elements as carbohydrates—carbon, hydrogen, and oxygen—their composition is more complex. The higher percentage of carbon and hydrogen and comparatively small amount of oxygen account for the higher fuel value of fats compared with carbohydrates. Whereas the carbohydrates are derived almost exclusively from plants, fats are the primary storage material of animals and thus are obtained from animal products to a large extent. Certain essential fatty acids are synthesized slowly or not at all in the animal body. Linoleic acid is the most important of the essential fatty acids, or unsaturated fats, that should be obtained from plant sources. Unsaturated fats are those which are not saturated with hydrogen; their molecular structure makes it possible for them to combine with more hydrogen. The saturated fats are those which have all the hydrogen they can take. Whole wheat, soybeans, peanut oil, and olive oil are among the good plant sources of fats.

Uses of fats and fat-rich foods are:

As a concentrated form of body fuel

As flavoring and to provide a lasting feeling of satisfaction

As a bearer of fat-soluble vitamins

The fuel value of fats is approximately 9 calories per gram, compared with 4 calories per gram for carbohydrates. A person who is trying to lose weight or to avoid adding excess weight should limit the intake of fatty foods. Uncertainty as to the desirable amount of fat in the diet is indicated by the failure of the Food and Nutrition Board, National Research Council, to state a definite allowance in the 1958 revision of *Recommended Dietary Allowances* (see page 242).

Bogert suggests that the person who tends to be overweight might well be advised to maintain the level of fat intake at about 25 per cent of daily caloric requirements [4]. Keys has recommended that Americans should reduce the amount of fat calories in the diet from approximately 40 per cent down to 15 per cent of the total calories and that saturated fats account for only 4 per cent rather than the present 17 per cent [28].

Inclusion of fats with other foods slows down the rate at which food leaves the stomach. This tends to delay the gnawing pangs of hunger, which appear so quickly after some meals. The limited supply of fats allowed on wartime rations in many countries during World War II was one of the most distressing wartime restrictions.

Foods such as eggs and sweetbreads are rich in fats and cholesterol, a substance that is deposited in the walls of arteries of some persons and tends to contribute to circulatory disorders. Cholesterol can be manufactured by the body from proteins or carbohydrates, but it is apparently more likely to be manufactured from fats. The American Heart Association, in a 1961 report, recommended that reducing the total amount of fat ingested and substituting a reasonable amount of vegetable oils and other polyunsaturated fats for saturated fats would help reduce the blood cholesterol level. It also concluded that evidence was not yet conclusive that lowering the blood cholesterol level would prevent atherosclerosis, heart attacks, and strokes [1].

PROTEINS

In addition to supplying carbon, hydrogen, and oxygen the proteins also provide our only source of nitrogen and small amounts of sulfur. Some of the proteins also contain phosphorus and iron. The proteins are found in adequate amounts in both the animal and plant kingdoms.

Proteins are essential constituents of the cells of all living tissues. The word *protein* is derived from a Greek word meaning "primary," which suggests its importance to life. Proteins are necessary for the body to build new tissues and repair those tissues which wear out. They are not stored in the human body as are carbohydrates and fats but must be supplied regularly by eating animal or plant foods which contain them. In addition to their function in building and repairing tissues, proteins are needed in manufacturing regulating substances, which control the complex functioning of the body. Excess amounts of protein serve in an additional capacity; they are converted and utilized as a source of energy. Approximately 10 to 15 per cent of the daily calorie requirement should be provided by protein foods [23].

Amino acids. Proteins are made up of substances called *amino acids*. More than 20 of these amino acids have been identified. Proteins are of different quality according to the combination of amino acids from which they are made. At least eight of the amino acids cannot be synthesized satisfactorily within the body but must be supplied directly from an external source. Proteins containing all these essential amino acids are referred to as *complete proteins*. Complete proteins provide all the amino acids needed by the body to manufacture the proteins required for growth and repair. Incomplete proteins must be supplemented by complete proteins to provide all the amino acids needed by the individual.

Animal and plant sources. Gelatin is the only incomplete animal protein. Because many plant proteins are incomplete, it is generally recognized that animal sources of protein are most satisfactory. It should be noted, however, that with careful selection an individual can obtain all the protein requirements without making use of animal sources [6].

In *A Daily Food Guide* the meat, fish, poultry, and egg group, which is the primary source of proteins, also includes some plant sources. Soybeans, dried beans, peas, and nuts or peanut butter are considered to be the best plant sources of proteins.

Protein requirements of the body. The greatest demand for protein comes during the periods of most rapid growth. During the first year of life, the protein requirement per kilogram of body weight is greater than at any other time. One must not forget, however, the maintenance requirement for protein, which persists throughout life. Table 9.6 lists the recommended protein intake for individuals, and protein values of selected foods are included in Table 9.5. When one ceases to grow, there is still a need for protein to repair or replace tissues.

Protein deficiency. In the United States, because there is an ample supply of animal protein food available, one finds few examples of extreme protein deficiency. In many of the underdeveloped countries of the world, however, where the population depends almost entirely upon plant sources of protein, there is a great deal of protein malnutrition. The disease is commonly referred to as *kwashiorkor.* Supplementing the diet with dried skim milk is an effective treatment for children with this condition.

MINERALS

The minerals required by the body are used for building and repair of body tissues and for regulating body activities. Some of the regulating functions are to [4, 8]:

Influence the contractility of muscles

Determine the irritability of nerves

Control the movement of fluids in the body

Aid in coagulation or clotting of the blood

Assist in the formation and functioning of digestive juices and hormones

Maintain the acid-alkaline balance in the body

Transport oxygen and carbon dioxide

Assist in all normal cell functions of oxidation, secretion, development, and reproduction

Calcium, phosphorus, iron, and iodine are the minerals most likely to be inadequately supplied in the diet. Relatively small amounts of sodium, potassium, magnesium, manganese, sulfur, chlorine, fluorine, and copper are required, but even in small amounts they serve important functions. Only traces of cobalt, silicon, nickel, aluminum, molybdenum, and zinc are found in the body tissues, and it is questionable that all of them are essential in the diet.

Calcium and phosphorus. Both calcium and phosphorus are required for proper bone and tooth development as they are the chief mineral constituents of these tissues. Calcium in the blood is essential for clotting, normal function of the nerves, and good muscle tone. Phosphorus is an essential constituent of muscles and nerves as well as blood.

Increased amounts of both minerals are required for the skeletal structure during periods of rapid growth. Likewise, the woman who is pregnant or who is producing milk to nurse an infant needs additional supplies of calcium and phosphorus. Marked effects of deficiencies are most likely to be noted during such times (see Table 9.6 for recommended daily allowances of calcium).

Calcium is unevenly furnished in foods, and calcium absorption from the digestive tract is poor compared with absorption of other nutrients. The best single source of calcium comes from milk and milk products. The second best source is green, leafy vegetables, but depending upon this source alone is not advisable because of the relatively small amounts of calcium compared with the large amounts available in milk. Dietary surveys have shown that of the mineral elements calcium is most likely to be inadequately supplied in the human diet.

Calcium utilization by the body depends primarily upon the presence of phosphorus and of vitamin D. Vitamins A and C, and perhaps other vitamins also, promote more favorable utilization of calcium. Phosphorus is amply provided in protein-rich foods and in milk products. A diet that includes these substances affords adequate amounts of phosphorus to meet one's needs.

The inclusion of recommended amounts of milk and milk products in the daily diet is advisable if one wishes to be assured of an adequate supply of calcium. Milk also supplies appreciable quantities of many of the other nutrients.

Iron and copper. The body is dependent upon iron and copper for the oxygen-transporting function of the blood. Hemoglobin in the red cells serves as the vehicle for carrying oxygen. Iron is a basic constituent of hemoglobin. Hemoglobin combines with oxygen in the lungs and transports it to the cells, where it is needed for the oxidation of fuel provided by the carbohydrates, fats, and proteins. It also carries carbon dioxide back to the lungs for elimination. Although copper is not a part of the chemical make-up of

Table 9.5 Nutritive values of the edible part of foods *

Food, approximate measure, and weight (in grams)			Water, per cent	Food energy, calories	Protein, g	Fat (total lipid), g	Fatty acid, g Saturated (total)
Milk, cream, cheese; related products							
Milk, cow's:							
Fluid, whole	1 cup	244	87	165	9	10	6
Fluid, nonfat (skim)	1 cup	246	90	90	9	Trace	—
Cheese, cottage, creamed	1 cup	225	78	240	30	11	6
Malted milk	1 cup	270	78	280	13	12	7
Eggs							
Boiled, shell removed	2 eggs	100	74	160	13	12	4
Scrambled, with milk and fat	1 egg	64	72	110	7	8	3
Meat, poultry, fish, shellfish; related products							
Bacon, broiled or fried crisp	2 slices	16	8	95	5	8	3
Hamburger, broiled market ground	3 oz	85	54	245	21	17	8
Steak, sirloin, broiled— lean and fat	3 oz	85	44	330	20	27	13
Chicken, ½ breast, fried	3.3 oz	94	52	215	24	12	3
Liver, beef, fried	2 oz	57	57	120	13	14	2
Pork, cured, cooked: chop, thick, with bone	3.5 oz	98	42	260	16	21	8
Haddock, fried	3 oz	85	67	135	16	5	1
Mature dry beans, peas; nuts; related products							
Beans, dry, red	1 cup	256	76	230	15	1	—
Lima, cooked	1 cup	192	64	260	16	1	—
Peanut butter	1 tbsp.	16	2	90	4	8	2
Vegetables and vegetable products							
Beans, snap, green, cooked in small amount of water, short time	1 cup	125	92	25	2	Trace	—
Cabbage, cole slaw	1 cup	120	84	100	2	7	1
Carrots, raw (5½ by 1 inch)	1 carrot	50	88	20	1	Trace	—
Celery, raw, outer stalk	1 stalk	40	94	5	1	Trace	—
Peas, green, cooked	1 cup	160	82	110	8	1	—
Potatoes, medium, about 3 per pound: baked, peeled after baking	1 potato	99	75	90	3	Trace	—
Tomatoes, raw, medium 2 by 2½ inches	1 tomato	150	94	30	2	Trace	—
Tomato juice, canned	1 cup	242	94	50	2	Trace	—

| Fatty acid, g | | Carbo-hy-drate, g | Cal-cium, mg | Iron, mg | Vita-min A value, IU | Thia-mine, mg | Ribo-flavin, mg | Nia-cin, mg | Ascorbic acid, mg |
| Unsaturated | | | | | | | | | |
Oleic	Lino-leic								
3	Trace	12	285	.1	390	.08	.42	.2	2
—	—	13	298	.1	10	.10	.44	.2	2
4	Trace	6	207	.9	430	.07	.66	.2	0
4	Trace	32	364	.8	670	.17	.56	—	2
5	1	1	54	2.3	1,180	.09	.28	.1	0
4	1	1	51	1.1	690	.05	.18	Trace	0
4	1	1	2	.5	0	.08	.05	.3	—
7	Trace	0	9	2.7	30	.07	.02	4.6	—
12	1	0	8	2.5	50	.05	.16	4.0	—
6	2	—	10	1.1	60	.03	.06	9.4	—
2	Trace	6	5	4.4	30,330	.15	2.25	8.4	18
9	2	0	8	2.2	0	.63	.18	3.8	—
3	Trace	6	15	.5	50	.03	.08	2.2	—
—	—	42	74	4.6	0	.13	.13	1.5	Trace
—	—	48	56	5.6	Trace	.26	.12	1.3	Trace
4	2	3	12	.4	0	.02	.02	2.8	0
—	—	6	45	.9	830	.09	.12	.6	18
1	4	9	47	.5	80	.06	.05	.3	50
—	—	5	20	.4	6,000	.03	.03	.3	3
—	—	1	20	.2	0	.02	.02	.2	3
—	—	19	35	3.0	1,150	.40	.22	3.7	24
—	—	21	9	.7	Trace	.10	.04	1.7	20
—	—	6	16	.9	1,640	.08	.06	.8	35
—	—	10	17	1.0	2,540	.12	.07	1.8	38

Table 9.5 Nutritive values of the edible part of foods (continued)

Food, approximate measure, and weight (in grams)			Water, per cent	Food energy, calories	Protein, g	Fat (total lipid), g	Fatty acid, g Saturated (total)
Fruits and fruit products							
Apple, raw, medium 2½-inch diameter	1 apple	150	85	70	Trace	Trace	—
Banana, raw, 6 by 1½ inches	1 banana	150	76	85	1	Trace	—
Orange, navel, California, 2⅘ inch diameter	1 orange	180	85	60	2	Trace	—
Frozen concentrate, undiluted, can, 6 fluid ounces	1 can	210	58	330	5	Trace	—
Grain products							
Bread:							
White, enriched, 3 to 4 per cent nonfat dry milk slice, 20 per loaf	1 slice	23	36	60	2	1	—
Unenriched	1 slice	23	36	60	2	1	—
Cake, chocolate, fudge icing, 1/16 of 10-inch-diameter layer cake	1 sector	120	24	420	5	14	5
Fig bars	1 fig bar	16	14	55	1	1	—
Corn flakes, plain, enriched	1 ounce	28	4	110	2	Trace	—
Doughnuts, cake type	1 doughnut	32	19	135	2	7	2
Macaroni, enriched, and cheese, baked	1 cup	220	58	475	18	25	14
Pie, apple, 1/7 of 9-inch diameter pie	1 sector	135	48	330	3	13	4
Fats, oils							
Butter, 64 pats per pound	1 pat	7	16	50	Trace	6	3
Margarine	1 pat	7	16	50	Trace	6	1
Thousand Island salad dressing	1 tbsp.	15	38	75	Trace	8	1
Sugars, sweets							
Fudge, plain	1 oz	28	5	115	Trace	3	2
Jellies	1 tbsp.	20	34	50	0	0	—
Granulated sugar	1 tbsp.	12	Trace	50	0	0	—

* Dashes show that no basis could be found for imputing a value although there was some reason to believe that a measurable amount of the constituent might be present.

hemoglobin, it is essential for its formation.

Iron may be stored by the body. Most of the iron not in the hemoglobin is found in the liver or the spleen, or where it is available for use when needed. Additional amounts of iron are found as a part of all cells of the body where it is required to stimulate the cells' vital processes [4, 6].

The standard allowance for iron is recommended in Table 9.6. Because only

SELECTING AND EATING WHOLESOME FOODS

Fatty acid, g		Carbo-hy-drate, g	Cal-cium, mg	Iron, mg	Vita-min A value, IU	Thia-mine, mg	Ribo-flavin, mg	Nia-cin, mg	Ascorbic acid, mg
Unsaturated									
Oleic	Lino-leic								
—	—	18	8	.4	50	.04	.02	.1	3
—	—	23	8	.7	190	.05	.06	.7	10
—	—	16	49	.5	240	.12	.05	.5	75
—	—	80	69	.8	1,490	.63	.10	2.4	332
—	—	12	19	.6	Trace	.06	.05	.6	Trace
—	—	12	19	.2	Trace	.02	.02	.3	Trace
7	1	70	118	.5	140	.03	.10	.3	Trace
—	—	12	11	.2	0	Trace	.01	.1	0
—	—	24	3	.5	—	.12	.03	.6	0
2	3	17	23	.4	40	.05	.04	.4	0
8	1	44	394	2.0	970	.22	.46	1.9	Trace
7	1	53	9	.5	220	.04	.02	.3	1
2	0	Trace	1	Trace	230	—	—	—	0
3	1	Trace	1	Trace	230	—	—	—	0
2	4	1	2	.1	60	Trace	Trace	Trace	2
1	Trace	23	14	.1	60	Trace	.02	Trace	Trace
—	—	13	2	.1	Trace	Trace	Trace	Trace	1
—	—	12	—	—	0	0	0	0	0

Source: Adapted from U.S. Department of Agriculture, *Nutritive Value of Foods*, Government Printing Office, Home and Garden Bulletin No. 72, Washington, September, 1960.

about 10 per cent of the iron in food is assimilated by normal adults, this allowance does not provide much margin for some persons. Women who have a heavy flow during menstruation and rapidly growing children may need to eat more foods that are rich in iron [4]. The best sources of iron are organ meats (liver and heart), egg yolk, whole grains, and dried fruits. Other foods, such as green, leafy vegetables, contain relatively high amounts of iron, but it is question-

DEVELOPING AND MAINTAINING HEALTH

Table 9.6 Recommended dietary allowances,[1] designed for the maintenance of good nutrition of healthy persons in the U.S.A.

Age, years	Weight, kg (lb)	Height cm (in.)	Calories	Protein, g	Calcium, g	Iron, mg	Vitamin A, IU	Thiamine, mg
Men								
25	70 (154)	175 (69)	3,200 [3]	70	0.8	10	5,000	1.6
45	70 (154)	175 (69)	3,000	70	0.8	10	5,000	1.5
65	70 (154)	175 (69)	2,550	70	0.8	10	5,000	1.3
Women								
25	58 (128)	163 (64)	2,300	58	0.8	12	5,000	1.2
45	58 (128)	163 (64)	2,200	58	0.8	12	5,000	1.1
65	58 (128)	163 (64)	1,800	58	0.8	12	5,000	1.0
Pregant (second half)			+ 300	+20	1.5	15	6,000	1.3
Lactating (850 ml daily)			+ 1,000	+40	2.0	15	8,000	1.7
Infants [4]								
0–1/12 [4]				See				
2/12–6/12	6 (13)	60 (24)	kg x 120	footnote	0.6	5	1,500	0.4
7/12–12/12	9 (20)	70 (28)	kg x 100	4	0.8	7	1,500	0.5
Children								
1–3	12 (27)	87 (34)	1,300	40	1.0	7	2,000	0.7
4–6	18 (40)	109 (43)	1,700	50	1.0	8	2,500	0.9
7–9	27 (60)	129 (51)	2,100	60	1.0	10	3,500	1.1
10–12	36 (79)	144 (57)	2,500	70	1.2	12	4,500	1.3
Boys								
13–15	49 (108)	163 (64)	3,100	85	1.4	15	5,000	1.6
16–19	63 (139)	175 (69)	3,600	100	1.4	15	5,000	1.8
Girls								
13–15	49 (108)	160 (63)	2,600	80	1.3	15	5,000	1.3
16–19	54 (120)	162 (64)	2,400	75	1.3	15	5,000	1.2

[1] Allowances are intended for persons normally active in a temperate climate. The allowance levels are intended to cover individual variations among most normal persons as they live in the United States under usual environmental stresses. The recommended allowances can be attained with a variety of common foods, providing other nutrients for which human requirements have been less well defined.
[2] Niacin equivalents include dietary sources of the preformed vitamin and the precursor, tryptophan. 60 milligrams tryptophan equals 1 milligram niacin.
[3] Calorie allowances apply to individuals usually engaged in moderate physical activity. For office workers or others in sedentary occupations they are excessive. Adjustments must be made for variations in body size, age, physical activity, and environmental temperature.
[4] The Board recognizes that human milk is the natural food for infants and feels that breast feeding is the best and desired procedure for meeting nutrient requirements in the first months of life. No allowances are stated for the first month of life. Breast feeding is particularly indicated during the first month

able that this iron is as readily available for use by the body.

Anemia is a condition in which the blood is unable to carry sufficient amounts of oxygen. Nutritional anemia is caused by an inadequate supply of iron in the diet, resulting in a lack of hemoglobin. The best insurance against nutritional anemia is to eat adequate amounts of foods that supply iron for bodily needs. Specific disease conditions likewise cause anemia. The treatment of

Ribo-flavin, mg	Niacin [2] mg equiv.	Ascorbic Acid mg	Vitamin D, IU
1.8	21	75	
1.8	20	75	
1.8	18	75	
1.5	17	70	
1.5	17	70	
1.5	17	70	
2.0	+3	100	400
2.5	+2	150	400
0.5	6	30	400
0.8	7	30	400
1.0	8	35	400
1.3	11	50	400
1.5	14	60	400
1.8	17	75	400
2.1	21	90	400
2.5	25	100	400
2.0	17	80	400
1.9	16	80	400

when infants show handicaps in homeostasis due to different rates of maturation of digestive, excretory, and endocrine functions. Recommendations as listed pertain to nutrient intake as afforded by cow's milk formulas and supplementary foods given the infant when breast feeding is terminated. Allowances are not given for protein during infancy.

Source: Food and Nutrition Board, National Research Council, *Recommended Daily Dietary Allowances*, NAS-NRC Publication No. 589, Revised 1958.

anemia is a medical problem because of the many possible causes other than insufficient iron intake in the diet.

Iodine. The fact that iodine constitutes only about 3 parts per million of the body weight does not minimize its importance. The striking effects of iodine inadequacy on the function of the thyroid gland provide sufficient evidence of the essential nature of this substance. Insufficient amounts of iodine cause a decreased production of thyroxin by the thyroid gland. The decrease in thyroxin results in a reduced metabolic rate. Enlargement of the thyroid gland to compensate for the reduced production of thyroxin is called *simple goiter*. Iodine in the diet will prevent such a condition. Other types of goiter or evidence of thyroid malfunction are not traced primarily to dietary inadequacy.

In some parts of the country the amounts of iodine in the drinking water or in the soil are insufficient to supply human needs. In such an area the regular diet may have to be supplemented. The use of iodized salt is generally accepted as being an economical and efficient way of providing for adequate amounts of iodine in the diet. Such use is especially important during adolescence and pregnancy.

Fluorine. Although fluorine is one of the mineral elements needed by the body in only minute amounts, its importance in the prevention of dental caries has been proved by a number of studies (see Chapter 7). The treatment of drinking water with sodium fluoride to raise the level to 1 part per million is recommended as the most effective means of providing individuals with the needed amount of this mineral element [6].

Other minerals. Because of the limited knowledge about the function of many of the other minerals and because of their availability in a typical diet, little need be said about these substances. Sodium, potassium, magnesium, iron, and calcium as basic or alkaline elements and phosphorus, sulfur, and chlorine as acidic elements are important in maintaining a normal acid-alkaline balance.

The body must maintain such a balance in order to live. Despite the misleading claims made for many products, the chemical balance of the body in terms of acid and base does not require the intake of particular neutralizing substances. The use of such substances is best left to the judgment of one's physician.

VITAMINS

Discovery of the existence of body-regulating substances, now called vitamins, marks an important milestone in the understanding of nutrition. The bombardment of advertising claims designed to establish the virtues of a particular vitamin preparation tends to distort their true value. The average person is often in a quandary as he attempts to determine how to satisfy his own need for vitamins. Many questions relating to individual requirements for vitamins are as yet unanswered, but essential facts are known, which are helpful to a person as he plans his diet.

The vitamins are required in extremely small amounts. They are essential for normal growth and for regulation of body activities. Animals, including human beings, are not capable of synthesizing some of the vitamins within their bodies and must depend upon foods to furnish them. The chemical make-up and the physiologic effect vary with different vitamins. It is difficult to generalize about vitamins except to indicate that they exert a regulating effect similar to that of the hormones produced by the endocrine glands and to that of minerals such as copper and iodine.

Vitamins are available in varying amounts in most plants used as food. Foods derived from animals also provide good sources of some of the vitamins. In addition, vitamin preparations provide an excellent source for supplementing the diet. In general, however, it is recommended that vitamin preparations be used only on the advice of a physician. Most individuals who select and eat a balanced diet have no need for supplementary vitamins [10]. There is no scientifically established evidence that additional doses of vitamins will increase general health or build up resistance to disease.

Vitamins are identified both by an alphabetical designation and by their chemical names. The alphabetical designations do not indicate the order in which these substances have been discovered. The terms *vitamin C* and *ascorbic acid* are used interchangeably, as are *vitamin B₁* and *thiamine,* and *vitamin B₂* and *riboflavin.*

Isolation of vitamins as pure substances makes it possible for research workers to measure the amount of a vitamin required to obtain a given nutritional response. Two units of measurement commonly used to designate the daily allowance of vitamins (see Table 9.6) are the actual weight in milligrams or the number of international units (I.U.). For most vitamins the amounts are stated in weight units such as milligrams. The recommended allowances in Table 9.6 are well above the minimum amounts required by the body, as these are standards designed to improve the quality of the diet of American people. *A Daily Food Guide* provides excellent help in selecting foods that provide adequate amounts of the various vitamins.

Vitamin insufficiencies rather than extreme deficiencies are typical of the American population. Scurvy from vitamin C deficiency and beriberi resulting from thiamine or vitamin B₁ deficiency rarely occur in the United States at present. The symptoms of an insufficient supply of vitamins are observed more frequently.

Fat-soluble vitamins. The fat-soluble vitamins are A, D, K, and E. The vitamins in this group are not all single substances. The identifying letter refers to a group of substances with a similar vitamin function. The fat-soluble vitamins are characterized by the presence of precursors, sometimes called *provitamins*. These substances are not active vitamins but are converted to vitamins in the body. Vitamin A, for example, has four precursors, of which beta-carotene is superior. The vitamin D precursor found in the skin is converted to vitamin D by the action of sunlight on the skin. An additional characteristic of the fat-soluble vitamins is the fact that they are stored by the body to a greater extent than are water-soluble vitamins.

Vitamin K plays an important role in blood clotting by aiding in the formation of prothrombin. Vitamin E apparently is an essential factor in reproduction, although its specific role is not known. Functions of other vitamins are listed below.

Water-soluble vitamins. Vitamin C and

Vitamin	Best sources	Functions	
Vitamin A	liver sweet potato spinach carrots cantaloup squash, winter dark green leafy vegetables	promote growth and repair of body tissues build general good health help maintain normal vision and healthy eyes help keep soft, smooth skin help maintain healthy mucous membranes of mouth, nose, etc.	The functions and important sources of vitamins. (Adapted from "Vitamins, Their Functions and Important Sources," National Live Stock and Meat Board.)
Thiamine (B1)	pork pork link sausage dried beans and peas liver lamb veal luncheon meat nuts, peas	help convert carbohydrates to energy help maintain good appetite aid in digestion and assimilation of food help the heart, nerves, and muscles function properly	
Riboflavin	liver poultry milk beef veal lamb pork luncheon meat oysters tongue fish cheese, cottage	help maintain good vision and healthy clear eyes build healthy skin and mouth tissues help use carbohydrates promote well-being and vitality	
Niacin	liver fish poultry lamb veal beef pork peanut butter pork link sausage luncheon meat	build and maintain healthy skin and tongue help use carbohydrates efficiently aid digestion help the nervous system function	
Ascorbic acid (Vitamin C)	orange grapefruit broccoli strawberries tomato melon dark green leafy vegetables cabbage liver potato	help maintain firm healthy gums help build and maintain bones, tissues, and blood utilize iron properly help build resistance to infection help heal wounds and fractures	
Vitamin D	fish liver oil liver milk (fortified) eggs	needed for calcium and phosphorus metabolism promote normal growth	

the B-complex vitamins are included among the water-soluble vitamins. Thiamine (B_1), riboflavin (B_2), and niacin, or nicotinic acid, are best known to lay persons.

WATER

Some of the main functions of water, which comprises approximately two-thirds of the body weight, include being a solvent for innumerable substances, serving as a vehicle for transporting nutrients and waste materials, aiding in the regulation of body temperature, acting as a cushion to protect organs from external shocks, serving as a lubricant to facilitate movement of the joints, and being a fundamental substance in building and repairing tissues.

The body uses water for its normal processes and excretes water as urine from the kidneys, with the fecal discharge from the intestinal tract, as perspiration from the skin, and in the air discharged from the lungs. The water needed by the body to replace what is used up or excreted is secured through the fluids that are drunk, the water contained in solid foods that are eaten, and water formed in the body tissues as a result of the combustion of foods.

The amount of water lost through excretion is regulated, to a degree, by the availability of water in the body. A scarcity of urine may be noted when fluid is cut down.

It is generally accepted that thirst is a satisfactory guide to adequate fluid intake for the normal adult person. It is, on the other hand, recommended that one drink five or six glasses of water per day to ensure sufficient amounts for normal functioning of the body [4]. Excess amounts of water are unlikely, as the water not needed is excreted by the body.

ROUGHAGE

Roughage, or vegetable fiber, is not an essential nutrient in the same sense as carbohydrates, fats, proteins, vitamins, minerals, and water. It does, however, have a regulatory function in eliminating solid waste material from the alimentary canal.

Because of the rather complete digestion and absorption of most of the nutrient substances, there is little residue left in the alimentary tract except for the presence of vegetable fiber, or cellulose. In the absence of this bulk, the amount of residue in the tract is so small that the stimulus to peristaltic action by muscles in the tract is inhibited and normal excretion is less likely.

Fiber is provided in a diet that contains recommended amounts of fruits, vegetables, and whole grains. The use of bran or other such substance is best left to the judgment of a physician, as harm can result from the excessive use of these substances.

Preparation of foods to conserve nutrient value

Despite widespread changes in processing food for home consumption, there is apparently no serious over-all loss in nutrient value. In foods where there is serious loss of nutrient value in preparation processes, steps have been taken to replace nutrients that one should expect

to receive from the given food. The indiscriminate addition of vitamins and minerals to foods is not permitted. Examples of fortification of foods recognized as desirable by the Council on Foods and Nutrition, American Medical Association, are not more than 400 units of vitamin D to a quart of milk, 15,000 units of vitamin A to a pound of margarine, iodine to table salt not in excess of 1 part of sodium or potassium iodide to 5,000 parts of salt, and the enrichment of white bread, flour, and cereal according to a prescribed formula. It is advisable to look at the label on grain products to determine whether or not the losses in milling have been replaced.

FOOD ADDITIVES

In addition to restoring or fortifying foods with vitamins and minerals on a controlled basis as indicated previously, there are numerous other examples of the use of chemicals in the preparation of food for human consumption. Table 9.7 includes examples of some of the common additives and the functions they serve.

The increase from approximately 400 additives in 1949 to almost 800 ten years later illustrates the rapid change taking place in the food industry [17]. Fortunately for the consumer, the use of chemicals in foods is not a haphazard matter but is subject to control by the Food and Drug Administration (see Chapter 10). The action taken by Arthur Flemming, Secretary of Health, Education, and Welfare, in 1959, to prevent the marketing of contaminated cranberries was one of the most dramatic examples of action to protect the consumer from possible danger due to additives in food products.

In addition to the examples listed in Table 9.7, numerous other additives, such as leavening agents, hardening agents, anticaking agents, propellants (for prod-

Table 9.7 Common food additives

Types of additives	Selected additives and their functions
Nutrient supplements	Potassium iodide (added to salt) to prevent simple goiter
	Thiamine, riboflavin, niacin, and iron to enrich grain products
	Vitamin A to margarine
	Vitamin D to milk
Nonnutritive sweeteners	Saccharin to replace sugar
Preservatives	Antioxidants to preserve fatty products
	Antimycotics to prevent mold in bread and fruit
	Sequestrants to prevent physical or chemical changes which affect color, flavor, texture, or appearance
Emulsifiers	Lecithin and propylene glycol to bakery foods, ice cream, and confectionery products for their effect on volume, uniformity, fineness of grain, smoothness, homogeneity, and keeping quality
Stabilizers and thickeners	Pectins, vegetable gums, gelatin, and agar-agar to stabilize and thicken ice cream, frozen desserts, chocolate milk, and some fruit juices
Acids, alkalies, buffers, neutralizing agents	Ammonium bicarbonate, tartaric acid, and sodium aluminum phosphate to control degree of acidity or alkalinity in foods such as soft drinks, butter, and baked goods
Flavoring agents	Amyl acetate, benzaldehyde, ethyl butyrate and methyl salicylate, and monosodium glutamate to flavor or season soft drinks, bakery goods, and ice cream
Bleaching agents	Benzoyl peroxide, chlorine, and oxides of nitrogen to speed up aging and bleaching of flour
Bread improvers	Ammonium chloride and calcium sulfate to serve as yeast foods and dough conditioners
Synthetic colors	Coal-tar colors to improve appearance of foods

ucts packed under pressure in dispensing cans), drying agents, and antifoaming agents, are in common use. The specific examples in the table are representative of the chemicals used [15, 29].

Pesticides. Pesticides are in widespread use to control weeds and insect pests, which interfere with production of crops on farms. The cranberry scare referred to above was a result of a weed killer used in the cranberry bogs. Tolerances have been set by the Food and Drug Administration for amounts of residue of pesticides that are permitted to remain on fruits and vegetables when they are shipped. Pesticides have played a major role in improving the yield of farm products so that more food is available to the consumer. Vigilance on the part of regulating agencies is essential, however, in order to prevent these chemicals from endangering the health of the consumer [15, 17].

Radioactive substances. Radioactive substances, strontium-90 in particular, are added to food by man in an indirect manner. As a product of atomic explosions, strontium-90 is scattered in the upper atmosphere and on the soil and plants, where it is taken up by plants along with the calcium they require.

Animals that eat the plants containing strontium-90 slowly accumulate this radioactive substance in their tissues. Man, who eats both the plants and the animal, also accumulates strontium-90 in his tissues. The amount of radioactive substances deposited in geographical areas varies widely. Therefore, the amount of strontium-90 in food varies from one locale to another and from time to time in a given locale [2, 13]. Fortunately, the strontium/calcium ratio decreases sharply as the substances pass from the cow's food to its body and then to the milk produced. The strontium/calcium ratio for meat is approximately one-fourth that in fodder, and the ratio in milk is only about one-tenth that in fodder [33]. When one considers the importance of milk in supplying calcium to meet nutritional needs, the lower ratio of strontium to calcium takes on added significance. Discovery in 1961 of a process which removes practically all of the strontium-90 from milk could eliminate this source of danger in case of heavy fallout.

Numerous studies have been made to determine the amount of radioactivity in food products and the extent of the build-up of radioactive substances in human beings. Permissible limits for amounts of strontium-90 have been determined; such limits may be subject to change as additional information is accumulated. It is apparent that steps must be taken to limit the amounts of strontium-90 and other radioactive substances to which man is exposed through contamination of his food supply.

FROZEN FOODS

Frozen foods provide an increasing source of food for Americans. Frozen foods handled according to recommended procedures for freezing and preparation for eating are safe, nutritious, and tasty. Frozen foods that are processed shortly after they are harvested lose little of their nutritive value. Individuals who rely on the fresh vegetables purchased in the market are in many cases buying produce that is days old, due to the marketing process. There can be considerable loss in nutrient value of food that is not eaten while it is fresh.

The convenience and satisfaction associated with frozen foods is reflected in increased usage—from approximately 6 pounds to 30 pounds annual per capita consumption from the end of World War II to 1960 [5]. The high retention of vitamin C and the improved flavor of frozen citrus juices along with their general availability make these concentrates a dependable source of one of the nutrients commonly lacking in American diets.

HOME PREPARATION

The loss of some nutrient content is preventable by the manner in which food is handled and prepared for home consumption. Failing to serve vegetables immediately after cooking, storing fruits and vegetables improperly, throwing away the greens and skins of vegetables, using large amounts of water in cooking, and overcooking of vegetables are some wasteful practices.

Converting food for body functions

The digestive system converts raw materials into substances that the body can absorb and use. A general understanding of the processes of digestion and elimination provides a sound basis for developing practices that promote proper functioning of the alimentary canal.

DIGESTION OF FOODS

Digestion of food is both mechanical and chemical in nature. The mechanical portion of digestion begins in the mouth, with the action of the teeth and the tongue serving to break the food into smaller physical components. Progressive constriction of muscles in the wall of the alimentary canal produces peristalsis, which serves to mix the contents thoroughly and to move them along.

The chemical phase of the digestive process is somewhat more complex. Enzymes in the digestive juices are involved, and each has a specific effect on the food (see Table 9.8). Chemical action is initiated in the mouth as salivary secretions mix with the food during mastication and begin the breakdown of carbohydrates.

The food passes down the esophagus into the stomach, where digestive juices are added and the mixture is reduced to a semifluid consistency by muscle action of the stomach. The digestion of proteins and milk is initiated in the stomach, and carbohydrate digestion is continued. The length of time required for foods to pass through the stomach into the small intestine is influenced by the nature of the food itself, as well as by emotional factors and physical activity. In general, the stomach requires three to five hours to empty itself following a meal. Fluids pass through the stomach in a matter of minutes. Carbohydrates tend to be emptied from the stomach more quickly than proteins, which in turn pass through more rapidly than do fats. Combinations of fats and proteins leave the stomach more slowly than does either of these nutrients alone. Persistent feelings of hunger, which cause some to overeat, can be relieved partially by eating foods that do not leave the stomach too quickly. Carbohydrates contain a rich supply of calories and by themselves do not satisfy hunger for a great length of time. Herein lies one of the reasons for those added pounds.

Bands of muscles, called sphincters, form valves at the upper and lower end of the stomach. The valve at the upper end normally prevents the acid contents of the stomach from moving back into the esophagus. At the lower end of the stomach the pyloric sphincter controls the flow of material from the stomach into the duodenum, the first section of the small intestine.

In the small intestine, food is acted upon by additional digestive juices. Some of these substances are produced by glands in the intestinal wall, and others are produced by special glands apart from the alimentary tract, the pancreas and the liver being two examples.

Digestion in the large intestine is continued by action of the digestive juices brought from the small intestine. There

Table 9.8   Digestion of foods

Place of digestion	Material digested	Digestive juices	Enzymes acting	Products resulting	Absorption
Mouth	Starch	Saliva	Ptyalin	Dextrins and maltose	None
Stomach	Starch				
	Protein	Gastric juice	Pepsin	Proteoses and peptones	None
	Casein in milk	Gastric juice	Rennin	Paracasein	None
	Fats and oils	Gastric juice	Lipase	Glycerol and fatty acids	None
Small intestine	Starch	Pancreatic juice	Amylopsin	Dextrins and maltose	None
	Dextrins Maltose	Intestinal juice	Maltase	Glucose	Glucose
	Sucrose	Intestinal juice	Sucrase	Glucose and fructose	Glucose Fructose
	Lactose	Intestinal juice	Lactase	Glucose and galactose	Glucose Galactose
	Proteins Proteoses	Pancreatic juices	Trypsin Chymotrypsin	Polypeptides Polypeptides	
	Polypeptides Dipeptides Peptones	Intestinal and pancreatic juices	Carboxypeptidase Aminopeptidase Dipeptidase	Amino acids	Amino acids
	Fats and oils	Pancreatic juice Intestinal juice	Steapsin Lipase	Fatty acids and glycerol	Fatty acids Glycerol

are no secretions of digestive enzymes into the large intestine.

Products of digestion. As a result of the digestive process, foods are converted into substances that the body is able to absorb. Carbohydrates are broken down into simple sugars. Fats are converted to fatty acids and glycerol. Proteins are reduced to their component amino acids. The vitamins and minerals are freed so they can be absorbed.

Conditions influencing digestion. Digestion of food is affected by a number of factors. One of the most significant factors is the nervous or emotional state of an individual. Anger, worry, fear, tension, and other emotional states disturb normal digestion by interfering with the secretion of digestive juices and by disturbing the muscular activity in the lining of the alimentary canal. Relaxing before a meal, maintaining a peaceful atmosphere during the meal, and avoiding tensions afterward contribute to better digestion.

While individuals should not believe old wives' tales about certain combinations of food being indigestible, they should understand that the digestion of some foods is more difficult and does take longer. The use of large amounts of fatty foods or foods coated with fat

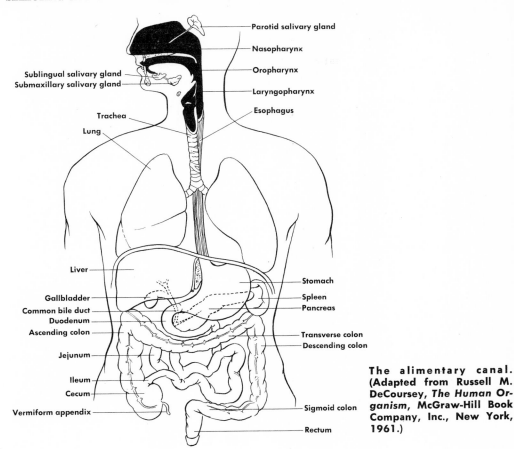

Parotid salivary gland

Nasopharynx

Oropharynx

Sublingual salivary gland

Submaxillary salivary gland

Laryngopharynx

Trachea

Esophagus

Lung

Liver

Stomach

Gallbladder

Spleen

Common bile duct

Pancreas

Duodenum

Ascending colon

Transverse colon

Jejunum

Descending colon

Ileum

Cecum

Vermiform appendix

Sigmoid colon

Rectum

The alimentary canal. (Adapted from Russell M. DeCoursey, *The Human Organism*, McGraw-Hill Book Company, Inc., New York, 1961.)

at one meal, protein foods that have been toughened by overcooking, and carbohydrate foods in which cellulose fiber has not been softened by sufficient cooking is likely to increase the difficulty of digestion. Eating such foods when overtired, after an illness, or when emotionally disturbed is more likely to create difficulties.

The properly nourished individual whose general state of health is good is less likely to have difficulties with digestion. Some unpleasant hours and even serious disorders can be averted by a sound, sensible regimen of eating.

ABSORPTION

The passage of food substances through the epithelial cells of the alimentary canal into the blood or lymph is called

absorption. Food is transported by these fluids to the various tissues where it is to serve its function as a source of fuel, for building and repair, or in the regulation of body activities.

Absorption occurs primarily within the small intestine, with little absorption taking place in the stomach. An exception to this is the absorption of alcohol, which explains the immediate effects of alcohol, particularly when one has not eaten for several hours.

Because of the length of the small intestine, the numerous folds, and the small, fingerlike villi that project from the lining of the intestinal wall, the surface available for absorption is extensive. Differences in the rate and degree of absorption due to variations in body build may be a factor in determining the ability to maintain normal weight. The movement of food as a result of peristaltic action brings it into contact with the lining of the intestine and facilitates the process of absorption.

The simple sugars and the amino acids are absorbed directly into the blood. The fatty acids and glycerol must be re-formed into tiny fat globules, which in turn are taken into the lympathic system. The lymph fluid eventually empties into the blood stream, and the fat products are distributed to the tissues, where they are utilized.

Absorption in the large intestine is confined to removing the excess amounts of water. The residue is left as a semisolid waste.

ELIMINATION OF WASTE

The fiber, or roughage, part of the ingested food remains as a major portion of the residue after digestion and absorption are completed. This residue passes through the large intestine and is eliminated as solid waste material called feces, or fecal matter. See Chapter 7 for additional information on elimination of body waste materials.

Disorders of the digestive system

It is a rare individual who does not at some time suffer from a disturbance of the digestive system. The pain or discomfort may be short-lived, or it may be a persistent or chronic ailment. The discomfort may be only mildly irritating, or it may be extremely painful. The degree of pain or discomfort does not necessarily indicate the seriousness of the disorder. Any abdominal pain which persists should be brought to the attention of a physician, who is best qualified to determine the cause and to recommend the treatment. Treatment that is effective for one disorder can be dangerous if used for another.

CANKER SORES

Many individuals suffer from canker sores in the mouth. They may be extremely painful and interfere with chewing and swallowing.

Canker sores are caused by a virus. Contributing causes include allergic reactions to foods such as walnuts and chocolate, gastrointestinal upsets, and emotional states. If the canker sores persist or recur, the individual should see his physician in order to determine the underlying cause.

INDIGESTION, OR DYSPEPSIA

Indigestion, or dyspepsia, is a symptom

of a disorder of the digestive tract. Simple indigestion is due to a functional rather than an organic condition. Functional nervous indigestion is a distressing condition frequently caused by faulty eating habits. Overeating, irritating substances such as alcohol, and emotional states are common causes of disturbances in function of the alimentary tract and the resulting discomfort of indigestion.

Advertisers do an effective job of convincing the consumer that he is suffering from an "acid stomach." This should not be difficult, because the contents of the stomach are normally acid in nature. Treatment of persistent indigestion by the use of preparations selected from the well-stocked shelf of the corner drugstore is dangerous. The assistance of a physician is required to determine and treat the cause and not just the symptoms. Ulcers, gallbladder disorders, cancer, and appendicitis can produce symptoms commonly associated with simple indigestion [7].

ULCERS

Peptic ulcers are associated with pepsin, an enzyme in the stomach digestive juices. Peptic ulcers are found in the stomach and also in the duodenum, or first part of the small intestine. Most of them are found in the duodenum, perhaps because the tissue lining this area is less resistant to the action of digestive juices. Few duodenal ulcers, but up to 10 per cent of stomach ulcers, become cancerous [34].

The exact cause of an ulcer is not known, but there are some contributing causes that apparently play an important role in the onset of the condition. Most persons who have duodenal ulcers tend to have higher gastric acidity than normal, but many who have extremely high concentrations of gastric acidity do not have such ulcers. Frequently it is the nervous type of person who has an ulcer, but many nervous persons do not develop the condition. More men than women, perhaps as high as ten times as many, are victims of this condition.

Despite the fact that the specific cause of ulcers is not understood completely, it is known that strong emotional tensions and high gastric acidity are associated with them. The gastric secretions literally eat the wall of the stomach or duodenum, and unless treatment is undertaken, a hemorrhage or perforation of the wall occurs.

Approximately one person in ten will have an ulcer at some time in his life; hence, it is important to be aware of warning signs and to seek medical care if such signs appear. Persistent indigestion or pain that tends to occur as the stomach becomes empty may indicate the presence of an ulcer. Treatment of ulcers is a medical responsibility, not a matter of self-diagnosis and drugstore remedies for an acid stomach. Fortunately, through diet and other treatment prescribed by a physician, most ulcers can be kept under control.

GALLBLADDER DISORDERS

Disorders of the gallbladder can produce symptoms such as heartburn, bloating after meals, nausea and vomiting, and, in some cases, pain in the upper right quadrant of the abdominal area. Because of the function of bile in the digestion of fats, the intake of foods rich in fats tends to aggravate the symptoms.

Disorders of the gallbladder require the care of a physician. In some cases the disorders respond to diet and medication; in others, surgery is necessary to correct the difficulty. In any case, early treatment of the condition is more likely to produce favorable results. Self-treatment of symptoms with liver pills or other such remedies seldom gets at the cause of the symptoms. It is much better to have a physician determine the cause and prescribe treatment before the disorder becomes severe.

CANCER

Cancer of the digestive tract accounts for more deaths than does cancer in any other organ or system of the body, for it is frequently undiscovered until it is too late to treat it effectively. Persistent indigestion or change in normal bowel habits may be the only early sign of cancer of the digestive tract. The importance of having a physician determine whether or not persistent indigestion is an early indication of cancer cannot be overstressed. A more detailed discussion of cancer is found in Chapter 12.

APPENDICITIS

Acute appendicitis—inflammation of the vermiform appendix near the juncture of the small and large intestine—produces symptoms similar to some other digestive disturbances. Severe abdominal pain may be felt in other areas of the abdominal cavity, but eventually the pain usually localizes in the lower right quadrant. Nausea and vomiting may occur as the condition becomes worse. Rupture of the appendix can cause peritonitis, which reduces the chance for recovery. Self-treatment for abdominal pain resulting from appendicitis, particularly if it involves the use of laxatives, can cause the appendix to rupture.

CONSTIPATION

Constipation is a condition in which excretion of fecal matter from the large intestine is delayed. Interference with the normal elimination of waste material results in considerable discomfort. In extreme cases of constipation, there is extensive irritation of the large intestine.

An estimated 6 out of every 10 Americans make frequent use of laxatives. Laxatives cost the American people approximately 148 million dollars during 1958 [16]. A variety of these products is too readily available on the drugstore shelf.

Laxatives produce their results in different ways. Some are drugs that stimulate peristaltic action of the muscles of the intestinal tract; some are substances that increase the bulk content by swelling up when combined with fluids; some contain salts to increase the fluid content; and others, such as mineral oil, soften the feces.

In most cases, laxatives do not get at the cause of constipation, called "our national neurosis" by one physician. They are used to treat symptoms, and their excessive use adds to the difficulties instead of eliminating them. The use of mineral oil interferes with absorption of fat-soluble vitamins in the intestinal tract. Drugs that stimulate peristaltic action can become habit-forming. Continued self-treatment with laxatives can very easily result in a delay in the diagnosis of a serious disorder of the digestive tract.

Proper elimination is promoted by a well-balanced diet, such as that suggested in *A Daily Food Guide,* sufficient intake of fluids, physical activity, good posture, and a regular time for bowel movement. In general, laxatives should be used only when recommended by a physician.

FOOD POISONING

Food-borne infections present a constant threat to health if there is careless handling of food during preparation or careless storing of food held over after preparation. The most prevalent type of food poisoning is the result of staphylococcal contamination of food from skin lesions or from respiratory discharge of a food handler. Cream fillings, custards, puddings, and casseroles that are kept unrefrigerated for several hours serve as excellent media for the growth of organisms, which produce toxins, which in turn cause gastrointestinal disturbances. Within a matter of 3 or 4 hours after ingestion of contaminated food, the victim experiences nausea, vomiting, diarrhea, and intestinal cramps. The duration of the illness is usually no more than a day and is frequently a matter of a few hours.

Outbreaks of food poisoning as a result of *Salmonella* organisms are more prolonged. The pattern of food contamination is much the same as with staphylococcal infections, and the symptoms are likewise similar but more persistent. Botulinus poisoning, or botulism, is a rare form of food poisoning now that foods are commercially processed. Low-acid foods such as beans, corn, beets, and asparagus have been the primary source of this type of poisoning when improperly processed in home canning. The toxin produced is one of the most potent poisons known, and mortality figures are about 65 per cent in botulism poisoning [6].

Other types of food poisoning include mussel and clam poisoning during certain seasons of the year, mushroom poisoning from inedible species, and ingestion of poisonous plants such as hemlock, Jimson weed, foxglove, and nightshade [6].

FOOD ALLERGIES

Food allergies are not necessarily allergic reactions manifested in the digestive system; they are due to an individual's reaction to an allergen contained in ingested food. Although many foods can cause allergic reactions, some of the most common offenders are wheat, milk, eggs, strawberries, nuts, and chocolate. For a more detailed consideration of allergies, see Chapter 12.

Summary

Early in life you were dependent entirely upon other persons to supply foods to meet your needs. Gradually, as you have matured, you have had more and more responsibility for providing the proper nourishment for your body. By the time you reach college age, you are able to exert a great amount of influence in the selection of foods, even though you may be dependent upon someone else to prepare and serve the food. In the final analysis, most Americans of college age and older have adequate financial resources to be properly nourished. If they are not, it is either because of lack of knowledge or because of failure to apply what they know. In this chapter information is provided to help an individual know what is best for meeting nutritional requirements.

An understanding of the more common dietary deficiencies, as indicated by nutrition studies, can be helpful to the person who is sincerely interested in avoiding deficiencies in his own diet. In addition, an understanding of common misconceptions about foods enables a person to make better selection of food products by helping him to detect misleading claims.

Particular emphasis is placed upon the problem of overweight. The causes, problems associated with excess weight, and guidelines for losing weight safely are discussed. Problems associated with underweight are also considered.

Fortunately, you do not have to be an expert in nutrition to select foods that will provide you with a balanced supply of the nutrients needed for energy, growth and repair, and regulation of body activities. By selecting from the four food groups as recommended in *A Daily Food Guide,* you can provide variety in your diet and at the same time secure needed nutrients.

Preparation can make a difference in the food value available. Foods properly prepared, both commercially and by the cook who prepares meals, retain most of the nutrients that they are expected to supply. Additives are being used in increasing numbers and amounts, but their use is controlled by Food and Drug Administration regulations in order to protect the consumer from possible harmful effects.

Included in the chapter is a discussion of the digestion of foods to convert them into substances that the body can utilize. In addition, there is a consideration of common disorders of the digestive tract, with certain recommendations for proper care in order to prevent serious complications.

Since eating is an activity that continues as long as a person lives, and may play an important role in both the length of life and the quality of living, it is essential that we understand and apply basic nutritional information in planning our daily meals.

Suggested readings

1. American Heart Association: *Dietary Fat and Its Relation to Heart Attacks and Strokes,* The Association, New York, 1961.
2. Arnold, James R., and E. A. Martell: "The Circulation of Radioactive Isotopes," *Scientific American,* 201:85–93, September, 1959.
3. Benson, Ezra Taft: "America's Nutrition Paradox: Want Amidst Plenty," *Today's Health,* 38:23–25, June, 1960.
4. Bogert, L. Jean: *Nutrition and Physical Fitness,* 7th ed., W. B. Saunders Company, Philadelphia, 1960.
5. Burr, Horace K., and R. Paul Elliott: "Quality and Safety in Frozen Foods,"

Journal of the American Medical Association, 174:1178–1180, Oct. 29, 1960.

6. Burton, Benjamin T. (ed.): *The Heinz Handbook of Nutrition,* McGraw-Hill Book Company, Inc., New York, 1959.

7. "But Is It 'Indigestion'?" *Consumer Reports,* 25:440–442, August, 1960.

8. Cooper, Lenna F., and others: *Nutrition in Health and Disease,* 13th ed., J. B. Lippincott Company, Philadelphia, 1958.

9. Council on Foods and Nutrition, American Medical Association: "Formula Diets and Weight Control," *Journal of the American Medical Association,* 176:439, May 6, 1961.

10. Council on Foods and Nutrition, American Medical Association: "Vitamin Preparations as Dietary Supplements and as Therapeutic Agents," *Journal of the American Medical Association,* 169:41–45, Jan. 3, 1959.

11. DeCoursey, Russell Myles: *The Human Organism,* 2d ed., McGraw-Hill Book Company, Inc., New York, 1961.

12. Everson, Gladys J.: "The Importance of Eating a Good Breakfast," *Food and Nutrition News,* 27:1, May, 1956.

13. "Fallout in Our Milk—A Follow-up Report," *Consumer Reports,* 25:64–70, February, 1960.

14. *Food Additives: What They Are/How They Are Used,* Manufacturing Chemists Association, Washington, 1961.

15. Food and Drug Administration, U.S. Department of Health, Education, and Welfare: *What Consumers Should Know about Food Additives,* Government Printing Office, Washington, 1960.

16. Hook, Charles W.: "Laxatives: A $148 Million Fraud," *Today's Health,* 38:30–31, October, 1960.

17. "How Pure Is Your Food?" *U.S. News and World Report,* 48:86–90, Dec. 7, 1959.

18. Kelley, Louis, and others: "Nutritional Evaluation of Food Purchased by 146 Urban Families during 1953," *Journal of Home Economics,* 48:355–358, May, 1956.

19. Lundberg, W. O., "Saturated vs. Unsaturated Dietary Fat in Atherosclerosis," *Food and Nutrition News,* 32:1, 4, April, 1961.

20. "More of the Facts You Should Know about Vitamins," *Consumer Reports,* 26:44–48, January, 1961.

21. Morgan, Agnes Fay (ed.): *Nutritional Status U.S.A.,* California Agricultural Experimental Station, Berkeley, Calif., 1959.

22. Mrak, Emil, "New and Improving Food Products," *Journal of the American Dietetic Association,* 36:578–580, June, 1960.

23. National Academy of Science–National Research Council, Food and Nutrition Board: *Recommended Dietary Allowances,* rev. ed., NAS-NRC Publication 589, Washington, 1958.

24. "Of Cranberries, Chickens, Lipsticks, and Black Jelly Beans," *Consumer Reports,* 25:96–98, February, 1960.

25. Ratcliff, J. D.: "Enzymes: Your Body's Amazing Chemists," *Today's Health,* 38:42–43, September, 1960.

26. "Strontium-90: A Special Hazard," *Consumer Reports,* 24:106–108, March, 1959.

27. "The Facts about Vitamins," *Consumer Reports,* 25:493–496, September, 1960.

28. "The Fat of the Land," *Time,* 77:48–52, Jan. 13, 1961.

29. The President's Science Advisory Committee: *Report of the Panel on Food Additives,* Nutrition Foundation, Inc., New York, 1960.

30. "The Strange Case of the Multi-million Dollar Food Supplement and the Frustrated Government Agencies," *Consumer Reports,* 25:550–554, October, 1960.

31. Trulson, Martha F., and others: "Food Fads vs. Professional and Public Education," in *The Role of Nutrition Education in Combatting Food Fads,* Nutrition Foundation, Inc., New York, 1959.

32. U.S. Department of Agriculture, Institute of Home Economics: *Food for Fitness: A Daily Food Guide,* Government Printing Office, Washington, 1958.

33. U.S. Department of Agriculture: *Food: The Yearbook of Agriculture, 1959,* Government Printing Office, Washington, 1959.

34. Vath, William R.: "Peptic Ulcers: Still a Medical Mystery?" *Today's Health,* 38:28–29, September, 1960.

35. Young, Charlotte M., and others: "What the Homemaker Knows about Nutrition," *Journal of the American Dietetic Association,* 32:429–434, April, 1956.

TEN

Selecting health products and services

FRAUDULENT CONSUMER HEALTH PRACTICES

LEGAL PROTECTION FOR THE CONSUMER

ORGANIZATIONS AND AGENCIES PROTECTING THE CONSUMER

EVALUATING HEALTH INFORMATION

SELECTING HEALTH PRODUCTS

SELECTING HEALTH SERVICES

RESPONSIBILITY OF THE INDIVIDUAL FOR CONSUMER HEALTH

You, as an American consumer, are confronted with a variety of attractively packaged and highly advertised health products to cure all possible illnesses, as well as to preserve and lengthen life. A multitude of quacks bombard the public with their services, which they guarantee to cure every disease from athlete's foot to cancer. Physical culture specialists, through a mail-order set of prescribed exercises, claim to be able to mold any skeletal frame into a body beautiful. Even more tempting are the aids to beauty, which are supposed to renew, restore, and invigorate one, and bring to light hidden powers of loveliness for women and manliness, including handsome features, for men.

Endless advertising, designed to ensnare each and every person, fills the daily paper and the weekly and monthly magazines. Advertising of health products and services is broadcast from coast to coast by radio and television stations, supplemented with billboards decoratively portraying a new, healthful, zestful life. Health information with quasi-scientific basis fills the atmosphere through every available medium. The opportunities for filling the need for health services and products is greater than ever before. At the same time, the dangers to life and the chance of financial loss, thwarted energy, and wasted time have increased proportionately.

Consumer health is but one aspect, though a significant one, of improving the quality of living. Health consumers are all people who use health products and services. This group includes the well, the sick, the young, the aged, the rich, and the poor. To be an intelligent consumer and to select products and services wisely, it is important for you to be concerned with answers to the following questions:

What are fraudulent health practices?

What protection do you, the consumer, have from quacks and nostrums?

What are the consumer organizations and agencies protecting you?

What are the sources of safe, reliable health information?

How can you critically evaluate health information and advertising?

How can you select health products and health services wisely?

How can you protect yourself and others from fraudulent practices undermining the individual and the group?

The information in this chapter is presented to help answer these questions.

Fraudulent consumer health practices

Quackery is the practicing of medicine by a faker or an incompetent person. Such an individual claims he has a cure-all or sure-fire method of restoring health. The quack preys upon the public, including the so-called intellectual class, by his adroit psychological suggestions. The dominating motive of the quack is to make money. It takes no special preparation or education to become a quack.

A *nostrum* is the product distributed by the quack. Usually, he sells it as a cure-all or sure-cure remedy. One thing certain is its worthlessness in the treatment of the disease or the condition for which it is sold. Legally, it is a patent or secret remedy sold directly to the public. Distinct and different from nostrums are proprietary chemicals or drugs. These are medicines whose composition or formula is protected by patent, owner control, or manufacture against free competition. They are used by medical doctors in the treatment of disease in addition to the drugs found in the pharmacopeias. The latter type drugs are produced by many manufacturers.

HISTORICAL EXAMPLES OF QUACKERY

Cure-alls are almost as old as history itself. It has been a weakness of all peoples through the ages to believe in a fountain of youth, an elixir of life that would free them from pain and restore youth and vigor. Certainly, the quacks prey upon this weakness of mankind as did P. T. Barnum. It is reported that the oldest nostrum, which later developed into a bona fide drug and still is in existence today, is called "hiera picra." This is a powder of aloes and canella, and dried juice of a common oriental plant.[1] Arab doctors, Greek practitioners in Rome, barbers, corn doctors, herbalists, the monastic doctors of the Middle Ages, and early English and American doctors used this drug, and quacks peddled an imitation of it.

One of the most colorful quacks in history was St. John Long of London, a handsome and clever Irishman. He was patronized by many fashionable and noble persons. He built up a reputation as one who could cure many diseases, particularly tuberculosis. His popular treatment consisted in applying a liniment made of turpentine, acetic acid, and egg yolk and inhaling a vapor. After reaping a fortune from his so-called tuberculosis cure, he died at the age of thirty-seven from pulmonary tuberculosis.

The grandfather of American quacks was Elisha Perkins, a physician who became an imposter in 1795 primarily because of the lure of lucrative returns. He discovered that pain was stopped when a metallic instrument was used to separate the gum from a tooth previous to pulling it. He decided that metallic substances influenced nerves and muscles. Therefore, he developed his famous metal tractors to influence the body when applied externally. The tractors consisted of two rods of brass and iron 3 inches long. One side was flat and the other half round. They were called Perkins Patent Tractors, cost 75 cents, and sold for $25 to $30. The purpose of the tractors, according to Perkins, was to draw the disease from the body by starting at the hairline and working back to the neck. He admitted this would not cure a headache caused by excessive drinking. He took his tractors to a session of Congress and sold a number to the distinguished lawmakers. However, he soon was exposed and forced to give up the sale of the tractors. Then he devised Perkins Medical Formula, a combination of vinegar and salt taken in tablespoon doses diluted with three parts of hot water, which was a sure cure for yellow fever according to Perkins. By a strange turn of fate he died of yellow fever in 1799. His work was carried on by his son, who fled to England, where he made a fortune from Perkins Patent Tractors.[2] The cases of Long and Perkins are two selected historical illustrations of quackery indicating fraudulent practices. Many more could be cited.

PRESENT-DAY PSEUDOSCIENTIFIC PRACTICES

Food, drug, and cosmetic racketeers are not past history but are prevalent in present-day culture.

The National Better Business Bureau announced in 1960 that, from the ratings of the complaints it received, "deceptive drug, device, and cosmetic advertising" was at the top of the gyp parade in that year. Among the major frauds perpetrated were cancer cures, arthritis and rheumatism cures, weight reducers, food fads, skin beautifiers, and baldness preventives. Most of these posed serious threats to health, even to life itself. Startling enough is the fact that these frauds increased to a large extent in comparison with the number of similar complaints in 1956 [24].

Cancer cures. One of today's most tragic rackets is conducted by the cancer quacks. Since the causes of cancer are not yet fully known to medical science, many opportunities are open to quacks to advertise their sure cures. These unscrupulous persons take in desperate persons who are grasping at any new hope for a cure.

The Hoxsey cancer cure is an example of this quackery. In 1956, on two differ-

---

[1] John A. Foote, "Medicine Fakes and Fakers of All Ages," *The National Geographic Magazine*, January, 1919, p. 69.

[2] Ruth Lamb, *American Chamber of Horrors*, Farrar and Rinehart, Inc., New York, 1936.

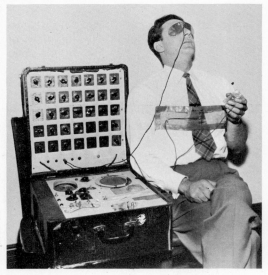

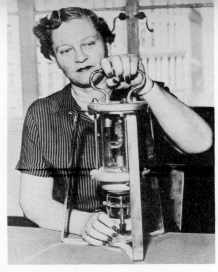

Another quack cancer device offered for sale for $10,000 was found by Federal inspectors to contain $1.60 worth of radium. Radium water from the machine was supposed to cure cancer.

Fake health devices, the products of quacks, are sold in a variety of forms to fleece the public. One of the worst devices is the Radionic Machine used by a naturopath. In the case shown here, the quack used his machine to diagnose a Food and Drug inspector's condition as cancer of the liver with 91 degrees of malignancy. The inspector previously had been pronounced in perfect health by a group of reputable physicians.

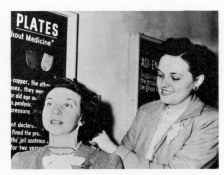

Then there is the Galvano Necklace, the string of beads and metal discs supposed to cure goiter. It probably will cure swelling of the wallet.

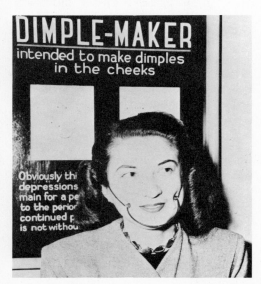

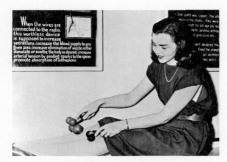

The gullibility of the public is demonstrated by the Dimple-Maker. Doctors report prolonged use might cause cancer, but will not produce new dimples or make small ones larger.

Here are two types of fake medical massages designed by a quack to prevent falling hair, headaches, constipation, and double chins. The Federal Food and Drug Administration has issued a statement that no therapeutic machine today manufactured for home use cures the basic cause of disease.

ent occasions the Federal courts determined that the Hoxsey medicines for internal cancer were worthless. Public warnings were issued by the Commissioner of Food and Drugs, Food and Drug Administration, to this effect. The Hoxsey treatment cost the patient $400, plus $60 in additional fees. This included a superficial examination at the Hoxsey Cancer Clinic at Dallas, Texas, or Portage, Pennsylvania, and treatment with pills and liquid medicine. The Food and Drug Administration found the pills and drugs to contain potassium iodide, licorice, red clover blossoms, burdock root, Stillingia root, berberis root, poke root, cascara sagrada, prickly ash bark, and buckhorn powder. Not one single verified cure of internal cancer was found in the investigation of the treatment, nor could any value be attributed to the medicine and pills in curing internal cancer. Thousands of persons were deceived by the false claims for the Hoxsey treatment over more than thirty years of promotion of this worthless cure before the exploitation of the public was halted in 1960.

Some types of cancer can be cured when detected early, but surgery, radiation, and chemical therapy are the only sure methods of treatment. Cancer is discussed further in Chapter 12.

The California Cancer Commission has disclosed many quacks and reports on typical cases. For example, the case is cited of a woman with breast cancer treated by a powdery substance supplied by a quack, which was supposed to kill the cancer cell. This person finally went to a medical doctor for treatment after she had spent nine months and all her life savings on the quack. By this time the cancer was not curable, since it had spread throughout her body.

Another example is that of a man with cancer of the bladder. This person was treated by a quack with an enzyme of the liver supposed to shrink cancerous tissue. Again, by the time he had gone to a reputable medical doctor who could have helped by X ray or surgery, he had wasted valuable time and his cancer was incurable [26].

After many such examples and with much work by the California Cancer Commission, the American Cancer Society, California Branch, and many other health organizations and interested persons, a state law was passed to outlaw the cancer quack. California became, in June, 1959, the first of the 50 states to pass legislation that prohibits the practice of quackery and provides penalties for lawbreakers. The law prohibits any person from treating cancer by the use of drugs, surgery, or radiation unless licensed to practice under state law. Violation of this provision constitutes unprofessional conduct under the State Medical Practice Act. First and second offenses are misdemeanors. The third violation and any thereafter are felonies. The law makes it mandatory for any method for diagnosing or curing cancer to be submitted to the State Department of Public Health for testing. Also, records must be kept of cancer treatments, which must be available at all times for investigation by state authorities [26].

Arthritis and rheumatism quackery. The Arthritis and Rheumatism Foundation [43] reports that sufferers from these two diseases are spending more than 250 million dollars each year, the major portion of which is going for worthless or dangerous drugs, devices, and treatments. The Foundation has estimated that there is an arthritic in every five families in the United States. These people become easy prey for the quack because there is no known cure for arthritis and because the affliction, by nature, comes and goes. The quack may receive full credit for relieving a condition that nature itself has taken care of temporarily.

The Foundation is making an all-out effort to provide the public with information that is accurate and reliable about arthritis and rheumatism. Until the specific cause or causes are discovered, only the symptoms can be treated to provide temporary relief from pain. The medical doctor can best prescribe treatment and care. He knows that aspirin, physical therapy, a hot-water bottle, or a long soak in a warm bath will bring relief. He knows, too, when these tried and proved procedures should be used and to what extent.

The Foundation has found that 14 out of 100 arthritics use a device such as a vibrator to relieve or attempt to prevent arthritis and rheumatism. The Food and Drug Administration has ruled that vibrators are useless and dangerous, and they are now declared illegal when promoted for the treatment or cure of arthritis.

Cases have been reported of radioactive minerals that have proved to be most cruel hoaxes. People have been enticed to sit in abandoned uranium mines for the price of $10 a day and to purchase so-called uranium-bearing dirt in pads or mitts, which upon examination contained nothing more than good Texas topsoil. Other sufferers have spent as much as $300 for worthless "Atomotrones," hailed as sure-cure devices. Other fake devices have been called Specto-Chrome, Oscilloclast, and Roto-View. The FDA found the latter to be nothing more than a blue plastic lampshade over a light bulb. The colored light supposedly had a curative effect [43].

Weight-reducing quackery. Reducing pills or appetite depressants, advertised as "dietless" reducing methods, are definitely on the increase, particularly mail-order diet plans. The American Medical Association and the Fraud Order Division, U.S. Post Office Department, have found these to be worthless or misleading. The serious consequence is that some people falling for these schemes are those who have conditions such as diabetes,

thyroid, heart, liver, and kidney diseases. Reducing without the advice and guidance of a medical doctor is particularly dangerous. But the advertising indicates that a famous movie actress diets by merely taking a few pills with no special eating. Also, according to the ads, a person can lose weight and eat all he wants by eating reducing candy or by eating a no-diet reducing wonder drug. The Fraud Order Division, U.S. Post Office Department, the Bureau of Investigation, American Medical Association, the Federal Trade Commission, the Food and Drug Administration, and, recently, a House of Representatives Subcommittee on Weight Reducers are all concerned with and working against fraudulent advertising and labeling practices in this area. The FDA warns against promoters that can shake fat off with vibrator, massage devices, and cosmetic creams that spot-reduce.

Losing weight is a difficult and serious process. Miracle or wonder diets and "fabulous formulas" just do not solve the weight-reduction problem. Hard work, great self-control, and expert supervision by a medical doctor are the safe way to reduce weight. This way the individual plans with his doctor a scientific program of reduced calories, together with appropriate exercise, both based on the individual's specific needs.

The discussion in Chapter 9 provides scientific information about proper diet, including weight reduction.

Food fads. Modern myths and superstitions about food are utilized by faddist operators to sell their product, particularly food supplements. There is little harm in the old superstition that fish is a brain food. However, there is danger when people are led to believe that garlic pills will correct high blood pressure or that grapes can cure ulcers and cancer. These superstitious beliefs are sheer quackery.

Food faddists commonly promote their wares by staging a health food lecture or by door-to-door selling. The fad-dists' lectures appear to be scientific, but there also is a strong mixture of pseudo-science and superstition, resulting in many half-truths. Their purpose, of course, is to sell their product, not to improve health. The door-to-door sales agents are adept at using the scare tech-nique to promote their vitamin, mineral, and herbal preparations. The FDA [3] lists four ideas used, each of which contains an element of truth but is false when all the facts are studied.

THE MYTH THAT ALL DISEASES ARE DUE TO FAULTY DIET. This usually refers to the premise that something is missing from the diet that can only be supplied if their food supplement is taken. In fact, few diseases resulting from dietary deficiencies are found in the United States.

THE MYTH THAT SOIL DEPLETION CAUSES MALNUTRITION. This myth is built on the theory that repeated cropping has impoverished the soil and that foods are therefore nutritionally inferior. Also, they state that chemical fertilizers poison the land and the crops. The remedy, according to the faddists, is that "natural" foods and the proper food supplements, which they sell, will provide the proper diet. There is no scientific evidence for these two theories. The FDA indicates there is no significant difference in the nutritive value of foods produced on different soils, with the exception of soils that lack iodine. The only disease associa-tion with a deficiency of soil or water is simple goiter due to lack of iodine in certain lands. The use of iodized salt corrects this deficiency.

THE MYTH OF OVERPROCESSING. Some food faddists overplay and exaggerate the fact that some methods of food proc-essing and cooking remove or reduce the vitamins and minerals contained in foods. Modern food processing pro-cedures are devised to preserve the needed nutritional values and to re-store them to foods. Adding vitamins and minerals as supplements to flour, bread, milk, and oleomargarine are ex-amples. Proper canning and freezing of fruits and vegetables are other illus-trations.

THE MYTH OF SUBCLINICAL DEFICIENCIES. A subclinical condition is one in which it is not possible to obtain any ob-servable evidence of a vitamin de-ficiency, but a deficiency is suspected. The myth is that anyone who has "that tired feeling" or an ache or pain is suffering from a subclinical deficiency and therefore needs to supplement his diet with additional vitamins and minerals. Almost every normal person at some time experiences a tired feel-ing, but this is not necessarily a sub-clinical deficiency. Your physician can diagnose a vitamin or mineral de-ficiency and prescribe proper treat-ment. One should question self-medica-tion with vitamins or minerals to cure diseases of the nerves, bones, blood, liver, kidneys, heart, or digestive tract. A much wiser plan is to visit a com-petent medical doctor.

Beauty quackery. The skin game is a most lucrative one for quacks. Beauty treatments and skin care have provided a fertile field for quacks for many years. Their nostrums consist of their claimed new discoveries, usually from Europe and endorsed by foreign doctors, that will make the skin young again, enabling the individual's face to appear younger rather than older. Hormones, vitamins, royal jelly, wrinkle-remover cream, turtle- and shark-oil creams—all have been advo-cated to restore youth, remove wrinkles, and add new beauty.

Emollient creams and oils will lubri-cate the skin and thus aid in smoothing out fine surface lines due to dryness. It is true that cold creams have been used

[3] Food and Drug Administration, *Food Facts vs. Food Fallacies*, FDA Leaflet 4, U.S. Department of Health, Education, and Welfare, Washington, July, 1959.

since Roman days. They are valuable for softening the skin, particularly if it is dry, and removing some dirt particles as well as serving as a lubricant. Special creams that claim to serve other purposes are merely nostrums and a waste of money.

Many people forget that health comes from within as well as without. As the common expression goes, beauty is more than skin deep. Health is not purchased in a jar from the local drugstore or from cosmetic counters. A balanced diet, fresh air and sunshine, proper rest, soap and water, a wholesome environment, and, if necessary, medical treatment will do more for the skin than cosmetic preparations. It is important to remember that the skin receives its nourishment from the blood stream. Creams and lotions cannot nourish the skin tissue from without or strengthen the facial muscles. No known external lotion or skin preparation will work miracles, such as preventing or removing wrinkles.

Baldness cures. There is no known cure for hereditary baldness, except a toupee to cover missing hair, and this is not always desirable. Baldness caused by an illness is best cared for by a competent dermatologist. But no amount of expensive treatments, lotions, drugs, or massages will grow hair. Frequent brushing and stimulating of the scalp and caring for the hair, particularly avoiding continual drying out of the hair, may help prevent premature baldness.

Devices and false claims. It was not many years ago that quacks depended on electricity and electric devices and claimed to bring new health to their gullible patients by means of electric shocks, shining lights, and magnetic fields. Today such instruments are in use, but not as extensively as formerly, for the modern quack has developed new machines to cure all diseases by means of "atomic energy" and "cosmic waves." Reputable physicians utilize X-ray and therapeutic machines as aids in the diagnosis and treatment of certain diseases. The quack builds machines designed to look like the approved devices and, in addition to treatment in his office with these fake machines, endeavors to sell or lease them for home use. No therapeutic machine today manufactured for home use cures the basic cause of disease [21].

Frauds occur in the sale of medicines today even though drug labels must tell a true story according to law. The smooth talk of salesmen or lecturers promises much more than is claimed on the label. Also, false claims are contained in booklets or brochures accompanying the drugs. The modern quack is still a part of the culture, and he is more subtle and clever than ever before.

The Director of the Bureau of Investigation, American Medical Association, gives five trademarks of medical quacks, who give themselves away [4]

1. When they guarantee quick cures.
2. When they decry the use of surgery, drugs or x-rays.
3. When they claim they have a secret or special machine or formula that cures diseases.
4. When they advertise by using case histories and testimonials.
5. When they claim medical authorities are persecuting them.

Legal protection for the consumer

Laws are one means of protecting the consumer. However, the common laws in America provide only slight protection against fraudulent selling of health products. Under the Uniform Sales Act, when there is a breach of warranty or breach of

[4] *Today's Health,* 37:71, August, 1959.

contract, the buyer can follow one of three procedures [52]: (1) refuse to accept the goods and cancel the contract; (2) keep the goods and sue the dishonest seller for damages; (3) keep the goods and insist on a deduction from the original price. These are not adequate protective procedures because the time and expense involved in suing or showing proof of the seller's fraud make this prohibitive in most cases. Also, consumers are loath to admit that they have been duped, and so they bear the financial loss. Since the common laws give insufficient protection, the consumer looks to statute law for aid. Through the statutes a number of governmental agencies have been established with the express purpose of protecting the consumer.

EARLY FOOD AND DRUG LEGISLATION

Congress passed its first legislation exerting control over drugs in 1848. This statute was concerned only with controlling importation of adulterated drugs into the United States. Soon, however, the adulteration of drugs in this country provoked attention to the extent that several states and the District of Columbia passed control measures. In 1906, Congress passed the Federal Food and Drugs Act governing the interstate commerce of drugs. The Food and Drugs Act made adulteration, which is the addition of inferior substances to products, illegal. It attempted to prevent the inclusion of harmful ingredients in foods and drugs by controlling branding, false statements, omissions of facts concerning the products, and the selling of products under assumed names. This was a serious effort to control quackery and nostrums through interstate commerce. As a part of the functions of the act, the Bureau of Chemistry, U.S. Department of Agriculture, made examinations of drugs. In the same year, 1906, the Federal Meat Inspection Act was passed. By this law all meat in interstate or foreign commerce was required to be inspected by the Bureau of Animal Industry, U.S. Department of Agriculture. By 1927, Congress established a law-enforcement agency known as the Food, Drug, and Insecticide Administration to enforce the 1906 act. In 1931 this agency became the Food and Drug Administration. Although the act was a great step forward, it lacked real enforcement powers and did not apply to many products. Because of numerous loopholes in the law the consumer was not adequately protected. Public interest called for better controls.

The Food, Drug, and Cosmetic Act. Congress responded to the public demand with a revision of the Food and Drug Act in 1938. This act was named the Food, Drug, and Cosmetic Act. It provided heavier punitive powers to prevent fraudulent practices and give better protection to the public.

The act defines "food" as articles used for food or drink for man or other animals. It includes chewing gum and articles used as components of food or drink. Certain health and sanitary safeguards are established to protect the consumer. For example, an illegal food is clearly defined as any food containing a natural or added substance that is injurious to health. The law declares food illegal that is filthy, putrid, or decomposed. Food labels must not be false or misleading and must actually represent the facts concerning the food. The required information must appear in a prominent position on the label. The Act prohibits traffic in new drugs unless they are tested and approved by the Food and Drug Administration. It was later amended so that drugs such as insulin, penicillin, and streptomycin must be from a batch certified by the Food and Drug Administration. Also, drugs must comply with one of three officially set standards: the United States Pharmacopeia (stamped U.S.P.), the Homeopathic Pharmacopoeia (marked H.P.), or the National Formulary of the American Pharmaceutical Association (labeled N.F.).

A section of the Food, Drug, and Cosmetic Act calls for the establishment of standards for foods to promote honest and fair dealing. As a result of this provision, certain standards have been adopted, which serve as official regulations to help carry out the law.

Three kinds of standards have been established: *standards of identity,* indicating what a given food product actually is; *standards of quality,* minimum specifications for tenderness, color, and freedom from defects; and *standards of fill of container,* informing the packer how full the container must be. The standard of identity states what the product is, the standard of quality provides for special labeling indicating that a product does not meet the standard, and the standard of fill assures that the consumer gets the quantity he pays for and puts an end to cheating the consumer by giving him less than the standard. Standards ensure not only quantity but also quality to the extent that the proper nutritional value must be present. The consumer is guaranteed uniformity of enrichment of flour, corn meal, macaroni products, oleomargarine, evaporated milk, rice, and other products.

In general, the act grants power to the Food and Drug Administration to control food, drug, and cosmetic traffic by issuing rules and regulations that have the force and effect of law. For example, criminal penalties for violations are increased; authority is given to establish minimum standards for foods and to prohibit traffic of all food injurious to health. Factory inspection of food, drugs, and cosmetics is authorized for interstate shipments, and truthful labeling of foods, drugs, and cosmetics is required.

New amendments to the Food, Drug, *and Cosmetic Act.* Several new amendments add to the functions of the FDA.

The Miller Pesticides Amendment of 1954 requires the FDA to establish and enforce tolerances for the safe use of all pesticides.

The Food Additives Amendment of 1958 requires the FDA to establish and enforce tolerances for the safe use of all additives used in foods.

The Color Additive Amendments of 1960 require the establishment and enforcement of tolerances for the safe use of colors used in foods, drugs, and cosmetics. This amendment deals with *all* colors and authorizes tolerances where necessary to ensure safe use of colors.

The Federal Hazardous Substances Labeling Act of 1960 requires the FDA to enforce uniform requirements for adequate cautionary labeling of packages of hazardous substances intended for household use. This amendment supercedes the caustic poison act of 1927. Thus, the provisions to control hazardous substances become a part of the Food, Drug, and Cosmetic Act. The new law applies to household substances that are toxic, corrosive, flammable, and radioactive.

Despite the number of provisions covered by the act and its amendments, the need for critical evaluation of products is still, to a great degree, left up to the consumer. This is an important reason for consumer health education today.

OTHER FEDERAL LEGISLATION PROTECTING THE CONSUMER

Three other acts designed to safeguard the health of consumers are closely related to the Food, Drug, and Cosmetic Act: the Tea Act, the Import Milk Act, and the Filled Milk Act.

The Tea Act became effective in 1897 and was last amended in 1920. It authorizes the annual establishment of standards of quality, purity, and fitness for consumption of all teas imported into the United States. If a lot, or chop, of tea imported does not meet these standards, it is rejected.

The Import Milk Act of 1927 was passed to protect the public health and promote the dairy industry of the United States. It prohibits the importing of milk and cream into the country unless the shipper holds a permit from the Department of Health, Education, and Welfare.

The Filled Milk Act of 1923 prohibits the interstate commerce of filled milk if it is adulterated or injurious to health or if its sale constitutes a fraud upon the public. Filled milk is defined as any milk or cream to which has been added, or which has been blended or compounded with, any fat or oil other than milk fat. Such a change in the product makes it an imitation or semblance of milk or cream rather than the true product itself [48].

STATE AND LOCAL LAWS PROTECTING THE CONSUMER

State and local communities have enacted their own laws to supplement and complement Federal legislation. At least 19 states have pure food and drug laws patterned after the Federal act. For example, the California legislature passed its own Pure Foods Act in 1939 patterned after the Federal act of 1938. The new act in California added provisions to the Health and Safety Code for control of food, drugs, and cosmetics, giving additional powers to the State Department of Public Health.

The new state of Hawaii, with its Hawaii Food, Drug, and Cosmetic Act is another example. Its legislation is administered by the Food and Drug Bureau of the State Board of Health.

Many county and city health departments, local public health units, and other official agencies at the local level protect the consumer's health every day. A few of the activities which these agencies undertake are inspection of food-dispensing establishments, meat inspection, milk inspection and pasteurization, supervision of the canning of food and the purity of the water supply, and the restriction of sale, possession, distribution, and use of narcotics and poisons.

Much of the effectiveness of the control of food, drug, and cosmetic traffic depends on the working relationships and the cooperation that exist among law-enforcement personnel of the Federal, state, and local agencies and private organizations. More effective control has resulted with improved legislation, similar legislation at each level, better-qualified personnel, and cooperative endeavor through better human relationships at each level. However, there is still room for great improvement in legislation and enforcement. Loopholes in legislation and enforcement make possible intensified activities of the quack and unscrupulous businessman.

Organizations and agencies protecting the consumer

It is reassuring to know that several governmental agencies, professional societies, and private organizations are assuming responsibility for the protection of the consumer. A brief description of some of these organizations and agencies is presented. For further information, consult references listed under Suggested readings.

GOVERNMENTAL AGENCIES

Governmental agencies enforce the legal measures protecting the consumer, perform research and testing functions to determine quality of products sold and shipped in interstate commerce, and set standards of quality for consumer products. The chief agencies on the Federal level include the Food and Drug Administration, the Federal Trade Commission, and the Post Office Department. On the state and on the local level, the public health department and some special food, drug, and cosmetics bureaus provide the protective services. The functions of the local official agencies are discussed in Chapter 15, pages 459–461. Attention at this point is centered on the activities of the Federal agencies.

The Food and Drug Administration. The function of the Food and Drug Administration is to enforce the Federal Food, Drug, and Cosmetic Act and thereby protect the consumer and law-abiding manufacturers and dealers. It does not have jurisdiction over advertising relating to foods, drugs, and cosmetics. Much of the work of the FDA is done in field stations, where some 625 inspectors visit factories and processing plants and look for samples of products that violate the law. Eighteen district offices maintain laboratories where samples of products are analyzed. Research laboratories are located in Washington, where work on the more difficult problems is done. Inspectors and chemists work together gathering evidence, which then is presented to the Federal courts for action against violators of the act. In 1961, 2,199 employees worked for the FDA. Some 823 employees work in Washington, while 1,376 are in the field.

Some typical criminal cases handled by the Food and Drug Administration in 1961 included convicting four officials of Texas and Missouri companies for selling $750,000 worth of sweetened water over a 1½-year period in place of fresh orange juice. The product sold was labeled "Fresh Orange Juice—As Nature Made It." FDA seized over 200,000 capsules of Dr. Taylor's Formula L, used for the treatment of cancer. In its court action the FDA alleged that Formula L was a new drug that had not obtained safety clearance through a new-drug ap-

plication required by the Food, Drug, and Cosmetic Act. In North Carolina the FDA seized bottles of sea water selling for $1.95 a pint and in Cleveland, sea salt for $1.50 a pound. Attached to the sea-water bottles was a booklet claiming that sea water was an effective treatment for arthritis and other diseases and that it helped prolong life. Furthermore, the bottle labels did not state its vitamin and mineral properties. Sea salt was misbranded and included reprints claiming the therapeutic value of sea water, which medical authorities long ago disproved. Sea water contains the same minerals as in ordinary foods, with the exception of iodine, which is available through iodized salt.[5]

Other criminal cases included such action as finding insects, insect fragments, and rodent hairs and filth in a candy company's candy bars, chocolate-covered raisins, and malted-milk balls. A shipment of coffee was destroyed because it contained wood, glass, sand, paint, metal, and bits of vegetation. One firm and its president were fined for shipping a "low-sodium" soup base for heart-disease sufferers. When analyzed, it was found to contain excessive sodium. A promoter of a food supplement was sent to jail for producing and selling his product, which claimed to ward off disease in healthy persons and cure cancer, diabetes, tuberculosis, and arthritis. In the fiscal year 1960, 26,311 factories and commercial warehouses were inspected. It is a goal of the FDA that factories and commercial warehouses may be inspected once in every 4 or 5 years.

In addition to providing over-all enforcement of the Food, Drug, and Cosmetic Act, the Food and Drug Administration[6] carries out the following functions

[5] Food and Drug Administration, *Report on Enforcement and Compliance,* U.S. Department of Health, Education, and Welfare, Washington, April, 1961, pp. 1–5.
[6] Food and Drug Administration, *Food and Drug Administration—What It Is and Does,* FDA Leaflet 1, U.S. Department of Health, Education, and Welfare, Washington, February, 1961, p. 2.

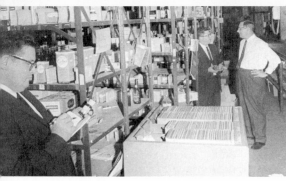

FDA inspectors check drug wholesalers to protect the public from possible labeling mix-ups.

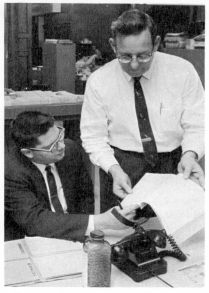

When an FDA inspector collects a sample, he also has authority under the Food, Drugs, and Cosmetics Act to examine shipping records.

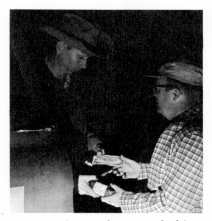

An FDA inspector disguised as a truck driver buys a drug that is available legally only on a doctor's prescription. This transaction is a part of FDA's undercover crack down on illegal traffic in amphetamine sulphate tablets (pep pills or bennies) and barbiturate capsules (goof balls).

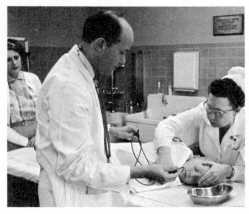

The New Hazardous Substance Labeling Act requires manufacturers to print a warning on the label telling of the chemical contents. This provision is designed to prevent a scene such as is depicted here with a doctor preparing to pump out the stomach of a boy while his mother watches anxiously.

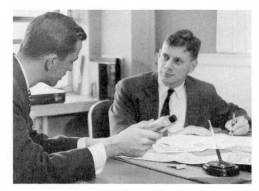

Legitimate business firms protect their own interests, as well as the consumer, by supporting better business bureaus. These bureaus answer queries and check complaints pertaining to all types of products.

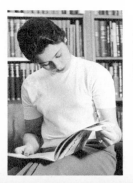

Consumer magazines distribute valuable health information to a wide reading public, and two consumer companies even conduct their own impartial testing and rating services.

in its job of policing the purity, quality, and labeling of foods, drugs, and cosmetics:

(1) Makes periodic inspections of food, drug, device and cosmetic establishments and examines samples from interstate shipments of these products. (2) Enforces the law against illegal sales of prescription drugs. (3) Checks the manufacturers' evidence of the safety of all new drugs (about 40 each month) before they are put on sale to the public. (4) Checks the manufacturers' proof of safety of colors for use in foods, drugs, or cosmetics, and where necessary establishes the amounts that may be used, and tests and certifies manufacturers' batches. (5) Checks the labeling and range of usefulness of therapeutic devices, and takes action against dangerous or bogus devices. (6) Tests all batches of insulin and five of the most important antibiotic drugs for purity and potency before they are sold. The manufacturers pay for such tests. (7) Issues and enforces regulations specifying the kinds and quantities of new food additives that may be used in or on food products. (8) Establishes the amount of pesticidal residues that may remain on food crops without injury to consumers, and polices shipments to see that residues are within safe limits. (9) Sets up standards which guarantee the composition and real value of food products in line with Congressional mandate to "promote honesty and fair dealing in the interests of consumers." (10) Checks imports of foods, drugs, devices, and cosmetics to make sure they comply with United States law. (11) Cooperates with State and Local officials in the inspection of foods and drugs contaminated by disasters, such as floods, hurricanes, explosions, and fires, and in the removal of dangerous items from the market. (12) Assists industry in voluntary compliance with the law, and in setting up controls to prevent violations. In addition, FDA enforces the Federal Hazardous Substances Labeling Act, which requires warning labels and antidotes to appear on household products that are toxic, corrosive, irritants, strong sensitizers, or generate injurious pressures.

Recent studies have called attention to serious deficiencies in FDA's manpower and material resources. In 1955, a Citizens Advisory Committee recommended the three- to fourfold expansion of the FDA in a five- to ten-year period and the improvement of facilities and equipment. A management consultant's survey in 1959, studying the field district system, recommended an increased number of resident posts, more supervisory inspectors and chemists, and, in general, an increase in the over-all field staff. In June, 1960, a committee reviewed the policies and procedures in approving new drugs. This committee recommended more statutory authority to improve its protective controls over drugs and antibiotics, to extend pretesting procedures to other drugs than the antibiotics, and to provide more funds and staff to strengthen its program and research projects [23].

The Federal Trade Commission. The purpose of the Federal Trade Commission is to prevent the free-enterprise system from being stifled or hindered by monopoly or corrupted by unfair or deceptive trade practices. The Commission enforces the Federal Trade Commission Act of 1914 and the Wheeler-Lea amendment of 1938. Originally, this act prevented price-fixing agreements, boycotts, combinations in restraint of trade, and other unfair methods of competition. The 1938 amendment gave the Commission jurisdiction over the false advertisement of food, drugs, cosmetics, and devices as well as over unfair and deceptive acts and practices. Such acts were declared by the amendment to be unlawful. False advertising is to be controlled by the Commission regardless of the medium used.

Since 1938, under its statutory responsibility, the Federal Trade Commission has issued an increasing number of cease-and-desist orders. Some complaints are registered through the Commission offices by the public and some by competitors. The names of the complainants are not divulged.

A special unit of the Commission maintains a continual survey of the advertisements by radio, television, newspapers, and other media. For example, some

4,000 radio and television broadcast stations are checked throughout the United States for false advertising.

When false advertising is disclosed, the Commission issues a formal complaint. The offender hears a written specification of charges, to which he must respond. If he contests, hearings are held. Findings of facts are made and a decision is rendered. If the advertising is proved false, a cease-and-desist order results and the offender must stop the practice. The order is subject to appeal in the courts. If it is not appealed, the order becomes final. Violators are subject to fines up to $5,000 for each violation. Penalties are assessed by the U.S. District Courts and are made in the name of the United States.

The FTC has issued complaints and orders based upon the dissemination of deceptive advertising through the U.S. mails or in interstate sale of drug preparations. It has acted against health fads and frauds with such products as vitamin preparations, minerals, and other dietary supplements when advertised as preventing or treatment for diseases. False advertising has been found advocating the superiority of natural vitamins over synthetic ones. The Commission has acted against books that have advertised to the general public descriptive regimens to prevent, treat, and cure heart disease, cancer, arthritis, and other chronic disorders. The efforts of the Commission cover the broad spectrum of health fads and frauds. The Commission's work is limited by the size of its staff and the ability of its workers to assemble evidence and prove that advertising claims are misleading [36].

The Post Office Department. The U.S. Post Office Department protects the consumer by preventing the use of the mails to perpetrate fraudulent schemes and the selling of nostrums. Postal inspectors are constantly on the lookout for fraudulent use of the mails. The consumer who discovers such a scheme should file a complaint. This greatly assists the Post Office Department. When evidence is discovered that the mails are being used to carry out fraudulent practices, a fraud order is issued against the individual or organization. The Department then requires the accused to answer the charges. Severe penalties are meted out to guilty persons.

PROFESSIONAL GROUPS

A number of professional groups are assuming functions designed to protect their members particularly, and the average citizen in general, with regard to consumer health. Chief among these professional organizations are the American Medical Association, the American College of Surgeons, the American Dental Association, home economic associations, better business bureaus, and the National Consumer-Retailer Council.

The American Medical Association. The American Medical Association is interested in the improvement of medical products for the use of the medical profession. It also is actively engaged in protecting the public as well as the medical profession against fraud and improper advertising of nostrums and proprietary medical products. Several committees of the association carry out these protective functions. The Council on Pharmacy and Chemistry judges on the basis of scientific and clinical study products that claim to have therapeutic value. The accepted products are discussed in the *Journal of the American Medical Association* and are included under the title, "New and Nonofficial Drugs." This section is revised and published annually. The Council on Physical Medicine investigates and reports on nonmedical apparatus and devices offered to physicians, hospitals, and the public. The Council on Foods studies and analyzes manufactured foods and makes known the findings to the medical profession regularly in the *Journal.* The Bureau of Investigation checks patent medicines, quacks, medical fads, and other phases of pseudo medicine. The results of the work of the various councils are most significant in protecting consumer health and, in turn, advancing the medical profession.

The American College of Surgeons. This is a professional society of surgeons in North and South America, which has as one of its purposes the development of standards for hospitals, hospitals services, and surgical products, such as surgical dressings. The work of the society constitutes a valuable contribution in protecting both surgeons and the lay public.

The American Dental Association. The American Dental Association is actively engaged in standardizing materials used in dental practice. One of its committees, the Council on Dental Therapeutics, passes on dental products, giving a seal of acceptance to those which meet the requirements of the council. The work of the council is primarily directed toward the dental profession, although its standardization of materials is a valuable guide to the consumer. The association publishes *Accepted Dental Remedies,* which includes the accepted products. In addition, research fellowships are provided by the association to members for work on dental materials at the National Bureau of Standards of the Federal government.

Home economics and nutrition groups. At least three groups, the American Home Economics Association, the Home Economic Education Branch of the U.S. Office of Education, and the American Dietetic Association, are working for the best interests of the consumer.

They are encouraging educational programs in schools and colleges. These programs are designed to provide students with an understanding of standards, grades of commodities, and services for individuals, families, and communities. The American Home Economics Association publishes a monthly *Journal,* a mimeographed edition called *The Consumer Education Service,* and a quarterly *Bulletin.* The Home Economic Education Service makes available to teachers, supervisors, and students numerous materials supplying information about commodities and services. One of the basic purposes of the American Dietetic Association is to combat food misinformation and quackery.

Better business bureaus. These bureaus are professional business organizations established to protect both the businessman and the consumer. Some 108 better business bureaus are located in the chief business centers throughout the United States. They are nonprofit organizations fighting frauds, promoting advertising accuracy, reducing unfair competition, and educating the public and its members. Their desire to improve the business world is a direct attempt to develop a better society in which to live. Businessmen and business firms support the bureaus through an annual subscription.

The local bureaus are affiliated with a national association, which acts as a coordinating body to promote the common welfare of all the bureaus.

The National Better Business Bureau functions on a nationwide scale, carrying out the same objectives as do the local bureaus. It handles inquiries and complaints and makes investigations on an interstate basis. It provides services to communities which do not have local bureaus.

A large number of publications are distributed by the bureaus as a part of their educational program for youth and adults. Such materials as *A Guide for Retail Advertising and Selling, Do's and Don'ts in Advertising Copy,* and the

Fact Booklet Series, including *Facts You Should Know about Health Quackery* and *Facts You Should Know about Accident and Health Insurance* are samples of their informative literature published to aid the public.

Any citizen may inquire about a firm or, if he wishes, file a written complaint of fraud with a bureau, free of charge. The bureau investigates, finds the facts through its own sources or cooperative activities of official agencies, such as the health department or the police department. Bureau officials contact the executives of the business firm, correcting the practice at this point, or, if necessary, taking more drastic action. When the case calls for it, the bureau publishes and distributes a special bulletin giving the name of the person and the type of malpractice. As a last resort, the case is presented to the law-enforcement agencies for punishment. Although the emphasis of the bureau activities is on prevention, when a fraudulent practice is found to exist, all the necessary steps are undertaken to stamp it out [5].

The National Association of Consumers. A nonpartisan, nonprofit, nontechnical national organization concerned with the advancement, protection, and welfare of all consumers in America is the National Association of Consumers. This organization, established in 1947 and reorganized in 1955, has its headquarters at Dickinson College, Carlisle, Pennsylvania. The NAC not only carries out its objectives nationally but assists local organizations to affiliate with it. Two such affiliates are the Consumer Conference of Greater Cincinnati and the St. Louis Consumer Federation. These local organizations promote the interests of consumers and help solve consumer problems in their respective cities. For example, the St. Louis Consumer Federation encourages consumers to make intelligent purchases of good products and provides meetings to discuss specific

problems, such as the hazards of food chemicals. The NAC publishes *Consumer News,* which gives authentic consumer information for its readers. The purposes and goals of this national organization are most noteworthy in promoting and protecting the interests of all consumers. Many of their problems are consumer health problems and, therefore, are of concern to us here [49].

The National Consumer-Retailer Council. From the experience of groups of consumers and retailers a need for a common meeting forum developed into the National Consumer-Retailer Council. Its basic purposes are educational, in respect to standards for consumers, manufacturers, and distributors. It provides information pertaining to labeling, use of truthful and factual information in advertising, establishing codes of ethics, and encouraging practices to reduce abuses of consumers or retailers.

The council's affiliate organizations include such organizations as the American Association of University Women, the American Home Economics Association, the General Federation of Women's Clubs, the American Retail Federation, the National Retail Dry Goods Association, the National Association of Better Business Bureaus, and the Association of Food Chains. Much of the work of the council is accomplished through committees, each of which serves as a forum on problem areas, such as informative labeling, grades and standards, and the like.

This is an important body, because it attempts to accomplish joint planning and action on mutual problems of buyers and sellers. It becomes a medium for collective bargaining between consumers and sellers. Considerable hope for greater consumer protection, for better business practices, and likewise greater security for the producer lies in the cooperative action of this council [52].

Private commodity testing and rating agencies. Two private organizations, supported by consumers with the avowed purpose of promoting consumer interests, have grown up in the United States since 1927. The organizations, in order of their establishment, are Consumers' Research, Inc., and Consumers Union, Inc. The primary purpose of these organizations is to provide their consumer members with accurate information about the purchasing of goods and services. Although the organizations are concerned with rating and testing all types of commodities, they give considerable attention to health products and services. In addition to rating and testing, they serve as spokesmen for the consumer and the consumer movement. As such they exert an economic and political force for this group.

Consumers' Research began as a consumers' club, founded by Stuart Chase and F. J. Schlink in 1927. It was incorporated in 1928 at Washington, New Jersey, as a membership corporation to provide unbiased information and counsel for the consumer. This independent research organization publishes monthly for its members *Consumers' Research Bulletin* and in September an *Annual Cumulative Bulletin.* Consumers' Research buys products in the open market, subjects them to scientific and engineering tests, and reports on quality and price without bias or prejudice. The rating of products and services is based on technical judgments and recommendations of the Consumers' Research staff, largely from its own tests and investigations. Occasionally, data are obtained from the Federal and state agencies, the professional societies, and other research bureaus.

Consumers Union, Inc., was established to tell consumers the truth about consumer goods and services and to permit consumers to make sound brand comparisons and intelligent selection of commodities. It was established in New York City as a nonprofit organization in 1936. Now it is the larger of the two major rating and testing organizations. It publishes for its subscriber-members *Consumer Reports* with a circulation of over 963,000 copies. In addition, the organization publishes an *Annual Buying Guide* in December of each year. The *Buying Guide* contains condensed information from the monthly issues of *Consumer Reports,* as well as new material not published previously.

One of the regular departments in both publications mentioned above is the health and medicine section, which is under the direction of a medical doctor. The ratings of products are made by technicians of the staff of Consumers Union or by consultants, free from bias, employed by commercial research concerns. Products are approved only after laboratory tests, controlled use tests, expert opinion, or experience tests. Consumers Union also draws heavily upon the test procedures and instruments developed by the government and other technical agencies.

Magazine testing and rating service. Two magazines representing the magazine testing and rating service are *Good Housekeeping* and *Parents' Magazine.* Both conduct a testing and rating service on a large number of goods.

Good Housekeeping has had its Good Housekeeping Institute and Investigation Service since 1901. After some difficulty with its seal of approval, it was discontinued in 1941. Since then a new seal is used which guarantees the merchandise. Replacement or refund of money is made by *Good Housekeeping* if the product is defective or not as advertised. *Good Housekeeping* makes no special ratings but offers a guarantee that a product bearing its seal does what it says it will do.

Parents' Magazine tests the products that are submitted to it for advertising. Two seals are available: a "guaranteed" seal, which means the magazine stands behind the product and is ready to refund the customer's money or replace the product if it is not as advertised; and a "studied and commended" seal, which provides the same guarantee to the consumer, but is preferred by some manufacturers since it denotes an excellent recommendation for the product. *Parents' Magazine* has no laboratories of its own, so it depends on commercial laboratories for its actual testing service [49, 52].

The contribution of testing and rating services. It is well to remember that none of the testing and rating agencies is infallible. They are not equipped financially or with laboratory facilities to test every item on the market. On the other hand, they are recognized as a type of organization whose primary purpose is the protection of the consumer. There is no question about their ability to improve the quality of products, to educate the consumer in choosing goods and services more wisely, to save the consumer money, and to form a consumer organization for a group attack on consumer problems. The results of the testing and rating service of these organizations can be used as one guide for the individual consumer in the intelligent selection of services and products.

Evaluating health information

Selection of reliable sources of health information and advice about health products and services is vital to consumer health and merits attention. With the advent of television, added to such media as the radio, magazines, newspapers, and billboards, the constant stream of health information reaching the average citizen is attaining flood-tide proportions. Health information should be appraised by scientific guides; that is, reliable and unreliable sources of health information should be differentiated by applying sound scientific criteria. Then a selection of the products and services needed should be made on the basis of the findings.

UNRELIABLE SOURCES OF HEALTH INFORMATION

Unsafe sources are:

Customs and superstitions of the culture that do not withstand the test of the scientific method

Information based on ignorance and prejudice

The expoundings of the quack or information devised by him for the consumption of the uneducated and gullible

Commercialized health information advanced for the sole purpose of selling a product regardless of its effect on the individual

Customs and superstitions. Many of the customs of our ancestors have helped materially in protecting, saving, and improving human health. The utilization by our forefathers of natural forces such as sunshine, sleep, rest, and invigorating work are good examples. On the other hand, many customs from early days are built on beliefs in magic or spirits or are based entirely on superstitions. Fortunately, with the progress of science and the increase of knowledge throughout the land, mythical customs and superstitions have waned, particularly the more serious ones. A belief in witchcraft, for instance, has disappeared from civilized society. No longer are the following beliefs held as they were at one time:

A baby will not grow if a hat is placed upon his head before he is a year old.

Illness of a child may be prevented by bathing him in greasy dishwater.

A sore throat is cured by drinking water out of a stranger's shoe.

You will not be sick the following year if

you dip your head in the ocean on January 1.

Sleeping with a dog prevents rheumatism.

Despite the great advance of scientific knowledge, however, customs and superstitions continue to exert an influence on the conduct of many. There is still belief in signs and omens. Charms are worn upon the person or affixed to the automobile to bring good luck and ward off disaster. The belief in lucky or unlucky circumstances is prevalent. The reading or telling of fortunes continues to be a profitable business and an expensive pastime. An interesting superstition pertains to the sneeze. In the early days of Greece and Rome the sneeze was an ominous sign and had to be counteracted by a protective saying. Today one frequently hears someone say after a person sneezes, "God bless you!" or the German version, *"Gesundheit!"* meaning "good health" [19].

Many such beliefs are trivial or minor. However, accepting superstitions and beliefs without critically appraising them can lead to poor health practices and needless expense. Since all untested beliefs are likely to be dangerous to health, every intelligent person should subject his health beliefs to the scientific method.

Ignorance and prejudice. Ignorance and prejudice are other unreliable bases for health information. It should be remembered that an adviser can be highly educated in the arts, languages, or history and at the same time be thoroughly misinformed and highly prejudiced in matters pertaining to health.

Health cults are frequently the result of ignorance or of narrow, one-sided education. The cultist is one who, regardless of education, training, and experience, claims to cure all disease. Also, he trusts but one dogma or particular belief. He exhibits a closed-mindedness, indicating extreme prejudice. His stock in trade consists of superstitions and a belief in magic and miracle cures.

Another example of blindness, ignorance, and prejudice is the individual who insists on self-diagnosis and self-treatment. The old adage, "He who hath himself for a doctor hath a fool for a patient," is more true today than ever before. Yet many are willing to stake their health and their very life on self-diagnosis and self-treatment. Many of the 5,000 yearly deaths in the United States from appendicitis are due to faulty self-diagnosis and self-treatment. Serious dangers threaten when persons making their own diagnosis purchase patent medicines and treat themselves. They are relying upon guesswork for diagnosis and upon possibly harmful, expensive products for cure of conditions that, for the most part, demand immediate expert medical attention. The gullible and ignorant every day are influenced by high-powered advertising and dramatic testimonials.

The quack as an unreliable source. Although the quack previously has been referred to, he must be included as an unreliable source of health information. The quack is the medical pretender whose silver tongue boasts of his achievements, who advertises in the daily papers or periodicals, cites the testimonials of cured patients, and promises miracle cures of such diseases as heart disease, cancer, arthritis, and kidney diseases. Quacks flourish for a number of reasons. Many diseases cure themselves after running their course, and the quack takes the credit for the work nature has performed. A large percentage of the population's ills are minor disorders due to nervous or emotional causes. The quack's fanfare, glib talk, soothing ways, mystic powers, and sure-cure elixirs provide needed confidence, sympathy, and a form of psychotherapy. Always, it is well to remember that the dominating motive of the quack is money, not the welfare of the individual.

Testimonials. Testimonials are the

backbone of nostrum advertising. They have an important commercial value due to the supposed experience of the testimonial writer. They serve as one of the best baits for prospective customers of the quack. There is no scientific value to the testimonial; it may have been purchased outright by the quack, written by him or his agent, or written in good faith by those who believe they have been or will be cured. In one investigation by the Post Office Department, 75 per cent of the testimonials came from deceased persons [8].

Bona fide medical testimonials are impossible to obtain, since it is unethical for any member of the American Medical Association to give a testimonial. The testimonial, then, is an unreliable guide for health information or products.

Commercialized health information. The health appeal in commercial advertising has developed tremendously within the last decade. This rise has been so marked that it is a definite part of the culture and has grown to big-business proportions. Appraisal of this type of health information is important because some commercial health information is desirable, while much is undesirable and unreliable. The reliable kind is that furnished by organizations whose primary purpose is to keep people alive and well. A good example of this type of organization is the life insurance companies, which are developing excellent health education materials for their policyholders, for school children, and for the general public.

A second type of commercial health information relates to health products such as household staples, clothing, foods, beverages, and the like. Such health information is furnished by advertising designed to sell a product, in which the health motive is used as the selling power. Breakfast cereals, milk, fruits and vegetables, enriched bread, and health shoes are illustrations of the products sold through an appeal to the health motive. The dangers from such advertising lie in the possibility of overemphasis, of distortion of the truth, and of misinterpretation by the public.

A third type of commercial health information concerns hygienic products, such as cosmetics and soaps with germicidal virtues and medicinal qualities, dentrifrices, deodorants, feminine-hygiene products, hair tonics, pimple creams, and the like. The greatest danger from information exploiting these products, and from one's using them, is the encouraging of harmful health practices. Furthermore, false health values are built up. Also of real consequence is the fact that purchasing such products relieves consumers of large sums of money annually.

A fourth type of information is furnished by the quack selling his nostrums. These hazards have been discussed previously [25].

The common method of communicating health information. John Peterson,[7] in talks to civic groups, has repeatedly stated: "The most common method of communicating health information is over the backyard fence." There is a great deal of truth in this statement. Time and time again the average American needing health information contacts a friend or neighbor for advice. At the college level, the friend or neighbor is a roommate, a fraternity brother, a sorority sister, a fellow club member, or a study partner.

The accuracy of the friend's recommendation will depend upon his preparation and experience and also on whether or not he has appraised critically the situation, the person, or the product he is recommending. Possibly he will operate entirely on ignorance, bias, prejudice, misinformation, or superstition. Possibly he will recommend another friend, a relative, or a product simply on an emotional basis.

Most well-meaning American citizens

---

[7] Director of the Health Division, Welfare Council, Philadelphia, Pa.

are eager to make diagnoses, prescribe, and even treat a friend or neighbor on the basis of their own past ills, and it is true that the intelligent quick thinking of friends has saved many lives. A sound procedure for the individual seeking the advice of a friend is to listen to his information, appraise it in the light of scientific criteria for evaluating health information, and check it with at least one other unquestionably reliable source.

CRITERIA FOR EVALUATING HEALTH INFORMATION

It is evident that some criteria for evaluating health information are needed. Before accepting health information or following health advice you should ask:

Who are the persons or organizations presenting the information?

What are their educational background and professional experience in the health sciences?

What reputation do they have in the community?

What are their motives? Are they to improve health and prolong life? Are they using the health motive as a sales appeal? Is the primary purpose to make money? Is there a subtle but consistent reference to money?

How is the information presented? In an educational, scientific manner? Or are the propaganda devices utilized, such as name calling, glittering generalities, transfer, testimonials, plain-folks appeal, card stacking, and band-wagon technique [40]?

RELIABLE SOURCES OF HEALTH INFORMATION

Specifically, the following individuals or agencies serve as examples of safe sources of health information that you might call upon readily, especially during your college years:

Your family physician, or a physician at your Student Health Service

An officer of your county medical society

or a physician to whom he may refer you

The health officer of your local—city or county—health department

The administrator or head of your community hospital

Your college health educator or health instructor

A religious counselor of your faith associated with your college or university or recommended by your dean of students, dean of men, or dean of women

The executive secretary of a local, state, or national voluntary health agency concerned with a health problem about which you desire accurate information, such as the local branch of the American Cancer Society for information regarding cancer or the relationship of cigarette smoking to lung cancer or the County Heart Association for information regarding heart diseases and the relationship of diet to heart disease

The Editor of *Today's Health* (535 N. Dearborn St., Chicago, Ill.) for an answer to a medical question from the American Medical Association's point of view. He will refer your question to the appropriate medical authority

Your county, state, or the American Dental Association (Director of Health Education, 222 E. Superior St., Chicago, Ill.) regarding dental health problems, including fluoridation

Your local better business bureau, or the National Association of Better Business Bureaus (Chrysler Building, New York, N.Y.) for information regarding protection from fraudulent business practices

Your area office or the Washington office of the Federal Food and Drug Administration for information about quackery or about how FDA protects the consumer

Your area office or the Washington office of the Federal Trade Commission for advertising abuses and rules and regulations governing health advertising

Your post office for information about mail-order quackery

Selecting health products

THE PROCESS OF SELECTING HEALTH PRODUCTS

Every consumer at some time or other buys a simple drug, cosmetic, or therapeutic device. Selecting the right health product appears to be a simple process until one discovers the numbers of brands, the varieties of sizes and shapes, the variations in weight, and the numerous price levels for each single item. Consumer confusion is the natural result. The easy way out is to take the clerk's advice, regardless of whether he has had thirty years' experience or whether it is his first day on the job. The person with discriminating judgment is not satisfied by this method. He wants to ask some questions, and he is willing to consider some guides to assist him in the selection process, for two reasons: protecting his health, and protecting his pocketbook.

GUIDES FOR SELECTING PRODUCTS TO PROTECT AND MAINTAIN HEALTH

The intelligent consumer:

Follows the advice of his physician and buys products prescribed by him, realizing that his supervision and recommendations are for the individual's best interests.

Does not permit pharmacists, druggists, or store clerks to prescribe health products.

Reads the label on products, and remembers that the Food, Drug, and Cosmetic Act requires the producer to tell the consumer the contents of the product, what it will do, how to use it, when to take it, and when not to take it.

Buys products bearing a seal of acceptance or a seal indicating a high-quality standard, and remembers that the American Medical Association and the American Dental Association, through their special committees, "accept" products meeting their standards. Recalls that the letters U.S.P., N.F., and H.P. mean that drugs meet the standards of the United States Pharmacopeia, the National Formulary, and the Homeopathic Pharmacopoeia.

Is critical of and does not buy drugs or devices offered as cure-alls or curatives for serious diseases, such as heart disease, cancer, tuberculosis, and kidney disease.

Is skeptical of products advertised by propaganda techniques.

Is skeptical of and refuses to purchase devices or machines that are claimed to cure disease and are offered for sale or lease for use in the home.

Reports frauds and suspected frauds in writing to the nearest office of the Food and Drug Administration or the better business bureau.

GUIDES FOR MAKING THE MOST OF THE HEALTH DOLLAR

The intelligent consumer:

Knows what is needed before buying. This means buying on the basis of need, not on impulse or to "keep up with the Joneses," to satisfy his vanity, or merely to take advantage of a bargain.

Compares values and checks the quality and purpose of the product and its design. "Shop and save" is a good motto, since prices may vary for the same item from store to store. The one-store buyer pays more.

Buys on the basis of standards in grade labels, in weights, in measures, drug standards, standards of identity, quality and fill of container. Utilizes the standards of the Department of Agriculture for qualities of canned fruits, vegetables, meats, butter, and eggs. Buys the cheapest brand meeting the grade A standard when there are several grade A products.

Buys on the basis of intended use. When standards are shown by grade levels, grades A, B, or C can be purchased wisely on the basis of intended use. For example, canned tomatoes, grade A, can be reserved for special occasions, since they are slightly higher priced. Grade B is of the same nutritional value but less perfect in size or appearance and is suitable for general use.

Buys from private brands. This is a particularly wise procedure in purchasing cosmetics and toiletries. Such products sold by a reputable dealer with U.S.P. or N.F. marked on the label can mean substantial savings over nationally advertised brands.

Buys the larger quantity. Larger sizes and quantities often result in savings.

Checks the cost per ounce of drugs and toiletries. Notes the savings in the long run.

Watches for buying opportunities. Appraising needs in advance and watching for regular and special sales save money.

Pays cash from cash-and-carry stores. Such firms operate for less and sell for less. On the other hand, however, paying cash at a credit firm does not result in savings.

Subscribes to a commodity testing service. Membership in one of the testing services, such as Consumers' Research or Consumers Union, Inc., provides information about the quality and price of products, which can result in substantial savings over a period of time [41].

Selecting health services

THE IMPORTANCE OF SELECTING A COMPETENT HEALTH ADVISER

One of the most vital factors in promoting and maintaining healthful living is choosing the proper health advisers. It is to these professional persons—the medical doctor (general practitioner, surgeon, medical specialist) and the doctor of dental surgery (the dentist, the dental specialist)—that a person entrusts his life and certainly the quality of his living. In discussing the student health service as a part of the college health program in Chapter 1 of this book, it was pointed out that the majority of colleges and universities throughout the country do not provide complete medical and dental services for the college group. As a result, many college students, on their own for the first time, are faced with the problem of selecting competent health advisers. If college students do have complete health service coverage during college, the prob-

lem is merely delayed until they establish their own homes after acquiring a college education.

The task of selecting the right health adviser is important because the human organism is the most delicate and highly interrelated and integrated of all mechanisms. Anyone who has studied the structure and function of the human body, even superficially, cannot help being awed by its delicate functions. When this complex organism is out of adjustment, for whatever cause, the most competent health adviser is needed. Preventive service is equally important to living a full life.

TYPES OF DOCTORS AND HEALTH SPECIALISTS

Because of the multiple use of the term "doctor," it is necessary to distinguish between those using this title. Originally, the term meant "teacher," and that meaning remains today when the title of Doctor of Philosophy or Doctor of Education is awarded with an advanced academic degree. From the medical point of view it denotes a person licensed to practice medicine. The dental profession calls the graduate of its schools, who is licensed to practice dentistry, a Doctor of Dental Surgery or Doctor of Dental Medicine. The osteopath, the chiropractor, the chiropodist, and the naturopath are representatives of other healing arts and may in some instances use the title "doctor." In selecting a health adviser, it is necessary to understand the various types of healing art and their theory and required training.

Medical Doctor (M.D.). The medical doctor serves as a counselor, to whom the individual can confide personal problems of adjustment as well as of physical well-being. However, the medical adviser is more than a counselor; he provides preventive services to protect total health. He gives continuous supervision to health needs, based on his findings in periodical health examinations, laboratory tests, and many subjective evaluations, which altogether give him a complete health history. When illness comes, he is able to stop pain and alleviate suffering. He offers medical care, including surgery, sufficient to rehabilitate the individual to a healthy state.

The medical adviser today realizes that he alone cannot furnish this complicated service. The task requires a team of well-trained personnel. The center on this team is a cooperative patient who works with, rather than against, the doctor's advice. The medical adviser, the quarterback, calls upon specialists when the condition warrants it. He arranges for hospitalization and nursing service. He is constantly in touch with consultants, technical assistants, and research workers. Also, he is working at all times with the public health officials in protecting and improving the health of the total community group.

The healing art of medicine is based on scientifically proved principles of preventing, curing, and alleviating disease. The medical doctor is carefully selected from among many students on the basis of scholarship, personality, character, and professional aptitude. He spends nine years in training under the careful supervision of leading scientists. The highest type of code of ethics governs his practice. Medical organizations at the local, state, and national level promote professional standards and offer opportunities for advanced study and continuous medical education.

Medical education in the modern medical school has a changed curriculum. A comparison of past and present programs shows the following: [8]

PAST

Formal, didactic programs
Barriers between basic science years (1 and 2) and clinical years (3 and 4)
Barriers between the various basic sciences
Many hours of required courses
Rigid four-year program

PRESENT

Conferences, seminars, and small-group teaching activities
Freshmen and sophomores participate in clinical work; basic sciences carried into junior and senior years
Interdepartmental teaching programs of neuroanatomy and neurophysiology and biochemistry, physiology, microbiology, and pathology
Scheduled free time for elective offerings
Interruptions of three to six months for research or elective work; one to three years may be devoted to graduate studies in basic sciences

In addition, there has been a rapid increase in student participation in medical research (10 to 50 per cent of the student body may be involved). New

[8] "The Changing Face of the Medical Curriculum," in *Patterns of Disease*, Parke, Davis and Company, Detroit, Mich., October, 1959, p. 3.

disciplines (comprehensive medicine, family care) use the community as a teaching laboratory.

Medical specialties (M.D.)[9]

† AVIATION MEDICINE. Concerned with the physiological, medical, psychological and epidemiological problems involved in present-day flying.

* ANESTHESIOLOGY. The study of anesthesia and anesthetics. (Anesthesiologist and anesthetist)

† CARDIOLOGY. Concerned with the study and treatment of heart disease. (Cardiologist)

* DERMATOLOGY. Concerned with diseases of the skin and skin manifestations of constitutional diseases. (Dermatologist)

† EPIDEMIOLOGY. Deals with the relationships of the various factors which determine the frequencies and distributions of an infectious process, a disease or a physiological state in a human community. (Epidemiologist)

† ENDOCRINOLOGY. Deals with the treatment of diseases arising from disordered internal secretions. (Endocrinologist)

† GASTROENTEROLOGY. Concerned with the stomach and intestines and their diseases. (Gastroenterologist)

† GERONTOLOGY. Study of the problems of aging in all their aspects—clinical, biological, historical and sociological. (Gerontologist) *Geriatrics* is one branch of the science of gerontology. The geriatrician is a physician who is concerned with preventing disease, prolonging life and promoting health for persons past middle life.

* GYNECOLOGY. Deals with diseases of the female reproductive tract. (Gynecologist)

* INTERNAL MEDICINE. Deals with diseases that cannot be treated surgically, or medicine as distinguished from surgery. (Internist) This also includes the allergist and the specialist in pulmonary disease.

* NEUROLOGICAL SURGERY. Deals principally with operations on the brain and the nerves distributed along the spinal cord. (Neurosurgeon)

* NEUROLOGY. Deals with diagnosis and treatment of diseases of the nervous system. (Neurologist)

* OBSTETRICS. Embraces prenatal care and all the problems of pregnancy and childbirth. (Obstetrician)

* OCCUPATIONAL MEDICINE. Deals with problems of industrial and occupational medicine. (Specialist in occupational medicine)

* OPHTHALMOLOGY. Concerned with diseases and disorders of the eye and vision. (Ophthalmologist or oculist)

* ORTHOPEDIC SURGERY. Concerned with the preservation and restoration of the function of the skeletal system, its articulations and associated structures. (Orthopedist or orthopedic surgeon)

† OTOLOGY. Deals with disorders and diseases of the ear. (Otologist)

* OTOLARYNGOLOGY. Gives special attention to diseases of the ear and throat. May use both medical and surgical methods. (Otolaryngologist)

† OTORHINOLARYNGOLOGY. Concerned with diseases of the ear, nose and throat. (Otorhinolaryngologist)

† OTORHINOLOGY. Deals with disorders and diseases of the ear and nose. (Otorhinologist)

* PATHOLOGY. Study of abnormalities of body tissues and fluids. (Pathologist)

* PEDIATRICS. Deals with diseases of children (usually up to sixteen). (Pediatrician)

* PHYSICAL MEDICINE AND REHABILITATION. Employs the use of physical agents (heat, cold, water, light, electricity, massage, manipulation, exercise and mechanical means) in the diagnosis and treatment of disease. (Physiatrist)

* PLASTIC SURGERY. Deals with the reconstruction of tissues, particularly soft tissues, to relieve disfigurements, deformities and malfunctions. (Plastic surgeon)

* PROCTOLOGY. Study of diseases of the rectum and anus; includes a considerable amount of surgery. (Proctologist)

* PREVENTIVE MEDICINE AND PUBLIC HEALTH. Emphasizes epidemiology, the prevention of disease and medical administration.

* PSYCHIATRY. Deals with diagnosis and treatment of mental disease. (Psychiatrist)

* RADIOLOGY. Deals with the application of x-rays, both to the diagnosis and treatment of disease. (Radiologist and roentgenologist)

† RHINOLOGY. Concerned with disorders of the nose. (Rhinologist)

* SURGERY. Deals with the treatment of disease, wholly or in part, by manual and operative procedures; has many subspecialties within field. (Surgeon)

[9] Prepared by Elena Sliepcevich and Mary Beyrer, The Ohio State University, in cooperation with Fred V. Hein, American Medical Association, 1960, * denotes a specialty having an American Examining Board approved by the Council on Medical Education and Hospitals, American Medical Association, and an Advisory Board for Medical Specialists; † denotes areas of subspecialization or fields of work under the American Board specialties.

* UROLOGY. Places emphasis on diseases of the genitourinary tract. (Urologist)

Related specialties. The following are specialists frequently confused with medical doctors:

CLINICAL PSYCHOLOGIST. One prepared to do diagnostic and psychotherapeutic work in a psychiatric clinic. He is required to have at least eight years of college and graduate education culminating in the degree of Doctor of Philosophy (Ph.D.). This is supplemented by at least one year's internship according to standards set by the American Psychiatric Association. Difficulty arises from the fact that the term "psychologist" is not protected or restricted by law. Anyone may call himself a psychologist and practice fraudulently upon the public. It is important to know that a qualified clinical psychologist must meet the above standards set by the American Psychiatric Association.

OPTICIAN. A mechanic skilled in making optical instruments and glasses. He fills prescriptions for glasses on the orders of ophthalmologists (oculists) or optometrists.

OPTOMETRIST (O.D.). One who is prepared to measure vision, fit glasses, and provide visual training of an optical or physical nature. He may treat visual defects and problems by prescribing glasses. He is not allowed to use drugs either in treating defects or in measuring vision, nor is he trained to perform surgery. Optometry is recognized in all states. It is a professional curriculum in colleges of optometry and in several colleges and universities. The four-year course is required for the B.A. or B.S. degree in optometry. Some colleges award the degree of Doctor of Optometry (O.D.). An examination is required before the optometrist is allowed to practice.

ORTHOPTIST. A technician trained and certified under the direction of the American Orthoptic Council to give visual training and eye exercises as prescribed by an ophthalmologist.

Dentists: Doctor of Dental Surgery (D.D.S.) or Doctor of Dental Medicine (D.M.D.). The dentist is concerned with the art and science of oral health. He is trained to treat the diseases of the teeth, jaws, and gums and to promote oral health as a part of general health. Dentistry has developed from a skilled art to a highly respected profession. Largely through the efforts of the dentists themselves standards of selection and training have been raised and sound professional ethics and conduct upheld. Procedures used in practice include diagnosis, health education, medicines, mechanical appliances, and surgery.

Soon the 43 existing dental schools will be increased to 50 in number to meet the demand for additional dentists. These schools provide training in fundamental sciences and practical experience in clinics, carry out experimentation and research, and offer postgraduate work. The dentist graduating from these schools approved by the Council on Dental Education, American Dental Association, must pass a state board examination before he is licensed to practice. However, states still vary in their laws governing the dental profession. Standards are adopted and upheld by the American Dental Association nationally and by state and local professional societies.

Some dental specialties include the following:

ORTHODONTIST (D.D.S.). A dental specialist who deals with the prevention and correction of irregularities of the teeth.

PERIODONTIST (D.D.S.). A specialist who treats the gums and parts of the mouth which help support the teeth.

PEDODONTIST (D.D.S). A specialist concerned with dental diseases in children, particularly with the treatment and prevention of tooth decay.

Doctor of Osteopathy (D.O.). A doctor of osteopathy is one who practices the healing art and follows the school of medicine and operative surgery that is based on the importance of the musculoskeletal system in total body health. It is a basic tenet of osteopathic medicine that man expresses his life through the primary machinery of the body; the musculoskeletal system, as directed by the nervous system. It considers that the musculoskeletal system interacts reciprocally with the other systems of the body. It influences their functioning and is influenced by them.

It is believed that an osteopathic lesion is a somatic component. The correction of a lesion is attempted by, and, when possible, achieved through, manipulative procedures that are osteopathic in origin and type. Osteopathy claims and administers all the procedures that have proved valuable in securing abundant health and in the prevention, diagnosis, and treatment of disease.

Osteopathy was founded by Dr. Andrew Taylor Still (1828–1917). Dr. Still believed that any malfunction or disalignment in body structure caused, or resulted from, ill health. He felt that realigning the functional parts along with other kinds of medication and treatment would help the body restore itself to a healthy state.

Osteopaths are licensed to practice osteopathic medicine and surgery in all states and have unlimited practice rights in 38 states and the District of Columbia. In 20 states and the District of Columbia, graduates of medical and osteopathic colleges take the same basic examination for state board certification in general medicine and surgery. The American Osteopathic Association is a member of the National Health Council. Doctors of osteopathy are permitted to serve as officers in the Department of Medicine and Surgery, Veterans Administration, and are eligible to be medical officers in the armed forces. Staff members of some county hospitals now include osteopathic physicians and surgeons.

There are six osteopathic colleges approved by the American Osteopathic Association. They are located in Kirksville and Kansas City, Missouri, and in Philadelphia, Los Angeles, Des Moines, and Chicago.

Osteopathic education requires at least three years in an approved undergraduate college or university. The standard curriculum of an osteopathic college requires 5,000 hours of instruction in four college years. The first two years are focused on the basic sciences, such as anatomy, physiology, chemistry, pathology, bacteriology, structural and physical diagnosis, toxicology, and pharmacology. The third and fourth years are referred to as clinical years, as the students serve as physicians under the supervision of their instructors. An additional year of internship is required in 1 of 90 osteopathic hospitals before the doctor of osteopathy becomes a practicing osteopathic physician. Three years of residency, two years of specialty practice, and passage of written, oral, and practical examinations are required before a doctor of osteopathy is granted a specialty [38].

Osteopathy is attempting to become a full-grown health profession. Osteopaths have established a creed similar to that of the medical profession, with similar educational requirements and similar specialties. They have developed their own hospitals and are now considering needed research to prove their theories of health and disease. With these and other parallels between the medical and osteopathic professions, an amalgamation of the two has been proposed. Each group nationally has opposed this, although in some states, regardless of national regulations against it, there have been close relationships, with joint consultations and unlimited practice rights.

In March, 1961, an amalgamation occurred on the state level between the California Medical Association and the

California Osteopathic Association. As a part of the amalgamation, the doctors of osteopathy were invited to become medical doctors, members of the California Medical Association, with the rights and privileges of medical doctors. In a sense, this consolidation constitutes the absorption of the osteopaths by the medical profession. It is on this point that the American Osteopathic Association has opposed the merger. However, with the precedent set, it is possible that other states might witness similar mergers between these two healing professions.

Regardless of the merger at the state level, the American Osteopathic Association continues to work for higher and better professional standards and to assure the uniqueness and respectability of osteopathy as a healing profession.

The American Medical Association, on the other hand, is reviewing its policy relating to a physician associating professionally with one who practices a different method of healing.[10]

Doctor of Podiatry (Chiropody) (D.S.C. or Pod.D.). In 1958, the National Association of Chiropodists changed its name to the American Podiatry Association. Podiatry and chiropody are considered to be synonymous terms by the Association, with a gradual shifting to the use of podiatry. A doctor of podiatry or surgical chiropody is professionally prepared to diagnose and treat the diseases, injuries, and defects of the feet. He is a specialist in caring for the feet in both health and disease. He is prepared to treat tumors, ulcers, fractures, skin and nail diseases, corns, calluses, and congenital and acquired deformities of the foot. In addition, he is trained to detect the symptoms of general body diseases occurring in the feet such as anemia, heart disease, diabetes, and kidney disease. The podiatrist refers such cases to the patient's family physician for treatment.

There are five podiatry-chiropody colleges approved by the Council on Education, American Podiatry Association. Two are located in Chicago and one each in San Francisco, New York, and Cleveland, Ohio. The Maurice J. Lewi College of Podiatry in New York offers the Doctor of Podiatry degree, and the four other colleges still confer the degree of Doctor of Surgical Chiropody. Entrance requirements include one year of college in three schools, whereas San Francisco and Lewi require two years. Four years of study are required for the degree. All five colleges offer an elective clinical internship to graduates so that requirements may be met for states holding to such standards for license to practice.

A number of hospitals have podiatrist-chiropodists as members, with their privileges defined in the hospital by-laws. General recognition is being given to this field as an ancillary to the medical profession [4].

Doctor of Chiropractic (D.C.). Chiropractic is a nonmedical form of healing. It is based on the belief that the nervous system controls all other systems and all physiologic functions of the human body and that interference with the nerve control of the systems impairs their functions and induces disease. The chiropractor treats his patient by use of the following procedures: [11]

(1) specific adjustment therapy to achieve normal nerve function; (2) nutrition and dietary guidance to restore normal chemical balance in the body and correct faulty nutrition; (3) physical therapy to help restore normal physiological functions of the body; and (4) counseling to help the patient achieve a proper balance between the mental, emotional, physiological and mechanical aspects of his person in order to get and keep normal health.

[10] Special Report of the Judicial Council to the A.M.A. House of Delegates, "Osteopathy," *J.A.M.A.* 177:774–775, September 16, 1961.

[11] Dewey Anderson, *The Present Day Doctor of Chiropractic,* Public Affairs Institute, Washington, 1956, pp. 5–6.

The National Chiropractic Association is improving educational standards and accrediting and approving chiropractic colleges. Eight colleges are recognized by the association, three have provisional accreditation, and three are not approved. A minimum of 4,400 hours of training and instruction is the standard of the association. It must be pointed out that not all doctors of chiropractic have had this standard of training and instruction. In 1956, all states, except New York, Massachusetts, Louisiana, and Mississippi, granted licenses to qualified doctors of chiropractic. The professional training required before being allowed to take the state license examination ranges from two school years of nine months each to four years, which is the standard in most states [2].

Doctors of chiropractic do not yet meet the same standards as osteopaths and medical doctors. It is encouraging that standards are being raised. Differences still exist, especially between medical doctors and chiropractors. This is true in respect to the over-all amount of study and preparation, in the quality of instruction, and in equipment and facilities available in medical schools as compared with chiropractic schools. A further difference exists in the treatment of diseases. The chiropractor does not have specialized knowledge or ability to cure infectious diseases or the serious degenerative diseases, such as heart disease and cancer. The chiropractor's treatment is to maintain and build up body resistance, to ease nervous tension, and to assure good nursing and diet. He is well qualified in adjustment therapy.

Doctor of Naturopathy (N.D.). Naturopaths are drugless healers similar to the chiropractors. These practitioners depend upon nature's forces, such as water, air, sunlight, electricity, exercise, rest, diet, and mental and moral science, for the cure of disease. Naturopaths believe that no one natural force can cure all diseases, and so the practitioner works out the best combination of these forces to suit the individual's case. A dozen or so naturopathic colleges award diplomas. Some of these schools award the Doctor of Naturopathy and the Doctor of Chiropractic degree as well. A high school education is required in some of the colleges and merely recommended in others. The faculty is similar in make-up to the faculty of chiropractic schools.

In recent years naturopaths have drifted from their dependence on nature's remedies to pursue more lucrative therapeutic methods, utilizing electrical treatment, violet ray, X ray, colonic irrigations, and the like. In certain conditions, such treatments are of some therapeutic value and can be compared with physiotherapy, conducted by trained physiotherapists under the direction of medical doctors. Other methods that may employ even more impressive-appearing machines or gadgets are sheer quackery and are expensive and time-consuming when competent medical care is needed.

CRITERIA FOR SELECTING HEALTH ADVISERS

If it is an important task to select health advisers, then it is necessary to establish criteria to aid in the selection process. The following are suggested as suitable for both medical and dental advisers:

Are they licensed to practice in the state in which they reside?

Are they graduates of approved medical or dental schools?

Are they members in good standing of local, state, and national professional societies?

Are they members of staffs of approved hospitals and clinics in the community?

Do they periodically increase their skill and extend their knowledge through professional conferences, meetings, and postgraduate studies?

Do they possess a wholesome personality that inspires confidence and interest in the individual and people in general?

Have they established a reputation for professional ethics, character, integrity, and dependable service?

Have they had a variety of professional experience to develop skills in providing medical or dental care?

PROCEDURES FOR SELECTING HEALTH ADVISERS

To apply the criteria suggested requires some time, thought, and effort. Yet all such time and trouble is well spent if competent advisers are selected. If you are away from home, it is wise to obtain references from the family physician and dentist with whom you have been associated. Former advisers are always glad to recommend competent physicians and surgeons and dentists in a new locality. The following suggestions are made for those who are not able to contact their former advisers or who are living under different circumstances:

1. Secure the names of competent medical and dental practitioners from two or more sources:
   a. The county medical and dental societies.
   b. The student health service.
   c. Approved hospitals in the community.
   d. The local health department.
   e. The nearest class A medical school or approved dental school.
   f. Educated, well-informed friends at the college or university or in the community.
2. Check professional membership by contacting the professional societies or their directories (found in most public libraries).
3. Check standing and reputation in the community by consulting educated, well-informed friends or acquaintances at the college or university or in the community.
4. Make an appointment with the doctor or dentist, and personally find out whether or not he inspires confidence and meets the established qualifications.

CRITERIA FOR SELECTING A MEDICAL-CARE PLAN

It is evident that many health insurance prepayment plans are in operation. The majority of these attempt to meet the medical-care problems of the public; however, as in other fields, some plans are not serving the best interests of the consumer. It is a wise consumer health practice to find out the details of a plan before one becomes a member, as has been pointed out. The following are suggested criteria for selecting a plan. These are high standards that are incorporated in present-day plans or are in the process of becoming operative.

An excellent prepayment medical-care plan provides [9]:

High-quality medical care by a family physician and coordinated services with specialists. Both family physician and specialists are affiliated with an approved hospital where there is competent nursing service.

Adequate medical care that will cover both acute and chronic diseases for the dependents as well as the wage earner.

Membership for the subscriber as an individual as well as through a group affiliation.

A choice of physicians for family doctor, with freedom to change when there is due cause.

Conveniently located service centers. A choice of hospitals on the accredited list of the American College of Surgeons and American Hospital Association.

A nonprofit or low-cost operating program.

Payment of fees on a family budgeting plan.

Remuneration for medical personnel sufficiently high to attract and hold competent physicians and surgeons interested in the practice of medicine and continued medical education.

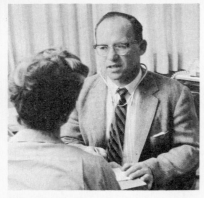

The family doctor is a wise source of health information and a reliable adviser concerning medical care plans.

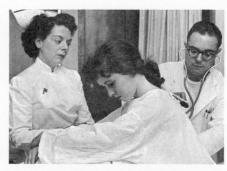

Blue Cross hospital-care plans and Blue Shield medical and surgical plans are contracted with the medical profession both by individuals and by groups.

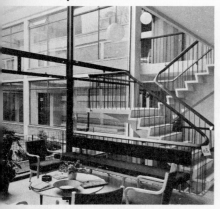

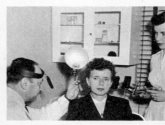

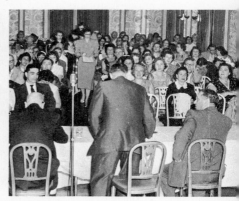

In sunlit medical centers, doctors associated with a major group health insurance plan provide diagnosis, treatment, and preventive health education for subscribers.

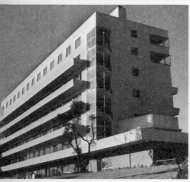

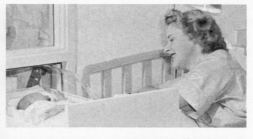

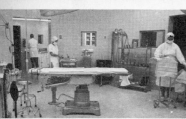

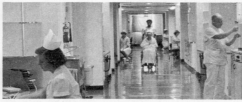

Modern facilities and many innovations, including a lying-in arrangement for mothers and new-born babies, and corridors restricted to patients and staff, are featured by another group health insurance plan.

Administrative responsibility for the operation of the plan under a group composed of physicians, subscribers, and civic-minded citizens. Medical standards of competence and performance to be determined by medical authorities organized for that purpose.

MEDICAL CARE

A variety of health services are necessary to promote and protect the health of the individual and group. In addition, when illness or defects cannot be prevented, competent health services are essential for diagnosis, treatment, care, and rehabilitation. All these personal services are classed as medical care [27]. Such medical care is furnished by the members of the medical profession who use clinics, hospitals, and other health facilities.

Each American family spent on the average $294 for medical care during 1959. This amount showed a 42 per cent increase over the previous five-year period. The highest sum was for the services of physicians, followed closely by expenditures for hospitals and for drugs and medications. The increases over the past five years have been due to high hospital costs, the result of increased wages and more employees per patient, and additional spending for drugs and medications. Another reason was due to general price increases in this period. This amount appeared to exceed an increase in the added use of health services. The comparative costs of 1957–1958 and 1952–1953 are shown in Table 10.1.

More than 16 per cent of all families reported a total yearly expense of over $500. This indicates the need for health protection against large financial amounts.

Should medical-care insurance be provided on a compulsory or a voluntary basis? For many years there has been more heat than light in the controversy. If the issue is closely examined, it is evident that there has been more progress than appears on the surface and that there are many points of agreement on both sides in the contest. Both sides agree that every individual has the right to adequate medical care, regardless of race, creed, or economic status. There is real agreement that a prepayment plan for medical care is both wise and desirable. Also, there is agreement among most parties that an insurance plan is the best type of prepayment plan. The basic point of disagreement is over the type and kind of insurance plan. One group led by organized labor, particularly the AFL-CIO, contends that a compulsory health insurance plan is the best means of providing medical care for all persons. On the other hand, the American Medical Association is the proponent of a voluntary system of health insurance sponsored and operated by them and by the American Hospital Association. An intelligent approach to the issue calls for a further examination of the pros and cons of both plans.

Compulsory health insurance. The supporters of compulsory health insurance believe that voluntary insurance for medical care, including hospitalization, does not meet the health needs of the citizens of the United States. It is argued by this group that a substantial portion of our population cannot afford medical care. Some 6 million persons or more receive public assistance and cannot pay

Table 10.1 The cost of health services in 1957–1958 and 1952–1953 compared, in cents

Service	1952–1953	1957–1958
Physicians	37	34
Hospitals	19	23
Drugs and medications	15	20
Dentists	16	15
Other medical goods and services	13	8

Source: Health Information Foundation, "Our Increased Spending for Health," *Progress in Health Services*, 9:4, February, 1960.

the costs of adequate medical care. Slightly higher in the financial scale but little better off from the standpoint of ability to pay for medical care are millions who are close to the level of public aid but who do not receive it. An estimated 100 million persons can meet the cost of minor illnesses and inexpensive care but cannot afford large or continuing medical costs [29].

Furthermore, advocates of compulsory health insurance believe their plan of paying for medical care works if it is coordinated with services already provided through public health programs. This includes the administration of insurance benefits by state and local public health agencies. Also, this plan including disability insurance would be coordinated with the present system of old-age and survivors' insurance. State and local health agencies would organize health services with physicians and hospitals. Negotiations and administering payment agreements would take place with representatives of insured persons and health personnel, all of whom are involved in the plan.

The plan for compulsory health insurance is based on the principle of the individual's ability to pay a percentage of his income, such as 3 to 4 per cent, for comprehensive health care. All the people of the nation would be covered, and comprehensive medical care would be available.

Those in opposition to compulsory health insurance argue that the quality of medical service would be seriously affected under a compulsory system. They believe that organized medicine would be controlled by government agencies and that the professional standards of the private practice of medicine would be lowered.

Voluntary health insurance. Voluntary medical-care plans are designed to assist the individual and his family in avoiding financial hardship when ill health or accidents occur. Through comparatively small

regular prepayments the unpredictable costs of medical and hospital expenses are partially or entirely covered. The acceptance of the prepayment health insurance principle took place in the 1930s when Blue Cross originated in Texas and spread rapidly throughout the country. This was the first stage in the development of prepayment plans, providing only for hospital services. The second stage resulted in the growth of in-hospital surgery plans. An example is Blue Shield. These plans were first organized in Michigan and California as contractual plans entered into with hospitals and physicians who provided the services.

The problems and issues during the 1940s revolved around the possibility of government-sponsored compulsory versus voluntary health insurance plans. How the range of voluntary health insurance services can be extended is the key question today. Specifically, the present issues are [7]:

Comprehensive benefits versus limited benefits

Salary versus fee-for-service payment for physicians

Group medical practice versus solo practice

Health insurance for the aged through social security versus individual coverage

The possibility of government-sponsored compulsory health insurance for the total population is definitely lessened as voluntary plans improve and provide more complete coverage. It is estimated that 137 million of our 178 million people in the United States were covered by some form of voluntary health insurance by the end of 1959.

Voluntary plans, their various types, and the way these plans are handled are the current concerns [32, 33]. Presented below is a brief description of representative plans. More detailed studies can be found in the Suggested readings.

Five types of health insurance protection are common in the numerous policies of insurance companies and Blue Cross and Blue Shield contracts written for individuals and groups:

Loss-of-income protection
Hospital-expense protection
Surgical-expense protection
Regular-medical-expense protection
Major-medical-expense protection

Loss-of-income protection is the oldest type of health insurance. Such policies are written for the family breadwinner, and by protecting against loss of earning capacity, they permit the family to pay rent, grocery, automobile, and other living expenses. Benefits usually begin a week or two after illness strikes and provide payments for a year or more, as a maximum. Deductible loss-of-income insurance that has a thirty-, sixty-, or ninety-day waiting period is inexpensive yet sound protection. Insurance to provide 50 per cent of regular salary is considered a good loss-of-income payment. It is not considered advisable to take out insurance that guarantees receiving more than 60 per cent of one's salary during illness.

Hospital-expense protection is the most popular protection for individuals and groups. Hospital benefits are commonly covered for a maximum period of 60, 90, or 100 days. These provide for room and board and other charges such as drugs, anesthetics, and operating room. More than half of those persons protected are dependents of the wage earner. By the end of 1959, some 75 million persons (55 per cent of the total number covered) were protected by insurance companies against hospital expenses, and 57 million persons (41 per cent) were covered by Blue Cross–Blue Shield and medical society plans. An additional 5 million persons (4 per cent of the total number covered) were enrolled in independent plans [32, 33].

Surgical-expense insurance, like hospital-expense protection, is written for both the wage earner and his dependents. More than half of those covered are dependents. Policies contain a list of fees payable for surgical operations, ranging from $50 to $200 or $500, depending upon the kind of operation. By the end of 1959, 72 million persons (57 per cent) were protected by insurance companies against surgical expenses, compared with more than 49 million (38 per cent) covered by Blue Cross–Blue Shield and medical society surgical plans. Another 6 million persons (5 per cent) were protected by independent plans for surgical services [33].

A more recent type of insurance is that protecting against *regular medical expenses.* This includes the cost of physicians' home calls or office visits, although some policies or contracts are limited only to hospital calls. Generally, payments from companies are not made for the first few calls with each illness, and an over-all maximum is stated for each sickness. At the end of 1959, 43 million persons (49 per cent of the total number covered) were protected by Blue Cross–Blue Shield and medical society plans for the cost of regular medical-care services. Better than 38 million persons (44 per cent) were covered by insurance company policies. Another 6 million (7 per cent) belonged to independent plans that included regular medical expenses.

A relatively new type of health insurance, which began in 1949, is *major-medical-expense protection.* This is commonly referred to as "catastrophic" protection. It provides payment against the exceedingly heavy medical and hospital bills and expenses resulting from disability and illness. These are expenses that might wipe out a lifetime of savings or throw one hopelessly into debt. Insurance of this type does not pay for small or minor medical expenses. The policyholder himself pays for these minor and more easily affordable medical expenses. Policies have a maximum limit on benefits payable, ranging from $2,500 to $10,000. Major medical insurance may be written with a deductible amount, similar to automobile insurance, to be effective for costs above $100 or $500 ranging up to $7,500 or as

292

high as $15,000. Another type calls for the insurance company to pay from 75 to 80 per cent of the expenses above the deductible amount, while the individual pays the remainder. Major medical plans are generally available at any desired level of coverage. This type of insurance is important because few persons can easily afford an unexpected medical emergency costing hundreds or thousands of dollars. Close to 22 million persons, by the end of 1959, held major medical policies. This was a gain of 26 per cent in the brief ten-year history of this type of insurance.

Regardless of the type of health insurance plan desired, one needs to investigate carefully before joining. Several hundred companies issue health insurance policies. A few of these are "fly-by-night" or disreputable companies. The major insurance companies with reputable agents offer sound plans.

Blue Cross hospital-care plans and Blue Shield medical and surgical plans have been mentioned above as illustrating plans that are contracted individually and by groups with the medical profession. Medical, surgical, and hospital care for the wage earner and surgical and hospital coverage for his family can be obtained from group plans. California Physicians' Service is such an example. California state employees, acting as a group, contract with the service, which is sponsored by the California Medical Association. Advantages are a continuing membership privilege after becoming a member regardless of status of health or job. No physical examination is required, one has a choice of his own doctor and hospital, and the service is honored throughout the world. The chief disadvantages are lack of comprehensive protection for the family members and out-of-pocket charges added over and above the prepayment costs. This second disadvantage refers to such payments as those for the first two visits to the doctor's office, and it includes additional charges by the physician if the sub-

scriber's salary is over a certain set ceiling. In line with the trend of the times, Blue Cross and Blue Shield are extending comprehensive coverage in some new contracts.

Two Washington state medical plans—the King County Medical Plan and the Okanogan County Plan—sponsored and governed by the medical profession provide comprehensive medical care and hospitalization coverage. The physicians are paid on a fee-for-service basis, with the fee schedule set by representatives of the medical profession. The subscribers have free choice of physicians; a large portion of the physicians in the counties belong to the plan. Physicians reported the standards and quality of medicine were high under the plans.

King County is the state's largest metropolitan area, including the city of Seattle. About 25 per cent of the county's population is enrolled in the plan. Okanogan County is a rural county with a population of approximately 30,000, of which about 7,000 are covered. These plans are unique in that they include home and office visits as well as surgery and other physicians' services: in other words, comprehensive coverage. The average total costs of health care, using the King County plan as an example, amounted to $335 per family annually. This included extended coverage for dependents. The average per capita cost was estimated at $96 for Boeing subscribers and $94 for other groups covered by the plan. These two plans serve as examples of the extension of broader benefits and health insurance coverage [31].

Group medical practice. The above prepayment medical-care plans are illustrative of those types in which the practice of medicine is continued on an individual basis. Group practice differs in that the doctors belong to a medical group. This is not to be confused with a consumers' group. In group medical practice there is a pooling of staff with a variety of specialists, and usually family doctors also, within the organization. In addition, there is a pooling of technical personnel, equipment, and facilities as well as business management. Such group practice cuts down on costs of operation. It provides special advantages of offering "on the spot" consultation and referrals in diagnosis and treatment, and it places emphasis on preventive medicine, keeping patients healthy, rather than purely curative treatment of diseases. Group medical practice has certain disadvantages as well as advantages. There has been opposition to group practice from organized medicine. This is now considerably less than was the case in the past. Medical men must be able to work together in the group as a team. Not all medical doctors believe in the importance of this method, nor are they pleased to work in this way. It is true, too, that lucrative solo practices have been relatively easy to build up during prosperous times. Group medical plans have been criticized, sometimes justly, because of poor doctor-patient relationships. The organizations today dispute this point, however.

Group practice definitely is on the upsurge. The continued large percentage of specialists, the opportunities for free time, for assistance, and for stimulating consultations with other doctors, and the convenience of working with all branches of medicine in one organization are all factors that have helped to boost group practice.

Two types of group-medical-practice organizations stand out in the present growth of this movement. The first is the type based on *fee-for-fee service*. The Mayo Clinic in Rochester, Minnesota [13], the Ochsner Clinic in New Orleans, the Lahey Clinic in Boston, and the Palo Alto Clinic in Palo Alto, California, are examples of private group practice centers offering teamwork medicine.

The second type of group medical practice is organized on *a prepayment basis for comprehensive coverage*. Three well-known examples of this type are the following: the Ross-Loos Clinic in Los Angeles (the pioneer in this type) [14]; New York City's Health Insurance Plan (HIP) [14]; the Kaiser Foundation Health Plan, formerly the Permanente Foundation Health Plan, located in San Francisco Bay area, Los Angeles area, the Portland-Vancouver area, and Hawaii [15].

Briefly, Ross-Loos offers comprehensive medical and hospital service at a low cost fee per person per month. Individuals, families, and consumer groups may enroll after each individual passes a physical examination. The Ross-Loos medical group is run as a partnership among the originators and 32 of the 115 staff doctors. Salaries are paid on a regular salary scale, with the partners sharing in the yearly profits.

HIP originated to care for the municipal workers of the City of New York. Now other New Yorkers in private industry and their families may join. HIP has 32 medical centers organized on a regional basis to provide its comprehensive medical services on a per capita plan. Choice of physicians occurs within each group. Most of the 1,000 doctors associated with HIP work on a part-time basis and maintain a private practice as well. The Medical Control Board responsible for this plan is working for a change to full-time group practitioners in the future. A unique feature of the plan is its Department of Health Education stressing education as one of its preventive aspects.

The Kaiser Foundation Plan operates as a nonprofit organization. It provides its subscribers and their families with complete medical service in the home, doctor's office, or hospital, including laboratory work and X rays, at a relatively low cost. Health education too is provided, especially for expectant parents. Individuals and organized groups may join on a prepayment basis. The subscriber may select a personal or family physician from the medical staff. In addition, he has access to specialists in every field. Some half million patients belong to this plan in California and Washington, obtaining service in 10 hospitals and 25 outpatient clinics staffed by approximately 500 full-time salaried doctors. The Kaiser plan represents one of the largest and most self-sufficient of the group-medical-practice plans at the present time.

Some dissatisfaction exists with certain group practice plans because of lack of complete benefits, with factors such as deductible plans, coinsurance, and additional out-of-pocket fees. Industrial workers are vocal on the need for more comprehensive coverage, as are many other consumers. This indicates the rising demand for medical-care plans that provide comprehensive benefits. Future plans will no doubt include wider benefits, since sooner or later the public achieves what it wants.

Medical care for the aged. A current issue in medical care of the American people relates to how medical protection can be best worked out for aged and future aged persons. In reality, the issue brings into focus the older controversy of compulsory versus voluntary health protection. The American Medical Association and various other groups, including the insurance companies, advocate voluntary health insurance. They are incorporating plans and suggesting approaches unheard of five years or so ago. On the other hand, President John F. Kennedy is pledged to, and has sent to Congress a bill providing for, medical care for the aged by increasing social security. In essence, this is a form of compulsory health insurance. Regardless of the result, the senior citizens now, and in the future, stand to gain by receiving greater protection at smaller costs to themselves.

Prepayment dental care. With the increase in prepaid medical care, there also has been considerable interest and experimentation in insuring against the costs of dental care. Those who have been most interested in dental health prepayment plans have been the labor unions, public health officials, some government groups such as the Farm Security Administration, cooperative groups, and, of course, the dental associations, as these plans might affect their standards and the practice of dentistry. A number of group plans have been developed and become operative. They include, as examples, the Group Health Dental Insurance, Inc., and the Dental Insurance Plan, Inc., both of New York City, and the prepaid group plan in Washington, D.C., called the Group Health Association, Inc. Some medical-care plans cover a portion of dental care, particularly oral surgery. There appears to be a number of limitations in relation to prepayment dental health plans, more so than is the case with medical care. It is expected in the future, however, that plans will be more widely available to provide for dental care of the most serious nature and highest cost, without which considerable hardship would result.

Responsibility of the individual for consumer health

Regardless of the present food, drug, and cosmetic legislation, the excellent work of governmental agencies enforcing legislation and conducting research, the many endeavors of the professional associations, and the nonprofit private consumer organizations and the social service work of private individuals, there is still much to be done to protect completely the health of the consumer and to solve the consumer problem.

You, as a consumer, cannot completely

solve the problem yourself, but your actions are important. You can make significant contributions if you:

Make sure you understand consumer health education as an integral part of the over-all consumer education movement.

Inform others about their rights and privileges as consumers, and the type of protection and safeguards presently available, as well as those needed in the near future.

Use discriminate judgment in purchasing products and services, since manufacturers are influenced by the actions of consumers. Each purchase counts in this respect.

Report frauds and suspected frauds to the proper authorities.

Support and work for improved legislation affecting the consumer on the local, the state, and the Federal levels.

Support and work for better producer-consumer relations, particularly better medical-care plans.

Summary

Health consumers comprise all persons, including college students, who use health products and services. The problem of consumer health is how to get maximum protection, value, and satisfactions from health information, products, and services. The intelligent consumer utilizes sound criteria based on scientific facts to evaluate health information and to select health products and services for the purposes of protecting his health and getting his money's worth.

Quackery, the practice of the healing art and the selling of products by a faker or an incompetent person, is nearly as old as history itself. The quack is still a part of the modern culture; in fact, he is more subtle and clever than ever before with his cure-all products and fake machines.

The consumer receives protection through Federal, state and local laws and regulations. The Federal Food, Drug, and Cosmetic Act of 1938 provides punitive powers to prevent fraudulent practices. It requires minimum standards and factory inspection of foods and prohibits traffic of injurious foods in interstate commerce. Truthful labeling of foods, drugs, cosmetics, and therapeutic devices is required by the Act. Many states have their own food, drug, and cosmetic acts patterned after the Federal legislation. Cities and counties have local regulations pertaining to food, drugs, and cosmetics. Loopholes in legislation and enforcement make possible intensified activities of the quack and the unscrupulous businessman.

Unreliable sources of health information include customs and superstitions, ignorance and prejudice, the expoundings of quacks, and some commercialized health information, particularly that produced for the sole purpose of selling a product. All health information pertaining to products and services should be appraised on sound scientific criteria, asking questions as, Who is the person or organization, and what are its motives?

Reliable sources of information comprise outstanding health authorities: your family physician, or your medical director of the student health service, or officer of your local medical society or your local health officer, your health educator; religious counselors who operate on a basis of ethics and scientific facts; scientific health organizations and agencies; and public and private consumer agencies working for the welfare of the individual and the betterment of society.

Selecting the right health product seems simple until one discovers the maze of brands, the varieties of sizes and shapes, the variations in weights, and the numerous price levels for each item. The person with discriminating judgment utilizes sound criteria to protect his health and his pocketbook. Suggested guides are formulated for the consumer's consideration.

Selecting competent health advisers, particularly when one is away from home or establishing a new home, is an important task. The medical doctor is recommended as an adviser who provides counseling services, complete medical care, and supervision, with the aid of many specialists and technical workers. Both medical and dental health advisers can be selected wisely by applying scientific criteria such as those outlined for consideration.

Medical care consists of all those personal services in the prevention, diag-

nosis, and treatment of disease and the rehabilitation of the patient. Specifically, medical care pertains to preventive services, such as the periodic health examination, immunizations, continuous health supervision in sickness and hospital care, and intelligent personal care of minor disorders and the administration of first aid.

It is your responsibility to assist in solving the consumer problem by understanding consumer health education and informing others; using discriminating judgment in purchasing products and services; reporting frauds and suspected frauds; supporting and working for improved consumer legislation; and supporting and working for better producer-consumer relations, particularly better medical-care plans.

Suggested readings

1. American Hospital Association, Blue Cross Commission: *Blue Cross Guide: A Summary of Group Enrollment Benefits, Rates and Regulations of Non-profit Blue Cross Service Plans,* The Commission, Chicago, 1956.
2. Anderson, Dewey: *The Present Day Doctor of Chiropractic,* Public Affairs Institute, Washington, 1956.
3. Becker, Harry: "The Changing Scene in Health Care Economics," *New York State Journal of Medicine,* 39:2044–2048, May 15, 1959.
4. Belleau, Wilfrid E.: *Podiatry-Chiropody as a Career,* Park Publishing Co., Milwaukee, Wis., 1959.
5. Better Business Bureau: *Facts You Should Know about Your Better Business Bureau,* The National Association of Better Business Bureaus, New York, 1959.
6. Beyrer, Mary K.: "How Reliable Is Health Information?" *Journal of Health, Physical Education and Recreation,* 27:11, April, 1956.
7. Brewster, Agnes W.: *Health Insurance and Related Proposals for Financing Personal Health Services,* U.S. Department of Health, Education, and Welfare, Washington, 1958.

8. Bureau of Investigation: *Testimonials,* American Medical Association, Chicago, 1940.
9. Campbell, Persia: *The Consumer Interest: A Study in Consumer Economics,* Harper & Brothers, New York, 1949.
10. Consumer Reports: *1962 Buying Guide Issue,* Consumers Union, Inc., New York, 1962 (yearly).
11. Cook, James: *Remedies and Rackets,* W. W. Norton & Company, Inc., New York, 1958.
12. Council on Foods and Nutrition: *Your Campaign Kit to Combat Food Faddism and False Claims,* American Medical Association, Chicago, 1959.
13. Deutsch, Albert: "Group Medicine (The Mayo Clinic)," *Consumer Reports,* 22:37–40, January, 1957.
14. Deutsch, Albert: "Group Medicine (The Ross-Loos Clinic, New York's HIP)," *Consumer Reports,* 22:83–86, February, 1957.
15. Deutsch, Albert: "Group Medicine" (The Kaiser Health Plan, and the Status of Group Medicine in the United States), *Consumer Reports,* 22:135–138, March, 1957.
16. Doyle, Kathleen C.: *Science vs Chiropractic,* Public Affairs Pamphlet 191,

Public Affairs Committee, New York, 1953.

17. "Exercising and Vibrating Machines," *Journal of the American Medical Association,* 170:966, June 20, 1959.

18. "False Advertising and Products for the Overweight," *Consumer Reports,* 24:612, November, 1959.

19. Fielding, W. J.: *Strange Superstitions and Magical Practices,* McGraw-Hill Book Company, Inc., Blakiston Division, New York, 1945.

20. Food and Drug Administration: *General Regulations for the Enforcement of the Federal Food, Drug, and Cosmetic Act,* Title 21, Part 1, U.S. Department of Health, Education, and Welfare, Washington, 1961.

21. Food and Drug Administration: *Read the Label on Food, Drugs, Devices, Cosmetics, and Household Chemicals,* F.D.A. Publication No. 3, U.S. Department of Health, Education, and Welfare, Washington, 1961.

22. Food and Drug Administration: *Leaflet Series,* Nos. 1, 2, 4, 5, 8, 10, 11, U.S. Department of Health, Education, and Welfare, Washington, 1961.

23. Food and Drug Administration: *Protecting Consumers of Foods, Drugs, and Cosmetics,* U.S. Department of Health, Education, and Welfare, Washington, 1961.

24. "Frauds and Gyps," *Changing Times,* 14:8–9, July, 1960.

25. Galdston, Iago: "Hazards of Commercial Health Advertisement," *American Journal of Public Health,* 21:242–248, March, 1931.

26. Garland, Henry L., and Henry La Cossitt: "California Outlaws the Cancer Quack," *Today's Health,* 37:30–31, 70–72, August, 1959.

27. Goldman, Franz, and Hugh Leavell: "Medical Care for Americans," *Annals of the American Academy of Political and Social Science,* 273:1–192, January, 1951.

28. *Health and Insurance Plans under Collective Bargaining, Surgical and Medical Benefits, Late Summer, 1959,* Superintendent of Documents, Washington, 1961.

29. *Health for the American People: A Symposium,* Little, Brown & Company, Boston, 1956.

30. Health Information Foundation: "Voluntary Health Insurance among the Aged," *Progress in Health Services,* 8:1–6, January, 1959.

31. Health Information Foundation: "Comprehensive Insurance for Physicians' Services: A Study of Two Washington State Medical Plans," *Progress in Health Services,* 9:1–6, June, 1960.

32. Health Insurance Council: *Nature and Types of Health Insurance: A Guide for the Practicing Physician,* The Health Insurance Association of America, New York, 1956.

33. Health Insurance Council: *The Extent of Voluntary Health Insurance Coverage,* The Council, New York, 1960.

34. Holbrook, Stewart H.: *The Golden Age of Quackery,* The Macmillan Company, New York, 1959.

35. "Hoxsey Cancer Cure," *Consumer Reports,* 21:303, June, 1956.

36. Irish, Frederick W.: "Activities of the Federal Trade Commission with Respect to Food, Drugs, and Related Products," *American Journal of Public Health,* 51:368–373, March, 1961.

37. Joint Meeting, The Nutrition Foundation with the Institute of Food Technologists, Northern California Section, Inc.: *The Role of Nutrition Education in Combating Food Fads,* The Nutrition Foundation, Inc., New York, 1959.

38. Keesecker, Raymond P.: *The Osteopathic Movement in Medicine,* American Osteopathic Association, Chicago, 1957.

39. Kursh, Harry: "Mail Order Quacks' Harvest: Dollars and Death," *Today's Health,* 39:30–31, 83–87, March, 1961.

40. Lee, Alfred M.: *How to Understand Propaganda,* Rinehart & Company, Inc., New York, 1952.

41. Margolius, Sidney: *The Consumer's Guide to Better Buying,* New American Library of World Literature, Inc., New York, 1953.

42. National Better Business Bureau: *Obesity Remedies,* The Bureau, New York, Apr. 10, 1959.

43. Public Affairs Committee: *The Arthritis Hoax,* Public Affairs Pamphlet 297, The Committee, New York, 1960.

44. Somers, Anne, and Herman Somers: "Coverage, Costs and Controls in Voluntary Health Insurance," *American Journal of Public Health,* 76:1–9, January, 1961.

45. Stanford Research Institute: *Chiropractic in California,* The Institute, Menlo Park, Calif., 1960.

46. "Symposium on the Group Purchase of Dental Care," *American Journal of Public Health,* 50:21–33, January, 1960.

47. Tabori, Paul: *The Natural Science of*

Stupidity, Chilton Company, New York, 1959.

48. Temporary National Economic Committee: *Investigation of Concentration of Economic Power,* Consumer Standards Monograph 24, Government Printing Office, Washington, 1941.

49. Troelstrup, Arch W.: *Consumer Problems,* 2d ed., McGraw-Hill Book Company, Inc., New York, 1957.

50. The National Osteopathic Foundation: *Focus on Osteopathic Education,* The American Osteopathic Association, Chicago, no date.

51. "What You Should Know about Health Insurance," *Changing Times,* 13:25–31, January, 1959.

52. Wilson, W. Harmon, and Elvin S. Eyster: *Consumer Economic Problems,* 5th ed., South-Western Publishing Company, Cincinnati, 1956.

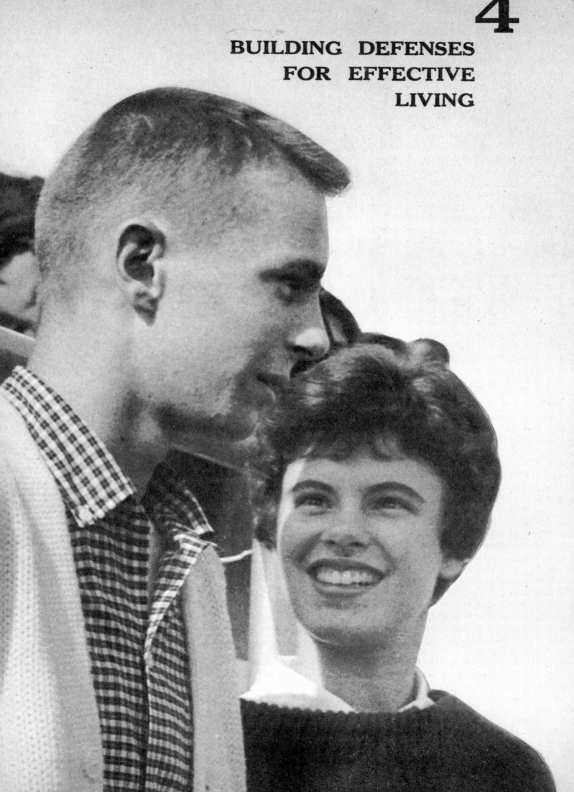

ELEVEN

Preventing and controlling communicable diseases

As more research is freeing mankind from disease, there is a cultural lag in disease prevention. This is characteristic of our way of life; we do not put into practice the scientific knowledge now available. Greater scientific progress has taken place in recent years in preventing and controlling communicable disease than in any other area affecting the health and welfare of man. These contributions have alleviated much suffering, prevented the loss of countless working hours, saved many persons from untimely deaths, and increased the life span.

Regardless of these remarkable advances, no single disease caused by microorganisms has been wiped out completely. More important to us immediately is that, because of our cultural lag, far too many illnesses, defects, and deaths occur that could be prevented.

An example of the lag is the almost total disregard for the consequences of the venereal diseases since medical discoveries have provided easy treatment for their control and elimination. The appalling increase in venereal-disease rates, particularly in the 15–24-year age group, has brought venereal diseases back as a major health problem. It has been reported in one study of 1,000 male VD patients that 800 had been infected more than once. Some 540 became infected for the first time between the ages of 15 and 19. Another study showed that more women are being infected today at the age of high school graduation than at any other age [1]. Many metropolitan areas across the nation reported in 1960 that 17 to 22 per cent of cases of venereal disease involved teen-agers.

College students are still affected much too often by the insidious or unsuspected occurrence of disease, usually at the most inopportune time. Communicable diseases such as tuberculosis are responsible for students' dropping out of college and postponing temporarily, and in some cases permanently, the college education they had planned. Each term, students are absent from important class activities and examinations because of illness. From a social point of view, illness upsets the best plans for the crowning social events and outstanding athletic contests, not to mention an occasional much-anticipated vacation period. Also, communicable diseases cut down ability to produce and to attain established goals. Another important fact is that such diseases, if not properly cared for, may lead to unnecessary complications or to more serious chronic and degenerative diseases. It must be admitted, too, that some college students do not develop an appreciation for effective living, free from disease, until they have experienced an illness. Other students, owing to lack of scientific knowledge, worry un-

necessarily about disease, the possibility of contracting disease, or how disease might affect them personally. Actually, you as a student are confronted with a great challenge. You are afforded opportunities for education and, in later years, research activities as never before in history. It is the young scientists of today who, more than likely, will provide information about the unknown factors in disease prevention and control.

There is emphasis on controlling respiratory diseases, which are the major cause of absenteeism from college classes as well as from industry. New viruses have been isolated and studied in the laboratory, and new laboratory techniques have improved classification and control of viral diseases. Viruses thought to be the cause of the common cold have been isolated, though much more needs to be known about these particular diseases. Constant vigilance over former epidemic diseases has prevented many modern epidemics, which in the past have wreaked such havoc with human life. New vaccines, particularly the multiple-type immunizations, appear to be the best weapon against the viruses.

Despite the great advances in disease prevention, there is much yet to be accomplished in scientific discoveries, human motivation and attitude formation, and application of knowledge and attitudes to individual health practices in order to solve the residual problem of communicable diseases.

The challenge to you as a college student is to understand fully the scientific information in this chapter and to apply to your program the principles of health education outlined in previous chapters, particularly Chapters 1, 2, and 3.

The information about communicable diseases is organized to help you answer the following pertinent questions:

What is the meaning of infection and disease?

What are the principles of disease prevention and control?

How are the principles applied to methods of control?

What are the common communicable diseases of the college age group?

How can the college student assume responsibility in the prevention and control of disease for himself and for others?

The modern concept of disease

In Chapter 1, health is defined as a positive quality of life enabling the individual to make successful personal and social adjustments in his environment. Disease, on the other hand, is a negative condition, a departure from a positive state of health.

To understand disease and the disease process, it is important to consider the forces that produce a healthy state free from disease, on the one hand, or a disease condition, on the other. These forces are: the individual, or *host,* harboring disease-producing organisms, the *specific agent* or agents that cause disease, and the *environment* in which the individual and the agents reside.

The biological concept of disease is that disease occurs when an imbalance exists between the host and the disease agents as they interact in the environment. The interaction of the host and the agents is directly related to, and depends upon, the environment in all its aspects—physical, biological, social, and economic. The environment includes climate, temperature, housing, sanitation, living organisms, and social stratification of people, as well as other conditions. It may influence the qualities and activities of either the host or the disease agents, tipping the scales in favor of one or the other, or it may help the two live together compatibly.

THE HOST-PARASITE RELATIONSHIP

The host affects the interaction process and the state of equilibrium among the forces through:

His powers within his body (his body defenses)

His heredity and constitution

His habits and customs

His age, sex, and race characteristics

His man-made means of increasing his resistance to agents

His powers to control these agents

The disease agents affect the interaction process and the state of equilibrium according to the following characteristics [17]:

Basic nature and characteristics, such as growth and reproduction, and toxic potential

Resistance to attack by body processes and against heat, cold, moisture, sunlight, and chemicals

Ability to gain access and adapt themselves to the host

Ability to cause tissue reaction in the host

Virulence or strength to cause a severe reaction

Reservoirs, or sources, in which they may be found

Means of transmission from reservoirs to the host

The influence on man of visible plants and animals is obvious and clearly understood. However, it is more difficult to realize the influence of microscopic plants and animals that are pathogens or disease-producing agents. These microscopic organisms infest man and live off him in a parasitic relationship. This relationship may have different consequences. The parasite may live off the host in such a way that both parties make satisfactory adjustments. This is referred to as a *symbiotic condition,* in which the infectious agent and the host live together without apparent ill effect on each other. An example of this is the carrier state, in which the individual himself is not affected visibly but is capable of transmitting disease-producing organisms to others, who in turn may be seriously affected. Another type is the lifelong association of host and disease agent, for example, herpes infection, which causes an inflammatory skin reaction producing small vesicles, or the coliform bacteria residing in the intestines of man. The parasite may infect the individual early in his development, and a perfect equilibrium is reached between the host and the agent [17].

In other conditions the parasite invades the host and causes severe illness and even death. The parasite may destroy its host and at the same time destroy itself. Also, it may be destroyed by the host or by the administration of products such as the antibiotics, which man has developed to counteract the invading organism. As man's knowledge increases, the balance swings more and more in his favor and against the disease-producing agents. Our statistics show that there is still need to extend and improve disease prevention and control methods.

DEFINITION OF DISEASE

The invasion of the host by the parasite is called *infection*. When the individual is infected, a struggle takes place between the organism and the body and its processes. The condition called *disease* results when, in the struggle between the organism and the individual, there is visible evidence of the interaction. That is to say, disease is the visible result of the unfavorable (for the host) equilibrium between him and the disease agent, in a particular environment. Disease may be defined, then, as *the visible reaction of the individual, the human host, to a parasite, an infectious agent, in a particular environment*. The visible reaction denotes a negative condition. The term itself signifies this, since it is a combination of "dis" and "ease," meaning "not at ease."

A *communicable* disease is defined by the American Public Health Association as:[1]

An illness due to a specific infectious agent or its toxic products, arising through transmission of that agent or its products from reservoir to susceptible host, either directly as from an infected person or animal, or indirectly through the agency of an intermediate plant or animal host, a vector, or the inanimate environment.

SIGNS AND SYMPTOMS OF DISEASE

The specific visible evidence for disease is the actual signs and symptoms. These serve to notify the individual and others that disease occurs in the body. The following are common symptoms:

Body temperature above 99°F
Chills
Diarrhea or constipation
Discharging nose
Dizziness
Excessive sneezing or coughing
Fatigue or lack of energy
Fever
Flushed face
Headache
Inflamed, watery, or "glassy" appearance of eyes
Nausea, vomiting
Pain—sharp, burning, dull, throbbing, knifing
Pallor—face, nail beds, eyes
Rash, "bumps," or other unusual condition of the skin
Restlessness
Shortness of breath
Sore throat
Sores or lesions
Swollen glands
Unexplained profuse sweating

EPIDEMIOLOGY

A brief explanation of the science of epidemiology and its functions aids in understanding disease. Epidemiology is concerned with the occurrence of dis-

[1] American Public Health Association, *Control of Communicable Diseases in Man*, 9th ed., The Association, New York, 1960, p. 11.

ease in groups of people. Many solutions to problems of communicable disease are made through this field, which pertains to all diseases, although its chief efforts are directed toward the communicable diseases.

Epidemiology is the study of the occurrence of disease through [37]:

Firsthand information from the bedside of the sick individual, the *clinical* approach

Controlled conditions in the laboratory, the *experimental* approach

Observation of disease under natural conditions of the population within the environment, the true *epidemiologic* approach

Epidemiology today views disease as a total process. The cause of disease involves more than a disease organism. The characteristics of the individual or the population attacked and the particular environment are important factors in the process. Therefore, in the prevention and control of disease, all factors must be brought into focus.

Principles of disease prevention and control

The foundation of disease prevention is the science of epidemiology. Therefore, the principles of disease prevention and control are observable in the actions of the epidemiologist and his associates. The epidemiologist is concerned with the series of events that makes disease possible, the disease process, and ways and means of controlling disease. He must be concerned with major forces previously mentioned: the individual who is host for the disease, the disease-producing organism or agent, and the related environment. Even today, it is not always possible to know all the factors about a disease. The epidemiologist by necessity is forced to determine the factors that are known about a particular disease. Armed with the available information, he looks for weaknesses in the disease-producing process where one or more procedures may be applied to prevent or control the disease.

The work of the epidemiologist is exemplified in a venereal-disease-control program. A case of venereal disease is reported to the health department. Immediately, the job of the epidemiologist is to determine the identity and the descriptions of the persons with whom the patient had contact. He also attempts to

find out the circumstances involving the contact. Such information includes the place, the date of exposure, and the relationship of the contact to the patient. While obtaining the information, the epidemiologist also tries to reeducate and reorient the patient. A third function of the epidemiologist is to follow up the contacts to find the source of infection. When found, this person is treated, and a source of infection is eliminated. During all steps of the epidemiologic study, reeducation and reorientation of patients and contacts are carried on as an important aspect of control and prevention.

The epidemiologist may discover the weak link in the disease-producing chain; however, he is not the only person involved in ultimate control. Prevention and control depend upon a team of individuals working together to guard the health of the community. These team members include the private physician, the health officer and his staff (epidemiologist or communicable-disease-control officer, sanitarian, public health nurse, and public health educator), research workers, and members of voluntary health agencies interested in the eradication of special diseases, as well as the average citizen.

THE INFECTIOUS-DISEASE PROCESS

When infectious disease occurs, it develops through several stages, as follows:

An *incubation* period, in which the organism is growing, multiplying, and overcoming the body processes

The *onset,* the stage in which signs and symptoms of the disease first appear

A *progressive stage,* in which the disease develops fully

The outcome will be either that the disease agents are victorious, resulting in the death of the individual and suicide for the invading organisms; or that the individual overcomes the disease and proceeds through a stage of convalescence and recovery.

An anonymous poem humorously pictures the interaction process between the host and the pathogenic organism:

What a Chance!

Cheer up!
You have two chances—
One of getting the germ
And one of Not.

And if you get the germ
You have two chances—
One of getting the disease
And one of Not.

And if you get the disease
You have two chances—
One of dying
And one of Not.

And if you die—Well,
You still have two chances.

The range between the extremes of no infection and severe infection is what is called an *infectious-disease spectrum.* The spectrum is comparable to the color spectrum showing the intensities and variations in colors. Actually, there are two spectra. The first is the spectrum of infection, which provides the over-all picture. The second is a disease spectrum, which is included within the broader spectrum of infection.

In the broader spectrum the range of infection is charted from no detectable effects (subclinical) to moderate and severe infections. The second spectrum, the disease spectrum, also has its range from extremely mild and mild to severe or fatal diseases.

Often the mild cases are the unrecognized infections in carriers or missed cases. These cases are more responsible for the spread of infection because they go unnoticed. The infectious-disease spectrum provides valuable information for the authorities concerned with prevention and control methods.

The infectious process progresses through a series of events as follows [5]:

A specific causative, or etiologic, agent, found in a suitable reservoir (man or animal) or source of infection, escapes from the source.

It is transmitted to a susceptible host.

It gains entrance into the new host.

After entering the host it develops sufficient numbers or virulence or both to overcome the resistance of the host. A breakdown at any one point in the series or chain of events means that the infection or disease does not develop. Information about this process is essential in the prevention and control of disease. Therefore, each factor in the process is discussed briefly.

CAUSATIVE, OR ETIOLOGIC, AGENTS

The agents producing infectious or communicable disease are minute microorganisms. For purposes of discussion, they are classified as bacteria, fungi, rickettsiae, viruses, protozoa, and metazoa.

Bacteria. Bacteria are one-celled plant forms belonging to the Schizomycetes class of organisms. They range in size from ultramicroscopic to those which are almost visible to the naked eye. However, none can be seen clearly without the aid of a microscope. Bacteria are found everywhere in nature. Most bacteria are

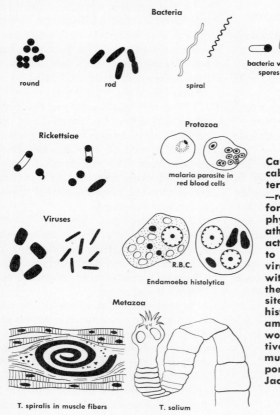

Causative agents producing communicable diseases (greatly enlarged). Bacteria: the three usual shapes of bacteria—round, rodlike, and spiral, also spore forms. Fungi: illustrated by Epidermophyton, one type of fungus causing athlete's foot. Rickettsiae: some characteristic shapes (note the similarity to bacteria). Viruses: two forms of viruses drawn from photographs taken with an electron microscope. Protozoa: the protozoon causing malaria, a parasite in red blood cells; and Endamoeba histolytica, the causative organism of amebic dysentery. Metazoa: a roundworm, Trichinella spiralis, the causative agent of trichinosis, encysted in muscle fibers; and Taenia solium, the pork tapeworm. (After a drawing by Jacqueline Tobian.)

nonpathogenic and do not cause disease; they do, however, play vital roles in the carbon and nitrogen cycles, particularly in the decomposition of waste materials. A relatively small number of bacteria are pathogenic, or disease-producing, microorganisms.

Bacteria exhibit one of three shapes. The rod-shaped bacteria are called *bacilli;* the round, spherical forms are *cocci;* and the spiral forms, resembling a comma or corkscrew, are *spirilla.* The bacilli are the causative organisms of diphtheria, typhoid fever, tuberculosis, and anthrax, to name several examples. The cocci cause pneumonia, gonorrhea, scarlet fever, and boils. The coiled variety of the spirilla are the causative organisms of cholera. The closer-coiled type are the spirochetes causing syphilis. The classifi-

cation of spirochetes is a disputed point. They are classified as bacteria, as protozoa, or in a separate classification of their own.

Bacteria reproduce rapidly by transverse or binary fission; that is, one cell divides in the middle to form two daughter cells. In favorable environments this occurs as frequently as every twenty to thirty minutes. At this rate and without interference, 1 bacterium could multiply into 500,000 within a short time. Approximately 2 billion may be contained in one drop of water [14]. Fortunately for man, many bacteria do not survive even when the conditions are favorable, and under unfavorable conditions they die quickly. Unfortunately for man, some bacteria produce spore forms that are especially resistant to heat, cold, chemicals, and other normally unfavorable environmental factors.

A spore form is a resting stage resulting from nuclear changes in the vegetative cell. The protoplasm shrinks, the cell wall contracts, and a heavier and more resistant cell wall forms. These changes cause the development of a dumbbell-shaped structure. In this state the bacteria can live almost indefinitely even in an unfavorable environment. When conditions again become favorable, the spore form may return to its vegetative state and continue its cycle, including the production of disease. Most spore forms are found in rod-shaped bacteria. Tetanus (lockjaw) and anthrax are caused by bacteria that form spores.

Fungi. Fungi, like bacteria, are plant forms that are both helpful and harmful to man. They, too, live almost everywhere on land and in the sea. They are classified by the botanist along with algae and lichens in the subdivision called Thallophyta. Fungi are spore-forming plants that include mushrooms, puffballs, yeasts, blights, smuts, rusts, rots, and molds. Pathogenic fungi attacking man are microscopic in size. Fungus infections of the skin, discussed more in detail later in the chapter, are prevalent and widespread. For example, athlete's foot and ringworm of the scalp are two common and troublesome fungus infections. Two more serious diseases caused by fungi are coccidioidomycosis, commonly called valley fever or desert fever, and histoplasmosis. Both diseases are often fatal in their acute forms. The spores of the fungus that causes coccidioidomycosis are found in the soil. People are infected when they breathe the the spores into their bodies with dust.

Fungi have a useful as well as a harmful side. On the positive side is the fungus Penicillium, the genus of molds from which the drug penicillin is extracted. Molds and their relatives constitute the greatest source of present-day antibiotics.

In the future, fungi may be more helpful than destructive to man as their activities are better controlled.

Rickettsiae. Rickettsiae are disease organisms named after their discoverer, Howard Ricketts. Ricketts described these organisms as the causative agents of two characteristic rickettsial diseases, typhus fever and Rocky Mountain spotted fever. He died of typhus during his studies. Rickettsiae are spherical or rod-shaped, resembling bacteria. In size they are between bacteria and viruses and are barely visible under the microscope. They are found in the tissues of man, other mammals, and insects and are transmitted by insects such as lice and ticks. Like viruses they are difficult to grow in laboratory media, although some strains have been cultivated in special tissue media.

Viruses. The virus is the smallest of all the causative agents and for this reason has been referred to as "the little bug that wasn't there." Viruses are not visible by means of the ordinary microscope. However, they can be seen with the electron microscope, or their presence may be determined in the laboratory by injecting material suspected of virus infection into a susceptible animal. Many viruses are so small that they pass through the smallest-pored porcelain filters used to retain bacteria. On the other hand, some viruses can be filtered out by small, dense filters, which allow only a few kinds of organisms to pass through. Some research workers believe viruses are autocatalytic bodies that injure a cell, with the result that the cell itself is stimulated to produce additional viruses of the same type. It is the general belief today that animal viruses are living but that some plant viruses may not be. It is safe to say that much is yet unknown about the nature of viruses. It is known, however, that viruses reproduce or are reproduced only within living cells. The cells of the chick embryo are a common virus medium used in experimental study in the laboratory. A characteristic of many virus diseases is production of a lasting immunity. Diseases in which an attack confers an immunity of comparatively long duration or a lasting immunity are smallpox, mumps, measles, poliomyelitis, and yellow fever. However, the common cold, influenza, fever blisters, and warts are virus diseases in which little or no immunity is produced.

Only recently has it been determined that some viruses, like some bacteria, do not necessarily cause disease. We may soon find out that viruses serve constructive functions in nature, but this is not yet proved, perhaps because viruses are so difficult to see. With the exception of the live-virus vaccines that confer immunity against diseases such as yellow fever, smallpox, and poliomyelitis the friendly viruses are beneficial to plants and to animals but not to man [19].

Human viruses can now be classified into six major families and a tentative seventh, with the recent discovery of several new viruses. The common cold viruses are those yet to be confirmed as a separate family. The family classes of viruses include the following:

The pox viruses, which, for example, cause smallpox.

The herpes viruses, responsible for chickenpox.

The arbor viruses, such as the virus causing yellow fever (arbor virus is a short term for "arthropod-borne virus," including those carried by mosquitoes and ticks).

The myxoviruses, which cause influenza and mumps (the prefix *myxo* comes from the Greek word meaning mucus; these viruses, characterized by mucus, cause the red cells to agglutinate, or clump together).

The adenoviruses, which commonly cause acute sore throat, or pharyngitis (the prefix *adeno* means "glands"; adenoviruses also cause acute respiratory

disease, which was first found in military recruits during World War II and subsequently in presently established military bases, where it was isolated and classed as a type of adenovirus).

The enteroviruses, smallest of all the known viruses and having some 57 varieties, which flourish for the most part in the intestines of man, although recently they have been traced to the respiratory tract. The most common example, as well as the most destructive, are the enteroviruses causing poliomyelitis. Enteroviruses include the Coxsackie viruses, which cause illness with fever. They are called Coxsackie because they were first discovered in children from Coxsackie, New York. Other enteroviruses are the ECHO viruses. ECHO stands for *enteric cytopathic human orphan* viruses. These viruses were thought to be "orphans" when first isolated in research done on poliomyelitis.

The common cold viruses, which may or may not be another family of viruses. Andrewes and his colleagues at the Common Cold Research Unit, Salisbury, England, claim that the common cold viruses, although related to enteroviruses, do not belong to any of the previously discussed families and could very well prove to be a separate family [2, 6].

Protozoa. Protozoa are one-celled animal organisms, the lowest of animal life, found in many thousands of forms. Only a few, twenty-five or so, are human parasites causing infectious diseases. Protozoa vary greatly in size; the smallest are comparable to the most minute bacteria, and the largest exceed the largest bacteria by many times. Like bacteria, they reproduce rapidly in a variety of ways, including both asexual and sexual reproduction. Usually, protozoa depend on an intermediate host for transmission. Strangely enough, an attack of a protozoan disease produces little, if any, immunity. Some protozoa develop a spore stage in which they form cysts. In this stage, similar to bacterial spores, they are capable of living for long periods of time. Three common human diseases caused by protozoa are malaria, African sleeping sickness, and amebic dysentery [14].

Metazoa. The metazoa fall in a broad, general classification of many-celled animals of higher organization. Metazoa include flukes, tapeworms, hookworms, trichinae, and insects such as the itch mite.

Flukes cause dysentery and other infections. Tapeworms, so named because they resemble a measuring tape, include pork, beef, fish, dog, rat, and monkey tapeworms. The adult tapeworm fastens itself by hooks in its head to the wall of the host's intestine, where it obtains its food from the host. While in the intestine, it lays eggs, which pass out of the body with the feces. The eggs are eaten by an intermediate host, such as a cow or hog. Larvae develop in the new host, bore through the wall of the intestine, and enter the blood stream. The blood stream carries them to the muscles, where they develop cysts. Human beings become infected when they eat the flesh of the infested cow, hog, or fish not sufficiently cooked to kill the cysts.

Hookworm is a disease caused by a parasite that is capable of piercing the skin. It is common in tropical countries where frost does not cover the ground. The hookworm attaches itself to the intestinal wall. There it injures the host by sucking blood, eating the epithelial tissues, and producing a toxin.

Trichinosis is the disease caused by trichinae, which are small, round worms. Man acquires the disease by eating infested pork not cooked sufficiently to kill the trichinae. The worms enter the small intestine. After a few days when the female eggs have been fertilized by the male sperm, the larvae pass into the blood stream and are carried to the muscles, where they become encysted. These cysts cause extreme muscular pain. While in the intestines, the worms cause gastrointestinal disturbances, which also can be severe.

Three bloodsucking lice cause disease in man: the head louse, the body louse, and the pubic, or crab, louse. Lice lay eggs, or nits, on clothing or at the base of body hair. The eggs hatch in about seven to ten days. Lice begin to suck blood from the host immediately after developing from the egg. They feed a number of times a day and more often at night when the host is quiet. They spread by direct contact, person to person, or by contact with infested personal belongings, including clothing.

The itch mite is an insect which burrows into the skin. It lays its eggs under the superficial layer and produces intense itching. Scabies, another insect disease, is also causd by mites. The female mite burrows into the horny layer of skin, remaining in her burrow until removed. Eggs are laid from which larvae hatch. They leave the burrow and enter the hair follicles. Here a nymph stage develops, and the nymph becomes an adult, either a male or an immature female. The entire cycle takes place in ten to fourteen days. Scabies is highly contagious, being transmitted by personal contact.

THE EFFECT OF MICROORGANISMS ON THE BODY

Much is yet to be learned about the struggle between the causative agents of disease and the body processes. It is already known that these microorganisms affect the body in the following ways:
They destroy body cells and tissues.
They cause mechanical injury.
They secrete toxins, or poisons.

Destruction of body cells and tissues. Many forms of bacteria, most of the viruses, the rickettsiae, and some protozoa and metazoa invade the tissues directly. For example, the hemolytic streptococci dissolve red blood corpuscles, and the staphylococci in boils injure the white blood cells. The tuberculosis bacilli destroy tissues extensively, gas bacilli in wound infections destroy muscle tissue, viruses kill cells, especially nerve cells, malaria parasites invade the body cells, and tapeworms and hookworms damage tissue and rob the host of food and blood.

Production of mechanical injury. Because of the rapid multiplication of micoorganisms from a few to billions in a few hours, the tissues of the body are affected by a material burden in some diseases. For example, the blood flow is altered, vessels are blocked, and the function of cells, tissues, and organs is interfered with and interrupted.

Secretions of toxins or poisons. Bacteria, particularly, secrete poisons, although other microorganisms such as some viruses, rickettsiae, and metazoa may also give them off. Bacteria release two types of toxins: exotoxins and endotoxins. Exotoxins (*exo* means "outside") are liberated poisons excreted freely by living bacteria and occur in most bacterial diseases. The bacilli causing diphtheria have a local effect, producing a sore throat as well as causing symptoms throughout the body by the freeing of toxins. In tetanus the toxin formed by the bacteria is liberated and carried by the blood stream to the nerve cells of the central nervous system.

The second type of toxin produced by bacteria, the endotoxins (*endo* means "inside"), are the result of the dead or killed bacteria themselves. This is sometimes referred to as the *effect of split proteins.* The toxin within the bacteria bodies, which are protein material, is released when the bacteria are split, or disintegrated. The bacillus causing typhoid fever is an example of this type.

SOURCE OF INFECTION

Since *source* means "origin" or "ultimate cause," *source of infection* means the "reservoir of infection," or place where the causative organisms live, grow, and multiply. There are two sources of infection: man and animals. Of these two, man is the more significant because human tissues are excellent media for the growth and development of microorganisms. Man then serves as a reservoir during an attack of a disease. Also, he may be a carrier during convalescence, that is, a temporary carrier, or a healthy carrier in a chronic state. Man may present an atypical case; examples are a walking case of typhoid fever, or an abortive case of infantile paralysis. In such situations the individual goes about his normal daily business but at the same time may spread disease. Most diseases are spread by personal contact, with an individual serving as the reservoir of the infectious agent.

Animals, likewise, are a source of infectious disease. A number of diseases are acquired by man from animals. Bovine tuberculosis is an example. Man is infected with this disease when the bacilli are transmitted from the cow through milk. Brucellosis, or undulant fever, is acquired by man from drinking the raw milk of infected cows or by handling the diseased animals. Rodents serve as a reservoir for plague, and dogs are the principal source of infection for rabies.

The natural environment, to a limited degree, also serves as a reservoir for infection. The soil and dust contain many pathogenic organisms, particularly spore forms. Soil and dust constitute the source of infection in coccidioidomycosis and in tetanus.

MODE OF PARASITE ESCAPE

As long as man or animals serve only as reservoirs, new infections do not take place.

Other factors are necessary for the transmission of disease. The next step in the infectious process is the liberation of microorganisms from the source. The escape of organisms depends upon their location in the body, the tissue in which they are reproducing, and available exits. The mouth and nose are exits through which infectious agents are expelled in sneezing, coughing, and expectorating. These exits expel infectious materials from tissues, for example, the respiratory tract, in which microorganisms readily grow and multiply. The intestinal tract serves as an exit through which feces transport disease-producing organisms, particularly bacteria. The urinary tract is comparable to the intestinal tract as a means of escape for disease-producing microorganisms. Surface lesions (open sores) likewise are means of exit; since they are readily visible, they are more likely to receive attention than are the normal body processes expelling causative organisms.

MODE OF TRANSMISSION

Information about the means by which microorganisms are spread from the source of infection to the susceptible host is invaluable for controlling communicable disease. Methods of transmission are related directly to the previously discussed channels of exit from the body. Microorganisms may escape from the sources; however, unless they are transmitted to a new host, infection does not spread. It is for this reason that knowledge of the mode of transmission is often the vital point of attack for those attempting to control disease.

There are two common means of transmitting infection: by *direct contact,* person to person; by *indirect contact,* by means of inanimate objects, by insects or other animal vectors, and through the air as a vehicle.

Direct contact is the most frequent method by which one individual infects another. Direct contact means actually touching the infected person or the source of infection or coming in close enough contact for transfer of the agent. Microorganisms expelled from the mouth and respiratory tract are transmitted through close contact, that is, by transmission of droplets containing disease-producing microorganisms through the air for a distance of 3 feet or less [4]. Colds, influenza, pneumonia, diphtheria, mumps, measles, chickenpox, smallpox, and tuberculosis are some of the diseases transmitted by this means. A few diseases are transmitted by direct physical contact, notably the prevalent venereal diseases, syphilis, gonorrhea, and chancroid.

There are several ways of transmitting infectious agents by indirect contact. Microorganisms are transmitted indirectly by vehicles of infection such as milk, water, other food, and inanimate objects, including articles of clothing and eating utensils. Typhoid fever, undulant fever, tuberculosis, and diphtheria are examples of diseases in which the disease-producing organism may be transmitted through milk. Typhoid fever, dysentery, and cholera organisms are spread through water. Trichinosis, typhoid fever, dysentery, and streptococcal infections are spread through food. The most dangerous inanimate objects are those which a number of persons handle frequently. The common drinking cup, public roller towels, and improperly washed eating utensils are classic examples.

Insects and other arthropods transfer microorganisms both mechanically and biologically. Flies and cockroaches may transfer disease-producing microorganisms on their feet, appendages, or by using their entire bodies as a mechanical means. The transfer is biological when the microorganisms undergo changes within the insect vectors. Such a process occurs in the female Anopheles mosquito carrying the protozoa causing malaria; in the *Aedes aegypti* mosquito in which the development of virus takes place, producing yellow fever; or in ticks harboring the rickettsia organism responsible for Rocky Mountain spotted fever.

ENTRY OF ORGANISMS INTO THE NEW HOST

Transmission of microorganisms to the new host is in itself not sufficient to produce infection. The microorganisms must gain entrance to the body before they can grow, multiply, and produce infection. The natural openings of the body—the mouth, nose, throat, urinary tract, and intestinal tract—are the main portals of entry. Any break in the skin also opens the way for infectious agents. A cut, an abrasion, an open wound, a scratch, a bite are all means of breaking through the protective mechanism of the skin. The individual himself causes some breaks. Another person, animals, or insects are responsible for other entries. Insect diseases result from insect bites, which make possible the entrance of the infectious agents. Fortunately, most infectious agents cannot penetrate the regular surface of the skin. One exception is the hookworm, which is able to pierce the soft skin between the toes or on the back of the hand. The mucous membranes may be directly infected by the gonococcus, causing gonorrhea. This is discussed further in the section on the venereal diseases.

In some instances the portal of entry determines whether or not infection takes place. Some microorganisms are not carried to the tissues where they grow and multiply unless they enter the right portal of entry for them. A dog bite which breaks the skin and deposits the rabies virus starts the infectious process, but the rabies virus in other portals of entry, the mouth, for example, does not lead to infection. Another example is the infectious agent causing dysentery. If deposited in an open break in the skin, it does not produce disease. But if the agent gains entrance through the mouth, is swallowed, and enters the intestinal tract, infection may result. The specific organisms are highly selective relative to portals of entry. They must use a portal of entry in the body that leads to a site in the body favorable to their growth and adaptation.

SUSCEPTIBILITY OF THE HOST

When microorganisms enter the new host, the struggle between the host and the microorganisms is set in motion in a similar manner to the contest that took place in the original host. The agents of infection may live, multiply, and produce infection or disease, in which condition the host is a susceptible person lacking *resistance,* the ability to ward off disease. Or the agents may live and multiply without producing disease, with the host becoming a carrier. Or the body defenses may overcome the infectious agents, in which condition the microorganisms are killed and the body increases its power of resistance.

Important to the epidemiologist and the physician is knowledge of the incubation period. This is the time during which the infectious agent is growing, multiplying, and producing disease, or, more specifically, it is the period from the entrance of the infectious agents into the body until the development of signs and symptoms. The incubation period varies according to the specific disease. In some diseases, for instance, syphilis, the disease is communicable during the incubation period. The period of communicability is that time during which the etiologic agent can be transferred from an infected person to another host or to another source of infection.

RESISTANCE

Resistance is a relative term, indicating the power of the individual's body mechanisms to defend against the invasion of infectious agents and to ward off their effects after they have entered the body. It consists of all the body mech-

Table 11.1 Classification of some communicable diseases by common portal of entry, causative organisms, and identifying characteristics

Disease	Characteristics
I. Portal of entry: respiratory tract	
A. Caused by fungi	
1. Coccidioidomycosis	Valley fever or desert fever, may resemble influenza
2. Histoplasmosis	Darling's disease, a systemic fungus disease
B. Caused by bacteria	
1. Diphtheria	Involvement of respiratory system, characterized by production of membrane and general symptoms
2. Leprosy	Chronic disease; certain forms are moderately communicable, with lesions commonly appearing in the skin and mucous membrane of nose and mouth
3. Meningococcal meningitis	Inflammation of the meninges or coverings of the brain
4. Pertussis or whooping cough	Spasmodic attacks of coughing and characteristic whoop
5. Pneumococcal pneumonia	Pulmonary inflammation, lobar and lobular
6. Hemolytic streptococcal infections	
a. Scarlet fever	Scarlatina rash characterized by sudden onset
b. Streptococcal sore throat	Septic or epidemic sore throat, acute tonsillitis
C. Caused by viruses	
1. Chickenpox	Acute and highly communicable disease with mild constitutional symptoms, characteristic rash
2. Common cold	Acute self-limited communicable disease of the upper respiratory tract
3. Infectious encephalitis	Inflammation of the brain caused by infectious agents or their toxins
4. Influenza	Acute highly communicable disease with characteristic fever, chills, with body aches and pains, and cough. Frequently in epidemics that vary in extent and severity
5. Lymphocytic choriomeningitis	Acute communicable disease with inflammation and infiltration of the meninges
6. Measles	Rubeola, acute and highly communicable disease characterized by catarrhal symptoms, spots, and rash
7. Infectious mononucleosis	Acute communicable disease affecting lymph glands, throat, or both
8. Mumps	Acute communicable disease characterized by local swelling of one or more salivary glands
9. Primary atypical pneumonia	Virus pneumonia, acute respiratory infection characterized by pulmonary infiltration, constitutional symptoms, and a variable course
10. Poliomyelitis (portals of entry: oropharynx and gastrointestinal tract)	Infantile paralysis, acute communicable disease affecting the central nervous system, sometimes resulting in paralysis
11. Psittacosis	Parrot fever, transmissible to man from parrots

Table 11.1 Classification of some communicable diseases (continued)

Disease	Characteristics
12. Rubella	German measles, mild but highly communicable disease with typical rash
13. Smallpox	Highly communicable disease characterized by sudden onset with fever, chills, headache, backache, and prostration; rash in several stages with frequent pitting or scar formation
II. Portal of entry: gastrointestinal tract	
1. Brucellosis	Undulant fever, acute bacterial disease with irregular fever, chills, sweating, and pain in muscles and joints lasting for weeks or months
2. Epidemic diarrhea of the newborn	Infectious diarrhea or nursery diarrhea
3. Amebic dysentery	Acute or chronic infectious disease caused by a protozoan, characterized by involvement of the large intestine and discharges of blood and mucus
4. Bacillary dysentery	Acute infectious disease caused by bacteria, characterized by abdominal pain, stools containing mucus, blood, and pus
5. Food poisoning	Contamination of food with bacteria or toxins
6. Food poisoning: botulism	Ingestion of toxin of *Clostridium botulinum*, characterized by encephalitis with involvement of eye and pharynx muscles
7. Salmonellosis	Acute condition following eating of food contaminated with bacteria, characterized by cramps, nausea, vomiting, diarrhea, and fever
8. Viral hepatitis	Infection of the liver
9. Paratyphoid fever	Similar to typhoid though of shorter duration
10. Trichinosis	Acute or subacute disease caused by infestation with *Trichinella spiralis*, characterized by muscle pain and fever
11. Typhoid fever	Acute communicable disease characterized by blood-stream invasion, involvement of lymphatics of small intestine, enlarged spleen, continued fever, rose spots
III. Portal of entry: mucous membrane or skin	
A. Direct inoculation	
1. Chancroid	Acute localized infection of genital region, characterized by ulcerated lesions
2. Gonorrhea	Characterized by purulent discharge: urethra in male; cervix, vulva, fallopian tubes, urethra in female; conjunctiva and rectal mucous membrane in either sex
3. Lymphogranuloma venereum	Virus venereal disease of lymph channels and nodes, genital elephantiasis, ulceration, and rectal stricture
4. Syphilis	Chronic venereal disease; characterized by primary infection followed by recurrent secondary manifestations, latent period, and serious crippling stage

Table 11.1 Classification of some communicable diseases (continued)

Disease	Characteristics
5. Ophthalmia neonatorum	Acute infection of conjunctiva in newborn infant
B. Direct or indirect inoculation	
1. Epidemic keratoconjunctivitis	Pinkeye, acute virus disease of the cornea and conjunctiva
2. Trachoma	Granular conjunctivitis, chronic disease of cornea and conjunctiva
C. Contact infection or infestation	
1. Impetigo	Skin infection characterized by formation of vesicles and crusts
2. Granuloma inguinale	Classified as a venereal disease, granuloma process of the genital and/or inguinal region
3. Pediculosis	Infestation of humans by lice, readily transmissible
4. Ringworm	Fungus infection of the skin
5. Scabies	Skin infection caused by burrowing action of female parasite
D. Inoculation by trauma	
1. Anthrax	Acute infectious disease involving animals, transferable to man
2. Cat-scratch fever	Result of bite, lick, or scratch of a cat, characterized by lesion and fever
3. Hookworm disease	Parasitic infestation, characterized by secondary anemia
4. Leptospirosis	Weil's disease, characterized by chills, fever, headache, vomiting, muscle pain, and the like
5. Tetanus	Acute infection characterized by spasms of neck, trunk, and muscles of the extremities
6. Tularemia	Acute disease of many vertebrate hosts, a plague-like disease of rodents; may be transmitted to man
E. Inoculation by bites of insects or insectlike organisms	
1. Malaria	Acute disease caused by a pathogenic protozoan transmitted by Anopheles mosquito
2. Rickettsial diseases	
a. Epidemic typhus fever	Acute infectious disease transmitted during epidemics from man to man by body louse
b. Rocky Mountain spotted fever	Acute infectious disease transmitted to man by ticks, characterized by fever, severe headache, bodily aches, and rash
c. Q fever	Acute respiratory illness accompanied by transient pneumonia
F. Inoculation by bites of lower animals	
1. Rabies	Acute infectious disease of animals caused by virus affecting the central nervous system, transmitted occasionally to man

Source: Adapted from Franklin Top, *Communicable Diseases and Infections*, 4th ed., The C. V. Mosby Company, St. Louis, 1960; American Public Health Association, *Control of Communicable Diseases in Man*, 9th ed., The Association, New York, 1960.

anisms that prevent the progress of invading infectious agents. The body lines of defense, such as the skin, the epithelial tissues, the stickiness of mucous membranes, the cilia of the nose, and the acidity or alkalinity of parts of the digestive systems, are all part of the power of the body to defend itself against disease. In addition to these, other characteristics of the body and environment contribute to resistance. For example, the state of nutrition, endocrine balance, fatigue, chilling and exposure to temperature, age, alcohol consumption, environmental factors such as climate, geographical locale, population density, sanitation, and socioeconomic conditions are factors affecting the body's resistance to disease-producing organisms. The body defensive measures or body properties form the barriers against the infectious agents trying to gain entrance into the body.

The first line of body defense. The skin, the protective covering of the body, plays a major role in the first line of defense. Although many kinds and varieties of infectious agents are found on the skin, it prevents their spread to the inner tissues where they can grow and develop readily. In general, microorganisms are unable to penetrate the skin unless there is a break in its surface, such as a cut or wound, which forms an unnatural opening. (Hookworms already have been cited as an exception to this statement.) Logically, then, most microorganisms gain entrance to the body through the natural openings.

Other defensive measures in the first line of body defense operate at these points. Each portal of entry is protected from the attack of infectious agents by mechanical protective means. For example, mucus, a sticky, thick secretion of the mucous membranes, lines the nose, the lungs, and the digestive tract. Mucus traps microorganisms when they come in contact with its sticky solution, much like flypaper catching flies [14]. Ciliated

cells in the upper passages in the lungs and nasal passages move microorganisms to areas where other defensive measures can act upon them. For illustration, the cilia in the bronchioles of the lungs push disease-producing microorganisms upward to the pharynx, where they are swallowed and destroyed in the digestive tract. Another accessory defensive measure is the filtering out of foreign materials in the nasal cavity by hairs. These hairs, by mechanical means, keep infectious agents from penetrating into the deeper tissues of the body.

Many microorganisms are destroyed in the stomach if they have passed through the mechanical barriers. The high acid content of the gastric juice serves to destroy or retard the growth of infectious agents and thus keeps large numbers of microorganisms from entering the intestinal tract. The intestinal tract in turn rids itself of microorganisms through its discharge of waste materials. In addition, the coliform bacteria, as symbiants, are helpful and necessary in digestion. Reflexes also are accessory aids to body defense. Coughing expels microorganisms from the respiratory tract, vomiting removes infectious material from the digestive tract, and the blinking of the eyes and eye secretions protect the eyes from bacterial growth.

The second line of body defense. If microorganisms evade the mechanisms of defense constituting the first line, then other measures are called upon to prevent the development of infection. The white blood corpuscles (cells) and antibodies together constitute the second line of body defense.

White blood corpuscles, also called *leukocytes* or *phagocytes,* are amebalike cells that surround and engulf microorganisms, digesting and killing them. This process is called *phagocytosis.* The term comes from the Greek words meaning "to eat" and "hollow vessel," or "cell." Phagocytes have the ability to change their shape and move about freely in the tissues. The leukocytes and lymphocytes are types of white cells. Leukocytes are the largest of the white blood corpuscles and the most numerous, composing about 70 per cent of the white cells [14]. The lymphocytes, located in the lymph nodes, are smaller types of white cells. Fixed phagocytes are cells that line the capillaries in the liver and spleen. They are larger in size than the leukocytes.

Antibodies are chemical substances found in the blood which combat microorganisms. The exact chemical nature and the method of production of antibodies are not known. It is believed, however, that when an antigen, a foreign protein substance, is introduced into the body, it causes the body to develop its own antibodies. There are several kinds of antibodies, each of which has a specific function. The lysins, or bacteriolysins, act directly on bacteria, dissolving them. Antitoxins are antibodies that neutralize the toxin produced by bacteria, such as the diphtheria bacillus. The precipitins precipitate the toxin or foreign protein, thus taking it out of solution. The agglutinins cause bacteria to clump together, aiding the white blood corpuscles in surrounding and engulfing them. The opsonins prepare bacteria for ingestion by the white blood cells.

In some diseases the white blood corpuscles play a greater role than do the antibodies, and in others the role of the antibodies is more important. These defensive mechanisms may also play reciprocal roles. Both are vital in the defense against disease. Recent experiments indicate that, in acute bacterial infections in which the struggle between the host and the bacteria is waged in an extracellular environment, phagocytosis is highly important. Phagocytes destroy bacteria by themselves when inflammation occurs; in this instance, the strands of fibrin formed in the clotting blood plasma aid the phagocytes, and the white blood cells use these strands to trap bacteria and engulf them. When viruses, some bacteria, and a few protozoa develop within cells, in intracellular infections, phagocytes are less effective. An example of the cooperation of white blood cells and antibodies is the host's fight against penumonia. Two species of microorganisms causing acute pneumonia are the pneumococcus and Friedländer's bacillus. These agents possess capsules, which serve as an armor against phagocytes. When the capsules are removed, the microorganism is suceptible to white blood corpuscles. Strangely enough, an antigen in the microorganism's capsule stimulates the formation of antibodies. These antibodies coat the microbes, which become opsonized, and make them more desirable for the phagocytes. When they are so prepared, the phagocytes are able to engulf and kill them. These antibodies are specific and react only to these types of antigen [34]. The defense in intracellular infections and chronic infections presumably is carried out by antibodies or processes at present unknown.

Defenses outside the body. Microorganisms are killed by natural forces existing outside the body as well as through the ingenious defensive mechanisms of the body. Drying kills pathogenic organisms except spores. Sunlight is effective in killing bacteria and their spores. Ultraviolet rays are used in some controlled areas as a means of killing microorganisms. High temperatures kill pathogens, as in the pasteurization of milk. Disease-producing organisms may be killed by other organisms, for example, bacteriophages. Bacteriophages are bacterial parasites, which also kill bacteria. However, they have not proved successful as therapeutic measures for combating disease. An unfavorable environment lacking food, warmth, or moisture causes bacteria to die readily. Chemical products include the antibiotics such as penicillin, erythromycin, streptomycin, Aureomycin, bacitracin, Chloromycetin, gramicidin, neomycin, and polymyxin. The antibiotics inhibit multiplication of or kill pathogenic organisms. Carbolic acid and creosote are among the many effective chemical disinfectants.

IMMUNITY

Immunity means a high degree of resistance in the individual, resistance sufficient to protect him against the usual invasion of disease-producing organisms. Immunity means absolute protection against disease. An immune person does not develop the disease under any circumstance. However, there are very few instances when an individual has an absolute immunity. Immunity among species (species immunity) illustrates this phenomenon. Man is never infected with distemper from dogs. On the other hand, dogs do not get measles. Immunity, as a high degree of resistance, must be considered to be a relative condition. It denotes the usual protection afforded the individual against a specific disease. Immunity is specific, in contrast to resistance. Immunity depends upon the aggregate of antibodies within the individual, and his own ability to produce antibodies quickly when an infectious agent or its products or components gain entrance into his body. To immunize is to increase the body resistance for one specific disease. Immunity may be active, artificially conferred (passive), or inherited.

Active immunity. Active immunity is developed naturally as a result of an infection, with or without evidence of the disease, or artificially by inoculation of the infectious agent. Active immunity is the specific resistance attained through the body's own efforts. The body does the work of developing its own antibodies in relation to a particular disease-producing organism. An antibody generator, commonly called an *antigen,* is the factor in the invading organism, with components or products that stimulate the body to produce specific antibodies. When sufficient antibodies are produced as a result of the antigen, the individual has developed his own immunity. This active immunity is relatively permanent. The exact duration of immunity is relative to the specific disease.

When immunity is acquired, whether as a reaction to infection or disease, the body develops sufficient antibodies to resist other attacks of this organism. Examples of diseases producing an active immunity through an attack of the disease are typhoid fever, scarlet fever, whooping cough, plague, smallpox, chickenpox, measles, German measles, mumps, poliomyelitis, and yellow fever.

Active immunity is attained artificially by injecting into the body modified organisms or their products. This modification occurs when the virulence of the disease-producing organism is attenuated (weakened), when the organism is killed, or when the effect of its product is reduced. In each case the virulence of the organism is weakened; yet the antibody-stimulating power still remains. The body produces its own antibodies, and an active immunity results.

The virulence of organisms may be reduced by many methods. Pasteur discovered one method when he inoculated fowls with old cultures of chicken cholera bacteria. Dried spinal cords of infected rabbits were found to have lost their pathogenicity; yet they provided immunity when introduced into a susceptible animal. Viruses may be weakened when cultivated in an unnatural host. For example, a strain of yellow fever virus was attenuated for man by introducing it into and through mice, and then it was used for human immunization. A second yellow fever virus strain was transferred through many tissue cultures, so that it became sufficiently attenuated for human inoculation, and is in widespread use today.

Injection of killed organisms is a

means of stimulating active immunity against many diseases. Phenol, formaline acetone, and merthiolate are widely used as killing agents. Heat is sometimes used; however, it may also diminish the immunizing power.

A potent immunizing agent may be derived from bacterial endotoxins and exotoxins. A combination of antitoxin produced in horses with the toxin to neutralize the lethal effect of the toxin renders it safe for immunization. Toxoids are toxins made nontoxic by heat, treated with formaldehyde, or precipitated by alum. Alum-precipitated substances are released slowly from the subcutaneous tissues and accomplish the same results as multiple injections of unprecipitated materials.

Passive immunity. Passive immunity may be produced either naturally as the mother transfers antibodies to the unborn child or artificially by inoculation of specific protective antibodies such as convalescent or immune serum or gammaglobulin. Passive immunity provides a high type of resistance but only for a short time—a few weeks or months. It may be referred to as the process of acquiring antibodies formed in another individual or animal. The tissues of the person receiving the immunity play no part in producing this degree of resistance.

Natural passive immunity is conferred to the child during the prenatal period, when the immune bodies in the mother's blood are transferred to the blood of the child by osmosis.

The widest use of artificial passive immunization is in the prevention and/or treatment of diphtheria, tetanus, gas gangrene, botulism, and scarlet fever. Antitoxin is manufactured by inoculating animals, usually horses, with the respective toxins or toxoids. Persons exposed to one of the above bacterial diseases may prevent or modify its development with prophylactic doses of antitoxin. Active immunization is given to fortify the temporary protection when possible. Antitoxin also is given as treatment to individuals with active cases of the disease. When it is administered early in the course of the disease, the antitoxin is effective in bringing about a rapid recovery. Passive protection is induced by transfusion of blood from a convalescent patient or by introduction of human immune globulin. This means of borrowing antibodies is a temporary protective measure against measles, infectious hepatitis, and poliomyelitis, to mention a few diseases.

Inherited immunity. The exact role of heredity in immunity is not definitely understood. Also, there is a confusion of terms used to describe this type of immunity. It is referred to as "natural immunity," as "nonsusceptibility," and as "inherited insusceptibility." Whichever term is desired, the important fact is that this type of immunity results from factors already present within the individual and is not due to any external stimulus. A previous reference has been made to natural immunity in which antibodies are present in the blood of the newborn. This immunity appears to decrease to a low concentration in the infant, and a higher concentration is developed in childhood lasting sometimes through to early adulthood.

Man has a natural or inherited immunity to many animal diseases. This is species immunity, previously mentioned on page 318. For example, man is not susceptible to infection from certain animal pathogens causing chicken cholera, canine distemper, and cattle plague. At the same time animals are immune to many human diseases, including measles, gonorrhea, syphilis, influenza, mumps, and whooping cough. The turtle does not develop tetanus, and the rabbit never has typhoid because the typhoid bacilli do not grow extensively within the animal's body.

Races within a species also possess a natural immunity to disease. For example, some authorities believe that American Indians and Negroes are more susceptible to tuberculosis than are white men. At the same time, the Negro is immune to malaria and yellow fever to a greater degree than members of the white race [35]. Natural racial immunity is believed to be established through natural selection, by which the susceptible die off in each generation, while the immune survive and reproduce. Natural individual immunity, that with which one is born, depends upon personal inheritance.

Methods of prevention and control

Charles E. Smith, Dean of the School of Public Health, University of California, describes the control measures of disease in terms of "the bridge between source and susceptible." In his discussion, he cites an epidemiologic analogy used by Neil McKinnon, of the Toronto School of Hygiene. In this analogy the infectious process is compared to two people on opposite sides of a stream with a bridge between them. The person on one side of the stream represents the source of infection. The person on the other side is the susceptible person. For disease to occur, infectious agents must escape from the source, make their way across the bridge, and enter and become established in the susceptible person [15, 33]. Successful control comes from finding the weakest link in the infectious cycle and applying effective measures. With this principle in mind, prevention and control measures can be directed at three points: eliminating the source of infection, breaking the lines of communication across the bridge, and protecting the susceptible and developing immunity, if possible.

ELIMINATING THE SOURCE OF INFECTION

If the source of infection for a communicable disease is known, the source may be destroyed or made noninfectious. Only in a few diseases can the source be destroyed completely. Bovine tuberculosis, plague, tularemia, anthrax, and rabies are examples [15]. The next alternative, applying to human sources, requires less drastic steps. In the first place, the disease must be reported to the health officer by the attending physician. Where no physician is available, any citizen can report the disease to the health department. Prompt reporting enables the health department personnel to muster all current knowledge about the source of the disease and to initiate control procedures immediately. A fence is built around the infected person by isolating him.

Isolation means separating the infected person from other persons for the period of communicability in order to prevent spread of the infectious agent to others.

In addition, the individual may be made noninfectious by treatment, as in the case of syphilis and gonorrhea by using antibiotics. The flow of infectious agents from the infected to the susceptible is stopped by means of disinfection. In concurrent disinfection, infectious material is disinfected as it is being produced or as soon as it is discharged from the infected individual. For example, paper tissues are used for nose and mouth discharges of tubercular patients, and these tissues are dropped into a paper disposal bag and then burned. Also, terminal disinfection is undertaken when the individual ceases to produce infectious material. Thus, when the tubercular patient ceases to produce tuberculosis bacilli, his personal belongings and inanimate objects within the physical environment are disinfected [4]. Burning, boiling, heating to a high temperature, scrubbing with hot, soapy water, sunning or exposing to light rays, and using chemicals are appropriate means of disinfection.

Quarantine means limiting the freedom of movement of persons exposed or suspected of exposure to communicable disease for the period of communicability. This includes any known contacts, members of the family, and any other exposed persons. The health department has specific rules for the length of the quarantine period, depending upon the particular disease. Recently, some health departments have liberalized quarantine regulations for contacts. Quarantine has been dropped in the case of whooping cough, with greater emphasis on isolation of the patient. Quarantine of poliomyelitis contacts has been modified from strict regulation to one left up to the judgment of the local health officer. A periodically revised guide for health departments in developing their regulations is the American Public Health Association publication, *The Control of Communicable Diseases in Man* [4].

New medical discoveries have added to the effectiveness of controlling sources of infection. Owing to contagious atypical cases, missed cases, and various carrier states, source control alone is not enough. Attack on disease must be taken from other points as well.

BREAKING THE LINES OF COMMUNICATION

Cutting the lines of communication from the source of infection to the host is an effective means of controlling the spread of disease. Such control is comparable to destroying the bridge crossing the stream between the source of infection and the susceptible person. Measures for cutting communication include purifying the water supply, sanitation of sewage and wastes, protection of food and milk supplies, and the destruction of intermediate hosts.

A general control measure is purifying the water supply. This procedure protects against the infectious agents carried by water that cause the water-borne diseases. Typhoid, paratyphoid, Asiatic cholera, and dysentery are examples. Water is purified slowly through plain sedimentation, an effect of the rate of flow by which many suspended materials settle to the bottom. Chemicals may be added to the water to coagulate the solid materials and speed sedimentation. Lake and reservoir waters are filtered as a means of removing bacteria. Small amounts of water can be disinfected by boiling for ten minutes or can be sterilized in thirty minutes [5]. The use of chlorine in the water is a standard means of disinfecting water for large-scale use.

Proper sewage disposal is an important means of controlling the spread of intestinal diseases. In rural areas sanitary excreta disposal consists in emptying wastes into a pit privy of 6-foot depth or in employing a septic tank, which is buried underground and has an adequate water supply under pressure [15]. Local and state health departments and the U.S. Public Health Service provide detailed plans for the construction of these sewage-disposal units. Urban communities use modern sewage-disposal plants employing physical, chemical, and natural devices for treating waste materials.

Means of breaking the line of communication for rat-borne diseases are ratproofing buildings, eliminating food and trash, placing circular metal disks on ropes mooring ships to docks, and destroying rats by poisoning, trapping, and fumigation [15].

The line of communication for diseases caused by metazoa is broken comparatively easily; thus trichinae are killed in pork when it is thoroughly

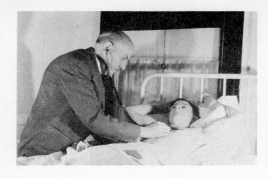

The source of infection is the individual harboring the disease-producing organisms. These agents are transmitted from him to others by any of several means. Below are examples of some agents and a few of the everyday situations in which transmission occurs.

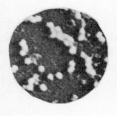
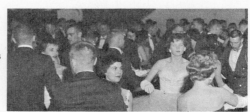

Influenza viruses are transmitted through direct contact.

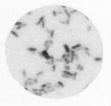
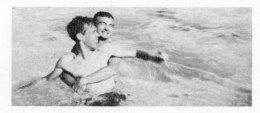

E. Coli are bacteria found in polluted water.

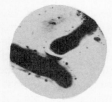
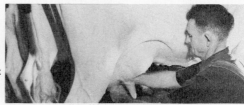

Bacilli causing tuberculosis may be transmitted through the milk supply.

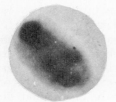
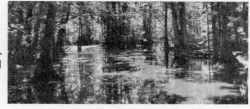

Rickettsiae, carried by ticks, serve as an example of organisms transmitted by insects.

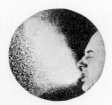
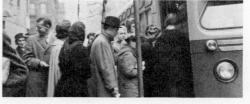

Cold viruses can be transmitted through the air.

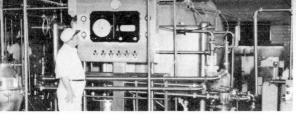

Cutting lines of communication from the source of infection to the susceptible person is important in controlling the spread of disease. Pasteurization is an example of an effective means. Other examples are shown below.

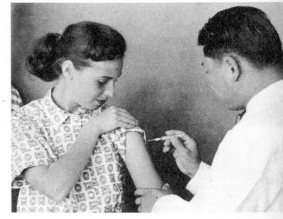

When immunizations have proved successful, they are the most effective measure for protecting the susceptible person.

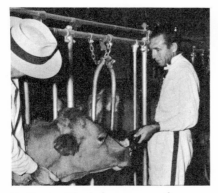

The line of communication may be broken by immunization or by isolating the source of infection . . .

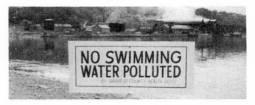

or by keeping the susceptible person away from the disease-bearing agent.

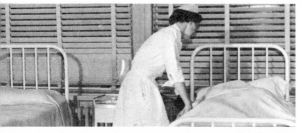

Testing cattle helps assure the community that disease is not being transmitted through its food supply.

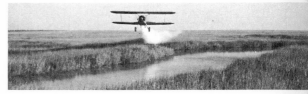

The line of communication may be cut by destruction of the vector and agent.

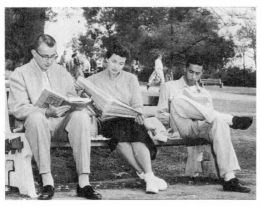

Rest, fresh air, recreation, and good eating contribute to a state of general good health.

Table 11.2   Schedules for immunization to communicable diseases

Disease	Immunization	Infants and Preschool	Children, 5–15
		Immunizations commonly used	
Smallpox	Active: attenuated virus, cowpox virus (calf lymph)	Vaccination during first year, preferably 12–14 months, either before DPT or at the time of last dose in series. Can be given at time of first dose of DPT-polio primary series.	Primary inoculation at any time. Revaccinate every 5 years, or at any time when exposed or during epidemic.
Diphtheria-pertussis-tetanus (DPT), with polio (either separate or combined)	Active: multiple or combined antigens; polio combined or separate	Starting at 1 to 2 months, four monthly intramuscular injections. Separate polio dose in different site. If series after six months, three injections only. If delay in giving an injection, no need to repeat previous injections.	First booster about 1 year after initial series (separate polio vaccine). Second booster at school entry. Third booster may be given at age 10 if pertussis prevalent.
Tetanus-diphtheria for adults, with polio (either separate or combined)	Active: multiple or combined antigens; polio combined or separate		If no previous tetanus-diphtheria immunization, two injections for those over 10 years of age.
Poliomyelitis (separate)	Active: Salk type of vaccine	At 2 months begin three injections with DPT at monthly intervals. Booster at 4-year intervals.	Booster 12 months after third injection. Subsequent boosters on advice of physician and new findings.
	Active: new Sabin type of oral attenuated-virus vaccine	Schedules not yet reported. Proposed immunization of all newborn babies, and community-wide immunization of largest possible number of susceptible persons; everyone under 40, during months of November to June.	
Measles (rubeola)	Enders attenuated Edmonston strain live-virus vaccine	Schedules not yet reported. Field trials proved effectiveness.	
	Passive: gamma-globulin; human immune serum globulin	Especially for children under 3 years. Not desirable for children above 3 years unless weak or suffering from another disease. Given within 6 days of exposure.	

Adults	Effectiveness
Same as previous column	Very effective
Tetanus-diphtheria for adults from 10 years on for boosters, as needed	Very effective
First booster 1 year after initial series; separate polio booster; subsequent boosters at 5- to 10-year intervals throughout life at same time as smallpox revaccination	Effective
Same as previous column	Effective
Same as previous column	Very effective
Same as previous column	
	Temporary protection

cooked, and hookworm cannot penetrate the feet if shoes are worn.

PROTECTING THE SUSCEPTIBLE

Destroying the bridge between the infected person and the susceptible host is only a partial answer, as was the case in source, or reservoir, control. Unfortunately, it is not always possible to control communicable diseases by cutting lines of communication. Therefore attention must be given to the third aspect of prevention and control: protecting the susceptible. The susceptible person can isolate himself, change his environment by leaving the area, use available protective devices, and increase his resistance.

The susceptible person can build a screen around himself to keep out flies, mosquitoes, and other insects, but this, too, is only a temporary, partially successful protective measure. He can run away from communicable diseases by traveling to other parts of the country or the world. However, disease-producing organisms know no boundary lines. With present-day means of transportation, no part of the world can be isolated completely, free from invasion by microorganisms. Quarantine at seaports and airports does aid in limiting the spread of infection, since it serves as a protective line of defense around geographical areas. In actuality, quarantine is more of a filter than an impregnable protective covering for the susceptible.

Immunization. The most effective protective measure for the susceptible host is increasing resistance through the body's defensive mechanism. This process changes a susceptible into an immune person. Though it is not possible to immunize against all communicable diseases, the list of diseases for which immunization can be obtained is steadily growing in number. Diseases against which the individual can be protected by either passive or active immunity are given in Table 11.2.

Table 11.2   Schedules for immunization to communicable diseases (continued)

Disease	Immunization	Infants and Preschool	Children, 5–15
		Immunizations commonly used (continued)	
Diphtheria	Active: alum-precipitated (ppt) toxoid or alum absorbed Passive: antitoxin	Suggested immunization: beginning at 3 months. Booster at 1 year or 18 months.	Previously inoculated: booster dose. Not previously inoculated: primary inoculation.
Pertussis (whooping cough)	Active: alum ppt or alum hydroxide absorbed	During epidemic: at 1–2 months at monthly intervals. Booster 1 year after and at 3 years.	Previously inoculated: booster dose. Not previously inoculated: primary inoculation; not advised after age 5.
Tetanus	Active: alum-ppt toxoid	Suggest multiple antigen preparation at age 3 months. Singly, two doses toxoid 1 month apart. Booster at 3 years and after injury.	Previously inoculated: booster dose at 3-year intervals and after injury. Not previously inoculated: two doses 1 month apart.
	Passive: antitoxin	Not used if person immunized as above.	
		Immunizations less commonly used	
Cholera	Active: killed spirilla	Mandatory for travel to or through many parts of the world; also for military service personnel and their dependents.	
Hepatitis, infectious	Passive: gamma-globulin	Of special value in epidemics, and in household contacts.	
Influenza	Active: virus weakened from chick embryos or killed by formaldehyde; polyvalent vaccine	Not generally recommended for infants and children under 12; annually at 12 years of age and over.	
Measles, German (rubella)	Passive: gamma-globulin		
Mumps	Active: attenuated virus, also killed virus	Not advocated at present.	
Plague	Active: attenuated virus, killed bacilli	Desirable for those traveling or residing in plague-infested areas.	
	Passive: antiplague serum		

Adults	Effectiveness
Toxoid if Schick test is positive	Very effective preventive measure Very effective at all ages; rarely used
Primary or booster inoculation not advised	Effective for appropriate ages
Same as previous column	Very effective protection
	Very effective after injury or exposure at all ages
Same as previous column	Of value, not absolute protection, temporary protection only; booster injections required every 4–6 months.
Same as previous column	Effective protection to those exposed; 6–8 weeks' protection
Annually for individuals or selected groups; two injections 2 months apart completed by November; booster each fall	Valuable only against specific strain or strains of virus; 60–75 per cent effective
For women exposed during first trimester of pregnancy	Doubtful and unpredictable, primarily prophylaxis; of little value
Suggested for physicians, nurses, and military personnel	Not widely used
Same as previous column	Temporary protection; reimmunization may be required every 6 months where plague is current hazard Temporary (3 weeks)

Effective control through immunization is possible for diphtheria, influenza (specific for epidemic strain), whooping cough, plague, poliomyelitis, rabies, Rocky Mountain spotted fever, smallpox, tetanus, typhoid, typhus, yellow fever, and measles.

New vaccines and other antigens for active immunizations against communicable diseases are continually being developed and improved. The most commonly employed vaccines or toxoids are applied against smallpox, diphtheria, pertussis (whooping cough), tetanus, and poliomyelitis. New protection is offered in multiple vaccines as in diphtheria, pertussis, tetanus, and poliomyelitis vaccine.

The new Sabin oral attenuated-virus vaccine against poliomyelitis has been tested successfully in field trials in Russia and in the United States and approved by the U.S. Public Health Service. It was expected to be manufactured and marketed by drug companies in 1962. However, this was delayed by Public Health Service standards until the manufacturer could prove no nonpoliomyelitis viruses were present in the vaccine. No such standard was required in the mass immunizations in Russia. The Sabin vaccine is expected to be less expensive, easier to administer, more effective, and longer lasting than the Salk vaccine. It is believed by some immunologists that this vaccine will completely wipe out poliomyelitis, which may be the first disease to be absolutely controlled.

The new Enders live-virus vaccine for measles has passed the severest tests. This new vaccine should prove effective for both children and adults providing an effective active immunization. A new adenovirus vaccine has been used but has been limited primarily to immunizing military recruits. It has proved to be about 90 per cent effective in this group. Immunization has lowered the incidence of influenza and has made it possible to prevent widespread epidemics. BCG con-

Table 11.2 Schedules for immunization to communicable diseases (continued)

Disease	Immunization	Infants and Preschool	Children, 5–15
		Immunizations less commonly used (continued)	
Q fever	Active	Not generally available.	
Rabies	Active: killed or atten-uated virus; Pasteur; Semple methods; hy-perimmune serum in severe exposure	Recommended when person is bitten by dog or other animal suspected of having rabies. Unless bitten on face or neck, vaccination delayed until animal ob-served for 10 days after bite; if animal is still alive, Pasteur treatment is unnecessary.	
Rocky Mountain spotted fever	Active: killed rickettsiae	Recommended for all individuals going into tick-infested areas where Rocky Mountain spotted fever is known to occur.	
Scarlet fever	Active: increasing doses of toxin (weakened) Passive: antitoxin, con-valescent serum	Not advocated for general community protection.	
Tuberculosis	Active: bacillus Cal-mette-Guerin (BCG), attenuated bacilli	World-wide program of mass vaccination promoted by World Health Organization. Desirability of use is controversial. Recommended for high-risk groups only in U.S.	
Typhoid and paratyphoid	Active: killed bacilli	Recommended in an epidemic or when residing or visit-ing in areas where diseases are prevalent.	
Typhus (louse-borne or flea-borne)	Active: attenuated vi-rus; for cow-type vaccine from chick embryo; for killed rickettsiae	Recommended for persons in contact with cases; may be offered to entire community.	
Yellow fever	Active: attenuated vi-rus, modified by growth on chick em-bryo	Mandatory for travel to or through many parts of the world; also for military service personnel and their dependents. Vaccination required every 6 years.	

Source: Based on data from American Public Health Association, *Control of Com-municable Diseases in Man*, 9th ed., The Association, New York, 1960; William C. Boyd, *Fundamentals of Immunology*, 3d ed., Interscience Publishers, Inc., New York, 1956; Howard F. Conn, *Current Therapy*, W. B. Saunders Company, Philadelphia,

tinues to be used for tuberculosis only with high-risk groups and is not recom-mended for mass immunizations in the United States. A search for a better vac-cine against tuberculosis still goes on in an attempt to find the ideal type, which will protect positive reactors (BCG does not) as well as those negative to the tuberculin test. Numerous immunizations are classed as less commonly used ones because they are not necessary except for persons traveling to or living in a par-ticular section. Rocky Mountain spotted fever and yellow fever are good ex-amples.

Prophylactic measures. The susceptible individual may be protected from de-veloping a disease, or the severity of attack may be lessened, by prompt pro-phylactic measures after the organisms have invaded the body. The use of

Adults	Effectiveness
For laboratory workers	Effective measure
Same as previous column	Effective measure
Same as previous column	Very effective protection
	Not widely used
	Effective for short period Not widely used
Same as previous column	Protection not complete
Same as previous column	Effective measure
Same as previous column	Effective though not absolute; prevalence and severity reduced; immunization seasonally and in presence of disease
Same as previous column	Very effective

1960 and 1961 editions; Franklin H. Top, *Communicable Diseases and Infections*, 4th ed., C. V. Mosby Company, St. Louis, 1960.

chemicals to prevent disease is a chemoprophylactic method of prevention. Atabrine taken by the susceptible individual protects against the malaria protozoan. Silver nitrate solution or appropriate antibiotic, such as penicillin, applied to the eyes of the newborn baby is highly effective against the gonococcus. The sulfonamides are a chemotherapeutic preventive and control measure against some diseases. They are effective against the pneumococci and the streptococci of meningitis. Specific serums are another prophylactic measure. For example, antitoxin may be given soon after exposure to diphtheria. Gamma-globulin (as well as the vaccine) administered after exposure to measles provides an effective protection. Gamma-globulin also is of special value against infectious hepatitis after exposure.

Antibiotics. Comparatively few antibiotics are effective in controlling disease, although the number is growing rapidly. Even the medical profession has difficulty keeping up with the new antibiotics, and for this reason only a few examples are given here. Penicillin, although very sensitizing, is one of the least toxic and most useful antibiotics. It is administered to combat pneumococci, streptococci, staphylococci, gonococci, and the spirochete of syphilis.

Streptomycin is successful against tularemia and against secondary bacterial infections occurring with pneumonia. It is most widely used against tuberculosis bacilli, although it is not absolutely effective against tuberculosis and it does produce a toxic effect on the nervous system. Less toxic is a variety identified as dihydrostreptomycin.

Chloromycetin is preferred to overcome the typhoid bacillus and the rickettsial infections, such as Q fever and Rocky Mountain spotted fever. Aureomycin, with its great penetrating power, is applied against rickettsial diseases, coccal bacterial diseases, and spirochetes that are resistant to penicillin. Terramycin, another drug produced from the Streptomyces earth molds, is proving effective against chancroid, amebiasis, brucellosis, and some rheumatic diseases. Two useful antibiotics made from bacteria are tyrothricin, used as an antiseptic in bandages and dressings and for upper-respiratory-tract infections, and bacitracin, for wound infections and upper-respiratory-tract infections.

Personal health and resistance. The susceptible individual can contribute to his powers of resistance by promoting and maintaining his general health. Proper diet, adequate sleep and rest, appropriate exercise, fresh air, and sunshine aid in developing general resistance to disease. Such resistance is of considerable importance against disease-producing agents causing pneumonia, tuberculosis, some streptococci infections, and some intestinal infections [15]. Nevertheless, the utilization of immunizations for specific diseases is paramount for increasing individual resistance.

Health education of children, youth, and adults through educational experiences in schools, colleges, and universities and in the community contributes to the prevention and control of communicable diseases. Scientific knowledge of control measures, together with positive attitudes and practices, is necessary for intelligent action. Cooperative action on the part of the individual citizen, the private physician, and the personnel of official and voluntary health agencies is the means by which successful prevention and control programs are made possible.

Some diseases pertinent to the college group

Space in this college health science text does not provide for a complete description of each communicable disease and the essential factors for controlling it. However, the basic principles and methods of preventing and controlling disease have been presented. These may be applied to any disease. A classification of common communicable diseases with a brief identifying description is included for general information in outline form in Table 11.1. For a fuller treatment of the reportable communicable diseases, the student is directed to the Suggested readings, particularly No. 4. In this informative handbook, each communicable disease is discussed in terms of means of identification, causative agent, source and reservoir of infection, mode of transmission, incubation period, period of communicability, susceptibility and resistance, occurrence, and methods of control.

A more detailed description of selected diseases pertinent to the college group is presented here. The diseases discussed are selected from studies of health needs and interests. Sutton's [2] study of health

needs shows that tuberculosis, the respiratory diseases (colds, influenza, pneumonia), and skin diseases are of great concern to the college age group. Recently, reports from student health services have indicated the increase and current prevalence of mononucleosis and infectious hepatitis. Lantagne's [3] study of health interests of college students reports that the venereal diseases ranked eighth out of 300 health topics, while poliomyelitis appeared twenty-third. The current upswing in venereal disease makes this of real concern. Pneumonia still ranks as a major cause of death. These relatively few diseases serve to illustrate the common diseases affecting the college age group.

TUBERCULOSIS

Tuberculosis clearly illustrates the present-day concept of prevention and control of communicable disease. In attacking this disease it is particularly important to know all the factors involved in relation to the agent of disease, the host, and the environment. Tuberculosis is definitely on the decline, yet it is still a

[2] Wilfred C. Sutton, "Determining the Health Needs of College Students," unpublished doctoral dissertation, University of California, Los Angeles, 1954.

[3] Joseph Lantagne, "An Analysis of Health Interests of 1,000 Junior College Students in California," *Junior College Journal*, 21:429–433, April, 1951.

serious disease. There has been a reduction in the number of cases among children and young adults and a marked drop in deaths from the disease, yet the average number of deaths for the past several years has been over 14,000 persons. Of the 178 million Americans on Jan. 1, 1960, 36 million were infected with tuberculosis. It is estimated that 156,000 new active cases will develop during 1960–1964 from the 20 per cent of the nation's population that is believed to be infected. Some 52,000 new cases will come from those who were not infected during this same period. Both the case rates and the death rates among nonwhites are nearly three times the rates among whites. Nonwhites make up one-tenth of the population and produce one-fourth of new active cases.[4]

Strangely enough, it is estimated that half the newly reported active cases of tuberculosis are in persons under 45 years of age. The Public Health Service estimates 2.2 million persons under 25 are infected. Also, 18 per cent of new active cases were in persons under 25. This number is important, because some of these young persons will break down and show active tuberculosis; they will be a source for new infections in the future. Stopping the infection among young persons will speed up the permanent elimination of the disease.[5]

Gertrude Huberty, M.D., Associate Physician, Student Health Service, University of California, Los Angeles, studied the problem of tuberculosis among college students. She found the incidence of active and arrested cases has dropped off sharply in the past twenty years. This decline in incidence of tuberculosis is no indication for relaxation of vigilance against the disease. It is estimated that about 10 per cent of the college population now harbor tubercle bacilli somewhere in their bodies [21]. In some of

these cases the disease will develop into active form during the college period. Vigilance also must be maintained against incoming students, new faculty, and other personnel who may have active cases. Huberty's findings in 1962 indicate that positive tuberculin reactors among foreign-born students appear to be approximately as high as 50 per cent. Also, it is evident that as the age of individuals increases, the percentage of positive reactors increases.

Tuberculosis may be spread as long as there is one person with the disease in a contagious form. Despite the tremendous gains made in controlling the disease, including the marked reduction in incidence and mortality, tuberculosis remains a major health problem throughout the world. This is due largely to its communicable nature and the vital importance of careful medical supervision and treatment of the infected person. It is predicted, however, that tuberculosis can be wiped out in the future if the present battle is continued on all fronts. National, state, and local tuberculosis associations are leading the fight through education, service, and research programs.

Recognition of tuberculosis. In primary or first infection, the tuberculosis bacillus causes a small lesion, or "spot," in the lung tissue after an incubation period of a month or more. The organism spreads to the lymph glands, causing them to enlarge and become inflamed. Often the infection is stopped at this point, as the host's resistance establishes an equilibrium with the tuberculosis bacilli.

In some cases resistance is not sufficient even early in the disease to bring about an equilibrium with the agent, and the bacilli travel in the blood or lymph stream to other parts of the body. Tubercles develop at these points. This traveling, or galloping, type of tuberculosis is called *miliary tuberculosis,* meaning that milletlike lesions are established throughout the body. Generally,

---

[4] Report of the Arden House Conference on Tuberculosis, *T.B. Control: The Big Push Ahead,* The National Tuberculosis Association, 1960, p. 17.
[5] *Ibid.,* pp. 7–9.

this primary type of tuberculosis heals itself without treatment. However, the invader may overcome the body defenses, and the disease then progresses to destructive pulmonary tuberculosis, and possibly death.

Reinfection tuberculosis, or the adult type, varies from insignificant tubercles, that do not progress, to a severe disease with great destruction of the lungs, which frequently results' in death. Reinfection occurs rarely when infected sputum is inhaled into the lungs, and more frequently when the bacilli from an infected gland invade a bronchial tube or bacilli from a lesion proceed into a blood vessel. This spread of the infective agent may also result in complications such as pleurisy and laryngitis. A state may develop in which the disease is active but not readily apparent for many years. The person with such a case belongs in a hospital or a sanitarium where he receives the best care and treatment and cannot spread the infection to others.

Tuberculosis can infect all the tissues and organs of the body. The most common site of infection is the lungs, which is characteristic of pulmonary tuberculosis. Other forms include tuberculosis of the bones and joints and of the intestines, kidneys, and meninges. Tuberculosis also attacks animals, as in bovine tuberculosis. Bovine tuberculosis is well controlled now in the United States by means of tuberculin testing of cattle, destruction of infected animals, and sanitary handling and pasteurization of milk.

Control of tuberculosis is aimed at three vital points, previously developed under Methods of Prevention and Control. These are discussed below.

Eliminating the source of infection. The source, or reservoir, of infection is both human and animal, the human source being by far the greater. The attack on the source is threefold:

Discovering patients as soon as possible after they become infectious by means of tuberculin testing, X-ray examinations, and routine examinations of contacts

Prompt placement of patients in institutions that provide isolation facilities for as long as the individuals remain infectious

Prompt and adequate treatment to make patients noninfectious; improved medical and surgical methods of treatment are important

All three measures of control must be utilized.

Cutting lines of communication. Transmission of tuberculosis occurs largely through continuous and intimate direct contact such as is characteristic of family relationships. Droplet infection through the air by means of coughing, sneezing, talking, and the like is considered a common method of transmission. Lines of communication can be cut by the following methods:

Isolating tuberculosis patients from susceptibles

Using good personal health practices, such as covering the mouth and nose with a handkerchief when sneezing or coughing and refraining from spitting in public places

Rinsing and scalding with hot soapy water dishes and other utensils handled by the infected person

Eliminating silica dust in quantities in industrial plants

Pasteurizing milk and milk products

Protecting the susceptible. The susceptible can be protected through specific measures as well. It is essential to provide healthy environmental conditions, such as good housing, adequate nutrition, suitable occupations, and freedom from physical and mental strain, and to furnish health education to children, youth, and adults.

Another method which may protect is the use of BCG to attempt to immunize the especially susceptible groups, such as doctors, medical students, nurses, hospital and laboratory personnel, and individuals in the tuberculosis patient's family who are naturally exposed, as well as persons in communities where tuberculosis is especially prevalent. BCG vaccine consists of a living culture of bovine tubercle baccilli of greatly diminished virulence. A world-wide program of mass vaccination is being promoted by the World Health Organization under the leadership of Danish investigators. It is estimated that some 60 million persons throughout the world have been vaccinated with BCG.

There are definitely two points of view regarding the use of BCG. The group that favors it believes that experience, observations, and a few well-controlled studies justify its use. They state that BCG vaccine under acceptable conditions administered to tuberculin-negative persons can be considered harmless. A relative degree of resistance to tuberculosis results from the vaccination. Protection is not complete, and it is not permanent. The incidence of tuberculosis is from four to seven times as prevalent among unvaccinated controls as among comparable groups who were vaccinated.

The other group, widely supported in the United States, believes that BCG vaccination has too many objections against it. For example, it destroys the value of tuberculin testing as a diagnostic means and as an index of tuberculosis control. Reliance on vaccination may result in the neglect of more effective tuberculosis control such as case finding and proper treatment. Treatment of childhood tuberculosis is so effective that mass vaccination is not needed with the relatively ineffective type of immunity resulting from the use of BCG [21].

An important need is for an improved vaccine that produces a greater immunity than BCG. Therefore, continued research is vital if the susceptible are to be fully protected.

Treatment. If control measures are ineffective and tuberculosis does develop, it is now possible to attack the tubercle bacilli directly with chemotherapy. Such treatment is best carried out where maximum facilities and expert medical care are available. It is still best provided in the hospital or sanitarium. When the patient's condition is satisfactorily stabilized, the period of hospitalization may be modified for some cases with home care. This needs to be carefully coordinated with hospital care during active stages of the disease. Of course, continuous supervision by a well-trained physician is essential. Adequate nursing care is vital too for effective recovery. Standard treatment includes bed rest in combination with prolonged chemotherapy. It is estimated now that, in an active case discovered at college in the early stages, proper treatment can be so effective that the student loses but one semester of college work. It is possible that he may return to the campus after the one semester's absence and continue under chemotherapy treatment. Such treatment changes the disease from a communicable to a noncommunicable state.

A plan of action to eradicate tuberculosis. A most significant conference to develop a plan of action for the eradication of tuberculosis was held at Arden House, Harriman, New York, Nov. 29–Dec. 2, 1959. This conference, called the Arden House Conference, was sponsored by the U.S. Public Health Service and the National Tuberculosis Association. Conferees were confident that with a sound plan and bold and decisive action tuberculosis could be completely wiped out in the near future. Some of their major recommendations include the following:

Treatment is the tool to make the big push ahead and control tuberculosis effectively. This calls for a widespread application of chemotherapy to sterilize the important part of the reservoir of tubercle bacilli that exists in the country in persons with active disease and those who have had active disease and were inadequately treated. Adequate treatment should be assured for all persons through the cooperative efforts of public health authorities and private physicians.

The tuberculosis control program should concentrate on those segments of the population which present the greatest tuberculosis problem.

Detection programs must be evaluated periodically to obtain maximum results.

Laboratory services must be provided so all physicians diagnosing and treating patients will have these essential services.

The criteria for the use of BCG vaccine are reaffirmed. It is important to overcome the differences in standards in using this vaccine in various countries. Also, the search for a better vaccine should continue.

A new skin test must be developed to detect new cases of tuberculosis. It should be one that can be applied and read by nonmedical personnel.

Recognition of the importance of current isoniazid prophylaxis is acknowledged, but a significant shortcut to eliminate tuberculosis is necessary so that greater effectiveness of the drug can be achieved or better drugs developed.

Expanded social research is needed to permit investigation of the social, psychological, and cultural factors affecting the incidence, detection, treatment, and rehabilitation of tuberculosis cases.

The challenge to eliminate tuberculosis is now more clearly apparent than ever before because of the Arden Conference [30].

MONONUCLEOSIS

Infectious mononucleosis, formerly called glandular fever, is now referred to as the "students' disease." On some college campuses it is called the "college disease."

It appears to be most prevalent in the age group seventeen to twenty-five, where indiscriminate kissing is characteristic of dating and courtship. Intimate oral contact and drinking from a common bottle are means of transmitting infectious mononucleosis. In actuality, it is by no means confined to college environments.

It is an acute communicable disease characterized by fever, sore throat, swelling of the lymph glands, fatigue, and loss of vitality. The symptoms frequently are vague and may resemble those of other communicable diseases, including the common cold. The causative organism is unknown, although a virus is suspected.

Little is known about the incubation period (probably varying between 4 and 11 days) and the period of communicability. A laboratory test of the blood serum and the white blood cells is necessary for the physician to make the diagnosis.

It is interesting to note that the disease does not spread throughout the general population in various age groups. It may strike one person in a family while other members of the family do not come down with clinical evidence of the disease. It is thought that perhaps other family members may have it in a mild form that does not produce disease signs or symptoms. It is possible, too, that such persons may be carriers of the disease.

Mononucleosis does not usually produce complications. However, there is always the danger of serious effects on the body unless there is early diagnosis and early treatment. The liver, the lungs, or the central nervous system may become involved, with symptoms such as headache, stiff neck, blurring of vision, and mental confusion. A typical skin rash over the trunk of the body has been reported. Jaundice symptoms indicate liver involvement. In such instances it is difficult to distinguish between mononucleosis and infectious hepatitis. As far as is known, these effects do not seem to

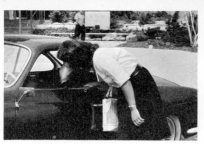

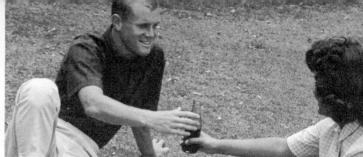

Although the complete nature of mononucleosis, the "students' disease," is not yet fully understood, it is known to be most prevalent in the age group seventeen to twenty-five, where indiscriminate kissing . . .

or other less direct forms of oral contact are likely to occur.

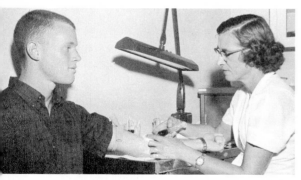

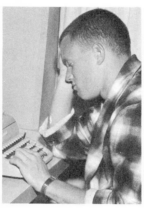

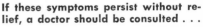

The signs of this disease are often the same as the symptoms of the common cold—fever, sore throat, or simply fatigue and listlessness.

If these symptoms persist without relief, a doctor should be consulted . . .

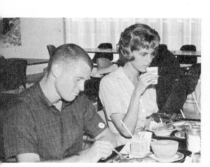

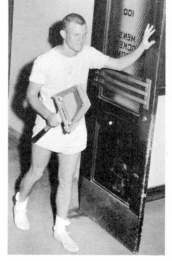

so that an accurate diagnosis can be made. An important part of this diagnosis is a laboratory test of the blood serum and the white blood cells.

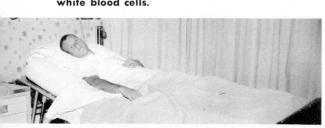

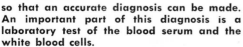

The most important factor in the cure of mononucleosis is rest in bed—a regimen which it may be necessary to continue for many weeks until the patient has completely recovered his strength and vitality.

cause permanent damage. They do, however, lengthen the period of recovery to a period of weeks or months.

There is no immunization for mononucleosis. An attack of the disease does not provide a permanent immunity; it may be contracted more than once. The degree of immunity is still undetermined. In general, mononucleosis is a mild disease, but it causes considerable discomfort and loss of time from one's regular duties. Because it is not usually a severe disease, few deaths result from it.

THE COMMON COLD

I am at this moment
Deaf in the ears,
Hoarse in the throat,
Red in the nose,
Green in the gills,
Damp in the eyes,
Twitchy in the joints,
And fractious in temper
From a most intolerable
And oppressive cold.

Charles Dickens [6]

Nearly all man's infectious diseases may become clinically manifest by symptoms that are often attributed to colds. Scarlet fever, diphtheria, and whooping cough may all begin as "kind of a cold." Q fever, influenza, psittacosis, and primary tuberculosis may simulate the symptoms of the common cold [2].

Man's most prevalent disease is the common cold. It is the No. 1 disease in the college population, as it is in the general population. The common cold is responsible for more loss of time from school, work, and recreation than all other diseases combined. Most people have at least one cold a year. A majority of the population suffer from three or more yearly. The over-all average for college students is estimated at three a year [20, 21].

[6] The Collected Letters of Charles Dickens, Chapman and Hall, Ltd., London, 1880, vol. I, p. 92; quoted in John Adams, *Newer Virus Diseases*, The Macmillan Company, New York, 1960 (frontispiece).

A cold is characterized as a self-limited, acute disease of the upper respiratory tract. Some colds affect the whole respiratory tract, producing some bodily discomfort, such as a headache and slight rise in temperature. Inflammation frequently is localized in the mucous membranes of the nose, sinuses, and throat. Signs and symptoms include congestion of the nose and throat, dryness, hoarseness, sore throat, coughing, and occasionally loss of voice. The nasal congestion is followed by a watery flow from the nose accompanied by sniffles and sneezes.

The common cold is mild in effect, but it is also serious because it may be the forerunner of secondary infections such as pneumonia, influenza, laryngitis, bronchitis, and sinusitis. The most significant role of the common cold is serving as precursor for serious diseases. As a self-limited infection, the cold usually lasts from two to seven days.

A cold is caused by one or more viruses. One theory is that a lowering of tissue resistance enables viruses to overcome the body's defensive mechanism and inflammation of the mucous membranes results. The complications are caused by streptococci, staphylococci, pneumococci, and influenza bacilli.

Colds are spread by direct contact from person to person. Coughing, sneezing, and even talking expel droplets into the air, and the virus is thus transferred to susceptible persons. Droplets may be carried through the air as far as 12 feet and may remain suspended in the air as long as three hours.

The incubation period is twelve to seventy-two hours. Colds may be transmitted to others before the symptoms develop fully. The period of communicability is in the early stages of the disease, usually one to four days.

Since 1958, the Common Cold Research Unit in Salisbury, England, has successfully grown and studied tissue culture and devised laboratory procedures for showing that viruses believed to be the cold virus are present. They have evidence that these viruses have multiplied without assistance from a human host. Their findings indicate these commonest of cold viruses differ significantly from all viruses previously isolated [6].

In addition, they have found, with the aid of human volunteers in their laboratories, that in not one instance does chilling alone produce a cold. Also, in several instances they determined that chilling plus inoculation with a cold virus actually produced fewer colds than inoculation alone. These findings are quite different from our previous beliefs and early experimental evidence [6].

Colds show a seasonal rise in prevalence beginning in October, followed by a depression and then an upswing, with the highest incidence occurring from December to April. Naturally, the lowest period is during the summer months.

Only a temporary immunity follows the attack of the common cold, which accounts for repeated colds during a year. No artificial immunity is effective against a cold. Vaccines made from bacteria, commonly referred to as "cold shots," have not proved successful. The preparation of an immunizing substance made from viruses is still in the experimental stage.

The effectiveness of antihistamines in controlling colds is known to have been exaggerated in popular articles. It is generally agreed that antihistamines have no important effect in preventing or diminishing the severity of colds. Since antihistamines produce ill effects in some people, it is wise to take them only on the advice of a physician.

The individual can protect himself from becoming infected with a cold by:

Avoiding as much as possible people with colds who are coughing, sneezing, or blowing their noses

Keeping up resistance by sufficient sleep, rest, recreation, and proper diet

Washing hands with soap and water before eating or handling food

Not employing towels, eating and drinking utensils, and toilet articles used by others

Keeping the head, back of the neck, and feet warm and dry

Avoiding drafts and sudden temperature changes (despite evidence from Salisbury, England)

Scheduling a regular medical examination for general physical checkup

It is important to take precautions in the early stages of a cold for one's own protection as well as for others'. Intelligent health practices include:

Getting as much rest as possible after one is exposed to a cold or feels a cold developing (going to bed during the first stages of a cold is an excellent practice, particularly if one has a fever)

Keeping warm and dry, avoiding undue exposure or indiscretion (one does not throw off a cold by strenuous exercise, or "working it out")

Eating light meals with nourishing food

Increasing the fluid intake by drinking plenty of water, fruit juices, soups, and the like

Protecting other people by staying away from them and by covering the nose and mouth with a handkerchief when coughing or sneezing

Blowing the nose carefully to avoid forcing infection into sinuses, eustachian tube, and middle ear

Calling a physician if a cold is severe, with chills, fever, aches, and pains throughout the body, or if it persists longer than usual

INFLUENZA

One of the most serious respiratory diseases is influenza, for it is able consistently to attack people of all ages throughout the world. Incidence frequently is highest in young adults. It is an example of a disease that has increased in virulence throughout the years, although since 1942 it seems to have become milder again. Influenza periodically has been epidemic in the United States from 1918 to the present time. Several tragic world-wide pandemics have occurred. One of the most dreadful was the 1918–1919 outbreak, in which there were some 20 million cases of influenza and pneumonia and approximately 850,000 deaths occurred.

Influenza is an acute disease of the respiratory tract that affects the whole body. It is characterized by a sudden onset, with chills, fever around 102° that may rise to 104°, headache, muscular pains, prostration, sore throat, and cough. Like the common cold, it paves the way for secondary infections caused by hemolytic streptococci and pneumonia. Most deaths are due to complications from pneumonia. Recovery is usual in four or five days.

The causative agent is classified in the myxovirus group of viruses. There are four different types of influenza virus, called influenza A, B, C, and CA. Influenza C and CA parainfluenza are rare varieties causing mild forms and are not as important as A and B. Influenza A breaks down into four different strains referred to as sets or families within this type. The A type has occurred in the Northern Hemisphere every year or so in epidemic form. These viruses have caused influenza on a world-wide basis since 1947.

In May, 1947, Asian influenza A virus was isolated. In 1957, it was identified as the responsible agent for the influenza epidemic of that year. This epidemic was first reported in Hong Kong and Singapore in April, 1957. From these points it spread to the Philippines, Japan, India, the United States, and other areas.

A vaccine containing the new Asian strain of type A was developed and proved safe and effective. It is the only preventive measure against the disease. Immunity against influenza is specific for each type and each strain. The virus of one type does not seem to produce antibodies against another type. This fact seems to be the reason for individuals

having second attacks in a year or two. For, according to serologic tests, an attack of influenza confers a relatively long-lasting immunity to the specific virus. The 1957–1958 epidemic proved to be the first time in history that physicians, public health workers, laboratory workers, and others were ahead of the influenza epidemic. The quick identification of the Asian A strain, the alertness of health personnel, and the stepped-up production of vaccine were significant factors in controlling the disease in the 1957 epidemic.

The B type is thought to have caused the epidemics of 1940 and 1946. One factor of the virus seems certain—it changes its form frequently. This factor increases the difficulty of controlling the disease.

Influenza is spread by direct contact, by droplet infection through the air, and possibly by inanimate objects contaminated with freshly soiled virus material. Sneezing, coughing, and talking are common ways of transmitting the virus from person to person. It quickly spreads from one part of the country to another and to other countries by modern means of transportation. The incubation period of influenza is short, ranging from twenty-four to seventy-two hours. The early stages are the most contagious periods.

Several studies of mass immunizations have shown the importance of immunization as a control measure in epidemics. However, because of the numerous strains of the virus and the necessity of having a particular vaccine for each strain, vaccination is not an absolute control procedure. One single vaccine that will be highly successful against all types is yet to be developed. Quarantine is not effective as a control measure during influenza epidemics. Prompt bed rest and good medical care are recommended measures for preventing serious complication and for early recovery.

The United States Influenza Information Center, National Institutes of Health, Bethesda, Maryland, and the

World Health Organization Influenza Center, London, not only are keeping up with the changing patterns of influenza viruses but are urging more rapid reporting of outbreaks and faster and better identification of influenza strains during epidemics.

PNEUMONIA

Pneumonia is the name given to several diseases characterized by inflammation in one or more lobes of the lungs. These diseases rank first among the communicable diseases in the list of the most common causes of death. Pneumonia ranked sixth in the ten leading causes of death in 1959 (see Table 12.1). All people are susceptible to pneumonia, although young children, the aged, and alcoholics are most susceptible. In the 15–34 age group there has been about a 95 per cent reduction in mortality rate since 1900. In 1959 the death rate per 100,000 was 185 for pneumonia and influenza combined.

The pneumonias are classified into three major types: Pneumococcal acute lobar pneumonia, bacterial pneumonia other than pneumococcal, and primary atypical pneumonia (virus pneumonia) [4, 35].

Acute lobar pneumonia. Lobar pneumonia is an acute infection, generally following some previous respiratory infection such as a cold or influenza. It is characterized by a heavy consolidation of lung tissue with leukocytes, serum, and red blood cells, together with a sudden onset of chill followed by fever, pain in chest, and cough. The air space of the lungs is filled so that breathing is seriously inhibited.

Pneumococcal pneumonia can be bronchial rather than lobar, particularly in children. In such cases, vomiting and convulsions are frequent symptoms. This situation also invalidates the older classification of pneumonia into lobar and bronchopneumonial types.

Pneumococcal pneumonia is a common disease affecting a large proportion of the population. No individual is exempt, for it is prevalent in all climates and seasons, although it most frequently occurs in winter and spring when cold, windy, changeable weather predominates.

It is caused by bacteria; the infectious agent is *Diplococcus pneumoniae*. Although there are some 75 different types of pneumococci, types I to XXXII cause 95 per cent of the cases. The organisms live and multiply chiefly in man. The infection is spread both by persons ill with pneumonia and by carriers, most frequently by the latter. High carrier rates precede epidemics. Transmission is by direct contact, through droplets, usually spread from carriers within a family, or indirectly through articles freshly soiled with nose and throat discharges of infected persons. The incubation period is believed to be from 1 to 3 days.

Resistance is generally high; however, this may be lowered through fatigue, chilling, exposure to wet and cold, and alcoholism. Immunity generally follows an attack and is highly specific for a particular type. Active immunization is possible but not considered practical.

Fatalities are prevented and greatly reduced by proper treatment. Chemoprophylaxis is effective with such antibiotics as penicillin and erythromycin and the sulfonamide drugs.

Bacterial pneumonia other than pneumococcal. The types of bacterial pneumonia are infections that produce an acute fever involving the lungs; they often occur along with other infections of the respiratory tract, such as colds, adenoviruses, and influenza, particularly epidemic influenza. These types of pneumonia are caused by several infectious agents. They include various pathogenic bacteria harbored in the mouth, nose, and throat, such as hemolytic streptococci, *Micrococcus pyogenes* var. *aureus*, the Friedländer bacillus, and *Hemophilus influenzae* [4].

Staphylococcal (micrococcal) pneumonia is rarely a primary disease. Rather it is secondary to staphylococcal infections in other parts of the body or to other infections of the lungs. It is similar to, and difficult to distinguish from, pneumococcal pneumonia. It is characterized by many small abscesses in the lungs, which consolidate into large ones. Because of the location of the abscesses and the speed with which they rupture, empyema (pus in the cavities) is a resultant complication. Untreated staphylococcal pneumonia is often prolonged and frequently fatal, in 30 to 60 per cent of cases. This disease is so dangerous that it requires immediate treatment in order to control it properly. The treatment is similar to that of pneumococcal pneumonia.

Preventive measures are also similar. They include good personal health practices to keep resistance high, avoiding crowded conditions in living quarters, and immunization against influenza to protect against primary infections.

H. influenzae is a common cause of primary pneumonia in children. It rarely produces pulmonary infection in adults unless another respiratory disease, such as influenza, is present. It is relatively easy to diagnose by isolating the organism from the respiratory tract or the blood or both. Drug therapy is effective treatment. However, it does have a fatality rate of approximately 40 per cent among untreated cases. It is particularly serious in children under one year of age. It has a 15 to 20 per cent fatality rate even with treatment [36].

Streptococcal pneumonia is not a common type. It usually is a secondary infection to pertussis, measles, or viral pulmonary diseases. It has a sudden onset, characterized by fever, chills, restlessness, cough, and blood-streaked sputum. An extensive bronchopneumonia develops, affecting the bronchioles of the lungs. The development of pus in the cavities is an early symptom. It is detected by early onset, filling of the pleural areas, and isolation of the streptococci. Penicillin or erythromycin usually produces a rapid cure, unless complications set in.

Friedländer bacillus pneumonia causes only a small portion of all the pneumonias. It resembles pneumococcal infection because of its quick onset with shaking chills, high fever, cough, and blood-tinged sputum. It generally attacks the upper lobes of the lungs rather than the lower ones. Its course is fast and possibly fatal, due to rapid tissue destruction. Chronic disorders predispose the lungs to this pneumonia organism. Early treatment is essential because of its rapid progress. Drug therapy other than penicillin, specifically combinations of the sulfonamide drugs such as streptomycin plus sulfadizine, has proved effective. The fatality rate is 20 to 25 per cent even with drug therapy. The importance of immediate treatment cannot be overemphasized [36].

Primary atypical pneumonia (virus pneumonia). Virus pneumonia, or primary atypical pneumonia, is a third type of the disease. It affects the small bronchiole tubes in a similar manner to bronchopneumonia. It is a scattered type of infection rather than complete congestion. Several viruses are thought to be the causative organisms. Cough, fatigue, muscle pains, chilliness, fever, and headache are common symptoms. It has a much longer incubation period than previously mentioned types, varying from seven to twenty-one days. Although virus pneumonia occurs in epidemic form, it is not so severe as the other two types. The death rate from virus pneumonia is very low. Another marked difference is its effect on the young adult group rather than on young children and aged persons. Important control measures include prompt reporting of the disease, immediate treatment by a competent physician, good nursing care, and disinfection of nose and throat discharges. Prevention includes previously mentioned factors such as good health practices.

POLIOMYELITIS

Poliomyelitis (infantile paralysis) is an acute, infectious, occasionally crippling disease caused by a virus organism. It affects those of all ages, but children from one to sixteen are more likely to develop it than adults. Older children and young adults appear to become infected more frequently now than formerly.

The incidence of poliomyelitis, particularly of the paralytic type, increased three-fifths more in 1959 over that reported in 1958. The paralytic cases comprised somewhat over 60 per cent, compared with a usual average of about 50 per cent. The failure of large segments of our population to become vaccinated is a large factor in the increased number of cases. In the age group 20–39 two-thirds have received fewer than three doses and more than half have received no vaccine at all. About one-third of the entire population under age 40 have not been vaccinated.[7]

Unlike the diseases previously discussed, poliomyelitis is most prevalent during the summer months.

The virus is found principally in the nervous tissues of the spinal cord and central nervous system. Occasionally it is found in the blood stream, the lymph glands, and the intestinal tract. Three types of poliomyelitis virus have been isolated. These are referred to as types 1 (Brunhilde), 2 (Lansing), and 3 (Leon). The virus causes lesions in the nervous system, destroying neurons in the motor areas of the brain and spinal cord. Bulbar poliomyelitis, in which the virus attacks the base of the brain, is the most serious type.

Early symptoms of the disease are headache, sore throat, fever, nausea, constipation, fatigue, listlessness, and pains or stiffness in the muscles, particularly in the neck. A spinal tap may have to be used to determine whether the symptoms are due to poliomyelitis or to some other infection.

The incubation period is three to twenty-one days—commonly seven to twelve days. The method of transmission is by direct contact and droplet spread through close association with infected persons. Milk has been found to be a vehicle of transmission in rare instances. The virus may be transmitted through the feces of infected persons.

It is known definitely that human beings are the reservoir of the virus. Individuals who have little or no illness may be carriers of the disease. Flies are proved to be carriers, since they have been found to be contaminated with virus material during epidemics. There is no reliable evidence that other insects, food, or water are media for transmitting the virus [4].

There appears to be a relationship between tonsillectomies and operations on sinuses, mouth, and nose, on the one hand, and the severity of subsequent poliomyelitis on the other. These operations are not recommended by many medical authorities during epidemic periods and months of high incidence except in vaccinated persons.

On April 12, 1955, an announcement was made, based upon nationwide field trials, that the poliomyelitis vaccine developed by Dr. Jonas E. Salk was safe and effective. Since that time efforts have been made to protect the entire public against poliomyelitis. This vaccine, which produces an active immunity against the disease, may have solved the problem of poliomyelitis prevention. Apathy of the public still remains an educational problem. Community organization for solving this problem is discussed in Chapter 15, pages 449–450.

Since certain lots of the early vaccine

[7] Metropolitan Life Insurance Company, "Recent Increase in Poliomyelitis," *Statistical Bulletin*, 40:1–3, September, 1959.

actually caused cases of polio, the National Poliomyelitis Surveillance Program was established in April, 1955. This program was designed to provide a clearinghouse for the collection, consolidation, and dissemination of all information concerning the poliomyelitis problems facing the nation. The Program is located in the Communicable Disease Center, Atlanta, Georgia. The first problems were to evaluate the safety of the vaccine and to measure its effectiveness.

The antibiotics are not yet a control measure for poliomyelitis. Quarantine is not recommended because many normal persons harbor the virus. Early detection of the disease, isolation of the infected person during the fever stage, concurrent disinfection of the patient's discharges as well as articles used, and immediate bed rest are effective control measures. Competent medical and nursing care, physical therapy, and rehabilitation of patients with disabilities are all important aspects of the care and treatment of poliomyelitis patients. Hot packs for early muscle soreness and spasm followed by reeducation of muscles, as practiced by Sister Elizabeth Kenny and others, is a successful method of treating symptoms. Respirators, or "iron lungs," are used in respiratory paralysis.

The Salk vaccine is not 100 per cent effective. It materially reduces chances of contracting paralytic poliomyelitis. The individual and family group need to be aware of recommendations for preventing polio.

The Surgeon General's Committee on Poliomyelitis (USPHS) recommended the following procedures in its January, 1961, meeting:[8]

Every unvaccinated person should be fully immunized against polio for his own protection. . . .

First priority should be directed to attaining complete and early coverage of the infant and pre-school group under 6 years of age.

Other children under 10 years of age and parents of young children are the next most important groups. . . .

When oral vaccines become available, every effort should be made to achieve total community participation in the immunization program on a single day or in a few consecutive days. . . .

All community sponsored immunization programs for the control of poliomyelitis should be planned and carried out in closest cooperation with private physicians and local medical societies.

Several other groups are vitally concerned with the control of poliomyelitis. The National Foundation, supported by the March of Dimes fund, is a voluntary health agency leading the fight for the eradication of poliomyelitis. The Sister Elizabeth Kenny Foundation is engaged in improving the treatment of the disease. Health departments, hospitals, and research centers also are assisting in efforts to conquer poliomyelitis.

THE VENEREAL DISEASES

Some eight diseases are classified as venereal diseases, three of which are important in the United States: syphilis, gonorrhea, and chancroid. Venereal diseases are so named because their common means of transmission is sexual intercourse. Specifically, they are diseases spread by mucous-membrane contact. The venereal diseases rank as one of the major social problems because of the resultant physical and mental suffering, sterility, destruction of life, cost to the public, decrease in production of goods and services from loss of time and inefficiency, and general effect on men, women, and children living in an environment where such diseases are present.

The Public Health Service has found that one-fifth of all reported cases of infectious venereal disease in the United States involve persons under age 20, and reported cases represent only a fraction of the actual number of cases. It is estimated that some 200,000 teen-agers acquire venereal disease each year in the

[8] U.S. Public Health Service, "Public Health Service Action in Poliomyelitis Control," U.S. Department of Health, Education, and Welfare, Communicable Disease Center, Atlanta, Ga., Jan. 23–24, 1961.

United States. In girls, more cases of venereal disease occur at 18 than at any other age. The proportion of all venereal disease cases in persons under 20 has increased significantly since 1957 [28].

In 1956, there was a slight increase in syphilis throughout the United States for the first time in eight years. By June 30, 1959, 29 states reported increases in primary and secondary syphilis and 35 states reported increases in gonorrhea. For the whole country, primary and secondary syphilis cases were up 23 per cent and gonorrhea, 8 per cent [28].

Syphilis. Syphilis rightfully is called the "killer" among venereal diseases. The exact mortality rate is unknown because so many cases are unreported. Syphilis is a direct or contributory cause of other diseases that result in death. It is a major cause of death in paresis, locomotor ataxia, apoplexy, and heart diseases.

Syphilis is caused by a spirochete, *Treponema pallidum.* This is a spiral organism that lives only a short time outside the body. It is easily killed by heat, drying, sunlight, and disinfectants. The spirochete is capable of entering the body through the normal ports of entry, through minute breaks in the skin, and directly through mucous membranes. It is not able to pierce the skin.

Sexual intercourse is the chief means of transmission, although direct contact with infected persons through kissing or a break in the skin may very rarely also transmit the spirochete. Indirect contact, as with toilet seats, hotel beds, library books, restaurant silverware, and the like, is seldom a means of transmission, since the organism lives only a short time in a dry environment.

A recently reported means of transmission of early infectious syphilis is male homosexual activity. During 1959, 292 persons in Los Angeles were reported as having primary or secondary syphilis. Some 89 of these persons were identified as having participated exclusively in homosexual relations. Among the persons who had sexual contact with the 89 exclusively homosexual patients, 93 were found to have syphilis. It is estimated that the major part of the increase in Los Angeles between 1955 and 1959 was due to homosexual transmission of infectious syphilis.[9]

The average incubation period is approximately three weeks, though it may last ninety days. The initial sign or symptom characterizing the first stage of the disease is the development of a chancre at the point of entry into the body. Usually this is a hard lump of tissue with firm edges. However, it may appear as an ulcerated sore with a thin secretion that becomes hardened after a few days. Both types are painless, with no general bodily symptoms. The chancre disappears of its own accord, whether treated or not. This gives the false impression that the disease is cured by the body defenses. The first stage is the most infectious.

The second stage of the disease develops some three to eight weeks after the disappearance of the chancre. In this stage bodily symptoms appear. There are possible fever, headache, swollen lymph nodes, small pink or white sores in the mouth and about the genital organs and anus, sore throat, loss of appetite, patch loss of hair, and a copper rash. Even these signs and symptoms may be extremely mild and so may be overlooked. This stage, too, is an infectious one, with the disease spreading through direct contact, including kissing.

Between the second and third stages a latent period occurs, which may last for several months or years. The spirochete is proceeding into the deep tissues of the body.

The third, or tertiary, stage is characterized by the development of gummas —firm, nodulelike tissue formed in practically any part of the body. The gummas often break down into destructive

[9] J. D. F. Tarr and R. R. Lugar, "Early Infectious Syphilis—Male Homosexual Relations as a Mode of Spread," *California Medicine,* 93:35–37, July, 1960.

ulcers. Also, in the third stage the disease grows progressively worse. For example, there may be involvement of the brain, resulting in paresis, a destruction of brain tissue; infection of the spinal cord, causing locomotor ataxia (tabes dorsalis); an attack on the heart and blood vessels, causing inflammation of the aorta and weakening of the blood vessel walls, resulting in aneurysms. In this stage the disease is least communicable.

Syphilis is not hereditary, but it is congenital. The spirochete may be transmitted by an expectant mother to her unborn child during pregnancy if she is not treated and rendered noninfectious.

Prevention and control measures for syphilis include the following [4]:

Health promotional measures: health education and sex education, preparation for marriage, premarital and prenatal examinations as part of general physical examinations, improvement of community social and economic conditions, including recreational facilities.

Suppression of commercialized prostitution and of sexual promiscuity.

Provisions for adequate early diagnosis following a plan,[10] such as the use of Venereal Disease Research Laboratories slide flocculation test on all serum samples as a screening procedure (nonreaction indicates the absence of syphilis), followed by the Reiter protein complement-fixation test for reactive or weakly reactive cases (to indicate past or present syphilis infection), followed by a *T. pallidum* immobilization test for the serum that shows a reactive or weakly reactive Venereal Disease Research Laboratories test and a nonreactive complement-fixation test result (a reactive or weakly reactive *T. pallidum* immobilization test indicates present or past syphilis infection. A nonreactive re-

[10] Charles M. Carpenter, James N. Miller, and Ruth A. Boak, "A Triple-test Plan for the Serologic Diagnosis of Syphilis—A Modern-day Approach," *New England Journal of Medicine*, 263:1016–1018, Nov. 17, 1960.

sult is a biological false positive one.)

Prompt treatment with penicillin to effect cure in the early stages, administered by private physicians or free clinics in health departments.

Intensive case-finding programs and tracing of contacts.

Control of patients with venereal disease in the transmissible stage.

Health education of the public as a means of prevention and control of early infections by providing scientific information and encouraging intelligent practices.

Gonorrhea. Gonorrhea is the commonest of the venereal diseases. Its frequency is two or three times that of syphilis. As with syphilis the exact number of cases throughout the country is not known. Many cases are not reported since persons infected with the disease are likely to be secretive about it; others do not know that they are harboring it. Medical authorities state that no other disease known to medical science has caused so much suffering and sorrow as gonorrhea.

Gonorrhea is caused by the gonococcus, a coffee-bean-shaped form of bacteria occurring in pairs. The gonococcus is easily distinguished with the aid of the microscope and appropriate stains. The organism grows and multiplies on mucous membranes. It affects the mucous membranes of the urethra (the urine duct or tube), vagina, uterus, fallopian tubes, and ovaries in the female, the rectum, and the conjunctiva —the delicate mucous membrane lining the eyelid and eyeball. Usually the gonococcus is contained in pus, a creamy-yellow discharge from the infected parts. It is important that this pus should not come in contact with other mucous membranes.

The most common form of transmission is sexual intercourse. By this means the genital organs are contaminated. It is possible to contaminate the eyes when soiled fingers or soiled materials transfer pus containing the gonococcus to the mucous membranes of the eyes. Also, the vaginal secretions from an infected mother may cause infection in the conjunctiva of the eye of a newborn baby. This is the reason for applying the 1 per cent solution of silver nitrate or a topical antibiotic to the eyes of every newborn baby. Towels or other articles contaminated with pus may be an occasional means of transmitting the infection. As with syphilis, the organism dies quickly outside the body.

The incubation period is one to fourteen days, usually three to five. In men, the urethra quickly becomes inflamed. There is a burning or stinging sensation at the time of urination, though it is well to note that this symptom may be due to causes other than gonorrhea. Pus is discharged from the urethra, and there is general discomfort such as fever, fatigue, and depression.

As a result of the inflammation, scar tissue forms in the urethra, distorting and constricting the passage and interfering with the flow of urine. If untreated, the gonococcus spreads to other genital parts, including the prostate, seminal vesicle, and epididymis. Sterility is a common result of infection of these organs. The urethra is often the first site of gonorrheal infection in women. The vagina and cervical canal of the uterus are the next to be involved, and the infection, if untreated, may progress to the fallopian tubes, causing intense pain. Inflammation of the tubes may lead to sterility.

Greater complications arise when the organism finds its way into the blood stream and to the heart. The valves of the heart may be damaged. Gonorrheal arthritis with high fever and intense pain results when the organism attacks the joints.

Measures for controlling gonorrhea are similar to those for syphilis. Avoiding contacts with the infected and prompt medical treatment with antibiotics are successful preventive and control measures.

Chancroid. Chancroid is a venereal disease associated with filth and poor health practices. It is less prevalent and less serious than either syphilis or gonorrhea. The rod-shaped Ducrey's bacillus does not live where soap and water are used plentifully. Chancroid is characterized by the appearance of one or more soft chancres, or ulcers, on or near the genitals or elsewhere on the body, whence it may be transferred to other parts if the discharge is spread by the hands or by soiled clothing. The disease sometimes resembles syphilis but has a short incubation period of three to five days. Both diseases may occur at the same time, with syphilis symptoms developing later. Chancroid is transmitted generally by sexual contact. As in syphilis, a break in the skin is necessary before the bacillus penetrates and sets up an inflammation. The first sign is a small sore on the affected part, which increases in size and ruptures through the skin, forming an ulcer. The sore is soft, spongy, and painful compared with the hard chancre of syphilis. Usually the penis in the male or the labia or vagina in the female is infected. The ulcers may damage these genital organs. Prevention and control measures are similar to those for syphilis and gonorrhea.

INFECTIOUS HEPATITIS

Infectious hepatitis is characterized as an acute infection with fever, nausea, malaise, abdominal distress, and enlargement of the liver, accompanied by jaundice in many cases. Most infections are mild, some are without jaundice, and some are recognized only by tests of liver function.

Infectious hepatitis has shown a marked increase in incidence in various parts of the country and a 37 per cent increase for the entire United States in 1960 compared with a previous five-year median. It is believed also that many cases were not reported as they may have been diagnosed as intestinal flu. Yet these cases are just as infectious as those clearly recognized. The disease is found most commonly among children and young adults, so it is of significance to college students. It has a seasonal variation, with greater incidence in autumn and early winter in the temperate zones.

Among the diseases for which morbidity data are collected throughout the country, only measles, streptococcal sore throat, whooping cough, tuberculosis, syphilis, and gonorrhea exceed infectious hepatitis in number of cases reported. At the same time, among these same diseases, infectious hepatitis ranks as the third cause of death, exceeded only by tuberculosis and syphilis.

The causative agent is a virus of hepatitis, not yet fully identified. It is transmitted generally through direct person-to-person contact and indirectly by contaminated water, food, and milk. Contaminated syringes, needles, and other instruments are another possible source of spread when sterilization is not complete. There is little evidence to show its spread through the respiratory route.

The virus is present in the feces and blood of infected persons during the incubation period. This is a long and variable period, from 10 to 40 days, usually about 25 days.

Preventive measures include good sanitation, good personal health practices, and proper technical procedures to prevent transmission by blood or blood products, including sterilization of equipment. Gamma-globulin offers good protection against the infection even as late as six days before the onset of disease. This is possible with the long incubation period. Gamma-globulin can be given routinely to persons known to have been exposed. There is no specific treatment fully recognized. Most patients recover with bed rest and high-calorie, low-fat diet [4, 35, 36].

SKIN DISEASES

The role of the skin as the first line of body defense already has been established. Because the skin is in contact with many disease-producing organisms and environmental irritants, it, too, is subject to a number of diseases. Diseases affecting the skin include erysipelas, scabies, pediculosis, cold sores, shingles, ringworm, and impetigo.

Tinea, or ringworm, is an example of a skin disease prevalent among college students. It is caused by a variety of fungus infections affecting the body in general, the scalp, and the feet.

Tinea pedis. Tinea pedis, or ringworm of the foot (epidermophytosis, athlete's foot), is discussed here because it is the most common of all fungus infections. Men are affected more often than women, undoubtedly owing to more profuse perspiration. The causative organisms are three fungi: Microsporon, Trichophyton, and Epidermophyton. After an undetermined incubation period, a lesion with a vesicle or vesicles appears on the soles of the feet, between the toes, and in some cases on the hands. The vesicle may break, discharging a watery fluid. Some forms are characterized by fissures in the skin followed by scaling. Once a fungus becomes established, it may become a stubborn chronic disease. Secondary eruptions similar to eczema also may occur along with the primary fungus infection. Such conditions are called *ids* and are believed to result from sensitive reactions to the fungi or the products of the fungi. Each type of fungus forms its own id. Vesicles may become infected secondarily with pyrogenic cocci, causing more serious conditions.

Recent experimentation shows that fungus infections are caused by decreased resistance of the human host to pathogenic fungi lying dormant on the skin rather than by contact with contaminated sources such as the floors of shower and locker rooms, shower stalls, or public bathing facilities. These experiments have demonstrated that persons clinically free from fungus disease of the feet still do harbor pathogenic fungi on their feet even though they have been carefully examined. Attempts were made in controlled studies actively to infect subjects free from the disease by exposure to masses of pathogenic fungi. Not a single case of fungus disease occurred within six weeks after exposure. The studies did prove that fungus disease developed because of the lowering of the defenses of the host, not as a result of contact with facilities or objects that have been blamed in the past. The investigators pointed out that the fungi cause disease on the feet in a manner similar to that of the staphylococci that cause boils. The staphylococci are present on the skin, and when the individual's resistance is lowered, boils can develop. These new studies add convincing evidence to the previous data, which have been used by some dermatologists during the last few years.

The data also indicate that past measures to prevent fungus disease are outmoded and new procedures are more effective. Any procedure that will raise or maintain the resistance of the individual's skin is important. The procedures suggested are [7]:

The use of well-ventilated or perforated shoes, especially during the hot periods of the year, to reduce moist conditions of the feet

The wearing of moisture-absorbing hosiery, such as wool and cotton socks rather than nylon, rayon, and other nonabsorbing materials

The continuous use of drying, mildly fungistatic foot powders, such as boric acid, tannic acid, talc, and other powders

The use of lamb's wool in the toe webs

The careful drying of the feet of persons who have an excess of sloughing-off skin between the toes

The frequent changing of shoes and socks when wet

The use of nonalkaline soapless detergents for washing the feet rather than ordinary alkaline soaps such as toilet soaps. There is no scientific evidence that foot baths placed at shower or swimming-pool entrances and exits assist in the prevention of fungus infections.

A new oral antifungal antibiotic, griseofulvin, is available in the United States. It was first isolated in England in 1939, but its use as an antifungal agent was not demonstrated until 1958. This oral preparation has the unique property of being absorbed into the blood stream and then deposited in the skin, hair, and nails, where it acts against fungi. The effect may take place slowly, over as long as a month or more, and continued treatment after lesions clear may be necessary. It has proved effective against Trichophyton, Epidermophyton, and Microsporon. There is not as yet complete agreement on its value against tinea pedis, and some side effects have been found. These include headache, nausea, diarrhea, and allergic skin rashes. However, in the future this may prove to be an important new control of athlete's foot [24].

Responsibilities of the college student

The student as a citizen in the college environment plays an important part in the modern program of preventing and controlling disease for himself, his living group, and his college community. After leaving college this same role should be carried out to a greater degree. As an intelligent citizen, the individual has opportunities to promote and protect his own health and that of his family and of his community, including the wider community of the state and nation. Today, with modern means of transportation, disease-producing organisms know no boundary lines. The possibility of the transmission of disease from any part of the globe is real. No area of this country or the world can be protected against disease by isolation. Rather, hope lies in cooperative action of citizens working with health personnel, research workers, and others for a comprehensive program of prevention and control of communicable diseases.

The college student can assume his individual and civic responsibility in the prevention and control of communicable diseases in a number of specific ways. For example, each college student should understand the principles and methods of preventing and controlling communicable diseases.

These factors include knowledge of the infectious process, the factors relating to the body's defensive mechanism, and the methods of control. These methods in the previous discussion were organized around ways of eliminating the source of infection, breaking lines of communication, and protecting the susceptible person. Also, the student needs essential information about the common communicable diseases in order to act intelligently when disease develops. Most important is to apply principles of prevention and control of disease in everyday health practices. Examples of such practices are the following:

Keep your general health and resistance to disease high through a balanced program of effective living including regular physical activity, adequate sleep and rest, proper diet, and a regular schedule for work and play. (Many other particular suggestions are made throughout the text.)

Protect yourself and encourage others to protect themselves, against the common communicable diseases for which immunization procedures are effective and available. Take advantage of immunizations for other diseases when traveling or residing in areas in which these diseases occur (see Table 11.2).

Recognize the common signs and symptoms of disease as they appear in yourself or classmates (see page 303).

Report to a physician at the student health service, a private physician, or the health department as soon as signs and symptoms of disease are apparent.

Have a medical examination at least once a year, or more frequently on the advice of the physician, to ensure optimum health status. Follow through on the findings of the examinations as prescribed by the physician.

Include the results of the medical examination as a part of your over-all personal health inventory.

Avoid exposure to disease, as suggested in the discussion on methods of prevention and control, pages 320–321. For example, prevent respiratory diseases such as colds and influenza by avoiding unnecessary contacts in crowded gatherings. Prevent venereal disease by avoiding direct contacts. Prevent pneumonia by taking care of colds, sore throats, and influenza, and avoiding undue exposure. Drink pasteurized milk to prevent septic sore throat, brucellosis, and types of tuberculosis. Drink from a purified water supply and make sure of proper sewage disposal in area of residence and on camping trips and outings to help prevent spread of intestinal diseases. Insist on proper screening of living quarters to provide protection from flies, mosquitoes, and other insects.

Secure competent medical advisers. Be protected with competent medical care through services of family physician, student health service, or medical-care plan as recommended by the college. (See suggestions on selection of medical advisers in Chapters 1 and 10.)

Select health products wisely and avoid self-medication as means of curing disease. (See suggestions in Chapter 10, pages 279–280.)

Participate in activities that help prevent and control communicable diseases through improved sanitation of personal living quarters as well as the total college environment. Such activities may include good housekeeping procedures, health education by means of committee action, personal endeavors, and cooperation with health personnel.

Summary

A cultural lag exists between scientific discoveries and application of this knowledge by the American public. This is one reason why no single disease caused by microorganisms has yet been wiped out completely. Additional efforts through medicine, public health, and education are being made to alleviate this situation. At the same time several communicable diseases are increasing in frequency. These include the venereal diseases, mononucleosis, and infectious hepatitis, to mention a few of concern to college students. Tuberculosis, influenza, and pneumonia still seriously affect the lives of many college students. Stepped-up efforts are being made to control these diseases as well as the common cold, to the extent that one or more of them may be completely eliminated in the near future.

Communicable diseases are defined as those diseases transmitted from person to person, either directly or indirectly. The modern concept of disease is expressed through the science of epidemiology, which shows the necessity of bringing all factors relating to prevention and control of disease into focus, including what is known about the host, the disease-producing organism or agent, and the related environment.

For the individual a knowledge of the principles of the prevention and control of disease is essential in order to understand disease and to assume civic responsibility. These principles are based on such items as the factors involved in the infectious process, the factors involved in the body's defensive mechanism, and methods of preventing and controlling disease.

Several communicable diseases selected on the basis of the needs and interests of college students have been discussed briefly. They include tuberculosis, mononucleosis, the common respiratory diseases, poliomyelitis, three venereal diseases, infectious hepatitis, and one fungus skin disease, athlete's foot.

The responsibilities of the college student are outlined for personal study and consideration. The student can develop his own resistance to disease through proper diet, adequate sleep and rest, appropriate exercise, and other wholesome health practices. He can participate in measures of control to protect himself and his family. Health education endeavors in school and community provide such opportunities for the individual and various groups. Modern control programs involve cooperative action on the part of individual citizens, the private physician, and official and voluntary health agencies in a team attack against communicable disease.

Suggested readings

1. Abramson, Martin: "V. D.—Return of an Old Scourge," *Today's Health,* 38:50, 82–83, December, 1960.
2. Adams, John M.: *The Virus Diseases,* The Macmillan Company, New York, 1960.
3. American Academy of Pediatrics: *Committee Report: The Control of Infectious Diseases,* The Academy, Evanston, Ill., 1955.
4. American Public Health Association: *Control of Communicable Diseases in Man,* 9th ed., The Association, New York, 1960.
5. Anderson, Gaylord W., and Margaret G. Arnstein: *Communicable Disease Control,* 3d ed., The Macmillan Company, New York, 1953.
6. Andrewes, Christopher H.: "The Viruses of the Common Cold," *Scientific American,* 203:88–102, December, 1960.
7. Baer, Rudolf L., and others: "Newer

BUILDING DEFENSES FOR EFFECTIVE LIVING

Studies on the Epidemiology of Fungous Infections of the Feet," *American Journal of Public Health,* 45:784–790, June, 1955.

8. Bolton, William: "Infectious Mononucleosis," *Journal of Health, Physical Education and Recreation,* 28:23-30, January, 1957.

9. Bower, Albert, Edith Pilant, and Nina Craft: *Communicable Diseases: A Textbook for Nurses,* 8th ed., W. B. Saunders Company, Philadelphia, 1958.

10. Burnet, Macfarlane: "The New Approach to Immunology," *New England Journal of Medicine,* 264:24–33, Jan. 5, 1961.

11. Carpenter, Philip L.: *Immunology and Serology,* W. B. Saunders Company, Philadelphia, 1956.

12. Conn, Howard F.: *Current Therapy,* W. B. Saunders Company, Philadelphia, 1960 and 1961 editions.

13. Dingle, John: "The Present Status of the Problem of the Minor Respiratory Diseases," *American Journal of Public Health,* 40:289, March, 1960.

14. Frobisher, Martin, Jr., Lucille Sommermeyer, and Raymond H. Goodale: *Microbiology and Pathology for Nurses,* W. B. Saunders Company, Philadelphia, 1960.

15. Hanlon, John: *Principles of Public Health Administration,* 3d ed., The C. V. Mosby Company, St. Louis, 1960.

16. Hilleboe, Herman E., and Larrimore, Granville W.: *Preventive Medicine,* W. B. Saunders Company, Philadelphia, 1959.

17. Leavell, Hugh Rodman, and E. Gurney Clark: *Preventive Medicine for the Doctor in His Community,* McGraw-Hill Book Company, Inc., Blakiston Division, New York, 1958.

18. "Major New Drugs of 1960, Part II," *Western Medicine,* 2:68–77, February, 1961.

19. Maramorosch, Karl: "Friendly Viruses," *Scientific American,* 203:138–144, August, 1960.

20. Metropolitan Life Insurance Company: "Recent and Future Mortality Trends," *Statistical Bulletin,* 41:1–3, June, 1960.

21. Meyers, J. Arthur, and others: "A Thirty-six Year Study of Diseases of the Chest on a University Campus," *Proceedings of the 34th Annual Meeting,* American College Health Association, Minneapolis, 1956.

22. *Modern Medicine Annual,* Modern Medicine, Minneapolis, Parts I and II, 1958, 1959, 1960.

23. Pelczar, Michael J., and Roger D. Reid: *Microbiology,* McGraw-Hill Book Company, New York, 1958.

24. "Present Status of Major New Drugs Introduced during 1960," *Western Medicine,* 1:10–19, 43–45, July, 1960.

25. Public Health Service: *V.D. Fact Sheet,* Publication 341, 16th revision, U.S. Department of Health, Education, and Welfare, Washington, 1959.

26. Public Health Service: *Immunization Information for International Travel,* Publication 384, U.S. Department of Health, Education, and Welfare, Washington, 1960.

27. Public Health Service: *Tuberculosis Chart Series,* 1960 ed., U.S. Department of Health, Education, and Welfare, Washington, 1960.

28. Public Health Service: *Venereal Disease in Children and Youth,* U.S. Department of Health, Education, and Welfare, Washington, 1960.

29. Public Health Service, "International Conference on Asian Influenza, National Institutes of Health, Bethesda, Maryland, February 17, 18, 19, 1960," *American Review of Respiratory Diseases,* 83, part II: 1–151, February, 1961.

30. Report of the Arden House Conference on Tuberculosis, Nov. 29–Dec. 2, 1959, "T.B. Control: The Big Push Ahead (Treament Is the Tool)," National Tuberculosis Association, New York, 1960.

31. Rivers, Thomas M., and Frank L. Horsfall, Jr.: *Viral and Rickettsial Infections In Man,* 3d ed., J. B. Lippincott Company, Philadelphia, 1959.

32. Rose, Anthony: "New Penicillins," *Scientific American,* 204:66–71, March, 1961.

33. Shepard, William P., and others: *Essentials of Public Health,* J. B. Lippincott Company, Philadelphia, 1948.

34. Smith, David T., and Norman Conant: *Microbiology,* 12th ed., Appleton-Century-Crofts, Inc., New York, 1960.

35. Top, Franklin: *Communicable Diseases and Infections,* 4th ed., The C. V. Mosby Company, St. Louis, 1960.

36. Weinstein, Louis: *The Practice of Infectious Disease,* Landsberger Medical Books, Inc., New York, 1958.

37. Winslow, C. E. A., and others: *The History of American Epidemiology,* The C. V. Mosby Company, St. Louis, 1952.

38. Yolli, Meir: "Animal Infections and Human Disease," *Scientific American,* 202:161–170, May, 1960.

TWELVE

Understanding chronic and degenerative diseases

The average life span of Americans has been increased to seventy years. As a result, more persons are surviving to the age when they are afflicted with the so-called chronic and degenerative diseases. Deaths resulting from "heart failure" are to be expected among men and women past the age of seventy. The fact is, however, that heart disease and other chronic and degenerative diseases disable or kill many persons at all ages, from infancy on. Even among individuals of college age, heart disease and cancer are among the five leading causes of death, and allergies and some types of rheumatism are frequent causes of disability. In addition, many college students discover that their parents and friends of their parents are in the age group afflicted frequently by diseases such as heart disease, cancer, diabetes mellitus, kidney diseases, and rheumatic diseases.

To comprehend the significance of the chronic-disease problem and to delay or prevent the onset of chronic and degenerative diseases, a person should be able to answer the following questions:

What diseases or disorders are considered to be chronic or degenerative?

To what extent do these diseases affect different age groups?

What factors contribute to the onset of chronic and degenerative diseases?

How can the individual assist his physician in the early detection and effective treatment of these diseases?

How can you support medical research, which is so vital to understanding and improving the means of controlling these diseases?

Although these questions cannot be answered completely, current evidence is presented, and research will continue to provide additional data.

The chronic- and degenerative-disease problem

Diseases that spread or are communicated from person to person are discussed in the preceding chapter. If we consider the meaning of "chronic" literally, some communicable diseases that persist for a long time are chronic in nature, such as tuberculosis. The diseases discussed in this chapter, however, are usually persistent or long-lasting but are not transmitted from person to person. The conditions may or may not be degenerative in the sense that the tissues are showing the effects of aging or wearing out, as is commonly suggested. It is important to understand that in many instances these diseases can be prevented or delayed in their onset and their effects decreased in severity.

CHRONIC AND DEGENERATIVE DISEASES AS A CAUSE OF DEATH

Mortality statistics provide evidence of the significance of chronic and degenerative diseases as a health problem. Data in Table 12.1 show that 6 of the 10 leading causes of death in the United States in 1959 were diseases of this kind. These diseases caused approximately 71 per cent of all deaths that occurred during 1959.

By comparison with the causes of death in 1900 in the United States, it is evident that, as communicable diseases have been brought under control, the chronic and degenerative diseases have increased rapidly as a cause of death. From Table 12.1 it can be seen that 4 of the 10 leading causes of death in 1900 were chronic and degenerative diseases, and they accounted for only 22.6 per cent of the total deaths during that year.

As a person ages, his tissues undergo changes that increase his susceptibility to the chronic diseases. However, these diseases are not, as commonly believed, a problem confined to older persons. The fallacy of such a belief is shown by the fact that two of the five leading causes of death in both the 5–14 and 15–24 age groups are chronic and degenerative diseases (see Table 12.2).

Table 12.1 Leading causes of death by rank, United States, 1900* and 1959

	1900				1959		
Rank	Causes of death	Deaths per 100,000 population	Per cent of all deaths	Rank	Causes of death	Deaths per 100,000 population	Per cent of all deaths
	All causes	1,719.1	100.0		All causes	941.7	100.0
1	Influenza and pneumonia	202.2	11.8	1	Diseases of the heart	366.3	38.9
2	Tuberculosis (all forms)	194.4	11.3	2	Malignant neoplasms (cancer)	147.1	15.6
3	Gastritis, etc.	142.7	8.3	3	Vascular lesions affecting CNS	108.3	11.5
4	Diseases of the heart	137.4	8.0	4	All accidents	50.7	5.4
5	Vascular lesions affecting CNS	106.9	6.2	5	Certain diseases of early infancy	38.5	4.1
6	Chronic nephritis	81.0	4.7	6	Influenza and pneumonia	32.5	3.5
7	All accidents	72.3	4.2	7	General arteriosclerosis	19.7	2.1
8	Malignant neoplasms (cancer)	64.0	3.7	8	Diabetes mellitus	16.0	1.7
9	Certain diseases of infancy	62.6	3.6	9	Congenital malformations	12.3	1.3
10	Diphtheria	40.3	2.3	10	Cirrhosis of the liver	11.0	1.2

* Rates for 1900 apply to the death-registration states only.
Source: "Trends in U.S. Mortality," *Progress in Health Services,* Health Information Foundation, vol. 10, no. 2, February, 1961, p. 4.

CHRONIC AND DEGENERATIVE DISEASES AS A CAUSE OF DISABILITY

Deaths alone do not show the extent of the chronic- and degenerative-disease problem. The resulting disability is of equal or greater importance. Some consequences of prolonged disability from chronic diseases are the suffering of the patient, the disruption of normal family living, the cost of medical care, and the loss in man hours of productive work.

The Department of Health, Education, and Welfare reported that in 1960 about 70 million Americans had one or more chronic conditions. An estimated 17 per cent of the population under 15 had one or more chronic conditions, 78 per cent at 65 and older, 83 per cent at 75 and older; 17 million persons were chronically limited to some degree in ability to work, keep house, or pursue outside activities; 4.5 million persons had trouble moving about or could not get around without help; and about 1 million persons were completely confined to their homes [38].

Although chronic and degenerative diseases are an important health problem at all ages, it is apparent that the longer a person lives, the more likely he is to be disabled or to die from the effects of one of these diseases. The chronic diseases seldom occur suddenly. They are usually slow and gradual in their onset. Individuals can do much while they are young to delay or prevent these diseases in their later years. You as a college student of today have many years ahead of you. You will, therefore, be likely to develop one or more chronic conditions. The extent to which you live a reasonably comfortable and productive life during your later years can be influenced considerably by what you do as a student and as a young and middle-aged adult.

Table 12.2   Leading causes of death in 5–14 and 15–24 age groups in the United States, 1958

Causes of death	5–14		15–24	
	Death rate per 100,000 population	Per cent of all deaths	Death rate per 100,000 population	Per cent of all deaths
All causes	45.8	100.0	106.4	100.0
Accidents	19.2	41.9	55.6	52.3
Malignant neoplasms	6.7	14.6	8.7	8.2
Congenital malformations	3.3	7.2		
Influenza and pneumonia	2.3	5.0		
Homicide			5.8	5.4
Suicide			4.7	4.4
Diseases of the heart	1.3	2.8	4.4	4.1

Source: Data from Department of Health, Education, and Welfare, Public Health Service, National Office of Vital Statistics, "Deaths and Death Rates for Five Leading Causes of Death in Specified Age Groups, United States, 1958," *Vital Statistics—Special Reports, National Summaries*, vol. 52, no. 7, Aug. 24, 1960.

The aging population

A thorough understanding of the problem of chronic and degenerative diseases invariably includes a consideration of changes taking place in the age composition of the population of the United States and the age of individuals afflicted by these diseases.

AGE COMPOSITION OF THE POPULATION

Pronounced changes in the age composition of the population of the United States have occurred during the past century. These changes are illustrated in the accompanying graph. The increase in the percentage of the population 45 and older was steady until it leveled off during the 1950s. The highest percentage of persons in the population 65 and older, however, was recorded in 1960. The current trend shows an increase in the under-5 age group since the lowest percentage was recorded in the 1930s and an increase in the 5–19 age group since the lowest percentage was recorded in 1950.

Among the factors that have changed the age composition of the population are reduction in infant mortality rates, improvements in disease control and prevention, increased life expectancy, fluctuations in birth rate, and reduction in immigration until it is now of little significance.

GERONTOLOGY AND GERIATRICS

This discussion leads to one of the significant problems confronting Americans in the 1960s: the problem of aged and aging persons and what is to be done for them. An obvious indication of concern is the proposals for medical-care plans for the elderly. Another indication is retiring persons at an arbitrary age of sixty-five or sixty-seven without considering their capacity to make an effective contribution to society.

The problem of planning for our population over 65 can no longer be delayed. Mere numbers make it imperative that something constructive be done. The estimated 16 million Americans who were over 65 in 1960 will be approximately 20 million by 1975. Not only will the

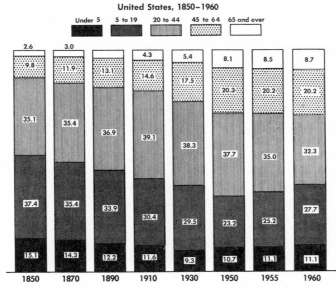

United States, 1850–1960

Under 5　5 to 19　20 to 44　45 to 64　65 and over

Per cent distribution of total population by age. (By permission from Metropolitan Life Insurance Company, *Statistical Bulletin*, 37:4, September, 1956; 1960 data: U.S. Department of Health, Education, and Welfare, *Health, Education and Welfare Indicators*, Washington, Jan., 1961, p. 1.)

number increase, but also life expectancy will increase [39].

Keeping people alive is not enough. Keeping them able to live usefully and happily is more important. *Gerontology* is concerned with the process of aging and the changes inherent in aging, particularly after maturation [10]. *Geriatrics* is a branch of medicine dealing with the process of aging and those diseases common to old age. Medical science has resolved some problems associated with aging, but a great deal remains to be learned and applied before man achieves his potential life span. The

White House Conference on Aging, held in January, 1961, was devoted to problems associated with aging, with recommendations for attacking and resolving these problems [39].

The life a person leads as a student and as a young adult can do much for him or against him as the years pass by. Health is a precious commodity, which enables an individual of any age to live most effectively. Individuals can benefit considerably by following the recommendations of the gerontologist and geriatrician and planning ahead to live long and well.

Diseases of the heart and circulatory system

Deaths from diseases of the cardiovascular system, the heart and blood vessels, increase in proportion to the effectiveness with which medical science is able to prevent deaths due to other causes. Therefore, evaluation of progress in controlling cardiovascular diseases on the basis of mortality rates alone is inaccurate. The age at which cardiovascular disease causes death and disability is an important criterion.

It is estimated that 10 million Americans have some form of heart disease and that 500,000 of these are under fifteen years of age. "Heart attacks," which annually kill many persons in what should be the prime productive years of life, demand the best attention that can be devoted to their prevention.

Cardiology, the medical specialty dealing with the detection and treatment of cardiovascular diseases, is relatively new. The effectiveness of present-day treatment is remarkable if one considers that most of the progress in control of heart disease has been made during the last quarter century.

The medical research worker and the physician have made important strides in solving heart-disease problems. Their continued efforts, along with efforts of cardiac patients in following the advice of their physician and efforts of potential cardiac patients in applying good health practices to maintain a high level of health, will help reduce heart-disease problems. An understanding of cardiovascular diseases and factors that contribute to their onset can be helpful to the potential cardiac patient—who could be almost anyone.

HEART DISEASE MEANS MANY THINGS

Heart disease is not a single disease. To say that an individual has "heart disease" without a more specific definition of the nature of the condition is somewhat like saying that he is ill. Many diseases involve the heart and blood vessels directly, and others exert a secondary effect on these organs. The classification of heart diseases into various types and kinds is recognized by authorities as one of the great medical advances. The identification of different diseases makes it possible for the physician to provide specific treatment for each, and more effective control results.

Different heart diseases are more prevalent or more likely to cause difficulty at one age than at another. During infancy congenital defects are the most frequent cause of death or disability due to heart disease. Congenital defects are imperfections in structure of the heart

or blood vessels at the time of birth. Infections, particularly streptococcal, are the primary cause of heart disease during school age and early adult life, but improved means of combating infections could almost eliminate this danger. Rheumatic fever is the most common specific cause of heart disorders during this period of life. Hypertension, or high blood pressure, is the cause of the greatest difficulty during the middle years of life, and coronary disease takes the heaviest toll during the later years. Arteriosclerosis (hardening of the arteries) is common in the middle and older age groups and frequently is associated with hypertension or coronary disease as cause of death or disability.

The fact that specific types of heart disease produce greater effects at different ages does not mean that they are not felt at other ages. Hypertension is not limited to the middle-aged, nor is coronary disease limited to the elderly.

CARDIOVASCULAR SYSTEM

The heart and the blood vessels, which make up the cardiovascular system, provide the pump and the pipes for circulating blood to the cells in all parts of the body.

The heart. The force that moves the blood throughout the body is provided primarily by a muscular organ approximately the size of a fist. It is estimated that all the blood in the body passes through the heart approximately every 90 seconds, even during rest [15]. The accompanying figure illustrates the structure of the heart and the pathway of the blood as it flows through the heart. The three layers of heart tissue (endocardium, myocardium, and pericardium) receive their own blood supply through a system of blood vessels, the coronary vessels, and not by absorption through the wall of the heart. Damage to any of the three layers of tissue or to the coronary blood vessels as a result of in-

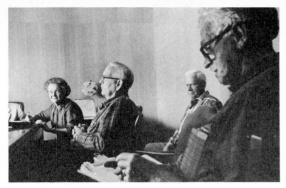

Old age must be recognized as a natural phase of human life. The advancements of science have lengthened the normal life span so that old age must be viewed as a time, not of loneliness or isolation . . .

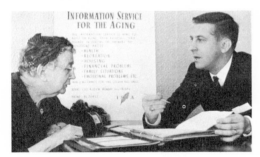

but of active seeking, and adjustment . . .

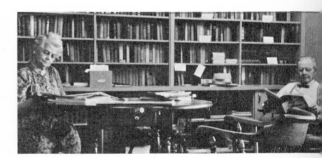

a time for sustaining old interests . . .

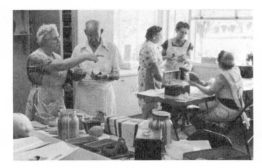

and developing new ones . . .

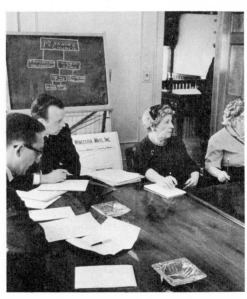

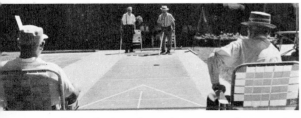

for enjoying the advantages of recreation and relaxation . . .

and making a continued contribution to one's community by participation in all forms of civic life.

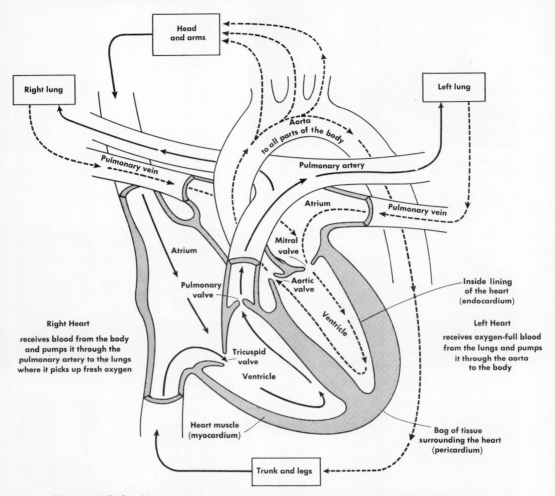

Head
and arms

Right lung

Left lung

Aorta
to all parts of the body

Pulmonary vein

Pulmonary artery

Atrium

Pulmonary vein

Mitral
valve

Atrium

Inside lining
of the heart
(endocardium)

Aortic
valve

Pulmonary
valve

Ventricle

Right Heart

receives blood from the body
and pumps it through the
pulmonary artery to the lungs
where it picks up fresh oxygen

Left Heart

receives oxygen-full blood
from the lungs and pumps
it through the aorta
to the body

Tricuspid
valve

Ventricle

Heart muscle
(myocardium)

Bag of tissue
surrounding the heart
(pericardium)

Trunk and legs

Diagram of the heart, which serves as a double pump. The right heart receives de-oxygenated blood and pumps it to the lungs, where it gives off carbon dioxide and receives a new supply of oxygen. The left heart pumps the oxygenated blood through the aorta, to be distributed by means of the arteries to all parts of the body. (American Heart Association and its affiliates.)

fection or injury may disrupt normal circulation.

Contraction of the left ventricle forces blood into the large arteries. This contraction, called *systole,* forces the walls of the arteries to expand. Relaxation of the ventricle walls, called *diastole,* relieves the pressure on the blood in the arteries and allows the walls of the arteries to contract and assist in the forward movement of the blood. The alternate expansion and contraction of the

arteries with each beat of the heart causes the pulse. Contractions of the heart chambers are controlled by the *sinoatrial node* (SA node) and the *atrioventricular node* (AV node). The SA node, called the *pacemaker,* is located in the wall of the right atrium, and the AV node is located in the septum between the atria, with branches extending down into the walls of the ventricles [15]. The average pulse rate of an adult male at rest is approximately seventy beats per minute and is slightly higher for an average female. Considerable variation from the average may be normal for a given individual. Some outstanding distance runners have had a pulse rate in the fifties or lower. The pulse rate is influenced by such factors as physical activity, nervous tension, venous return of blood to the heart, smoking, and endocrine secretions (thyroxin from the thyroid and epinephrine from the adrenals).

The blood vessels. The blood is carried to the various parts of the body by the arteries. It exchanges its food and oxygen supply for waste materials from the cells through the thin walls of the capillaries and returns to the heart through the veins.

The three layers in the walls of the arteries make them stronger than the other blood vessels. The smooth lining of epithelial cells allows blood to flow freely, the smooth-muscle fibers of the middle layer permit control of the caliber of the vessels through their ability to contract and relax, and the outer layer of connective tissue provides elasticity and added strength. Thickening and hardening of the walls with aging reduces the ability of the arteries to expand and contract. Roughening and scarring of the smooth lining of the arteries cause a slowing down of the flow of blood.

The tiny, thin-walled capillaries are the "end of the line" for the blood, which has been moving away from the heart. These minute vessels enable the blood to reach all the living cells, which require food and oxygen and which have waste materials to eliminate. From the capillaries the blood flows into the veins and then back to the heart. The veins have thinner walls than do the arteries and, in addition, have valves at frequent intervals along their course. The valves help to overcome the force of gravity, which inhibits the return of venous blood from the lower part of the body. Interference with normal venous flow of blood

may result in injury to the valves and eventually in varicose veins.

Blood pressure. The pressure required to circulate the blood is measured by using an instrument called a *sphygmomanometer*. The physician wraps the elastic cuff around the patient's upper arm and inflates the cuff to stop the flow of arterial blood. When air is released from the cuff until the blood pressure is sufficient to allow blood to flow through the arteries, the physician is able to detect the flow by listening with the stethoscope on the artery below the cuff. He reads the amount of pressure in millimeters either by the height of a column of mercury or by means of a needle on a dial. This reading of the pressure at its highest point is called *systolic pressure*. When more air is released from the cuff, the distinct beat sound disappears as the flow of blood in the artery becomes smoother. The point at which the beat disappears is called the *diastolic pressure*, or lowest level of pressure in the artery.

A reading of 120/80 means a systolic pressure of 120 and a diastolic pressure of 80. The normal range of systolic pressure is about 110 to 140, and the diastolic range is 70 to 90. Average blood pressures of healthy persons accepted for ordinary insurance are shown in Table 12.3. Studies indicate, however, that normal pressure for some individuals may be outside the range suggested for average persons. The difference between systolic and diastolic is the pulse pressure.

Blood. Blood makes up about one-thirteenth of the body weight. An individual weighing 150 pounds has approximately five to six quarts of blood. It is composed of formed elements, the red blood cells, the white blood cells, and platelets, suspended in a fluid called *plasma*.

The plasma portion of the blood is approximately 92 per cent water, in which organic salts and other substances are

Table 12.3 Graduated average blood pressures among persons accepted for ordinary insurance during 1935–1953, by sex and age at issue

Age, years	Men		Women	
	Systolic, mm	Diastolic fifth phase, mm	Systolic, mm	Diastolic fifth phase, mm
15–19	117	71	114	70
20–24	119	73	115	72
25–29	121	75	117	73
30–34	122	76	118	74
35–39	123	77	120	75
40–44	124	78	123	76
45–49	126	78	126	78
50–54	128	79	128	79
55–59	130	79	131	80
60–64	132	80	134	81

Source: *Build and Blood Pressure Study*, Society of Actuaries, Chicago, October, 1959, vol. 1, p. 30.

suspended or dissolved. They include food products such as glucose, amino acids, and cholesterol; waste products, such as urea, uric acid, creatine, and ammonium salts; inorganic chemicals, such as calcium, sodium, and other minerals needed by body tissues; and hormones.

The red cells, *erythrocytes,* contain hemoglobin, which enables the blood to carry oxygen. An insufficiency of red cells, or of hemoglobin in the cells, results in a condition known as *anemia.* New blood cells are continuously produced in the red marrow of the bones, and old red blood cells are destroyed at a rate of about 10 billion per hour by the liver and spleen. The life span of red blood cells is approximately 120 days. The number of red blood cells, approximately 5 million per cubic centimeter for males and 4½ million for females, remains relatively constant under normal conditions. Determination of the red blood cell count and measurement of the hemoglobin content of red blood cells provide the physician with information about certain illnesses.

The white blood cells are of several types, of which leukocytes and lymphocytes are the most common. Leukocytes are formed in the same area of the bone marrow as are the red blood cells. The lymphocytes are formed in lymphatic tissue. The white blood cells are less abundant than the red; the normal range is 5,000 to 10,000 per cubic centimeter. Their life span is eight to ten days. The functions of white blood cells in combating communicable diseases is extremely important, as was indicated in Chapter 11.

The primary function of the more than a trillion platelets in the blood of an average person is to form clots. The clotting process is essential in controlling blood loss due to hemorrhage. Studies suggest that the platelets may have other significant functions not yet clearly understood [42].

Disorders or diseases that interfere with the normal function of any of the constituents of the heart, blood vessels, or blood have a corresponding effect on health.

CONGENITAL DEFECTS

It is estimated that between 30,000 and 40,000 children are born each year in the United States with congenital heart defects and that 75 to 80 per cent of them can be helped by surgery [6]. Some of the causes of such defects are not known. However, some of the contributory causes are known and can be prevented. It is known that if a woman has an attack of German measles early in pregnancy, her child may be born with a defective heart or with other defects. Protecting the mother's health during pregnancy decreases the likelihood of serious defects in the child.

Congenital defects in the structure of the heart or blood vessels can result in an insufficient supply of blood to the lungs for aeration or to the organs of the body. Some of the more common defects, which are serious enough to require correction and which can be treated by surgery, are patent ductus arteriosus (an open passageway between the pulmonary artery and the aorta); ventricular septal defect (an opening between the ventricles); atrial septal defect (an opening between the atria); coarctation of the aorta (a narrowing or constriction of the aorta); aortic and pulmonary stenosis (narrowing of one of the heart valves); and the tetralogy of Fallot (a combination of ventricular septal defect, overriding aorta, pulmonary stenosis, and enlarged right ventricle) [6].

RHEUMATIC FEVER

Infections in other parts of the body can cause disturbances in heart function. Even though decreases in mortality have been encouraging, rheumatic fever remains as the greatest danger to the heart of the school-age person. Rheumatic fever is a general systemic disease, which may or may not cause damage to the heart.

Cause. Although the immediate cause of rheumatic fever is not entirely clear, the disease process is initiated by beta-hemolytic streptococcus infection of the upper respiratory tract. The symptoms of rheumatic fever sometimes are observed after such an infection. It is generally believed that an allergic reaction to the streptococcal infection is the cause of rheumatic fever. The part that hereditary susceptibility and environmental factors play in the onset of rheumatic fever is not known definitely but is being explored by research workers.

Unfortunately, one attack of rheumatic fever does not protect against future attacks but instead makes the patient more susceptible. The danger of recurrences makes it essential that the first attack be recognized and the damage minimized.

Detection. Frequently the symptoms of rheumatic fever are mild, and damage to the heart is slow in appearing. Some of the symptoms that may indicate the presence of rheumatic fever are loss of appetite, fatigue or weakness, slight persistent fever, and pain in the muscles or joints. Appearance of such symptoms in a young person, especially following throat infections or colds, should be brought to the attention of a physician.

Rheumatic heart disease, which results from rheumatic fever, generally consists in damage to the endocardium and scarring of the valves of the heart. Damage to the valves permits blood to leak back into the auricles from the ventricles. The leaking of blood during contraction of the ventricle can be heard by the physician through his stethoscope. He is also able to detect sounds associated with stenosis, or narrowing of the openings that allow blood to flow through the heart. Unusual heart sounds are called *murmurs*. Some are referred to by physicians as *innocent* or *functional* murmurs. Heart sounds of this type may be normal for a given individual. Functional murmurs may be temporary conditions, which disappear after a time.

In addition to listening to heart sounds, the physician makes use of X ray and the fluoroscope to determine the size, shape, relative position, and action of the heart. The electrocardiogram records the electric impulses associated with the contraction and relaxation of the heart muscles; these tracings may provide evidence of malfunction.

Even the blood provides information for the physician. A blood sedimentation test—measurement of the rate and extent to which red cells settle to the bottom of a blood sample—is of value in diagnosis.

Prevention. Prevention of rheumatic heart disease is based primarily upon prevention and early treatment of the streptococcal infections that can cause rheumatic fever. Penicillin has been used effectively by physicians to prevent and to treat "strep" infections.

Medical care in early stages of rheumatic fever, as well as later, is essential in preventing serious complications. Complete bed rest and proper diet are prescribed by the physician. Complete rest during acute stages of the actual disease reduces the burden on the heart and decreases the likelihood of permanent damage. Measures helpful in preventing and controlling heart damage as a result of rheumatic fever also are helpful in controlling subacute bacterial endocarditis, a disease that formerly was usually fatal.

Those who have recovered from an attack of rheumatic fever are advised to maintain their physical vigor through a balanced program of rest and activity and by eating proper foods. In addition, they are advised to avoid exposure to respiratory infections and to seek medical attention in case of exposure. Prevention and control of streptococcus infections are more readily accomplished since the discovery of penicillin.

HYPERTENSION—HIGH BLOOD PRESSURE

Of the conditions affecting the cardiovascular system, hypertension is one of those most talked about and least understood by lay persons. *Hypertension* means high blood pressure, or pressure above normal. It is important to note that blood pressure varies with individuals and with the same individual at different times. Emotions such as fear, anger, and worry cause blood vessels to constrict, and the blood pressure is thus increased. Many individuals have high blood pressure most of their lives and seem to suffer little or no ill effects. Others have blood pressure above normal associated with serious complications. Worrying about blood pressure adds to the difficulties by increasing the pressure.

Blood-pressure problems are an individual matter. Actually, high blood pressure is a sign or symptom rather than a disease. The associated conditions, as in the arteries or kidneys, determine the seriousness of the hypertensive condition.

Causes. There are a number of causes of hypertension. Page suggests four categories of causes [29]:

Those resulting from kidney diseases

Those due to endocrine disorders, such as a tumor of the adrenal gland

Those due to vascular disorders, such as obstruction of the aorta

Those resulting from neurogenic factors

High blood pressure not associated with any other disease or for which the cause is unknown is called *essential* or *primary* hypertension. Although the exact cause of essential hypertension is not known, suggested contributory causes include:[1]

1. Heredity—people whose parents had high blood pressure are more likely to develop it than are those whose parents did not.
2. Emotions—an excessive rise in blood pressure as a result of emotional stress may result in continual high pressure for some "hyperreactors."
3. Body chemistry—malfunction of some organ may start a chain of chemical events that results in raised blood pressure.

Secondary hypertension designates

[1] American Heart Association, *High Blood Pressure*, The Association, New York, 1957, pp. 5–6.

high blood pressure due to malfunction in some organ. The kidney is thought to be a factor in causing secondary hypertension by producing an enzyme that acts on a blood constituent to release *angiotensin*. This substance is thought to cause high blood pressure because, when injected into human beings, it raises blood pressure more than any other known substance. Fortunately, the kidney also has the ability to control the enzyme action through the function of the tubular cells [29].

Although hypertension is more frequent among older persons, it may occur at any age, even in babies. The average age of onset is in the thirties. The overweight person and the individual with a short, stocky build have a higher incidence of essential hypertension than does the person of average weight and tall, slender, narrow-chested build.

Effects. High blood pressure indicates that the heart is required to exert greater effort in order to circulate the blood. The amount of resistance determines the size of the pump needed. The increased resistance that the heart must overcome may result in enlargement of the heart muscle. It is possible for a strong heart to become enlarged and be uninjured by increased pressure over a period of years. A weak heart is unable to cope with the additional demands.

The increase in pressure not only adds to the burden on the pump but also places extra strain on the pipes, or blood vessels. Strong, elastic arteries can withstand the added strain for many years. Weakened or nonelastic arteries are less able to withstand the pressure. Changes in the structure of blood vessels associated with hypertension may result in an insufficient supply of blood to organs. The organs that are most frequently and most seriously affected by hypertension are the heart, the brain, and the kidneys.

High blood pressure does not always

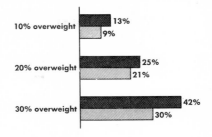

OVERWEIGHT SHORTENS LIFE

EXCESS* MORTALITY FROM ALL CAUSES

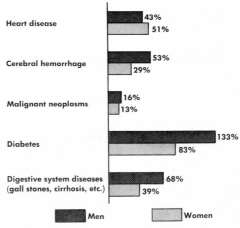

EXCESS MORTALITY DUE CHIEFLY TO HEART AND CIRCULATORY DISEASES

EXCESS* FOR PRINCIPAL DISEASES AMONG PERSONS ABOUT 20% OR MORE OVERWEIGHT

*Compared with mortality of standard risks (mortality ratio of standard risks = 100%)

Overweight and Its Prevention, Metropolitan Life Insurance Company, 1960.)

cause symptoms that can be detected by the individual. There may be general symptoms, such as headache, dizziness, lightheadedness, and vertigo, which can be due to some other condition. The cause should be determined by a physician. The diagnosis of high blood pressure can be made accurately only by measurement with an instrument such as the sphygmomanometer. Regular medical examinations enable the physician to detect changes in blood pressure and other signs that indicate the onset of hypertension.

In preventing complications from high blood pressure, it is important to follow the advice of the physician regarding kind and amount of physical activity, diet, use of tobacco and coffee, rest, control of weight, and control of emotions.

ARTERIOSCLEROSIS

Arteriosclerosis, hardening of the arteries, may be associated with high blood pressure, coronary diseases, and apoplexy, which are common among older persons.

Arteriosclerosis occurs to some extent in everyone who survives long enough. However, it is more common in men than in women, it affects men approximately ten years earlier than it affects women, and it tends to occur earlier in persons with diabetes.

Arteriosclerosis is the result of degenerative changes in the middle layer of the artery wall and a fibrous overgrowth of the inner lining. The result is a loss of elasticity and contractility. In atherosclerosis, a form of arteriosclerosis, a fatty substance, cholesterol, is deposited on the inner lining of the artery. The deposit eventually blocks the flow of blood in the artery, with serious or minor consequences, depending upon the location of the block. See pages 235–236 for discussion of cholesterol in the diet.

A number of factors are associated with the development of arteriosclerosis, including heredity, hypertension, lack of exercise, stress, sex, and diet [7, 20].

CORONARY HEART DISEASE

Coronary heart disease is a result of changes in the arteries supplying the heart and a subsequent interference with the blood flow. The heart muscle, like any other muscle of the body, needs a supply of oxygen and food and must eliminate waste products. Insufficient blood supply to the heart muscle produces more dramatic and severe results than does the same insufficiency in other muscles.

Some persons, the minority, die as a result of the first attack of coronary disease. Wright suggests that the mortality rate is between 5 and 15 per cent. Many individuals apparently have mild myocardial infarctions, blockages of coronary blood vessels, which are unrecognized [30]. A high percentage of persons not only survive the first attack but are able to enjoy many happy and useful years. The chance for recovery depends upon the extent of the damage, the ability of the body to repair or compensate for the damage, and a sensible program of healthful living.

Angina pectoris. Angina pectoris is a symptom of disturbance in the coronary circulation. Pain results because the heart muscle is deprived of its normal supply of oxygen. The pain of angina

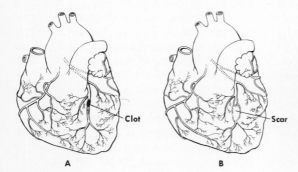

A coronary attack. (A) Four days after attack white cells are clearing away the dead tissue; scar tissue is beginning to form at the edges of the damaged area (just below the clot). (B) Eight weeks or so later tough scar tissue has formed. (Adapted from *Heart Attack*, rev. ed., American Heart Association, New York, 1959.)

A   B

pectoris has characteristics that help identify it. "Strangling in the chest" is a frequent description. The pain occurs under the breast bone and may radiate out to either arm, although the left arm is affected more frequently. Pain from angina pectoris may be mild or severe, depending somewhat upon the extent of interference with the coronary blood supply.

Coronary thrombosis. A blood clot which remains stationary is called a *thrombus.* Coronary thrombosis is a closing or blocking of a coronary artery by a blood clot. If the stoppage involves a large branch of the artery, the individual is likely to die quickly. If it involves a small branch, the circulatory system sometimes is able to overcome the difficulty by means of collateral circulation, making use of other blood vessels. This ability to compensate for blockage of one vessel is a fine example of the adaptability of the human organism.

The heart muscle fibers whose blood supply is cut off undergo changes. Some of the fibers die. Over a period of time the damaged fibers are replaced by scar tissue, and the wound is healed. Until the healing process is completed, there is danger of hemorrhage in the area. Resting the whole body decreases the amount of work required of the heart and, in turn, reduces the strain on the injured area. By avoiding excessive strain during the healing process, an individual increases his chances of living a comparatively normal life thereafter.

STROKE, OR APOPLEXY

Stroke and *apoplexy* are terms commonly used to indicate cerebral hemorrhage. Strokes may cause death immediately, or they may be so mild as to escape detection. The extent of the damage depends upon the amount of bleeding and the area of the brain involved. Individuals with arteriosclerosis and hyper-

Hemorrhage

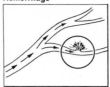

The wall of an artery of the brain may break, permitting blood to escape and thus damage the surrounding brain tissue.

Thrombosis (clot formation)

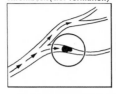

A clot of blood may form in an artery of the brain and may stop the flow of blood to the part of the brain supplied by the clot-plugged artery.

Embolism (blocking of a vessel by a clot floating in the blood stream)

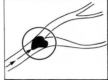

A clot from a diseased heart or, less commonly, from elsewhere in the body may be pumped to the brain and stop up one of the brain's arteries.

Compression (pressure)

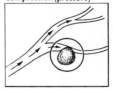

A tumor, swollen brain tissue, or a large clot from another vessel may press upon a vessel of the brain and stop its flow of blood.

Spasm (tightening and closing down of the walls of an artery)

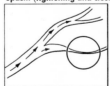

An artery of the brain may constrict and thus reduce the flow of blood to an area of the brain. If the spasm is of short duration permanent damage does not necessarily occur.

Interference with blood supply to the brain. (*Cerebral Vascular Disease and Strokes,* U.S. Department of Health, Education, and Welfare, pub. no. 513, 1958.)

tension are more susceptible to strokes and may suffer a series of them over a period of years.

In addition to damage to brain tissue due to hemorrhage, damage may result from loss of blood supply to an area of the brain by a blockage of blood vessels. The blocking may be due to the formation of a clot (a thrombus), the lodging of an embolus (a foreign body, such as a portion of a clot which breaks loose and travels in the blood vessels) or pressure on arteries due to brain tumor.

The paralysis of facial, arm, or leg muscles on one side of the body is a frequent result of a stroke. Pressure on the brain due to hemorrhage or damage to the nerve cells causes paralysis. If the damage to the brain tissue is slight and the blood is gradually reabsorbed, permanent damage may be slight. When brain cells are destroyed, they do not regenerate and the paralysis is permanent. In addition, personality changes sometimes result from damage to an area of the brain.

In addition to causing nearly 200,000 deaths in the United States each year, strokes, or vascular lesions of the central nervous system, cripple many persons and are a leading cause of admissions to state mental hospitals.

PSYCHOSOMATIC ASPECTS OF HEART DISEASE

Anxiety is an important aspect of heart disease. The frequency of death from heart disease and the importance of this organ generate anxiety about its function. Complaints about symptoms referred to the heart region are perhaps more common than heart disease itself [40].

Some of the common symptoms of heart neurosis are:

Pain, likely to be felt when at rest and in the left side where the heart is thought to be

Rapid and irregular heartbeat

Shortness of breath, not associated with effort

Weakness and fainting utilized to control the environment

Fatigue without evidence of organic disease

It is important to note that these same symptoms for different reasons may indicate organic heart disease.

The problem of heart neurosis is a real one, which should receive the best medical care as well as understanding on the part of the patient, his family, his physician, and his nurse.

VARICOSE VEINS

Varicose veins are most commonly a disorder affecting vessels near the surface of the legs. The characteristic protruding appearance of the dilated veins is a result of damage to the valves and a thinning and weakening of the walls of these vessels. The enlarged veins cause an unsightly appearance and may result in considerable discomfort to the individual. In prolonged and advanced cases ulcers may result.

It is possible that there is a hereditary tendency involved in the development of varicosity, but in general the cause is considered to be primarily a mechanical factor. Interference with the normal return of venous blood from the lower extremities creates undue pressure, which in turn can result in a breakdown of the valves and damage to the walls of the veins. Some of the common contributing causes appear to be occupations which require heavy lifting and prolonged standing, constricting clothing, chronic constipation, and pregnancy.

Prompt treatment under the direction of a physician can reduce the discomfort and danger involved. Elastic stockings or bandages to create external pressure, regular exercise, weight reduction of an overweight individual, injections, surgery, and elimination of the factors causing mechanical interference may be required to overcome the problem [37].

PROGRESS IN CONTROLLING HEART AND CIRCULATORY DISEASES

Despite the fact that diseases of the heart and circulatory system are the most common cause of death in the United States, significant progress has been made in treating and preventing some of these diseases. The electric pacemaker, which can be surgically implanted to compensate for the failure of the SA node to regulate heart contractions; new sections of arteries made of nylon to replace defective vessels; surgical treatment to remove obstructions from coronary arteries and relieve angina pectoris; surgery to correct congenital defects of the heart and blood vessels; cardiac massage, including a procedure for applying external pressure rhythmically over the sternum or breast bone, to stimulate heart action temporarily when the heart stops; drugs to reduce the clotting tendency that causes obstructions in blood vessels in some persons; drugs that reduce hypertension—these are some of the newer advances, which offer hope in further reducing morbidity and mortality rates of diseases of the heart and circulatory system.

Kidney diseases

Nephritis and *Bright's disease* are terms commonly used to designate kidney disease. Bright's disease is named for Richard Bright, an English physician, who demonstrated in 1827 that albumin in the urine indicated the possible presence of kidney disease. "Nephritis" means an inflammation of the nephrons, or filtering units of the kidneys. Nephritis and nephrosis (noninflammatory diseases of the kidneys) rank fourteenth among the leading causes of death in the total population [26].

KIDNEYS

Two bean-shaped organs, each weighing about ⅓ pound and each containing upward of 1 million filtering units, are responsible for removing the end products of protein digestion and other waste products from the body. Complete failure of this filtering system causes death. Partial failure results in an impairment of function which sometimes makes itself known by changes in the amount of urine passed, changes in the composition of the urine, edema (excess accumulation of fluid in body tissues), backache, and general fatigue.

The filtering units in the kidneys are called *nephrons*. Each nephron consists of a minute, cuplike chamber called *Bowman's capsule* and a tubule. The tubule follows a winding pathway ending in the collecting chamber of the kidney, where the urine accumulates and then passes through the ureters to the bladder. Blood comes into the nephrons under high pressure as it passes rapidly from the aorta into the renal artery and thence to the filtering chamber, or capsule. In these chambers the renal artery divides into a network of capillaries, the glomeruli. The surface provided by the many small blood vessels allows fluid to pass into the chamber surrounding the blood vessels and thence into the tubule. It is estimated that about fifty gallons of fluid pass from the blood into the tubules each day [33]. As the fluid passes down the 1½-inch length of the tubule, reabsorption of useful materials takes place and the waste materials continue through the tubule into the collecting area of the kidney. From the blood that passes through the kidneys each day, only about 1½ quarts of fluid is removed and eliminated as urine. Urine normally contains urea, uric acid, and creatinine, which are end products of protein metabolism in the body. In addition, sodium chloride, potassium, calcium, and magnesium salts, and phosphoric and hydrochloric acid are found in varying amounts. Urine normally is slightly acid in reaction, although the effect of diet may cause it to become slightly alkaline. The bulk of the urine is water, which carries the solid waste materials.

The selectivity of the nephron in reabsorbing substances needed by the body and eliminating harmful substances can be disturbed by various disorders. Failure of the kidney to eliminate harmful substances produces the symptoms mentioned earlier.

Among the common disturbances of normal kidney function are:

Blockage of the ureters by "stones," which form when mineral salts such as calcium phosphate are precipitated

Loss of selectivity of nephrons as a result of inflammation, thereby permitting the excretion of protein substances normally retained, retention of harmful substances normally excreted, and retention of water, producing edema

Production of substances that affect the vascular system and cause a type of hypertension

CAUSES OF KIDNEY DISEASES

Some factors that cause disturbances in kidney function are infections, poisoning (mercury or lead, for example), toxic effects of widespread body burns, toxemias associated with pregnancy, and tumors.

Considerable burden is placed upon the kidneys by infection in other parts of the body. Infected teeth and tonsils and other infections, seemingly remote, mean additional work for the kidneys, which must eliminate toxins produced as a result of such conditions. However, the normal kidney is able to carry an extra burden in most circumstances because of the abundance of filtering units. This abundance of nephrons is demonstrated by the fact that an individual is able to live and remain in good health with only one kidney.

Occasionally, poisons or toxins accumulate too rapidly, and the nephrons are unable to perform their function as rapidly as they should. The accumulation of waste material in the blood stream as a result of kidney insufficiency produces general systemic poisoning, called *uremia*.

DETECTION OF KIDNEY DISEASES

Some symptoms of kidney malfunction can be detected by the individual. The passage of excessive or inadequate amounts of urine, blood in the urine, backache in some instances, or puffiness of body tissues may indicate that kidney function is impaired. Regardless of the cause, anyone with such symptoms should visit a physician. The physician can use numerous tests to determine the nature and extent of kidney disease.

One of the most valuable means of detecting kidney disorders is by an analysis of the urine to determine its chemical composition as well as its specific gravity or density. Examination of the urine includes testing to discover the degree of alkalinity or acidity and determining whether or not it contains albumin, sugar, pus or blood cells, sediment, or casts. Urinalysis is a routine procedure in most examinations conducted by a physician because the urine provides information about malfunction of other organs of the body beside the kidneys. Albumin, a simple protein substance found in many animal and vegetable tissues, is present in the blood as a part of the blood protein. Normally the urine is practically free of albumin. The presence of albumin does indicate possible malfunction of the nephrons, but additional tests must be made to confirm the cause.

Bacteriologic examination of the urine to determine the nature and extent of any pathogenic (disease-producing) organisms is an extremely important aspect of a complete urinalysis. The presence of casts in the urine is another clue to nephritis. Casts are small, threadlike masses of protein material formed by an accumulation of such material in the tubule of the nephron. Different types of casts can be detected by the laboratory technician.

X-ray pictures provide information about size, shape, and position of the kidney; by use of liquids that are opaque to X rays the physician obtains information about the internal structure of the kidney. In addition, harmless dyes are injected into muscles or veins, and the time required for their passage is measured to determine the ability of the kidney to excrete materials. Fortunately, instruments such as the cystoscope and catheters may be used to approach the renal pelvic cavity without resort to surgery.

On the basis of information gathered by means of the above procedures, the physician is able to direct treatment at the specific cause of the difficulty. The individual must realize that proper diet, adequate rest, and control of infections in the body are important in both pre-venting and treating kidney diseases. In addition, the individual should avoid self-medication with drugs advertised as increasing the amount of urine. Such diuretic substances can be dangerous in some kidney disorders and should be used only when prescribed by a physician.

Machines to serve temporarily as artificial kidneys and kidney transplants offer hope in combating kidney disorders. The artificial kidney functions by having blood pass through a filtering machine and then back into the circulation. A kidney transplant from a fraternal, not an identical, twin was successful, and the patient has survived in good health for a period of eighteen months [33].

Cancer

The chances of surviving cancer are improving at the rate of approximately 1 per cent per year, according to the National Cancer Institute. Among persons who have developed cancer since 1950, the survival rate for five years or more has been 37 per cent [22]. The American Cancer Society reports that approximately one out of two cancer patients could be saved with early detection and proper treatment. It is estimated that 6 out of every 24 persons will have cancer and that of this number 2 are being saved, 1 dies who could be saved, and 3 die of cancer that cannot at the present time be controlled [4].

The 85,000 victims who die needlessly each year are evidence of the importance of information about cancer in order to assist in early detection and to appreciate the need for complete cooperation with one's physician in detection and treatment. A study by the American Cancer Society of 1,100,000 adults showed that 80 per cent did not see their doctor about symptoms commonly associated with cancer [36].

Cancer is the second leading cause of death in the United States, accounting for more than 15 per cent of all deaths in the total population. Because malignant growths are more frequently found in older persons, the death rate is likely to continue to be high as the number of older persons in the population continues to increase. Cancer is not limited to the elderly, however. It is the second leading cause of death in the 5–24 age group as well.

WHAT IS CANCER?

Cancer is a name used for a group of diseases which have the common characteristic of abnormal cell growth. *Malignant neoplasms* and *malignant tumors* are other terms used to designate this abnormal cell growth. "Neoplasm" or "tumor" means a new growth; "malignant" defines the growth as being harmful. Malignant tumors have the ability to grow and to spread from the original site to other parts of the body. This ability to spread to other tissues and establish new growth centers is called

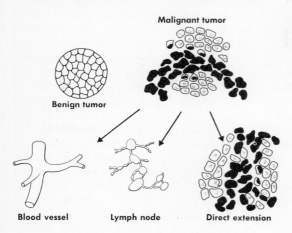

Malignant tumor

Benign tumor

Blood vessel   Lymph node   Direct extension

Benign tumors are localized; malignant tumors spread to other parts of the body. (Adapted from *A Cancer Source Book for Nurses*, American Cancer Society, New York, 1956.)

metastasis. They rarely cease growing of their own accord but must be stopped by external means. Benign tumors are harmless in the sense that they do not spread to other parts of the body but are localized. They may, however, be harmful to the extent that they interfere with normal functions in the local area of the body.

Normal cell growth. Normal cell growth is an orderly process. The individual develops from a single cell to a mature adult person. As he develops through infancy, childhood, and adolescence, the growth of different body tissues speeds up and slows down in a regulated manner. Finally the individual reaches his maximum height, but growth and repair of the various body tissues continue in order to maintain the efficiency of the organism. Millions of cells are destroyed and replaced each day. An example of the normal replacement of tissue is the healing of an incision or cut on a finger. The replacement of destroyed cells continues until the wound is healed, and then replacement or growth of cells ceases.

When man is able to solve the secret of what starts and stops the normal growth of cells, he undoubtedly will have the answer to the riddle of abnormal cell growth, which occurs in cancer.

Cancer does spread. Control of cancer at the present time is based on detecting the malignant tumor before the abnormally growing cells break from their original site and establish "colonies" elsewhere in the body. Metastasis occurs by direct extension to adjacent tissues, by spreading through the blood stream, and by transfer of cells through the lymphatic system.

Once metastasis occurs, treatment is relatively ineffective because of the difficulty of locating all the new growth centers and destroying them.

Cancer cells are different. Cancer cells differ from normal cells. Diagnosis of cancer is based upon detection of abnormal cells by microscopic examination of suspected tissue. The pathologist, a medical specialist, is able to detect malignant tissue by this means, which is called a *histologic test*.

Cancer in the different tissues of the body is differentiated as follows:

Sarcoma, a malignant tumor of connective tissue (bone, muscle)

Carcinoma, a malignant tumor of epithelial tissue (skin, membrane linings, and glandular structures)

Melanoma, a malignant tumor arising in the pigment cells

Lymphoma, a tumor affecting lymphatic tissues (Hodgkin's disease and lymphosarcoma)

Leukemia, a malignant tumorlike disease of the blood-forming tissues, causing abnormal growth of the white blood cells

CAUSES OF CANCER

Unfortunately, an exact cause of cancer is not known. Instead, it has been established that there are a number of contributing or predisposing factors. Examples of the predisposing causes of cancer include cancer of the bladder among aniline-dye workers; cancer of the bone in luminous-dial painters; cancer of the skin in asphalt workers; cancer of the scrotum among chimney sweeps; cancer of the cheek in natives of India, the East Indies, and the Philippines who chew betel nuts; cancer of the lungs in chromate workers; cancer of the blood due to ionizing radiation; cancer of the lip associated with the heated stem of the pipe of smokers; cancer of the skin among individuals exposed excessively to the rays of the sun; and melanoma arising in a pigmented mole irritated by friction from a belt, suspenders, or brassière strap [22]. It should be understood that not all persons exposed to the above factors develop cancer, but a relationship between incidence and the predisposing causes has been established.

In addition to the examples mentioned above, other factors have been suggested as being significant predisposing causes of cancer. Hormones apparently are involved in some types of cancer, but the specific relationship has not been established. Heredity is believed by many lay persons to be a strong factor in the occurrence of cancer, but the opinion of experts indicates that, over all, the role of heredity is limited [2].

Irradiation with X rays, radium, and radioactive isotopes is a proved means of destroying cancer cells, but there is a danger of causing cancer by excessive exposure to radiation. For example, the chance of radiologists' developing leukemia is greater than for other physicians or for white males of comparable ages. Because of this danger, workers who are exposed to radiation are provided with all possible safeguards. The extent of the danger from the fallout of radioactive substances produced by testing atomic and hydrogen weapons is not clearly established. Some individuals have become alarmed by the increased strontium-90 in milk, but the consensus of authorities has been that the milk is still safe to drink. (See page 248).

There is no conclusive evidence to show that cancer is caused by organisms that spread from person to person. In other words, cancer is not contagious or communicable. There is an interest in the possible role of viruses as a cause of cancer and as a deterrent to the growth of cancer cells, but findings indicate that, if they are involved, they do not function in the same role as in the contagious diseases such as measles or poliomyelitis. Virus as an inciting factor in some types of cancer in animals has been established, but in human beings the evidence is inconclusive.

The relationship of diet to cancer is being studied. Best evidence would seem to suggest that omissions from the diet may be a contributing factor in some instances. The lack of vitamin B in the diets of natives of South Africa and Java and the occurrence of a type of liver cancer is an example [11]. Possible danger from additives to food is being considered, and restrictions on specific additives will result as studies produce any evidence of danger. The cranberry incident of 1959 illustrates government efforts to protect the consumer.

Tobacco has been one of the most controversial of the possible causes of cancer. Statistically a relationship has been established between heavy smoking and the occurrence of lung cancer. The cause-and-effect relationship is, however, subject to disagreement. See the discussion of cancer of the lung for additional information.

COMMON SITES OF CANCER IN THE BODY

The frequency with which cancer occurs in specific organs differs between the sexes. Table 12.4 gives comparative data by sex and site. Cancer of the digestive tract (esophagus, stomach, large intestine, and rectum) accounts for more than one-fourth of cancer cases in men. The two most frequent single sites are the skin and the lungs. For women the breast and genital organs are the site of nearly one-half of cases. The skin and digestive system are also among the more common sites in women.

Cancer of the skin. Skin cancer can be cured in 95 per cent of cases if proper treatment is undertaken in the early stages. Skin cancer is visible to the naked eye and therefore can be detected early enough to allow for effective treatment. However, each year approximately 4,000 persons die of this type of malignant condition simply because they fail to observe the growth or because they

Table 12.4 Percentage of cancer incidence in the United States by site and sex

Site	Males	Females
Skin	14	10
Mouth	4	1
Respiratory system	18	3
Breast		25
Digestive tract	29	23
Urinary system	6	3
Genitals	14	23
Leukemia and lymphomas	8	5
Other	7	7

Source: American Cancer Society, *The Hopeful Side of Cancer*, The Society, New York, 1960, pp. 8–9.

delay in seeking medical assistance until the cancer has metastasized. The skin is an organ, and any condition that affects it can have an effect on other organs of the body. To assume that a growth on the skin cannot cause severe damage or even death is but to invite disaster if the growth is malignant.

Moles or skin blemishes which increase in size or undergo changes of any kind should be examined by a physician. Self-treatment or treatment by a quack is dangerous because of the delay in correct diagnosis if the mole becomes malignant. Fortunately most moles do not become cancerous. The type of mole most apt to develop into a malignant tumor is dark brown or bluish black and slightly raised. This type of mole, if irritated by the clothing, may show signs of growth after being dormant for years.

Any skin sore or lesion that resists normal healing and persists longer than usual should be referred to a physician. He is best qualified to determine the nature of the growth or lesion and to prescribe the best treatment.

Cancer of the lung. Cancer of the lung has become one of the most significant cancer problems in the United States due to its rapid rise as a cause of death and because of the relationship of cigarette smoking to its occurrence. The following statement by the American Cancer Society indicates the nature and extent of the problem: [2]

In 1959 the death rate from lung cancer among men in the United States was over 10 times as high as it was in 1930. The disease is now one of the most common and most lethal of all forms of human cancer. This tremendous increase in number of deaths and the reported association of cigarette smoking with lung cancer has led the American Cancer Society to pursue an aggressive program of research on lung cancer and to disseminate

[2] Warren H. Cole, "Statement of American Cancer Society on Cigarette Smoking and Lung Cancer," *Journal of the American Medical Association*: 172:1425, Mar. 26, 1960.

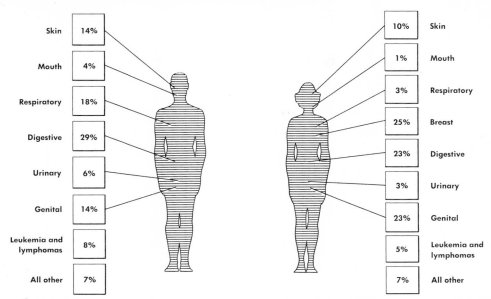

Skin	14%
Mouth	4%
Respiratory	18%
Digestive	29%
Urinary	6%
Genital	14%
Leukemia and lymphomas	8%
All other	7%

10%	Skin
1%	Mouth
3%	Respiratory
25%	Breast
23%	Digestive
3%	Urinary
23%	Genital
5%	Leukemia and lymphomas
7%	All other

The diagram indicates the incidence of cancer according to the site of the disease and the sex of the victim. (*The Hopeful Side of Cancer*, American Cancer Society, November, 1960.)

new evidence bearing on the subject to the medical profession and to the public. . . .

The strong association between cigarette smoking and lung cancer has been established by an extraordinarily large amount of evidence. Twenty-eight studies have indicated that a history of smoking is more common among lung cancer patients than among those without the disease. Three follow-up studies of smokers and nonsmokers have demonstrated that the death rate from lung cancer among cigarette smokers is about 10 times as great as among nonsmokers. Epidemiologic studies indicate also that cigarette smoking is associated with about 75 per cent of all cases of lung cancer. The incidence of the disease increases with the amount of cigarette smoking, and no threshold below which lung cancer will not occur has been identified.

The fact that the association is one of cause and effect is well supported by several types of evidence. For example, in experiments condensates of tobacco smoke have produced cancers on the skin of mice and rabbits. After experimental exposure of mice to tobacco smoke or its condensates, abnormal cellular growths have been reported on the mouse bronchial epithelium, in tissue cultures, and on the cervix. Cilia, one of the lung's major defenses against inhaled particulate matter, have been shown to be paralyzed by tobacco

smoke. At least 10 chemical agents that have been identified in cigarette smoke have caused the development of cancer in laboratory animals. Studies of pathological changes in bronchial tubes of smokers have shown that abnormal cellular changes in the bronchi of the lung increase in degree and frequency as the amount of cigarette smoking increases and that in nonsmokers these changes are scarcely present at all.

Some studies indicate that cigarette smoking is not the only causative factor in lung cancer. Certain occupational causes are recognized, and other factors such as air pollution have been implicated. The evidence indicates that the development of most cases of lung cancer is a complicated process in which cigarette smoking is the major controllable, though possibly not the only, factor. . . .

The American Public Health Association has suggested that, if the present trends are not reversed, nearly one million children who are now in school will die of lung cancer before they reach the age of seventy [3].

Only 4 per cent of men and 8 per cent of women who develop lung cancer survive; hence, it is extremely important to take all possible steps to avoid suspected causes of lung cancer and to seek the assistance of one's physician in early detection [22].

If the highest possible survival rate of lung-cancer patients is to be achieved, early detection is vital. A persistent cough, persistent hoarseness, coughing up blood, and obscure chest pains indicate that the individual should see his physician. These symptoms can, but probably do not, indicate the presence of cancer in the respiratory tract. In any case the diagnosis should be made by a physician and the symptoms treated by him.

Cancer of the digestive tract. Cancer of the digestive tract causes many deaths because it is difficult to detect in its early stages.

Some of the more specific symptoms are:
Difficulty in swallowing food
Persistent indigestion or a vague uneasiness after eating
Persistent change in bowel habits, toward either diarrhea or constipation
Bloody discharge from the anal opening or black or tarry stools
Bleeding from the anal opening can be caused by hemorrhoids (commonly called piles). Self-diagnosis of hemorrhoids is especially risky because it may mean delay in detecting the presence of cancer in the rectum or lower part of the digestive tract. The danger of hemorrhoids, a form of varicose veins, should not be minimized. They are a common ailment, which can be treated to prevent serious complications.

Regular medical examinations are essential for early detection of malignant tumors of the digestive tract. Loss of weight, anemia, and fatigue should indicate a special visit to a physician.

Cancer of the breast. Breast cancer is rare in men and common in women—about one-fourth of all cancers in women. As a result of the educational campaign to inform women about breast cancer, many lives are being saved. However, cancer of the breast still causes thousands of needless deaths each year.

An early indication of breast cancer is a lump. The lump is painless in most cases, at least in the early stages of growth. Most lumps of the breast are not cancerous, but they should be examined by a physician as soon as they are detected. Other signs that may indicate the presence of a malignant condition are alteration in shape of the breast, elevation or retraction of the nipple, puckering of the skin, bleeding or discharge from the nipple, or a swollen lymph node or gland in the armpit. Cancer of the breast frequently is associated with the menopause. Women undergoing this change should be alert to detect symptoms noted above. Single women have higher death rates from breast cancer than do married women. Nursing a child is believed to reduce chances of breast cancer.

Cancer of the female genital organs. The reproductive organs are a common site for malignant conditions in women. Over 10 per cent of the total number of cancers in women occur in the cervix. Fortunately, cancer of this area of the uterus is relatively easy for a physician to detect and, if treated adequately in its early stage, responds more readily to treatment than any of the major forms of cancer [14].

The most important sign is irregular or abnormal bleeding from the vagina. However, in many cases, such bleeding does not occur until the growth is in its advanced stages. Therefore, it is important for a woman, particularly from about thirty-five years of age on, to have regular examinations.

Cancer of the male genitourinary tract. Cancer of the genitourinary tract accounts for approximately 20 per cent of all cases in men. The prostate gland is more likely to be the site of cancer than is any other organ in the male genitourinary tract. It is estimated that as many as 20 per cent of all men past fifty-five years of age develop cancer of the prostate but that most cases remain symptomless and unrecognized [11].

The most specific symptom indicating possible cancer in the genitourinary tract is the presence of blood in the urine. In addition, any change in normal habits of urination is reason for consulting a physician.

Leukemia. Leukemia, cancer of the blood-forming organs, occurs at all ages. Acute leukemia is the most common type of cancer found in children and causes nearly 2,000 deaths per year in children under 15. The incidence of leukemia is increasing faster than the population increase.

In most cases of leukemia there is a great excess of white blood cells; counts up to 800,000 per cubic centimeter instead of a normal 5,000 to 10,000 are not uncommon. In some cases there is no increase, and in some cases there may be a decrease. One index of the presence of leukemia, however, is not the number of white cells but the proportion of immature cells, which can be detected readily by microscopic examination.

Leukemia may be acute, as it is most commonly in younger persons, or it may be slow in developing and producing symptoms. Chronic myeloid leukemia usually occurs after the age of twenty-five, and chronic lymphatic leukemia occurs later in life [1]. In any case, there is no known cure, although patients with chronic lymphatic leukemia have survived ten to twenty years. Palliative drugs have offered some hope by delaying the effects of leukemia. Among the substances being used are steroid hormones (ACTH), antimetabolites (substances similar to those required for cell metabolism but having different metabolic effects), and cytotoxic substances (damaging to all cells but more damaging to

leukemic cells). With extensive research being conducted, it is likely that many patients now being kept alive by palliative measures will someday be cured.

MEANS OF DETECTING CANCER

Control of cancer depends upon early detection. Current means of treating cancer are effective only if they are used early. Therefore each individual should arrange regular examinations by his physician, observe common symptoms that might indicate the presence of a malignant tumor, and report such symptoms to his physician.

Common symptoms. Early symptoms may or may not be detected easily.

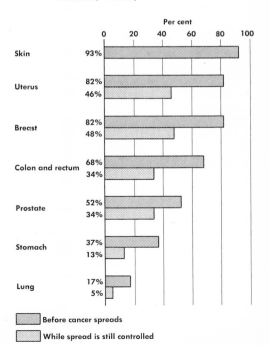

How early detection helps increase five-year survival rates. The chart does not show survival rates for advanced cancer, which is virtually incurable, or rates for earliest discovery, which are close to 100 per cent. (1961 Cancer Facts and Figures, American Cancer Society, California Division, 1961.)

Per cent

| | 0 | 20 | 40 | 60 | 80 | 100 |

Skin 93%

Uterus 82% / 46%

Breast 82% / 48%

Colon and rectum 68% / 34%

Prostate 52% / 34%

Stomach 37% / 13%

Lung 17% / 5%

▨ Before cancer spreads

▨ While spread is still controlled

BUILDING DEFENSES FOR EFFECTIVE LIVING

Unfortunately, pain is seldom an early sign of cancer. The following danger signals are stressed in the educational campaign carried on by the American Cancer Society [2, 4]:

Any sore that does not heal
A lump or thickening, in the breast or else-where
Unusual bleeding or discharge
Any change in a mole or wart
Persistent indigestion or difficulty in swallow-ing
Persistent hoarseness or cough
Any persistent change in normal bowel habits

The appearance of any one of these symptoms may mean cancer, or it may mean some other condition. The individual cannot make the diagnosis for himself. He should not put off visiting his physician until more symptoms appear. Delay may be fatal.

Diagnosis by a physician. The physician has at his disposal various means for determining whether a growth is present and, if so, whether it is malignant. These means include:

Observing and feeling for growths
Microscopic examination of secretions from the lining of the respiratory and genital tracts
X-ray pictures of inaccessible areas of the body
Microscopic examination of suspected tissue

The so-called pap smear test, named after Dr. George Papanicolaou, is an effective early detection procedure for cancer of the female reproductive organs. It should be a routine part of regular annual examinations of the female.

Research studies are attempting to discover a simple, inexpensive means of detecting the presence of cancer through blood tests or some other means. A means of early detection will be a major step in reducing deaths from cancer.

TREATMENT OF CANCER

There are three ways to treat cancer: by surgery, by radiation, and by chemo-

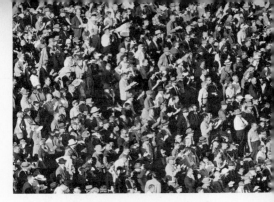

Of every twenty-four people, six will be afflicted with cancer.

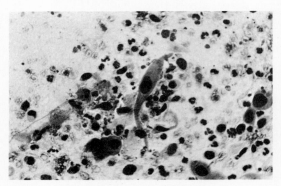

In the all-important detection of malignant cells . . .

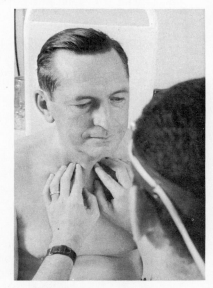

medical examination by one's physician . . .

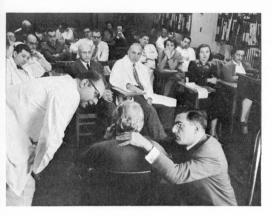

or at a reputable clinic is the first essential step.

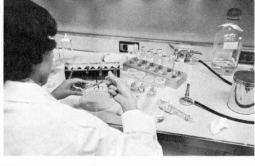

Tissues suspected of malignancy are then subjected to a laboratory test. If the presence of the disease is confirmed . . .

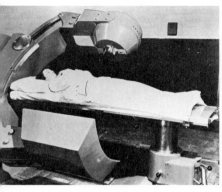

a method of therapy—surgery, radiation, or chemotherapy—is decided upon, and treatment is begun.

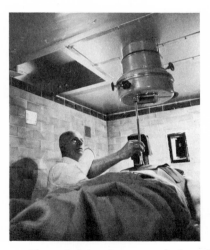

Through intensive research, knowledge about this disease is growing. It is through this knowledge that new resources for combating it may be discovered, and a higher percentage of lives saved.

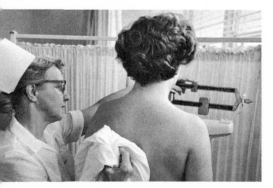

The absence of any recurrence of malignancy over a five-year period is considered a reliable indication of cure.

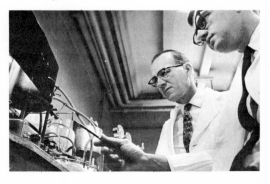

therapy. The desired result in each case is the complete destruction of malignant cells with as little damage to normal cells as possible. Surgical procedures are used to cut away the cancerous growth and in this way prevent metastasis. Radiation, which has been in use for cancer treatment for about fifty years, destroys the malignant cells where they are. Chemotherapy is more commonly used to inhibit or control abnormal cell growth when the cancer is inaccessible.

All cancers do not respond to the same type of treatment. Surgery may be the treatment of choice in one type of cancer, and radiation or chemotherapy may be more effective in others. When surgery is performed, a biopsy specimen is usually examined at once by a quick-freezing and staining process to confirm the malignancy. Radical surgery may be employed, in which considerable tissue around the malignant growth is removed in order to eliminate any cells that might have migrated through the nearby lymph system.

Radiation is used, in one form or another, with about six out of every ten cancer patients. Radiation, by knocking positively or negatively charged particles out of atoms that make up cells, produces chemical and biological changes that destroy cells. It is fortunate that radiation seems to be more destructive of the rapidly multiplying, immature cancer cells than of normal cells. Radiation, however, will destroy normal cells as well if there is too much exposure. It has been found that some types of cancer cells are unaffected by radiation in doses safe for the surrounding normal tissue. Two general types of radiation are used: X rays and radioisotopes [31].

Improved techniques of concentrating the effects of radiation from points outside the body have greatly increased the value of radiation [31, 32]. Advances in science have made it possible to make radioactive substances artificially. This has helped reduce the expense of radium, which was the original radioactive substance used in cancer treatment. Beaming radioactive waves from outside the body requires X rays and substances such as radium, cobalt-60, and cesium-137. The latter three are used in a pack, or bomb, which encloses the radioactive substance and directs the rays through an opening, or cone. In some instances radioactive substances are placed within or directly on the body. The use of radioactive iodine in the treatment of cancer of the thyroid is an example. The radioactive iodine is picked up by thyroid tissue wherever it is in the body; for this reason it may be helpful in diagnosis as well as treatment.

Intensive research has resulted in the discovery of a number of chemicals that have been used experimentally against malignant growths with varying degrees of success. Among the substances are hormones (estrogen used for cancer of the prostate gland), cell poisons (some 40 compounds including nitrogen mustards used against chronic leukemia), metabolic antagonists (antimetabolites, which starve cancer cells by interfering with life processes) [31]. Research and experiments with vaccines offer some hope of an effective anticancer vaccine for some types of cancer.

Even though treatment is started early, the physician is cautious about claims for cure. Only if the patient is free from recurrence for a five-year period is the malignant condition considered to be arrested. Following this five-year period regular examinations are essential, because of the possibility that the cancer may recur near the same site or in other parts of the body. Recovery from cancer does not confer immunity against subsequent malignant conditions.

Despite the claims made by many persons outside the medical profession, there is no evidence that unorthodox treatments have cured cancer. Cancer quacks take advantage of fear and igno-rance and are a distinct menace. The great danger in seeking the advice of quacks is that proper treatment is de-layed until it is too late.

Preventive methods are used in some occupations where workers are likely to be exposed to irritants predisposing to cancer—shielding for radiologists, for ex-ample. Great strides are being made in cancer research, and cancer detection centers are increasing in scope and value. The most important steps in control of cancer must be made by the possible cancer victim—regular examinations and early reporting of possible danger signs.

Diabetes mellitus

Diabetic persons occupy important posi-tions and take part in nearly every phase of life. Doctors, lawyers, political leaders, businessmen, professional athletes, and laborers are represented. It has been only since the discovery of insulin in 1921 that diabetes could be effectively treated. The average age at death of diabetic persons has been raised until it is only a few years less than that of nondiabetics. The significance of this is appreciated more when one realizes that at the turn of the century such patients had an aver-age life expectancy of approximately three years after onset of the disease.

Diabetes remains as a major health problem in the United States despite improvements in treatment. It is eighth among the leading causes of death. It is estimated that there are nearly 3 million diabetics in the United States, of which number almost half are undetected [34].

WHAT IS DIABETES?

Diabetes results when the pancreas, an endocrine gland located near the stomach, fails to supply a sufficient amount of the hormone insulin. As a result of the in-sufficient supply of insulin, the storage of sugar in the liver in inhibited, the formation of sugar from glycogen stored in the liver is speeded up, and the utilization of sugar by the tissues is de-pressed.

As a consequence of these changes, the following symptoms occur:
The blood sugar level is abnormally high.

The kidneys excrete sugar in the urine. The excretion of sugar results in an ex-cessive loss of salt and water.
Increased utilization of protein and fat sources of heat and energy is required to compensate for the inability of tissues to oxidize sugar.
The system is poisoned by products of incomplete combustion of proteins and fats.

Cause. No single factor causes diabetes mellitus. In some persons, specific in-jury due to infection or the presence of growths causes the islets of Langerhans in the pancreas to produce insufficient amounts of insulin. In others, the onset of diabetes is gradual, with many factors contributing to its development.

Heredity is recognized as an important factor in diabetes. If both parents are diabetic, all children may develop dia-betes; if one parent is diabetic, the child has a 50 per cent chance of developing diabetes; if neither parent is diabetic but there is diabetes in both families, the child has a 25 per cent chance of de-veloping the disease; if one parent is free of the disease and there is no family history of diabetes, the child should not develop it [34]. A pair of simple reces-sive genes apparently are responsible for most cases of diabetes.

Obesity is a contributing factor. The American Diabetes Association points out that 20 stout persons develop dia-betes for every thin person. Studies show that over 80 per cent of diabetic patients who were forty years of age or older when they developed diabetes were overweight prior to the onset of the disease [21, 34]. Whether or not overeating causes diabetes in an individual who does not have an inherited susceptibility has not been clearly established. There is little doubt, however, that the strain placed on the islets of Langerhans of a susceptible person by overeating is a contributing factor.

Although more than four-fifths of cases of diabetes develop after the age of forty-five, diabetes is not limited to older persons. Women are more likely to develop diabetes than are men. After the age of forty years, a woman has about one-third more chances of developing diabetes than a man has. It is not known whether the increased rate for women is due to differences in eating habits, glandular changes during menopause, or some unknown factor or factors.

DETECTION

Diabetes can be detected by the physician in its beginning stages before symptoms are apparent to the individual. Regular physical examinations, including urinalyses, provide the opportunity for early detection. In addition, the appearance of the following symptoms may indicate the onset of the disease.

Symptoms. An increased output of urine may be the first indication that diabetes is present. The increase occurs because the kidneys eliminate excess amounts of sugar that accumulate in the blood. The demand for fluid to aid in the elimination of excess sugar causes an increased feeling of thirst. Owing to the inability to oxidize sugar properly, the tissues lack an adequate energy supply. The result is a constant feeling of hunger. The use of protein and fat supplies as a source of energy results in weight loss. There is also a tendency to tire easily.

Other symptoms appear in varying degrees of intensity. The person may be annoyed by excessive itching, he may begin to notice a change in vision, and he may discover that wounds do not heal readily.

Screening tests. Because of the estimated 1 million or more undetected cases of diabetes in the United States, attempts are being made to screen large numbers of persons. Effective screening can detect undiagnosed cases and also some prediabetic individuals. It has been found that mothers who give birth to big babies, over 10 pounds, are more likely to develop diabetes. Careful testing of these women would aid in early detection and more effective control.

The work of the American Diabetes Association and other interested groups and persons should receive the fullest cooperation of citizens. Through education and widespread screening projects, which they support, many complications of diabetes are being reduced.

CONTROL

Under the supervision of a competent physician, diabetes is the most readily controlled of the chronic diseases. Diabetic persons are fortunate compared with victims of some other chronic diseases, because diabetes can be treated effectively. When the diabetic person is able to maintain relatively sugar-free urine and to prevent other symptoms, the diabetes is said to be controlled. However, diabetes is not cured in the sense that a communicable disease is cured. Regulation of diet, exercise, and insulin must be maintained, or symptoms of the condition appear once again.

Oral drugs, the sulfonylureas, have been in general use since 1957. They have been effective in 80 per cent of cases in which the patient was over forty at onset of the disease but less effective in cases with an earlier age of onset [34]. The sulfonylureas, Orinase and Diabinese, and a new drug Phenformin (DB1) have some distinct advantages in convenience and simplicity from the patient's standpoint. It is important, however, to recognize that care must be exercised in their use and that the user should be under the supervision of a physician.

COMPLICATIONS

Before insulin became available, diabetic coma ranked as the primary cause of death in diabetic cases. Diabetic coma occurs when the individual does not have enough insulin. As a result, products from the incomplete combustion of proteins and fats cause acidosis, which is fatal if untreated.

Overdoses of insulin will cause a reaction, or "insulin shock." Since the individual suffering from insulin reaction may exhibit symptoms of intoxication, an identification card indicating that he is diabetic saves him considerable embarrassment and may avert a real disaster. A physician should be called immediately if diabetic coma or insulin reaction is suspected.

Rheumatism

Rheumatism and rheumatic diseases are commonly accepted as synonymous terms to indicate any of a number of painful disorders in which the principal symptoms are related to the joints or to their anatomic supporting structures [9]. Rheumatic diseases are not among the newer afflictions of mankind. The Java man, who lived some 500,000 years ago, and the Neanderthal man, of 25,000 years past, were both victims of rheumatic diseases.

The problem of rheumatic diseases in the United States is illustrated by the estimated 11 million persons who are afflicted with arthritis or some other type of rheumatic disease. More than 4 million persons, over half of them under the age of 45, are victims of rheumatoid arthritis. Victims of arthritis are being cheated of more than 250 million dollars every year as a result of misrepresentations made by promoters who claim cures. Annual loss in work days totals 115 million for arthritis victims. Lost wages are approximately 700 million dollars each year [8, 9, 35].

Although there are many rheumatic diseases, only rheumatoid arthritis, osteoarthritis (degenerative joint disease), gout, and rheumatic fever are discussed in the following pages.

RHEUMATOID ARTHRITIS

Rheumatoid arthritis is a systemic disorder that produces general symptoms, but the primary concern is joint changes that result from the disease. Rheumatoid arthritis is found in all parts of the world, although it is more common in temperate climates. Although it may strike at any age, it is more likely to occur between the ages of twenty-five and fifty. Women victims outnumber men approximately three to one.

There have been many hypotheses as to the cause of rheumatoid arthritis, but as yet the cause is not known. Among the suggested possible causes are infection, endocrine imbalance, hypersensitivity, and faulty adaptation to either physical or psychic stress, but evidence to support any of these is not conclusive [8].

The onset of this disease is gradual in approximately four out of five victims. In the early stages there may be vague and fleeting joint pains and joint stiffness upon awakening in the morning. Such symptoms may persist for weeks before the disease progresses to a more acute stage. In its early stages only one joint or several may be involved.

During acute stages of the disease general ill health and an elevated temperature may be present. It has been found, however, that extensive joint changes may take place in healthy, robust individuals.

Destruction of tissues resulting in swelling and deformity are the characteristic signs of a person with an advanced case of rheumatoid arthritis. Swelling, inflammation, and eventual loss of articulation of the affected joint result in partial or almost complete disability for some victims.

The importance of seeking medical advice when the early signs of possible rheumatoid arthritis are noticed cannot be stressed too much. Early diagnosis and treatment can play an important role in modifying the disease process and reducing the danger of disability. Even though there is no specific treatment for curing rheumatoid arthritis, treatment by a qualified medical adviser can do much to reduce suffering and prevent loss of mobility.

As indicated earlier, quacks find arthritis victims particularly susceptible to misleading claims. Some of the suggested treatment is beneficial but expensive, some is expensive and of no value, some is harmless in itself but dangerous because of the delay in seeking qualified medical advice, and some is dangerous because the condition is aggravated by improper treatment.

Generally accepted treatment measures are: general measures (diet, rest, controlled exercise), drug therapy (aspirin is the preferred drug in most instances), physical therapy, steroid therapy, orthopedic measures, and psychotherapy [8]. Treatment should be under the direction of the qualified medical adviser who can make the most effective use of treatment for each individual.

OSTEOARTHRITIS

This disease is most likely to be found in older persons who are overweight and have faulty posture or poor muscle tone.

Joints literally show signs of wearing out because of the burdens placed upon them. Joint injury is a factor that contributes to the onset of osteoarthritis. The weight-bearing joints are affected by the conditions mentioned above. As a result, the knees, ankles, hips, and vertebrae frequently are altered by this degenerative process.

X-ray examinations of a joint affected by osteoarthritis show calcium deposits or bony outgrowths. The cartilage at the joint shows signs of aging. These permanent changes in joint structure produce some pain and stiffness and result in enlarged, knobby joints.

Osteoarthritis, or degenerative arthritis, responds to treatment and is not, in most cases, the crippler that rheumatoid arthritis is. With early recognition and treatment of the condition, the prognosis for this disease is much more favorable.

GOUT

Gout is a rheumatic disease, found more commonly in some families than in others. Approximately 95 per cent of victims of gout are men, and in most cases they are past thirty years of age. Individuals who develop gout have a higher than normal amount of urates (salts of uric acid).

The joint tissues of hands and feet are most often affected by the deposits of urates. The big toe is frequently the particular joint affected. Attacks of gout tend to recur unless proper treatment is instituted. Physicians have effective means of treating acute attacks of gout and also for controlling uric acid excretion, thus eliminating the irritation that brings on the attack of gout [8].

RHEUMATIC FEVER

Rheumatic fever is a major rheumatic disease. Because the damage to the heart is the most serious consequence of rheumatic fever, this disease is discussed earlier in the chapter in connection with heart diseases.

OTHER RHEUMATIC DISEASES

Among other rheumatic diseases of some consequence are:

Collagen diseases (systemic lupus erythematosus, scleroderma, dermatomyositis)

Arthritis due to infection (acute infectious arthritis, gononcoccic arthritis, arthritis and spondylitis due to tuberculosis, syphilitic arthritis)

Nonarticular rheumatism (tenosynovitis, bursitis, fibrositis, psychogenic rheumatism)

IF ONE HAS RHEUMATISM

Any symptoms indicating possible involvement of the joints in some disease process should be brought to the attention of a qualified medical adviser. Competent assistance is needed in order to diagnose the condition properly and to institute treatment to relieve suffering and interrupt the progress of the disease. Despite many claims made through advertising media, there is no "magic means" of treating the rheumatic diseases.

Allergies

An allergic person who is sneezing, wheezing, or itching is one of the most miserable individuals in the world. It is unrealistic, however, to consider the reaction as only a temporarily annoying condition. It is suggested that one of the nation's major health problems is being neglected until allergy is recognized as a lifelong condition causing impaired efficiency in mild cases and a serious economic drain on families in more advanced forms [16].

Among the allergic complaints are hay fever, asthma, hives, eczema, allergic rhinitis, gastrointestinal upsets, headaches, and eye inflammations. It has been estimated that more than 24 million Americans are afflicted with a major allergy. Additional evidence of the extent of the problem is that antiallergic drugs were eighth among all prescriptions filled in the United States during the period April–July, 1959, and that they made up 50 per cent of all prescriptions filled [16].

WHAT IS AN ALLERGY?

Allergic reactions are of many different types, depending upon the substance precipitating the reaction and the body tissues involved. The reactions vary considerably, but the basic process is essentially the same in all cases. The reason why some individuals are allergic and others are not has not been clearly established, but there is evidence of a hereditary tendency or predisposition.

Allergens. The chemical substances responsible for allergic reactions are called *allergens.* Allergens are antigens that induce the body to develop specific antibodies (see Chapter 11, page 318). The antibodies produced by the reaction of body tissues to antigens from disease-producing organisms serve a definite protective function. The antibodies produced by the reaction of body tissues to allergens do not serve a protective function. Instead, they in turn react with additional amounts of the same allergen to release histamine, which produces the typical allergic results.

Although allergens for a long time were thought to be exclusively protein in nature, it has been demonstrated that other chemical substances are capable of causing allergic reactions.

How do allergens enter the body? Allergens make their way into the human organism by different routes. An individual who is constitutionally predisposed to allergic reactions may become sensitized by inhaling or breathing, by ingesting or swallowing, by injection, by contact with a particular allergen, or by bacterial infection in the body.

Allergens taken in through the respiratory tract include dusts, mold spores, animal danders, and pollen from a variety of plants. Hay fever is an allergic reaction in the nasal membrane resulting from exposure and sensitization to allergens of this type. Hay fever affects 7 or 8 million Americans each year [5]. Hay-fever symptoms may make a seasonal appearance when due to pollens, an irregular appearance when due to animal dander (dog, cat, horse) that the person contacts only occasionally, or a regular appearance when due to house dust. Symptoms of hay fever include obstruction of nasal passages due to swelling of membranes, nasal discharge, and sneezing.

Allergens, whether they enter the body through the respiratory tract or by other means, may produce their effect in the bronchial tubes and cause asthma. It is estimated that about one of three hay fever victims develops asthma. The asthmatic person has difficulty in breathing because of the constriction of the bronchial tubes. He may make a wheezing sound as he breathes, and he is likely to discharge sputum by coughing as the attack begins to terminate. The symptoms tend to vary with individuals. They may be mistaken for other conditions, especially in children.

Immune serums obtained from animal sources can produce an allergic reaction when injected into individuals. Because of the danger of extreme allergic reactions, the patient is commonly tested before such serums are used. The replacement of serum treatment by the sulfonamides and antibiotics reduces the danger from this source. However, these drugs themselves can cause an allergic reaction. With some persons the reaction is so severe that the use of these drugs is dangerous and must be avoided. Individuals who are allergic to penicillin may be advised to wear a tag warning against the use of penicillin in case of injury.

Allergies resulting from ingestion of foods are common. The results may be simply a feeling of discomfort, or they may be definite and pronounced. Hives, eczema, asthma, and migraine headaches are sometimes symptoms produced by allergic reaction to foods. Wheat, milk, eggs, nuts, fish, peas, beans, potatoes, and cocoa are some of the foods most likely to produce allergic reactions.

Poison ivy causes a distinct and severe allergic reaction in some persons as a result of contact of the oily residue from the plant with the skin. First exposures serve to sensitize the person, and subsequent exposures produce the characteristic inflammation of contact dermatitis. Failure to develop the allergic reaction following an exposure is not definite proof of immunity. Instead, it can mean that the individual is being sensitized and that through additional exposures he may develop the reaction. Other plants, various chemicals, metals (mercury in particular), and dyes used in clothing are some of the common offenders which produce allergic reactions through contact with the skin.

SOMETHING CAN BE DONE

Detecting an allergy is not always a simple matter, even for the physician, and self-diagnosis is likely to result in error. Fortunately, the family physician or the allergist has at his disposal the means for determining whether or not an allergy is present, the substances responsible for the allergy, and effective means for relieving or curing the condition. Early treatment for allergies is important because of the danger of developing more severe types of allergic reactions.

Determining the cause. Once a diagnosis of allergy has been made, it is essential to discover all the substances causing the reaction. A detailed health history, a thorough study of the patient's environment, and allergy testing are tools used to determine the specific allergen or allergens. Testing for sensitivity by means of skin and mucous-membrane tests is effective in most instances, although it may take a long time to complete the extensive number of tests to be made. The tests are based on the fact that the sensitized individual has developed antibodies, which react locally with allergens being injected.

Avoiding the allergens. Avoiding the allergens responsible for producing the allergy is an important method of treatment. Unfortunately, this method is not always practical. A vacation away from his home area for a period of time during the pollen season may be practical for one person and impossible for another. Devices for filtering the air coming into the home are effective for relieving the symptoms for some individuals.

Food allergies are alleviated by planning a diet that avoids the particular foods responsible for the allergy. Unless the person is allergic to a number of foods, the elimination of such foods from the diet is the most successful treatment available. In most cases careful planning of substitute foods allows the proper balance of nutrients to be maintained.

If the source of the allergen is the household pet, either cat or dog, the most effective procedure for avoiding exposure is to find a new home for the pet. Recognition of poison ivy and care in avoiding exposure to it provide the most practical control measure for most persons.

In some instances, avoiding the allergen is difficult or even impossible. Fortunately, there are other methods which can be used effectively in cases where exposure is certain.

Building up resistance. The basic principle of building up resistance is an active immunization process. Prepara-

tions of the offending substance are injected underneath the skin in increasing quantities. After a time a tolerance is developed, which permits ordinary exposure without the allergic reaction. Unfortunately, all allergies do not respond to this type of desensitization. The physician determines whether or not this treatment is effective for specific individuals. In general, this protection lasts only for a limited period and may have to be repeated.

Relieving symptoms. Relieving symptoms is only a stopgap measure, and the continued treatment of an allergy by relieving the symptoms is not always recommended by a physician. There are effective means for relieving allergies that endanger life or cause extreme discomfort.

The use of preparations for constricting blood vessels in the nose to reduce nasal discharge may be effective, but the indiscriminate use of nose drops is not recommended and may be harmful. Many individuals simply add to their difficulty by using commercial preparations without seeking the advice of their physician. Antihistamines, which provide relief from the symptoms of some allergies, can produce dangerous reactions in some persons.

WHAT LIES AHEAD?

Many of the answers to allergy problems are not known. Some allergies defy the best efforts of specialists to discover the cause or to provide relief. Studies indicate close relationship between allergies and many disease conditions affecting mankind. One factor slowing down allergy research is lack of funds. The third-place ranking of asthma and hay fever among the chronic diseases in the United States testifies to the nature and extent of the problem [5]. In comparison with the amount of money spent on other types of research and on relieving symptoms, the amount made available for research on allergies is lagging far behind.

Cystic fibrosis

Cystic fibrosis (C/F) is a generalized disorder of the exocrine, or duct, glands, which secrete sweat, tears, mucus, and saliva. It is one of the most common and at the same time one of the most serious chronic diseases affecting children. The condition most often affects the pancreas, the lungs, and the sweat glands.

Interference with the flow of enzymes from the pancreas disrupts the normal digestion of food and may result in mucus plugs obstructing the intestinal tract. C/F may also cause a thick mucus to fill the lungs and obstruct breathing. It may, in other instances, cause such profuse sweating that the sodium supply of the body is depleted and profound shock may be the result.

The high sodium content of the sweat of a victim of cystic fibrosis is the basis for a simple but effective test which enables the physician to make a rapid diagnosis and to provide for early treatment. During the 26 years since the disease was recognized in 1936, significant steps have been taken to control its serious consequences. Research has provided a source of the enzyme lipase, which is lacking in the victim of C/F of the pancreas. A daily supply of lipancreatin, taken with every meal, at a cost of approximately 50 cents per day, provides the victim with the enzyme essential for the digestion of fats.

Cystic fibrosis is considered to be a hereditary disorder, probably due to a recessive gene transmitted by each of the victim's parents. It has been estimated that the problem gene may exist in approximately one of every 50 adults; the result is approximately 6,000 new victims of the disease each year [13].

Chronic diseases affecting the muscles and nervous system

MULTIPLE SCLEROSIS

Multiple sclerosis is a chronic disease in which the myelin sheath of nerves is destroyed and replaced with scar (sclerotic) tissue. It is called "multiple" sclerosis because it is likely to affect many parts of the nervous system. It is estimated that more than 500,000 persons in the United States are afflicted with multiple sclerosis and closely related diseases [27]. It was from multiple sclerosis that Lou Gehrig, a baseball immortal, died at the age of thirty-seven.

Symptoms vary with individuals, but the general symptoms listed by the National Multiple Sclerosis Society are [28]:

Partial or complete paralysis of parts of the body

Numbness in parts of the body

Double or otherwise defective vision, such as involuntary movements of eyeballs

Noticeable dragging of one or both feet

Severe bladder or bowel trouble (loss of control)

Speech difficulties, such as slurring

Staggering or loss of balance (MS patients often erroneously are thought to be intoxicated)

Extreme weakness or fatigue

Prickling sensation in parts of the body ("pins and needles")

Loss of coordination

Tremors of hands

The onset of multiple sclerosis is limited almost entirely to the years between twenty and forty. Symptoms may appear at irregular intervals over a period of years, may persist to a minor degree, or may appear and progress rapidly. Life expectancy is approximately that of the general population.

Although there is no clearly established treatment for curing the condition, good medical care enables many patients to continue to live a happy and productive life. Research being conducted under the auspices of the National Multiple Sclerosis Society, the National Institute of Neurological Diseases and Blindness, and other interested groups offers much hope to victims of the disease.

CEREBRAL PALSY

Cerebral palsy is a condition in which the person is not able to control voluntary muscles effectively because of damage to the motor area of the central nervous system. The United Cerebral Palsy Association estimates that approximately 550,000 persons have cerebral palsy [25]. The condition is inherited in 10 per cent or more of cases [17]. The cause is damage to the motor areas of the brain as a result of such factors as birth injury, Rh incompatibility between mother and fetus, disease conditions such as German measles during the first third of pregnancy, anoxia (lack of sufficient oxygen), trauma, or head injury following birth, and congenital malformations. Prematurity is considered one of the chief predisposing factors.

Injuries to different parts of the motor area of the brain may produce different symptoms. The most common kinds of cerebral palsy on the basis of effect on the victim are spastic, athetoid, ataxia, tremor, and rigidity. It is possible for an individual to have mixed symptoms. The spastic individual is characterized by muscle tenseness or excessive contraction of muscles. The athetoid individual lacks control and has many involuntary, unorganized movements. The spastic and athetoid cases account for more than three-fourths of the victims. Ataxia is a disturbed balance or sense of equilibrium; this type of paralysis is most usually acquired rather than congenital [12]. Tremor is a trembling or rhythmic pattern of uncontrolled movements. Rigidity indicates a stiff and rigid condition due to muscle contractions. One or more of the limbs or parts of the body may be affected by these symptoms.

Some of the possible ways in which the number of victims of cerebral palsy can be reduced include [12, 17]:

Developing healthy and informed potential mothers

Protection of the health of expectant mothers through good diet and prevention of infections

Reduction in the number of premature deliveries

Safe delivery and adequate care of premature infants

Prevention or quick reduction of neonatal anoxia

Control of Rh incompatibility

Prevention of accidents in infancy and childhood

The fact that an individual is a victim of cerebral palsy does not mean that he is below normal in intelligence. Mental handicaps may be associated with cerebral palsy, but many victims are average or above average in intelligence. It is important to understand that proper treatment and the correct type of educational activities can be extremely beneficial to the cerebral-palsied individual.

EPILEPSY

Individuals with epilepsy, a disorder of the nervous system, may have greater problems with misinformed fellow citizens than they have with the disorder itself. The epileptic may have normal or superior intelligence and be a successful and well-adjusted member of the community. In spite of this, if he should have a seizure, the reaction of misinformed friends, neighbors, fellow employees, and his employer can make his adjustment difficult.

The epileptic seizure is produced by a sudden, violent, disorderly discharge of brain cells. A severe seizure can be most disconcerting to bystanders, but a mild seizure may go undetected. Development of the electroencephalograph (EEG), which provides a record of the activity of brain cells, has made it possible to determine that some individuals have abnormal brainwave patterns. An estimated 10 to 12 per cent of the total population are "latent" epileptics [18]. Many of these persons go through life without seizures if no precipitating factor is present.

Types of seizures. Grand mal is a generalized seizure in which the individual loses consciousness, the body stiffens, jerking movements of the whole body are observed, labored breathing occurs, and there may be loss of control of the bladder. *Petit mal* is less severe and may be no more than a brief interruption of consciousness observed as a blank stare or a rapid blinking of the eyes. The psychomotor attack may be seen as a series of movements that seem to have a purpose but are unrelated to the situation—chewing motions and smacking the lips. Focal seizures start in one part of the body and may be limited to that area or may spread and become general seizures of the grand mal type.

Causes of seizures. Lesions of the brain and conditions that disturb brain function by interfering with biochemical processes are the two general causes of seizures. Lesions of the brain include those due to faulty development of brain tissues or cerebral vessels during fetal life; tumors, chronic abscesses, or blood clots due to trauma; infections producing inflammation of the brain or its coverings (meninges); cerebral vascular disease; and degeneration of brain tissues leading to atrophy. Conditions, other than lesions, altering the biochemical function of the brain include conditions limiting the supply of oxygen and/or sugar. In some instances no primary cause is discovered, but the EEG may show a diffuse cerebral

dysrhythmia. These cases are referred to as *idiopathic* (of undetermined cause). The age of onset of seizures generally varies with the cause. It is estimated, for example, that 70 per cent of idiopathic cases start before a person is twenty years old [18].

Treatment. Fortunately, seizures alone rarely cause death, mental deterioration, or disorders in personality. Even more fortunately, it should be noted that proper treatment, which usually includes drug therapy, by a qualified physician can prevent the occurrence of seizures in a majority of epileptic patients. Improvement in understanding the disease and attitudes toward the epileptic can make adjustment easier.

MUSCULAR DYSTROPHY

Muscular dystrophy is a chronic disease which causes the muscles to weaken and waste away. Although the exact cause of the disease is not known, muscular dystrophy is not contagious. The disease is found in all parts of the world and it occurs at all ages. The Muscular Dystrophy Associations of America indicate that more than two-thirds of the estimated 200,000 victims in the United States are between the ages of three and thirteen years [24].

The wasting away of the muscles is progressive, and there is no known treatment for stopping the progress of the disease. In muscular dystrophy the nerves are not affected as in multiple sclerosis and most other types of paralysis or muscle weakness. The gradual wasting away of the voluntary muscles of the body reduces the ability of the victim to move about. In addition, if the muscles which enable one to breathe are affected, serious problems arise even with a common cold.

In the most common form of muscular dystrophy (pseudohypertrophic type) the onset is usually between the ages of three and ten, and the course of the disease tends to be more rapid than with other types. This type is hereditary, due to a recessive gene, in approximately one-third of cases, and it affects about three times as many males as females [24]. Other types are more likely to affect a certain part of the body, usually occur later in life, and are about equally divided between the sexes.

Since the first emphasis on research in the early 1950s, there has been increased interest in learning more about the disease. The establishment of the Institute of Muscle Disease in New York has provided a major impetus in research, and continued emphasis on research by the Muscular Dystrophy Associations of America offers hope that the cause of this crippler will be determined and that effective means of treatment will be established.

Summary

Diseases of the heart and circulatory system, cancer, diabetes, kidney diseases, rheumatism, allergies, cystic fibrosis, and diseases of the muscles and nervous system are chronic and degenerative diseases, which kill or disable many persons in the United States. Early detection is essential for effective control of the diseases. Both the individual and the physician have responsibilities for the early detection of these diseases and for delaying their onset.

The college student reading about chronic and degenerative diseases may tend to feel that they are a long way off for him. He may wonder whether he can do anything about them if he wants to. As has been pointed out in respect to a number of these diseases, they may not be too far off and some things *can* be done. Information in many other chapters of this book has implications for delaying, preventing, and controlling chronic and degenerative diseases.

Application of the recommendations concerning good adjustment and the developing and maintaining of good mental health is extremely important not only for its own sake but also in many chronic conditions. A proper diet today is important now and also for your future. One aspect of diet, a surplus of calories and the resulting excess weight, is perhaps most significant in respect to chronic diseases. The unwise use of stimulants and depressants has many potential hazards; the danger of lung cancer associated with smoking is one example. Physical activity and physical fitness can be depended upon to pay dividends in delaying the onset of some chronic conditions.

Chronic diseases are not isolated conditions that have little relation to total living; rather, they are part of, and a consequence of, living. How you live today can dictate how well you live tomorrow.

Suggested readings

1. American Cancer Society: *Leukemia,* The Society, New York, 1959.
2. American Cancer Society: *Answers to 101 Questions about Cancer,* The Society, New York, 1960.
3. American Cancer Society: *Shall I Smoke?* The Society, New York, 1960.
4. American Cancer Society: *The Hopeful Side of Cancer,* The Society, New York, 1960.
5. American Foundation for Allergic Diseases: *Hay Fever and Other Allergic Disease,* The Foundation, New York, 1960.
6. American Heart Association: *If Your Child Has a Congenital Heart Defect,* The Association, New York, 1960.
7. American Heart Association and National Heart Institute: "A Decade of Progress against Cardiovascular Disease," *Congressional Record,* Mar. 5, 1959.
8. American Rheumatism Association: "Primer on the Rheumatic Diseases," *Journal of the American Medical Associ-*

ation, 171:1205–1220, Oct. 31, 1959; 171:1345–1356, Nov. 7, 1959; 171:1680–1691, Nov. 21, 1959.

9. Arthritis and Rheumatism Foundation: *Questions on Arthritis,* The Foundation, New York, 1960.

10. Birren, James E.: *Handbook of Aging and the Individual,* The University of Chicago Press, Chicago, 1959.

11. Cameron, Charles S.: *The Truth about Cancer,* Prentice-Hall, Inc., Englewood Cliffs, N.J., 1956.

12. Cardwell, Viola E.: *Cerebral Palsy: Advances in Understanding and Care,* Association for the Aid of Crippled Children, New York, 1956.

13. Conniff, James C. G.: "C/F: Mystery Menace at Bay," *Today's Health,* 39: 42–43, Aug., 1961.

14. "Cytological Screening Techniques," *Journal of the American Medical Association,* 172:165–166, Mar. 12, 1960.

15. DeCoursey, Russell Myles: *The Human Organism,* 2d ed., McGraw-Hill Book Company, Inc., New York, 1961.

16. Dees, Susan C.: "Chronic Allergy—Crippler and Killer of Children," *Journal of Chronic Diseases,* 12:326–339, September, 1960.

17. Denhoff, Eric, and Isabel Pick Robinault: *Cerebral Palsy and Related Disorders,* McGraw-Hill Book Company, Inc., 1960.

18. Duggens, Virginia A.: *Epilepsy: Its Causes, Effects and Treatment,* Federal Association for Epilepsy, Inc., Washington, 1959.

19. Earle, Howard: "What You Should Know about Your Kidneys," (Interview with David P. Earle), *Today's Health,* 39:52–54, June, 1961.

20. Gilbert, Philip: "Can Heart Attacks Be Predicted," *Today's Health,* 38:36–37, December, 1960.

21. Joslin, Elliott P.: *Diabetic Manual,* Lea & Febiger, Philadelphia, 1959.

22. McGrady, Pat: "Some Highlights of the 4th National Cancer Conference," *Cancer News,* 14:3, Fall, 1960.

23. Metropolitan Life Insurance Company: "Fifty Years of Health Progress," *Statistical Bulletin,* 42:1–12, January, 1961.

24. Muscular Dystrophy Associations of America: *Muscular Dsytrophy—The Facts,* The Association, New York, 1960.

25. National Institute of Neurological Diseases and Blindness: *Cerebral Palsy: Hope through Research,* U.S. Department of Health, Education and Welfare, Washington, 1960.

26. National Office of Vital Statistics, Public Health Service: "Mortality from Each Cause: United States, 1957–59," *Vital Statistics—Special Reports: National Summaries,* U.S. Department of Health, Education and Welfare, Washington, vol. 54, no. 1, Apr. 12, 1961.

27. National Multiple Sclerosis Society: *Tackling a Mystery—the Story of Multiple Sclerosis,* The Society, New York, 1958.

28. National Multiple Sclerosis Society: *SOS for Multiple Sclerosis,* The Society, New York, 1959.

29. Page, Irvine H.: "High Blood Pressure: How Dangerous Is It?" *Today's Health,* 38:60, 65–67, June, 1960.

30. "Prevention and Control of Heart Disease," *American Journal of Public Health,* 50, part II: 1–34, March, 1960.

31. Public Health Service: *Treating Cancer: Surgery, Radiation, Chemotherapy,* U.S. Department of Health, Education and Welfare, Washington, 1960.

32. "Radiation's Other Face: The 'Bomb' That Can Heal," *Today's Health,* 38:38–39, January, 1960.

33. Ratcliff, J. D.: "Your Body's Master Chemists," *Today's Health,* 38:59, December, 1960.

34. Seeman, Bernard: "What You Should Know about Diabetes," *Today's Health,* 38:50–51, January, 1960.

35. *The Arthritis Hoax,* Public Affairs Pamphlet 297, Public Affairs Committee, New York, 1960.

36. "The Cancer Prevention Study," *Cancer News,* 14:8, Fall, 1960.

37. U.S. Department of Health, Education, and Welfare: *Varicose Veins,* Government Printing Office, Washington, 1959.

38. U.S. Department of Health, Education, and Welfare: *Health, Education and Welfare Indicators,* Government Printing Office, Washington, January, 1961.

39. U.S. Department of Health, Education, and Welfare: *The Nation and Its Older People: Report of the White House Conference on Aging, January 9–12, 1961,* Government Printing Office, Washington, April, 1961.

40. Weiss, Edward: *Anxiety and Your Heart: The Psychosomatic Aspects of Heart Disease,* American Medical Association, Chicago, 1960.

41. "Your Heart: The Perpetual Motion Pump," *Today's Health,* 38:23–28, January, 1960.

42. Zucker, Marjorie B.: "Blood Platelets," *Scientific American,* 204:58–64, February, 1961.

THIRTEEN

Understanding depressants and stimulants

DEPRESSANTS AND STIMULANTS DEFINED

BEVERAGE ALCOHOL

TOBACCO

DEPRESSANT DRUGS

STIMULANTS

The American public is contentedly consuming more kinds and quantities of stimulants and depressants than at any time before in its history. Right or wrong, this is undeniably an expression of a way of life during the last half of the twentieth century— an expression which costs the American public over 25 billion dollars annually. Americans are heavy consumers of stimulants and depressants such as coffee, tea, cola beverages, tobacco, alcoholic beverages, and some narcotics.

A substantial number of people, including college students, lack either the ability or the interest to distinguish between the serviceable and the harmful commercial forms of depressants and stimulants. Many are influenced by new testimonials, advertising, and opinions of so-called authorities on these products. When compiled, these data become a formidable array of truth, half-truth, and untruth. They either reinforce attitudes and practices already formed or increase the perplexities of those who find it difficult to discriminate.

As has been previously indicated, college students consider stimulants and depressants a major concern, one of the important health factors. Lantagne found that this area, which he termed "habit-forming substances," was rated the first interest of college students.[1] It was even ahead of mental health and family health.

The subsequent discussion is presented to assist the student in making an intelligent appraisal of depressants and stimulants and answering the following questions:

What are stimulants and depressants?

What are the properties of alcohol, tobacco, and narcotics?

How do these various products affect the body?

What are the problems created by undisciplined use of these products?

What decisions should be made concerning the use of stimulants and depressants?

Depressants and stimulants defined

For purposes of this discussion, depressants may be defined as *substances that produce relaxation, profuse perspiration, reduced ability to move and think, and reduced action of the vital organs of the body.* Acetylsalicylic acid, bromide, barbiturates, chloroform, ethyl alcohol, ether, and opium and its derivatives are typical depressants.

Stimulants may be defined as *substances that produce the opposite effect from depressants.* They also serve to irritate body tissue. Nicotine,[2] caffeine, cocaine, Benzedrine, tannic acid, and theobromine are typical stimulants.

However, such classification means

little unless one can identify these products or substances in their commercial form. Table 13.1 should help in such identification.

In order to report the amount and kind of stimulants and depressants the American public is consuming, it will be necessary to depart, temporarily, from specifics and to study four principal groups:

Beverage alcohol (depressant)

Tobacco (both stimulant and depressant)

Narcotics (depressant)

Benzedrine and "stay-awake" substances (stimulants)

Beverage alcohol

Historically, the drinking of beverage alcohol is a very old custom. Its first appearance probably occurred simultaneously in many parts of the world. When primitive peoples first caused grain mash, fruit mash, mare's milk, or palm-tree sap to ferment, an ingredient

was discovered that became evident to the consumer and to the observer alike. It gave to the consumer temporary pleasure and to his community unhappiness. The drinker believed he had the answer to his feelings of fatigue and anxiety. His inhibitions were released. He became aggressive and delighted in fighting. As a result of this type of behavior, it became necessary to develop controls for both the manufacture and the consumption of alcoholic beverages.

---

[1] Joseph E. Lantagne, "An Analysis of Health Interests of 1,000 Junior College Students in California," *Junior College Journal,* 21:429–433, April, 1951.

[2] Nicotine first acts as a stimulant, then becomes a profound depressant.

Table 13.1   Substances which depress or stimulate

Product	Depressant	Stimulant
Brewed liquors (beer)	x	
Distilled liquors (brandy, gin, rum, whisky)	x	
Wines (dry, fortified, heavy, light, sparkling, sweet)	x	
Elixirs (cordials, crèmes, liqueurs)	x	
Nicotine	First stimulant, then depressant	
Acetylsalicylic acid	x	
Barbiturates	x	
Bromides	x	
Chloroform	x	
Demerol	x	
Ether	x	
Heroin	x	
Marihuana	x	
Morphine	x	
Opium and derivatives	x	
Benzedrine		x
Cola beverages		x
Cocaine		x
Coffee		x
Maté		x
Tea		x

TYPES OF DRINKERS

Haggard and Jellinek define the *moderate drinker* as one who does not seek intoxication and does not expose himself to it. He drinks for the mild sedative effects. Beverage alcohol is not a necessity to his daily living, nor does it become a major item in his budget [9].

The *intemperate drinker* extends the limits of moderation and purposely exposes himself to the intoxicating effects inherent in alcohol. Intemperate drinkers are called *inebriates*. The inebriate may follow any of four patterns of drinking: normal excessive, symptomatic, stupid, and alcoholic addiction [9].

The normal (occasional) excessive drinker is motivated essentially by the feeling of well-being produced. He drinks because he enjoys it. Symptomatic drinkers are those who drink because of mental deviations. Stupid drinkers are those who drink because of low mental ability and because they cannot rise any higher in their periods of leisure. An alcoholic addict is one who has no control over his desire for alcohol; he cannot stop drinking. He is so frequently intoxicated that he does not lead a normal life [9].

There was a time when it was believed that the desire to drink alcoholic beverages was transmitted biologically. Today it is accepted that the desire is acquired.

The reasons commonly advanced for drinking are that ethyl alcohol helps to reduce tensions, it acts as a tranquilizer with social approval, it is a fast way to ensure a "happy time," it is a ready antidote for bankrupted conversation, it seems to bolster courage even among friends, and it is expected and accepted socially. Remember these are the reasons drinkers give for drinking. They may be sound reasons, or they may be merely rationalizations.

Table 13.2   Facts about drinkers

Type of drinker	Occasion and frequency	Reason for drinking	Effects of alcohol
I. Occasional:			
Medicinal	For minor physical ailments such as a cold or toothache	To reduce physical discomfort	Drug action like that of aspirin
Social	Holiday or family celebration	Custom, tradition	Mild animation or gaiety
II. Frequent:			
Medicinal	Prescribed for some heart or artery ailments	To reduce physical discomfort or anxiety	Sedative action
Dietary	With certain foods or dining occasions	Flavor	Minor increase in satisfaction with meals
Social	Depends on number of social affairs—maybe one to three times weekly	Custom, relaxation	Mild animation or gaiety, conversational ease
III. Regular:			
Dietary	Frequent or daily use with meals	Custom, considered important in diet	Minor, except to increase enjoyment of food
Social	Several times weekly or less	Considered important in social relations	Feeling of physical and psychological well-being, mild animation or gaiety
IV. Alcohol-dependent	Daily whenever possible, but not to avoid meeting responsibilities of life	Limited personal assets; to find satisfaction in drinking, to remove tension	Dulls feelings of inferiority, frustration, and personal failures; blocks possibility of emotional growth; intoxication may occur
V. Alcoholic:			
Regular	Frequent, sometimes daily, intoxication	Dissatisfaction with self or environment	Major changes in behavior
Periodic	Drinking sprees at intervals		Indication of a severe emotional illness

Source: Raymond G. McCarthy, *Facts about Alcohol*, Science Research Associates, Inc., Chicago, 1951, pp. 32–33.

THE CONSUMPTION OF ALCOHOL

Not including the illegal liquor consumed, it has been estimated that the American public drank 231 million gallons of whisky, 3 billion gallons of beer, and 500 million gallons of wine in 1960 [8].

The editors of *Changing Times* estimate that about 75 million persons in this country over fifteen years of age use some form of alcoholic beverages. Mark Keller, editor of the *Quarterly Journal of Studies on Alcohol*, advanced an "educated guess" that 67 per cent of the adult population in this country use alcoholic beverages.

All authorities agree that alcoholism in the United States is increasing. In 1945, the estimate was 2,876,000 alcoholics; in 1960, the figure was 5 million.

THE PROPERTIES OF BEVERAGE ALCOHOL

If the student is to make wise decisions in matters of beverage alcohol, he should be familiar with some facts about its properties.

Brewed liquors. Perhaps the most commonly used alcoholic beverages are the brewed liquors. This group comprises liquors such as beer, ale, porter, and stout, made from cereal grains.

Distilled liquors. Brandy, gin, rum, and whisky comprise the distilled liquors. Until 500 years ago, these drinks were unknown. To satisfy the increasing demand for a drink stronger than beer and wine, brewers developed the process of distillation.

Brandy is distilled from fermented grapes or other fruits. It was probably the first of the hard liquors to be distilled. Its alcohol concentration is usually 100 proof, or 50 per cent alcohol. Gin is a colorless distillation from fermented rye. Like brandy, it is usually 100 proof. Rum is also 100 proof. Because molasses is the base for rum making, no malt is necessary. Grains such as corn, rye, or barley are used to produce whisky. Modern as well as ancient wine making involves primarily the natural fermentation of sweet fruit juices. Liqueurs, cordials, *crèmes,* and the like are elixirs, or sweetened alcoholic beverages.

EFFECTS OF ALCOHOL ON THE BODY

Research reveals, in part, what happens when beverage alcohol is taken into the body. In spite of the fact that extensive time and effort have been allotted to the study of alcohol and its physiologic effects on tissue, there are still many gaps to be filled. It is thought that alcohol passes directly from the stomach or intestines into the blood stream. It requires no digestion. A few minutes after ingestion, it can be found circulating in the blood, and it continues to circulate throughout the body until it is oxidized or eliminated by the lungs or kidneys. Once in the stomach, alcohol causes an increased flow of digestive fluids. This is probably due to the fact that it sets up a chemical action as it passes through the walls of the stomach.

Because beverage alcohol is oxidized and energy is liberated, it is sometimes classified as a food. It is, however, a mistake to classify alcohol with such important foods as proteins, fats, carbohydrates, vitamins, and mineral salts. Its chief value is to yield approximately 7 calories per gram. It cannot create new tissue, nor can it repair injured tissue. It has no protective or regulating functions as have vitamins and minerals. Hence, alcohol should never be recommended as a food.

It is not uncommon for heavy drinkers to suffer from malnutrition and constipation, probably because they tend to be careless about their diet and ingest little or no roughage. Diarrhea may also result because of excessive intake of fluids or oils used in flavoring such drinks as gin.

Man does not build up an immunity to alcohol. It takes exactly the same amount of alcohol to kill a nondrinker as to kill a chronic alcoholic.

Alcohol causes small blood vessels in the skin to expand, thus permitting larger quantities of blood to flow close to the surface, creating a feeling of warmth. Much body heat may be lost. This can be dangerous to health, especially in cold weather.

When large amounts of alcohol are ingested in a short period of time, the liver becomes enlarged and inflamed. After the alcohol is oxidized, the liver returns to normal functioning with no apparent injury. The serious pathologic conditions of the liver frequently found in some alcoholics are thought to be produced by malnutrition rather than by direct action of alcohol [9].

Perhaps the most obvious physiologic effect of alcohol is its effect on the brain. Because of the rich supply of blood flowing to that organ, alcohol reaches it rapidly and affects it markedly. For example, reaction time is lengthened; there is an obvious loss of inhibitions; the optic center is dulled, and vision is distorted; and the centers which control muscular coordination become affected. When the concentration of alcohol in the blood reaches 0.4 or 0.5, it acts as an anesthetic and causes unconsciousness. Should the concentration increase, the cardiac and respiratory centers can become affected and death may follow.

Beverage alcohol has no value in curing snake bites or head colds. It should never be used by one who is suffering from shock. Shock is primarily a state of extreme depression, and since alcohol acts as a depressant, their combined effects are likely to produce very serious results.

After large amounts of alcohol have been drunk, there is a definite disturbance in body chemistry. This tends to bring on a hang-over, with headache, thirst, and fatigue. The headache is caused by disturbance in the liver and by impurities found in alcoholic beverages. The thirst comes from dehydration, which is produced by a shifting of the water within the body cells to the extracellular areas. The fatigue probably results from loss of sleep, tensions, undernourishment, and careless living in general.

Alcohol has a narcotic effect on the function of all body tissue. It can be direct or indirect, immediate or delayed.

On the cells of the nervous system the inhibitory action is direct and is nearly six times as great as on other body cells. This is probably caused by the large lipoid content of the nerve cells which attract and hold alcohol readily. Like other fat solvents, alcohol can pass from the blood of the mother through the placenta and into the blood stream of her unborn baby [7].

In acute intoxication, the brain is congested with excessive fluids. This causes a reduction in oxygen, which can have serious effects. All living tissues, especially nerve cells, require a constant supply of oxygen. A reduction is likely to bring about a destruction of nerve cell groups and permanent damage to brain tissue.

Excessive use of alcohol also creates a vitamin deficiency with its attending disorders. For example, deficiency in thiamine results in beriberi. Niacin failure produces pellagra. A lack of vitamin B can bring on hemorrhagic encephalopathy. Cirrhosis of the liver with its harmful increase of fibrous connective tissue is usually the result of malnutrition. It can be caused by chronic alcoholism [9].

The ingestion of beverage alcohol has a disturbing influence on the effectiveness of general anesthetics used at the time of surgery. This makes the chronic alcoholic and the intoxicated individual more of a surgical risk than other patients. Some physicians advise the postponement of surgery until this deficiency can be corrected [7].

The following diseases are closely associated with the excessive use of beverage alcohol [9]:

POLYNEUROPATHY. Burning sensation in the soles of feet, pain in legs, difficulty in walking.

WET BERIBERI. Swelling of legs, swelling of the heart, so-called "beer heart."

DRY BERIBERI. Excessive mental states of anxiety.

"ALCOHOLIC" PELLAGRA. Spotty reddening

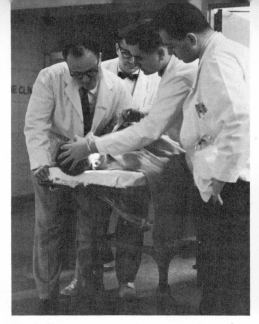

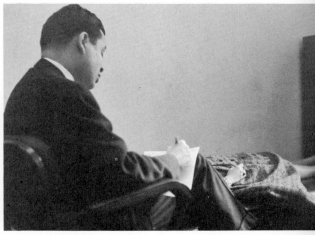

Alcoholism causes growing concern in modern society. An increasing number of problem drinkers find their way to hospitals and organizations for special help. It is now recognized by medical authorities . . .

that alcoholism requires the same careful treatment as any other emotional disorder. Psychotherapy . . .

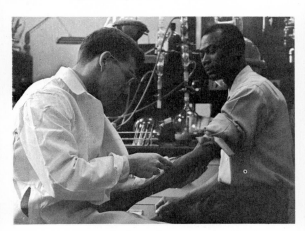

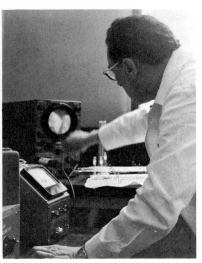

and drug therapy are effective elements in programs of study and treatment. In some clinics . . .

intensive research is in progress. Hospitals and treatment centers . . .

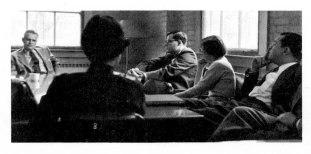

depend heavily on the psychiatric team. It is this group of specialists that help the alcoholic overcome the personality difficulties which drive him to the intoxicant.

of the skin. The tongue, lips, gums, and palate may take on a scarlet hue, and ulcers may develop.

CIRRHOSIS OF THE LIVER. Increase in fibrous connective tissue.

PNEUMONIA. Chronic alcoholics are more susceptible.

The following physical conditions are often associated with the use of beverage alcohol [9]:

TUBERCULOSIS. Any association between tuberculosis and inebrity results not from direct action of alcohol but from neglect of hygienic conditions often characteristic of the families of inebriates.

VENEREAL DISEASE. Those who are intoxicated become irresponsible and are more frequently exposed to venereal infection.

INFANT MORTALITY. Mortality of children is much higher in alcoholic families than in temperate families, in fact, nearly twice as high, probably owing to environment [9].

FEEBLEMINDEDNESS, EPILEPSY, AND MENTAL DISORDERS. Such states are more frequent in the offspring of abnormal drinkers than in the offspring of those practicing moderation or abstinence. Alcohol does not make for poor heredity, but many alcoholics come from groups that have poor heredity. The offspring inherit the defects of the parents; and the defects may predispose to alcoholism.

PERSONALITY AND ALCOHOL

There is no evidence to show that an emotionally mature person—that is, one who gets on well with his fellows, who has a sense of security, who accepts responsibility, who handles his problems well, and who is interested in his position as a citizen of the community—is likely to become addicted to the use of beverage alcohol. He may drink, but the appeal is limited; alcohol is not used as an escape, nor does it become an important item in his budget. There is evidence, much evidence, to show that the emotionally immature person—that is, one who does not face issues squarely, who seeks ways of escaping responsibilities, who feels insecure and lacks faith in himself—often seeks pseudo security in drinking. Such immature action actually puts to sleep the very forces that could be of greatest help.

Ethyl alcohol is often classified as a crude form of anesthetic [7]. The physiologic reactions of one undergoing anesthesia are not difficult to recognize. Because ethyl alcohol acts primarily on the brain and the central nervous system, the behavior of the individual ingesting such alcohol undergoes change. In mild intoxication, there appears a wide variety of behavior changes. In profound intoxication, the variations are slight. Early Asian philosophers described it by saying: [3]

When the evil one gave man alcohol he added the blood of a fox, a wolf, and a pig. Thus when man takes beverage alcohol into his body and becomes mildly intoxicated, his voice is smooth like velvet, his words are soft and oily, and his eyes are sharp like the fox's. When he is well under the influence of alcohol, he becomes cruel like a wolf and when he is in the state of severe drunkenness, he becomes filthy as a swine.

Modern observers are more factual and scientific in reporting behavior changes. For example, behavior common to mild intoxication may be classified as follows [9]:

1. Mild intoxication.
   a. The emotional expressions are heightened and expanded.
   b. The individual has a feeling of complete well-being and a notion that the time has arrived for the solution of all his problems.
   c. He shows great interest in his immediate environment.
   d. Motor expressions become overvigorous and he tends to be aggressive.

[3] Howard W. Haggard and E. M. Jellinek, *Alcohol Explored*, Doubleday and Company, Inc., New York, 1954, p. 114.

2. Moderately severe intoxication.
   a. There is no doubt that the individual is intoxicated.
   b. There is an inhibitory effect upon his senses.
   c. He cannot concentrate, and his thinking is superficial.
   d. He repeats over and over again a single thought (overemphasis on one idea).
   e. He is incapable of using sound judgment.
   f. There is a gap between his feeling of competence and his ability to perform.
   g. His behavior may take a violent turn.
   h. There is an obvious failure of muscle coordination.
3. Severe drunkenness.
   a. The individual has lost control over thought, perception, muscular action, speech, and vision. From this stage, it is easy to pass into unconsciousness and even death.

A significant contribution of experimental psychology to the studies of alcoholism reaffirms the conclusion that ethyl alcohol is a depressant and not a stimulant. As a depressant, it inhibits all body processes.

Much has been written on mental diseases brought about by excessive drinking, and many case studies have been made of them. Most authorities in the fields of psychology, sociology, and medicine agree that prolonged drinking may produce one or more of the the following mental disorders [9]:

SIMPLE ALCOHOLIC DETERIORATION. The important symptom is a degeneration of the ethical sense; that is, the individual shows a progressive tendency toward brutal behavior to those with whom he has the closest association.

CHRONIC ALCOHOLIC DETERIORATION WITH PSYCHOSIS. Chief among the symptoms are the increasing fits of rage and delusions.

PATHOLOGIC INTOXICATION. These reactions are not commonly observed. The individual's control over his emotions has diminished to the vanishing point. Suicides are frequent among individuals in this classification.

DELIRIUM TREMENS. This is a mental disorder occurring in about 4 per cent of compulsive drinkers. It appears to be the end result of ten to fifteen years of excessive indulgence in alcoholic beverages. The chief symptom is an increasing activity of the entire body; the head, tongue, face, fingers, and legs tremble. Various types of hallucinations occur. The condition may last for as many as five days and usually is not fatal.

KORSAKOFF'S PSYCHOSIS. This mental disorder is characterized by failure in memory. The individual spends most of his time trying to fill in the gaps.

ALCOHOLIC PARANOID STATES. This condition, brought on by excessive drinking, is not uncommon. The chief symptom is feelings of persecution, arising from the most harmless acts of others. This state is exceedingly dangerous. Many murders have been committed by individuals suffering delusions of persecution.

ACUTE ALCOHOLIC HALLUCINOSIS. Individuals in this classification are probably showing early symptoms of schizophrenia. The drinking of beverage alcohol is largely symptomatic.

If a person drinks for a bracer, or to escape worries and troubles, or when he feels blue, or the first thing in the morning, or if he feels uncomfortable unless he has had a drink, or if he often drinks alone, it is time to call a halt and seek ways and means of controlling the practice.

REHABILITATION OF ALCOHOLICS

The first and most important move in controlling compulsive drinking is to recognize it as a problem that one cannot solve alone. The drinker must recognize the need for help, which can come from a variety of sources, namely, physicians (psychiatrists), clergymen, clinics, and through group therapy such as that offered by Alcoholics Anonymous. Alcoholics Anonymous is a comparatively new movement and a highly successful one. Its unique contribution is made when the individual adheres closely to twelve all-important steps. An interpretation of these 12 steps has proved highly successful in rehabilitating both men and women who want to be helped [1].

Scientists look upon the alcoholic as a mentally and physically ill person. They believe he can be cured to the extent that his desire for alcohol can be arrested. An effective start toward the rehabilitation of the alcoholic is to identify his personality difficulty or the situation which made alcohol so attractive. From that point treatment becomes a matter of reeducation, of sound medical care, of good nutrition, of security and love.

A person seldom becomes an alcoholic alone, nor is his recovery from alcoholism accomplished in isolation. He needs the help and encouragement of those who are dedicated to his welfare—his family, his friends, and his associates [9, 14].

Whereas drug therapy is only one approach to the rehabilitation of the alcoholic, it is a reliable resource during the acute stages of his treatment. The medical profession has found a variety of drugs which are helpful. Antabuse, citrated calcium carbimide, promazine, and cetadiol are used with varying degrees of success. Antabuse, used extensively in Europe, has not found much favor in this country. It is considered too dangerous, and its power to cure is questionable. Citrated calcium carbimide likewise can guarantee no safe usage or permanent results. Promazine (Sparine) [4] given to alcoholic patients in the hospital relieves the distressing symptoms that accompany recovery from acute alcoholic intoxication. Cetadiol,[5] for relief from the hang-over effects of intoxication, helps patients to eat and sleep well during the first twelve hours of treatment whereas without it they do not begin to do so for seventy-two to ninety-six hours.

Promazine and cetadiol have proved useful for immediate and effective relief from the symptoms of acute alcoholism. These two drugs are of value to that extent only.

The so-called cure, or arrested desire for drinking, is as varied and complicated as are the conditions and situations that produce the alcoholic. In short, there is no one cause of alcoholism, nor is there one cure for it. Perhaps the best single answer to the problem is prevention. To help people make successful adjustments to their personal and social problems, to make known to all what science knows about alcohol, alcoholism, and the alcoholic, and to provide rehabilitative treatment for the present victims of alcoholism will go far in controlling this serious health problem.

ALCOHOL AND TRAFFIC ACCIDENTS

Is it safe to drive after drinking beverage alcohol? This question was asked a group of 500 college freshmen.[6] The answers were revealing: 15 per cent said, "Yes, unless you are drunk—there is no reason why you cannot drive if you are careful"; 2 per cent said, "One or two cocktails are O.K., but no more"; 33 per cent said, "It is safe to drive after consuming two or three cans of beer"; 40 per cent said, "Let your experience be the judge—if you start to drive and find you are not sure of yourself, stop"; 10 per cent said, "If you have been drinking, don't drive."

The study was informal. Out of this group of 500, few were prepared to give

[4] E. H. Mitchell, "Treatment of Acute Alcoholism with Promazine (Sparine)," *Journal of the American Medical Association*, 161:44-45, 1956.

[5] C. H. Campbell and H. G. Sleeper: "Cetadiol in the Treatment of Hospitalized Alcoholics," *American Journal of Psychiatry*, 112:845, 1956.

[6] Lloyd E. Webster, unpublished study.

a statement based on established fact. The majority expressed an opinion that they thought it was safe to drive if the indulgence in alcohol was mild. Unfortunately, the most dangerous driver on the highway is the person who takes his automobile out believing that the small amount of alcohol he has drunk makes him a more skillful driver. The laboratory, the clinics, and the record books have all proved this thinking to be wrong.

The brain is the first organ to be noticeably affected by alcohol and the last to be free from its influence. The Harvard School of Public Health, experimenting with a subject who had been given an amount of alcohol equal to eight highballs over a period of four hours, found that the subject became intoxicated, with a blood alcohol level of 0.15 per cent, in two hours. He maintained this level for nine hours and after 14 hours had a blood alcohol level of 0.09 per cent, which is too high to consider him a safe driver [20].

Bjerver and Goldberg,[7] Swedish scientists, after meticulous research both on the highway and in the laboratory, concluded that the drinking of three bottles of beer having 4 per cent alcohol by volume caused a deterioration in the driving of experienced drivers of between 25 and 30 per cent. They also reported on a test to determine the ability of the eye to distinguish a flickering light and a test to determine the blink reflex. The subjects consumed between 100 and 130 cubic centimeters of distilled spirits containing 40 per cent alcohol by volume. The result showed a deterioration of 34.2 per cent on the flicker test and 35.0 per cent on the blink-reaction test. These scientists concluded that the part played by alcohol in causing traffic accidents is greater

than that which appears on official statistical records. They further concluded that the threshold of impairment of driving ability is an alcohol concentrate of 0.035 to 0.04 per cent in the blood.

The National Safety Council of this country believes all persons having a concentration of alcohol in the blood above 0.15 per cent to be unsafe drivers. It appears that the zone between 0.05 to 0.15 per cent concentration of alcohol in the blood might be considered a questionable one for safe driving [9].

ALCOHOL AND CRIME

Studies indicate a close connection between the drinking of alcohol and crime. A high percentage of all persons committed to state penal institutions have a history of drinking or were under the influence of alcohol at the time they committed their offense. The identification officer of a large state reformatory notes that the average age of the new arrivals in this institution is twenty-two years and also that nearly 50 per cent of those he interviewed said that alcohol was the actual cause of their crime. There are, of course, many factors involved in crime. Statistics do not prove or disprove a cause of crime. The important point is that alcohol is associated intimately with many acts of violence. Such a fact warrants more than the passing attention of students.

ECONOMIC LOSSES CAUSED BY BEVERAGE ALCOHOL

The two chief causes of arrest by police officers in the United States are traffic violations and being intoxicated in public. Over 70 per cent of the cost of maintaining the 4,000 jails in this country each year is for taking care of 90,000 men and women who have been drinking. This amounts to 27 million dollars annually.

It is difficult to give an accurate estimation of the total economic losses due to alcohol. Many factors are not acces-

---

[7] K. Bjerver and Leonard Goldberg, "Effects of Alcohol Ingestion on Driving Ability," *Quarterly Journal of Studies on Alcohol,* 1:1–20, March, 1950.

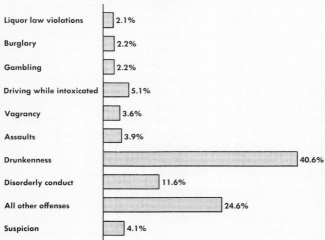

CATEGORIES OF CRIME
in 1,500 cities in the United States

Liquor law violations	2.1%
Burglary	2.2%
Gambling	2.2%
Driving while intoxicated	5.1%
Vagrancy	3.6%
Assaults	3.9%
Drunkenness	40.6%
Disorderly conduct	11.6%
All other offenses	24.6%
Suspicion	4.1%

Survey of 1,500 cities showing drunkenness as the cause of more than 40 per cent of all arrests. Add to this the 7.2 per cent of those attributed to drunken driving and liquor law violations, and the total would be nearly one half of all arrests. To this total can be added many of the disorderly conduct and vagrancy offenses as well as a portion of almost every other offense shown. (*Listen,* American Temperance Society, Washington, November-December, 1960, p. 2.)

sible for study. For example, an accurate accounting of a traffic accident must take into consideration the following:

Loss of time from job

Repair of automobile or its replacement

Repair to city property

Cost of hospitalization and medical care

Cost of litigation—insurance adjustments

If there is a death, many of the items just listed, plus funeral expenses

Because there is no central reporting, these important facts are seldom recorded. Further, there is a need for studies to determine losses resulting from fires set by careless drinkers and also deaths and accidents occurring in industrial plants where alcohol is involved. Few, if any, reliable studies have been made covering all these details. Needless to say, when these studies have been made, they will show that the total sum lost because of alcohol is huge. Spalding and Montague have given a conservative estimate of 2,400 million dollars annually; probably it is much more.

BEVERAGE ALCOHOL AND BUSINESS

Part of an assignment to freshman men registered in a university health education course was to interview men and women who had attained leadership in

motion pictures, transportation, the steel industry, department stores, the oil industry, government, law, medicine, dentistry, education, engineering, and religion. One of the twenty-five questions asked in the interview was, Of what significance is the drinking of beverage alcohol to success in your business? Ninety-nine per cent of the people interviewed stated that the use of beverage alcohol played no role in achieving success in their fields.[8]

Most businessmen make it apparent that, when one is entrusted with the responsibility of the welfare of his fellows or is in charge of precision instruments or of dangerous machinery, he does not drink—at least not on the job. Railroads do not permit drinking among their personnel while on duty. Commercial air lines make it grounds for dismissal if a pilot indulges in any form of drinking within twenty-five hours before a flight.

In his lectures and discussions at the Yale School of Alcohol Studies, E. M. Jellinek emphasized the point that industry loses heavily each year because of the drinking practices of the workers.

[8] Lloyd E. Webster, unpublished study.

He believes that, of the 1 million workers who are more than moderate drinkers, each is likely to lose twenty or more days annually from his job. This is a staggering loss of man-hours. It is estimated that industry would stand to gain over 1 billion dollars a year if workers who drink would avoid indulging while on the job and would control their drinking practices so that the familiar hangover does not take its heavy toll of absenteeism.

BEVERAGE ALCOHOL AND THE COLLEGE STUDENT

Bacon and Straus, in a study of the drinking practices of 17,000 American college youth in 27 colleges, found that four out of five college men who drink began their drinking before entering college and 65 per cent of the college women who drink began before entering college. They concluded that the probability that college students will drink at all is closely related to the practice of their parents. Ninety per cent of the college men who drink and 83 per cent of the college women who drink came from homes where both parents drink [2].

Further, the study shows an interesting correlation between family income and drinking. For example, where the annual income is $10,000 or over, 86 per cent of the men and 79 per cent of the women drink. Where the income is under $2,500, 66 per cent of the men and 30 per cent of the women drink.

There appears to be a difference in the type of beverage most frequently used by the students answering the questionnaire. Seventy-two per cent of the men preferred beer. Forty-two per cent expressed a preference for distilled liquors, but only 21 per cent could afford to purchase them. Forty-one per cent of the college women who were studied drank beer, but only 17 per cent preferred it. The preferred drink for the woman students was wine.

Perhaps the most striking finding of the study was the fact that customs and attitudes of college students with regard to drinking are already well determined before matriculation.

The college men and women who do not drink are challenged often by their colleagues to do so. They are asked to drink as a symbol of fellowship. Sometimes the appeal is to learn how to appreciate appropriate wines with food. They are urged to drink at initiations. Some feel that drinking is necessary to acquire status; others drink as a symbol of rebellion against school and home authority. In spite of this wide range of motivations, there are many men and women on the campus who do not drink. Apparently they have established their fellowship and status without the benefit of alcohol.

The fact that beverage alcohol is a depressant, that it can interfere with basic nutrition, that it can produce an impressive array of physical and mental disorders, that it can cause a variety of accidents, that it contributes to much crime and unhappiness, and that it is a constant threat to efficiency and progress in industry should be sufficient reason for the college man or woman to consider its consumption wisely or to abstain.

Tobacco

The smoking of tobacco is a very old practice. Archaeologists have found a variety of implements in the ruins of early cultures—Anglo-Saxon, Chinese, and Roman—which indicate that people even before the first century were using some form of mixture and implements for transmitting smoke through the nose and mouth for pleasure.

The present-day use of tobacco probably had its inception among the Indians of America. Early explorers of the

Americas who observed the practice and returned to Europe with Indian pipes and tobacco were Captain Philip Amadas, Captain Arthur Barlow, Sir Francis Drake, Sir John Hawkins, and Sir Walter Raleigh.

After 1600 the use of tobacco in Europe and elsewhere became widespread. Opponents of the new practice sprang up everywhere. Smoking was denounced by the clergy, by medical men, and finally by the rulers of England, Turkey, and Russia. King James of England wrote *A Counterblaste to Tobacco,* which condemned smoking. Amurath IV of Turkey prohibited the use of tobacco and sentenced all smokers to death. Tsar Michael of Russia ordered that all men and women found guilty of smoking were to have their noses cut off. In spite of these vigorous and cruel efforts to stamp out smoking, it continued to flourish, and today, in the United States, it is estimated that 75 per cent of the men and 40 per cent of the women use tobacco in some form. Of this group, 53 per cent of the men and 25 per cent of the women are regular smokers.

Over 3 million pounds of tobacco are produced annually in this country. In 1916, the American public smoked 25 billion cigarettes. In 1959, the figure had risen to 475 billion cigarettes annually. Increases in cigar smoking and the chewing of tobacco and the use of snuff follow a similar trend. This rapid growth in the use of tobacco and its products has been accelerated by extensive advertising plus new smokers. When it was established that there is a positive relationship between lung cancer and the use of tobacco, the number of smokers gradually declined. However, with the advent of the filter, there has been an upsurge in cigarette sales. It is not unusual for a tobacco company to spend several million dollars annually to advertise over television and radio, in motion pictures, and in newspapers and magazines. Much of the advertising should not be taken seriously. For ex-

ample, the Federal Trade Commission [9] reports:

Scientific evidence in the record establishes that there is no significant difference in the acid in the tobacco used in the manufacture of popular brands of cigarettes or in the smoke therefrom. Furthermore, contrary to claims made in advertising, there is no difference in the effect of the acidity on the persons smoking any of the popular brands of cigarettes.

Testimony of medical witnesses, as well as reports of tests and experiments conducted by chemists, establishes the fact that there is no significant difference in either the tars and resins or the nicotine in the smoke from all the leading brands of cigarettes. The testimony of medical experts also establishes the fact that the smoke from all the leading brands is irritating to the mucous membrane of the respiratory tract and that the differences in the chemical constituents of different brands of cigarettes, as shown by reports of tests, are so slight that the smoke from one brand of cigarettes is no less irritating than is the smoke from other brands.

No manufacturer attempts to remove all the nicotine from the tobacco. To do so would destroy the tobacco for commercial purposes.

The smoke from all the leading brands of cigarettes contains throat irritants "in essentially the same quantities and degree." There is no known practical process by which the nicotine, tars and resins in the tobacco leaf "may be removed or substantially reduced" without at the same time denaturing the tobacco and rendering it unsatisfactory for use in the manufacture of cigarettes.

In cease-and-desist orders, the Federal Trade Commission [10] had further directed the major tobacco companies to stop claiming

That smoking cigarettes encourages the flow of digestive fluids or that it aids digestion in any respect.

That smoking cigarettes relieves fatigue.

That smoking does not affect or impair the "wind" or physical condition of athletes.

That such cigarettes or the smoke therefrom will never harm or irritate the throat, nor leave an aftertaste.

That the smoke from such cigarettes is

[9] Federal Trade Commission, Orders 4827, 4795, and 4922, Washington, 1950–1951.
[10] *Ibid.*

soothing, restful or comforting to the nerves, or that it protects one against nerve strain.

That their cigarettes are less acid than other popular brands of cigarettes.

That their cigarettes offer throat protection.

That their cigarettes are less irritating to the throat than competing brands.

That their tobacco is better and higher priced than the tobaccos used in competing brands of cigarettes.

That one has protection against coughing in smoking their brand.

That their brand of cigarettes has twice as many exclusive smokers as have all other cigarettes combined.

That the superiority of their particular brand is recognized by eminent medical authorities.

That the throats and mouths are as fresh and comfortable and the breath as pure and sweet after a day of smoking their cigarettes as in the morning.

The American Medical Association conducted a series of tests to determine how much, if any, nicotine was removed from the main stream of cigarette smoke by filter-tips. The conclusion was: [11]

Filters are responsible for removing very little of the total nicotine in the smoked portion of the cigarette. The bulk of the nicotine, about 75 per cent in the case of the "regular" cigarette, is lost in the side stream or is destroyed by the burning coal.

Advertisers often claim that there is a low percentage of nicotine in the mainstream smoke if filters are used. However, American Medical Association reports state that this is misleading, "that widely divergent values can be obtained from the same analytical data by choosing different bases for the calculations." [12]

WHY PEOPLE SMOKE

In spite of the fact that tobacco can become a sizable item in the budget, that it may be a contributing factor in the cause of serious physical ailments, and that it can become a fire hazard, millions of people smoke, with thousands of new converts springing up each year. In 1945, Finnegan [13] summarized the reasons for this popularity as follows:

1. Nicotine craving.
2. Optical perception of the smoke.
3. Agreeable smell and taste.
4. Manipulation and sucking of cigar or cigarette somewhat resembling the influence of the nipple on the infant.
5. Pleasurable irritation on the laryngeal and tracheal sensory branches of the pneumogastric nerve.
6. Relief of tension.
7. Stimulation.
8. Sociability.
9. Gives people something to do.
10. Permits one to do "nothing" gracefully.
11. Satisfies a desire or craving.
12. Sense of "grown-upness."
13. Feeling of self-confidence.
14. Pyromania.
15. Pleasure.

Today the reasons for smoking remain unchanged. Once the practice of using tobacco has been established, it is difficult to stop. This was attested to during World War II by the long lines in front of stores selling a limited supply of cigarettes. Arutzen observed the strength of the practice or habit among the Germans during 1946–1947. At that time tobacco was rationed; men were allowed 40 cigarettes a month, and women were allowed 20. In order to obtain something to smoke, the majority of men and women preferred to go without food in order to have money to buy cigarettes.

WHY PEOPLE DO NOT SMOKE

Not all people smoke. Throughout the country perhaps 60 per cent of the adult women and 25 per cent of the adult men do not smoke. Their reasons are: [14]

Education (knowledge of harmful effects)

Religion (contrary to church doctrines)

[11] Walter Wolman, "A Study of Cigarettes, Cigarette Smoke, and Filters," *Journal of the American Medical Association*, 152:917–920, July 4, 1953.
[12] *Ibid.*

[13] J. K. Finnegan, "The Role of Nicotine in the Cigarette Habit," *Science*, 102:94, July 27, 1945.
[14] Laurence E. Morehouse, University of California, Los Angeles, unpublished material.

Expense
Fire hazard
Lack of desire

THE EFFECTS OF SMOKING ON HEALTH

It is possible to prove that smoking brings about some permanent change in well-being. In the case of beverage alcohol, the social and physical reaction can be readily observed. In the case of tobacco, one may have to resort to the laboratory to determine what, if any, action substances within the tobacco plant have on the body.

The chief toxic element resulting from combustion of tobacco is nicotine. It is an oily substance and is poisonous. There is enough nicotine in one cigar to cause quick death to an adult should he receive the full concentrated dose into his circulatory system. Tobacco smoke contains not only nicotine but carbon monoxide, pyridine bases (collidine, a stronge irritant), hydrocyanic acid, and ammonia. When absorbed into the body through the smoke, nicotine first stimulates the cerebrum and autonomic nervous system and then acts as a depressant. Beginning smokers and those who have smoked too heavily at any one time may suffer dizziness, nausea, diarrhea, and, in some cases, excitement and insomnia.

Pyridine bases are local irritants. Hydrocyanic acid interferes with the normal oxidation process in body tissue. Ammonia is a local irritant. Carbon monoxide, having a high affinity for hemo-

Mortality ratios by number of cigarettes smoked per day. The death rate of men smoking regularly at a rate of less than one-half pack per day is 34 per cent higher than the death rate of men who never smoked. The death rate of men smoking from one to two packs a day is 96 per cent higher than the death rate of men who never smoked. The death rate of men smoking two packs or more a day is 123 per cent higher than the death rate of men who never smoked. (Adapted from C. Cuyler Hammond and Daniel Horn, *Smoking in Relation to Death Rates*, from a report to the Annual Meeting of the American Medical Association, New York, June, 1957.)

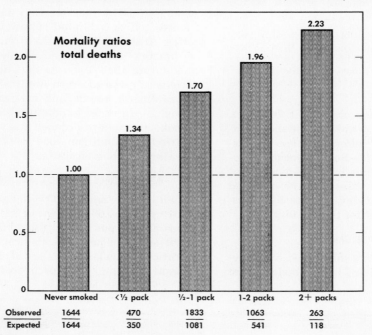

	Never smoked	< ½ pack	½-1 pack	1-2 packs	2+ packs
Observed	1644	470	1833	1063	263
Expected	1644	350	1081	541	118

globin of the blood, can interfere seriously with blood oxygenation. The amount of nicotine and its companion substances in tobacco smoke varies because of variations in the soil and in methods of processing the leaf. For example, no two cigarettes in the same brand contain the same amount of nicotine. The so-called denicotinized cigarette made from tobacco leaves is largely a myth. At present, there is no satisfactory method of substantially reducing nicotine and at the same time maintaining a high quality of tobacco for the manufacturing of cigarettes.

The amount of by-products that enters the body in smoking depends upon several factors: the size of the cigarette, the pack of tobacco within a given cigarette, dryness of the tobacco, and the rate at which the cigarette is smoked. The shorter and thicker the cigarette, the more nicotine passes out with the inhaled smoke. The looser the tobacco within the cigarette, the more available becomes the nicotine. The drier the tobacco, the greater the amount of nicotine. The faster the cigarette is smoked, the greater the amount of nicotine.

Tobacco smoke taken into the mouth deposits its substances on the mucous membrane lining of the nose, mouth, and throat for absorption into the blood stream. When smoke is inhaled, the coverage is large and absorption of nicotine may be as much as ten times greater than when it is not inhaled. A cigarette smoked down to the butt end gives a higher percentage of nicotine than one discarded earlier.

There is no scientific evidence to support the belief that cigarette paper contains harmful substances.

Many scientists have tried to determine whether there is any relationship between efficiency of animal tissue and the use of tobacco. Most agree that some change takes place when tissue is exposed to the by-products of burning tobacco. However, this change varies with the sensitivity of the individual to tobacco smoke. It is also possible that an immunity to the effects of tobacco may gradually be acquired if the practice of smoking persists. Following are some of the reactions to smoking which have been accepted by those investigating in the field [3].

The heart rate increases as much as 20 beats per minute. This may last for 10 to 20 minutes after the smoking ends. This increase results from a stimulation of sympathetic ganglia. Blood pressure, both systolic and diastolic, is elevated. Blood flow in the peripheral vessels is decreased, causing the temperature to drop slightly in fingers and toes. The coronary flow of blood in the heart muscle appears to be reduced. Blood sugar level is raised.

Further it has been noted that after smoking one to two cigarettes some individuals develop vasospasms of the small arteries of the fingers, toes, cheeks, nose, and ears. This condition is called Raynaud's syndrome and may lead to serious vascular conditions such as Buerger's disease.

A study [15] conducted at Johns Hopkins University Hospital used the ballistocardiograph, a device that records the stroke volume of the heart as a means of calculating heart output. Of the 190 coronary patients studied, 48.9 per cent showed abnormal ballistocardiograms after smoking. Of the 282 normal people tested, only 7.5 per cent registered abnormalities.

Strober [16] of the Medical Corps, United States Air Force Reserve, made a similar study with similar findings. He took ballistocardiograms of 2,736 normal men from eighteen to sixty-five years of age, after smoking. Fifteen per cent of the group, mostly younger men, showed a 20 per cent increase in their heart rate.

[15] F. W. Davis and others, "The Ballistocardiograph Cigarette Test: Further Observations," *American Heart Journal*, 51:167–169, February, 1956.
[16] Murry Strober, "Effect of the Dock Cigarette-Smoking Test on the Ballistocardiogram," *Journal of the American Medical Association*, 161:1061, July 14, 1956.

The incidence of abnormality, however, increased nearly 30 per cent in individuals over thirty years old.

The relationship between Buerger's disease, or thromboangiitis obliterans, and the use of tobacco has been well established. The disease is painful and repulsive but seldom fatal. Because of heavy smoking the arterial flow in the small arteries slows and eventually stops, thus plugging the vessel. All body tissues need fresh freely flowing blood to survive; when the arteries fail to deliver fresh blood, these tissues become gangrenous and die. This condition is most likely to occur in the hands and feet; however, it is not limited to the extremities. Wynder reports cases where arms and legs of patients with Buerger's disease have had to be amputated to save the life of the patient. He also notes that the progress of the disease stops upon the cessation of smoking and recurs when smoking is resumed.

A person who has been injured often asks for a cigarette. Caution should be used granting the request. In a tobacco-sensitive person, smoking may cause irreparable damage to blood vessels associated with the injury. Spasms within these vessels and vasoconstriction can increase the trauma. Research studies indicate that premature births are twice as great for smoking mothers as for nonsmoking mothers [6].

Tobacco smoking and physical performance. For many years tobacco smoking has been considered to have a definite effect on athletic performance. It has been reported that the exact knowledge of the effect of tobacco on athletic performances is inadequate.

Much more research is needed on the problem. However, two series of experiments with subjects performing on a bicycle ergometer showed that abstinence from smoking for one week caused improvement in tobacco-sensitive subjects and had no effect on nonsensitive ones. Since a relatively large proportion of an athletic team may consist of tobacco-sensitive men, the nonsmoking rule is a wise precaution.[17] The effect of tobacco smoking on physical performance may depend on individual differences to the extent that no uniform effects can be shown. Future studies will no doubt be made on this problem.

TOBACCO AND LONGEVITY

The first serious study on the relationship between length of life and the use of tobacco was conducted by Pearl in 1938. He concluded that the death rate for excessive users of tobacco was higher than for the nonsmokers for all ages up to seventy years. Since this early approach to the problem of longevity and smoking, other studies have been made showing similar findings. For example, Hammond and Horn[18] report that death rates among men who smoked cigarettes regularly is higher than among those who do not use tobacco. The rate for men smoking less than half a package of cigarettes a day is higher than for nonsmokers. The men consuming one or more packages a day have a death rate more than twice that of nonsmokers.

It is the belief of many investigators that smoking a pack of cigarettes or more a day can result, for some individuals, in the loss of as much as ten years from their normal span of life. That is, they may be physiologically ten years older at a given age than they would have been had they not smoked.

From these studies it would seem that longevity is adversely influenced by the habitual use of tobacco.

TOBACCO AND LUNG CANCER

Both clinical and statistical studies have established a positive relationship be-

[17] Peter V. Karpovich and C. J. Hale, "Tobacco Smoking and Physical Performance," *Journal of Applied Physiology,* 3:573–636, April, 1951.

[18] E. Cuyler Hammond and Daniel Horn, "Smoking in Relation to Death Rates," from a report delivered at the Annual Meeting of the American Medical Association, New York, June 4, 1957.

UNDERSTANDING DEPRESSANTS AND STIMULANTS

tween lung cancer and the smoking of tobacco.

In 1928 studies suggesting the possibility of the relationship between lung cancer and smoking were recorded. Since that period epidemiologic surveys conducted in several parts of the world have verified this conclusion. For example, studies in England and Wales indicate that after forty-five years of age the chances of developing lung cancer are in proportion to the amount one has smoked. Hill and Doll,[19] two British health authorities, summarized the results of 17 investigations conducted in United States, Finland, West Germany, Holland, and Switzerland with the point that there is much more lung cancer among smokers than among nonsmokers.

In this country most scientific investigators have reached the conclusion that lung cancer is more likely to be found among heavy smokers than among nonsmokers [3, 6].

Dr. Leroy E. Burney,[20] former Surgeon General, U.S. Public Health Service, writing in the *Journal of the American Medical Association*, concluded:

It is a statutory responsibility of the Public Health Service to inform members of the medical profession and the public on all matters relating to important public health issues. The relationship between smoking and lung cancer ·constitutes such an issue and falls within this responsibility of the Public Health Service.

[19] A. B. Hill and R. Doll, "Lung Cancer and Tobacco," *British Medical Journal,* 1:1160, May 19, 1956.
[20] Leroy E. Burney, "Smoking and Lung Cancer," *Journal of the American Medical Association,* 171:1829–1835, Nov. 28, 1959.

The Public Health Service believes that the following statements are justified by studies to date: 1. The weight of evidence at present implicates smoking as the principal etiological factor in the increased incidence of lung cancer. 2. Cigarette smoking particularly is associated with an increased chance of developing lung cancer. 3. Stopping cigarette smoking even after long exposure is beneficial. 4. No method of treating tobacco or filtering the smoke has been demonstrated to be effective in materially reducing or eliminating the hazard of lung cancer. 5. The nonsmoker has a lower incidence of lung cancer than the smoker in all controlled studies, whether analyzed in terms of rural areas, urban regions, industrial occupations or sex. 6. Persons who have never smoked at all (cigarettes, cigars or pipe) have the best chance of escaping lung cancer. 7. Unless the use of tobacco can be made safe, the individual person's risk of lung cancer can best be reduced by the elimination of smoking.

Doll,[21] reporting on a study of lung cancer and smoking in England, indicates that the death rate from cancer of the lungs is more than twenty times higher among heavy smokers than among nonsmokers. He further notes that those who smoke cigarettes show a higher mortality from cancer of the lungs than do pipe smokers.

In summary, the student who smokes should take into consideration the following evidence:
There is a positive relationship between cigarette smoking and cancer of the lungs [12].
Lung cancer is the leading cause of cancer death among men [12].

[21] Richard Doll, "Lung Cancer in Smoking," *Royal Society of Health Journal,* 77:247–250, June, 1957.

Table 13.3. Cases of lung cancer expected to develop per 1,000 smokers and 1,000 nonsmokers (white males forty years of age)

Source of data	By age 80		By age 70		By age 60	
	Smokers	Nonsmokers	Smokers	Nonsmokers	Smokers	Nonsmokers
Sadowsky et al.	48	10	30	7	12	4
Wynder and Graham	50	3	32	2	13	1
Doll and Hill	45	5	29	3	11	1

Source: Ernest L. Wynder, *The Biologic Effects of Tobacco,* Little, Brown & Company, Boston, 1955. (From S. J. Cutler and D. B. Loveland.)

If the present trend in smoking continues, 1 million students now in school will die of cancer before they are seventy years of age [12].

Eighty per cent of lung-cancer victims have a history of smoking the equivalent of two packs a day for twelve and a half years or longer [19].

A filter cigarette gives about the same amount of tars and nicotine as an unfiltered cigarette [3].

There is a high relationship between smoking and cancer of the larynx, bladder, and esophagus; gastric ulcers; cirrhosis of the liver; and cerebral vascular lesions [3, 15].

Depressant drugs

In discussing the use of beverage alcohol and tobacco, it is important to appraise all the scientific facts faithfully, so that the millions of consumers of these products, as well as those who abstain, can be accurately informed of their effects. This is even more important in the case of habit-forming drugs, whose use is governed by law. Public opinion vigorously opposes the use of these drugs except as prescribed by the medical profession. At present the law in most states is so strict that even physicians are not granted a free hand in writing prescriptions for them.

Depressant drugs act on the central nervous system and, in turn, affect all the physiologic processes of the body. They have no curative value. They are used primarily for purposes of escape, such as relief from pain, unpleasant memories, and insommia.

Typical of the depressant drugs are the barbiturates, chloral hydrate, bromides, marihuana, and heroin. Opium and its derivatives are also depressants. Opium comes from the *Papaver somniferum* poppy. It has many useful functions in medicine. Its illegal use, however, has brought nothing but suffering and great harm to mankind. The chief alkaloid from opium is morphine, from which codeine and heroin are derived. Codeine's chief use is in medicine, and it is not considered important as a habit-forming drug. It is a white crystalline alkaloid and is used as a substitute for morphine.

BARBITURIC ACID

Of all the sedative and depressant drugs of the nonopiate class, the most commonly used by the average adult are the barbiturates. This group of sedative, sleep-producing drugs, of which there are at least 20, was first synthesized in Germany in 1863. By 1882 the first hypnotic barbiturate, called *barbital,* was ready for the public market. Fifty-eight years later the demand for the derivatives of barbituric acid had reached 70 tons a year in this country alone. As the tempo of life increased, so did the demand for barbiturates. By 1950 the American public was consuming over 300 tons annually. Since that date the consumption rate has risen steadily, and it continues to rise. This is fair evidence that a portion of the American public should take a serious look at its mental well-being.

Under proper medical supervision, the barbiturates serve a useful purpose. However, to use these drugs indiscriminately as an easy, quick, readily available method of reducing conscious activity of the brain is very unwise. The danger in using barbiturates lies both in long-continued use and in overdosing. If the drugs are used to a greater extent than prescribed by a physician, acute or chronic intoxication results. A person intoxicated by barbiturates is likely to consume more of the drug than he realizes, and the result is usually fatal. In most major cities of the United States the number of deaths attributed to over-dosage has increased from 400 to 1,300 per cent in an eight-year period.

Barbituric acid compounds are taken in either capsule or pill form. Upon prescription, they may be purchased under a variety of names, such as Sodium Amytal, Allonal, barbital, phenobarbital, Seconal, Nembutal, Tuinal, and Veronal. When a reputable physician prescribes one of these compounds, he does so for a specific purpose and usually permits only 2 to 12 capsules or pills per prescription. Once the prescription has been completed, it cannot be refilled except on written permission of prescriber. This is in accord with legislation, in all states. However, this law is broken many times by addicts who appeal to unscrupulous physicians or who make their purchases on the black market.

Because some physicians treat the law rather loosely and unprincipled or un-informed pharmacists make available barbiturates for a price, the danger inherent in the use of barbiturates by the public is very real.

CHLORAL HYDRATE

This synthetic drug, sometimes called "knockout drops" or "Mickey Finn," is a strong sedative. It is bitter and has an unpleasant taste. The usual therapeutic dose produces five to ten hours of sleep. Larger doses will cause longer sleep and may lead to coma and death. The drug is not widely used by the medical profession. At times criminals have used chloral hydrate to render their victims unconscious. In their hands or in the hands of any unskilled persons the result is likely to be fatal.

BROMIDES

Sodium bromide, a white odorless powder, a depressant on the central nervous system, is widely used by persons needing a sedative or a sleep-producing drug. Prolonged use of the drug can result in a serious impairment of health. Overdos-ing causes bromism, in which there is a breaking out on the skin, appetite for food is lost, speech is affected, memory is impaired, the pulse is slow, and the reflexes are diminished. Taking bromides usually results in a psychic dependence, not a physical reliance. A person does not build up a tolerance to bromides, and he may develop some unpleasant toxic reaction to an accumulation of the drug in his body.

MARIHUANA

Marihuana is a renegade hypnotic drug, outlawed by both medicine and law. Its action on the body is unpredictable. Swallowing a small amount of the smoke may leave one person unaffected but produce serious personality changes in another. Marihuana is one of the oldest of the drugs used for narcotic purposes. Ancient history records the use of hemp plants (hashish) in Arabia and in Persia. Over 4,000 years ago, Persian outlaw bands were given hashish when their raids called for rashness and cruelty. These criminals were known as hashish users. The English word "assassin," meaning "killer," stems from this term.

By the year 1545, the hemp plant was being grown in Brazil primarily for the purposes of making rope. Soon the Brazilians began smoking the dried tops of the hemp plant. This practice spread north, and before 1600 it was widespread among the Indians of Mexico. It was here that the plant became known as mari-huana. By 1920, marihuana smoking had spread farther to the north, and for the first time the American public became aware that it was being used in this country. The practice became so wide-spread that by 1937 the Marihuana Act was passed by Congress. This act forbids the importing, manufacturing, producing, compounding, selling, prescribing, administering, or giving away of marihuana in any form, including the seeds.

As previously stated, the effect of marihuana on the individual is unpre-

The first and most vital step in cure of the individual addicted to narcotics is the desire to be helped by qualified medical authorities.

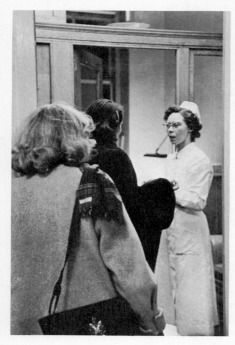

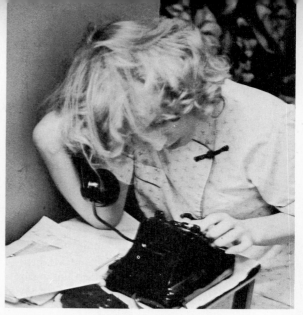

Even after the addict makes the decision to submit to hospitalization, there is a long and difficult struggle ahead.

Once the individual recognizes the seriousness of the decision to fight against drugs, there may be a serious loss of will power.

The process of withdrawal from drugs aims at ultimate removal of narcotics from the patient's system . . .

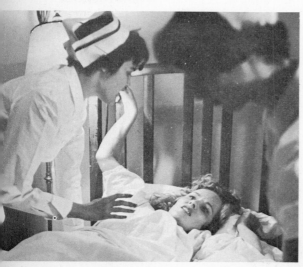

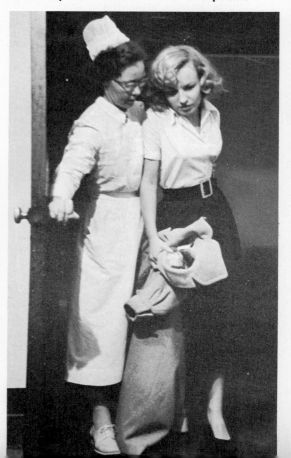

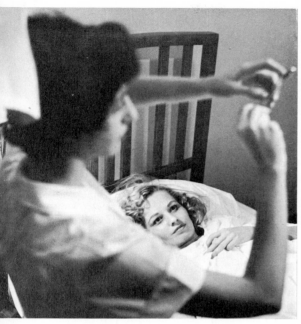

but the traumatic experience of withdrawal must at times be eased by reduced doses of narcotics administered to the patient.

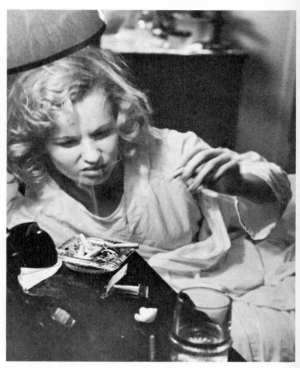

Although these weaker doses of the drug afford temporary relief . . .

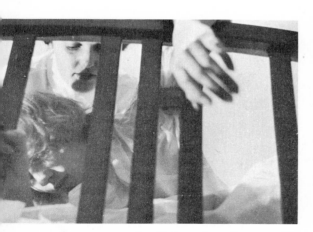

the ravages of withdrawal continue as the patient is finally forced to exist entirely without narcotics.

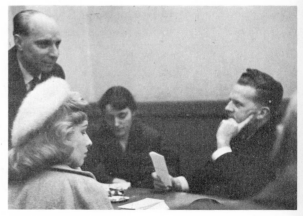

The strength to endure without drugs is a hard-won achievement for the rehabilitated addict, who lives always in the shadow of being enticed again into "the habit."

dictable. Some can smoke it without apparent reaction; for others, it may lead to heroin addiction. It is not difficult to recognize someone who has recently been smoking marihuana. Usually the eyes are bloodshot, the speech is rapid and high-pitched, the breath has an odor of marihuana (it is sometimes said that marihuana smells like musty hay), and the throat will be so dry it may be difficult to expectorate.

Marihuana itself does not compel people to commit crimes or to be sexually promiscuous; it does, however, make them irresponsible and may release inhibitions, with the result that laws are broken. Reactions to marihuana are similar to reactions to over indulgence in beverage alcohol. The drug provides an initial feeling of stimulation followed by drowsiness and full or partial coma.

Marihuana is psychologically habit-forming. Some success has been had in breaking the habit by treating the underlying condition that made the drug so attractive. Perhaps the most sinister problem in relation to marihuana smoking is that it is a steppingstone to the use of heroin.

HEROIN

Heroin, a habit-forming drug, is a morphine derivative (diacetylmorphine). It is a white, bitter crystalline powder. At one time it was used by physicians as a sedative. Today, it is illegal to use it or to manufacture it.

Those using heroin either sniff it or inject it into the blood stream. The effects are similar to those of morphine. The individual finds himself greatly elated. He loses his sense of pain. He forgets unpleasantness and for a few hours appears to be at peace with the world. As soon as the body fluids have neutralized the heroin, which takes 3 to 6 hours, the addict needs another shot. An addict of a year's standing or more requires between $25 to $75 a day to satisfy his desires. Heroin is sold illegally in 1-grain capsules, usually at $5 a grain.

Addiction to heroin often follows closely upon the repeated use of marihuana and is a rapid and vicious process. Within a few weeks, one can become a full-fledged addict—a "main liner." Placing the needle in a large vein of the arm gives a fast, jolting reaction. Usually the first four or five shots cause illness. It is at this point that the individual is most susceptible to efforts to turn him away from the drug. After two to four weeks of injections, the body builds up a tolerance, and the desire or ability to stop is lost. When an addict is deprived of the drug, he suffers the agonies of withdrawal pains. They are very real and are caused by dehydration of the body. The only temporary release is another shot or administration of methadone.

The heroin addict is a pitiful specimen. His face has a gray pallor. He is restless, nervous, and suffers auditory and visual hallucinations. He is constipated and malnourished. His appetite for food is unstable. He is a sick person —mentally, morally, and physically.

There are two Federal government hospitals in the United States where drug addicts are treated. They are located at Fort Worth, Texas, and Lexington, Kentucky. The personnel of these hospitals believe a high percentage of the patients can be cured. One of the great dangers in the cure is that only one shot can return the "cured" individual to addiction.

Stimulants

Stimulating drugs temporarily excite those who use them. They heighten nervous irritability and make one tend to be more alert and less inclined to sleep. The drugs of this class which are most likely to be used are Benzedrine and cocaine. The latter is used by addicts only.

COCAINE

This crystalline alkaloid, methylbenzoyl-ecgonine, is made from coca leaves. Pizarro, in 1537, was the first to note its effects as he observed the Indians of South America chewing the leaves. By 1855, cocaine had been extracted from the coca leaf by German scientists. Its chief use in the United States is for local anesthetics. Because it is habit-forming, science developed procaine (Novocain), a powerful non-habit-forming drug, which is taking its place. However, cocaine is still used as a local anesthetic and for treatment of diseases of the eye and the nose. The unstable person who becomes addicted to cocaine finds short-lived exhilaration by injecting the drug into his veins or sniffing it up his nose. The "kick" soon gives way to feelings of fear and hallucinations. Cocaine is a dangerous drug; once a person is "hooked," he is powerless to stop using it. Personality changes, such as paranoia delusions and intense excitement, often lead to spontaneous and unwarrantable acts of violence and death. The addict is unable to differentiate between hallucinations and reality. His mental apparitions force him to "protect" himself from those (imaginary, of course) he believes would harm him. His actions are purely defensive but often result in great harm to innocent people.

BENZEDRINE

Amphetamine or Benzedrine sulfate, sometimes called "benny" or "pep pill," is a white powder closely related to epinephrine. Benzedrine has an exhilarating effect on the body and for that purpose is widely used by those who need a crutch. It tends to increase alertness, promotes initiative, reduces appetite, and creates an all-round feeling of well-being.

Benzedrine is taken in pill form and by nasal inhalers. To protect addiction-prone individuals state laws have been enacted making it necessary to have a physician's prescription before purchasing the drug in pill form. Benzedrine inhalers have also been replaced by the less potent Benzedrex inhalers. An overdose of Benzedrine can cause serious illness and death. Students have frequently asked if Benzedrine pills would give them greater physical and mental efficiency. There can be no sound yes or no answer to this question. The normal person is likely to find that after taking Benzedrine he has little desire to sleep; his blood pressure rises; his respiration and pulse rates increase; his visual acuity improves; his physical processes are stimulated; and fatigue appears to be delayed. There is usually a letdown following this stimulation. These reactions are more intense in women than in men. However, not all people are stimulated by Benzedrine; there are normal individuals who have a feeling of depression and dizziness.

In light of these points it is unwise for a student to resort to Benzedrine unless it is prescribed by a reputable physician. Scholastic excellence is more likely to be achieved when a balance is established between periods of work, rest, relaxation, recreation, and sleep. Add to this, wholesome food and drink, and one possesses a success formula superior to any concoction known to pharmaceutical skill.

OTHER STIMULANTS

Research gives no dictum on other stimulants, such as cola beverages, coffee, and tea. Findings on the effects these products have on the human body are considered as trends in research data and not as final evidence.

Caffeine. The stimulant common to cola, coffee, tea, and maté is caffeine. In most cases of normal indulgence, caffeine tends to retard fatigue and aids in rapid recovery from "that tired feeling." As yet, science has not produced evidence to show that moderate ingestion of drinks containing caffeine is harmful to the normal adult.

Table 13.4.   Addicting drugs

Drug	Cause emotional dependence	Cause physical dependence and withdrawai illness	Create tolerance or a need for bigger doses
Sedative or narcotic drugs (relieve pain, cause mental and physical inactivity, have a numbing effect, produce sleep, and in larger doses cause stupor, coma, and death):			
Opium and its products: morphine, heroin, codeine, Dilaudid, metopon, Pantopon, paregoric, laudanum	Yes	Yes	Yes
Synthetic substitutes for morphine: Demerol, methadone	Yes	Yes	Yes
Barbiturates, "sleeping pills": Luminal (phenobarbital), Amytal, Nembutal, Seconal, barbital, Pentothal	Yes	Yes	Yes
Bromides: Nervine, Neurosine, sodium bromide, potassium bromide, triple bromides, Bromoseltzer	Yes	No	No
Marihuana—Indian hemp, "reefers," "muggles"	Yes	No	No
Stimulant drugs (cause sleeplessness and excitement): Cocaine	Yes	No	No
Benzedrine-type drugs: Benzedrine (amphetamine), Benzedrex, Dexedrine, Tuamine, Desyphed Tablets	Yes	No	No

Source: Victor H. Vogel and Virginia E. Vogel, *Facts about Narcotics*, Science Research Associates, Inc., Chicago, 1951.

The United States Navy, Office of Naval Research, collaborating with Tufts University, Institute for Applied Experimental Psychology, has gathered together interesting research data about the effects of caffeine on physiologic functions. The results of the study indicate that caffeine affects certain functions in the following ways:

CIRCULATION. The pulse is increased 5 to 10 per cent 30 minutes after drinking coffee. Blood pressure is increased about 5 per cent.

RESPIRATION. There is little or no effect on the rate of respiration.

SLEEP. One to four grains of caffeine has no appreciable effect on the sleep of most normal people. Five to six grains produces a marked disturbance in the sleep of most individuals.

TEMPERATURE. Caffeine has little effect on body temperature.

DIURESIS. Before tolerance of caffeine has been developed, there is a marked increase in the amount of urine.

GENERAL WELL-BEING. Four or more grains of caffeine can produce dizziness, a feeling of numbness, headache, indigestion, diarrhea or constipation, and irritability in many people.

MOTOR EFFECT. Caffeine usually increases motor response.

SENSORY EFFECTS. It is believed that sensory responses are favorably affected.

HIGHER MENTAL PROCESSES. Small amounts of caffeine, that is, amounts under four grains, have a more favorable effect on the mental processes than do large amounts.

It appears from the foregoing data

that small amounts of caffeine cause but slight reactions in normal individuals. However, large amounts of caffeine may produce unfavorable reactions such as indigestion, heartburn, dizziness, headache, irritability, insomnia, numbness of extremities, and peripheral coldness. It has been found that drinks containing caffeine taken on an empty stomach or late in the evening have more general effects than if taken in the forenoon or with food in the stomach.

Summary

The legal and illegal use of depressant and stimulant drugs is increasing throughout the world. Depressant drugs taken internally cause the consumer to relax and to perspire noticeably; his ability to move and to think is inhibited; and there is a marked reduction in the function of his vital organs. Stimulants taken into the body have the opposite effect from that produced by depressant drugs.

The drinking of beverage alcohol is a very old custom. Primitive people drank primarily during community gatherings. Today beverage alcohol is used by at least 75 million persons in the United States. The annual consumption of alcoholic drinks in this country approaches 231 million gallons of whisky, 500 million gallons of wine, and 3 billion gallons of beer. Drinkers of alcoholic beverages are found in all socioeconomic levels. They have been classified as occasional, frequent, regular, alcohol-dependent, and alcoholic. An excessive use of beverage alcohol often results in serious physical, mental, and social problems for the consumer.

Man has used tobacco in some form for many centuries. The annual consumption of cigarettes in the United States is well over 475 billion. This immense popularity is due in part to advertising, imitation, desire for sociability, need of relief from tension, and the fact that, once the practice has been established, it is very difficult to break.

The toxic elements in tobacco smoke can seriously affect the body. Excessive use of tobacco may injure heart tissue, may disturb circulatory action and vision, and may impair physical and mental efficiency.

In 1959, the U.S. Public Health Service declared in an official statement that a positive relationship exists between the smoking of cigarettes and the development of lung cancer.

Research reports by reliable scientific groups question the value of filter cigarettes as adequate protection against harmful tars and nicotine in tobacco smoking.

The use of depressant drugs such as heroin, barbituric acid, bromides, and marihuana is increasing in this country. Marihuana is particularly dangerous in that its use often leads to heroin addiction. Heroin, a morphine derivative, is addicting, and its use can result in complete mental, moral, and physical breakdown.

Stimulating drugs such as benzedrine and cocaine are taken to give temporary excitement to the consumer. The most popular drug in this class is benzedrine, sometimes called "pep pills." A benzedrine addict may develop serious physical reactions. Although cocaine addiction is less common than other habit-forming drugs, cocaine is very dangerous to use. Once a person is "hooked," he is powerless to stop using the drug. It lowers his resistance to disease and often results in early death.

Stimulants of the non-habit-forming class are cola beverages, coffee, and tea. The facts concerning the effects of these products on the human body indicate trends and are not final evidence.

Suggested readings

1. Alcoholic Anonymous: *An Interpretation of the Twelve Steps of the Alcoholic Anonymous Program,* Coll-Webb Co., Minneapolis, 1959.
2. Bacon, Seldon, and Robert Straus: *Drinking in College,* Yale University Press, New Haven, Conn., 1953.
3. Beaven, Winton H.: "Injurious Effects of Tobacco and Alcohol," *Health Education Journal,* 24:14, November, 1960.
4. "Cigarettes," *Consumer Reports,* 25:13–21, January, 1960.
5. Cooley, Donald G.: "The Story of Tranquilizers," *Today's Health,* 78:32, November, 1960.
6. Cornfield, J., and others: "Smoking and Lung Cancer," *Journal of the National Cancer Institute,* 122:173, 1959.
7. Courville, Cyril B.: *Effects of Alcohol on the Nervous System of Man,* San Lucas Press, Los Angeles, 1955.
8. Ewen, Edward T.: "More People Drink, But Less," *The New York Times Magazine,* May 14, 1961, p. 53.
9. Haggard, Howard W., and E. M. Jellinek: *Alcohol Explored,* Doubleday and Company, Inc., New York, 1954.
10. Hammond, E. Cuyler, and Daniel Horn: "Smoking and Death Rates: Report on Forty-four Months of Follow-up of 187,783 Men," *Journal of the American Medical Association,* 166:1294–1308, Mar. 15, 1958.
11. Hewitt, Donald W.: "Alcohol and Crime," *Life and Health,* 55:16, November, 1960.
12. James, Walter G.: "Teen-age Smoking and Lung Cancer," *Journal of Health, Physical Education and Recreation,* 31:25, November, 1960.
13. Jellinek, E. M., *The Disease Concept of Alcoholism,* Hillhouse Press, New Haven, Conn., 1960.
14. King, Albion R.: *Basic Information on Alcohol,* Cornell College Press, Mount Vernon, Iowa, 1960.
15. Lieb, Clarence W.: *Don't Let Smoking Kill You,* Bonus Books, Inc., New York, 1957.
16. Ochsner, Alton: *Smoking and Health,* Julian Messner, Inc., Publishers, New York, 1959.
17. *Planning for Alcohol Education,* California State Department of Public Health, Feb. 16–19, 1960.
18. Root, Lin: "They Stay Awake to Die," *Today's Health,* 38:32, October, 1960.
19. "Smoking and Lung Cancer," *New England Journal of Medicine,* 262:417, Feb. 25, 1960.
20. Whitman, Howard: *Our Drinking Habits,* Division of Alcoholic Rehabilitation, State of California Department of Public Health, Berkeley, Calif., 1960.
21. Zappella, David: "Psychological Effects of Alcohol," *California's Health,* 18:25–28, Aug. 15, 1960.

FOURTEEN

Living safely in our time

RADIATION PROBLEMS

FALLOUT SHELTERS

CIVIL DEFENSE

SAFETY EDUCATION

CAUSES AND PREVENTION OF ACCIDENTS

SAFETY IN RECREATION AND SPORTS

AUTOMOBILE SAFETY

FIRE PREVENTION

FIRST AID

ACCIDENT INSURANCE AND LIABILITY

As a result of rapid and unique developments in science and inventions, man has created an imposing list of hazards to his life and well-being. Learning how to live safely with these hazards both in the college environment and elsewhere is a challenge to students and to the institution of higher learning they attend. Living safely in our times, in other words, living safely in the Space Age, means that the American public must be better

419

informed about safety hazards current in the world today. For example, radioactive fallout offers a formidable health hazard; increased speed creates transportation hazards of mounting proportions; increased leisure time allows greater participation in recreation and sports, with possible accidents; and there is always the problem of home and farm accidents. To ensure an adequate understanding and appreciation of living safely and to develop a sound functional approach to safety practices, students in health education should be able to think and act intelligently about such current questions as:

What is meant by radiation and how harmful is it to mankind?

Is it possible to limit exposure to radiation?

How effective are fallout shelters?

How important are civil defense and defense mobilization plans?

What are the principal accident hazards to college students and how can these hazards be reduced?

What are the chief causes of accidents in the home and how can they be prevented?

What information should the student have about first aid to the sick and injured?

How important is it to have the protection of accident insurance?

The following presentation makes no attempt to give all the answers to these questions, but discussion of various aspects of these important problems should help you to increase your understanding and to act more wisely.

Radiation problems

When man created the atomic bomb, he provided a temporary deterrent to a "hot war" and a threat to the physical well-being of mankind. Scientists the world over are concerned not only with protecting their respective nations against possible foreign aggression by stock-piling atomic bombs but also with ways and means of protecting against radioactive fallout resulting from atomic explosions. The Atomic Energy Commission estimates that up to 1958, when the great powers agreed to stop bomb testing, 90 million tons of fission yield had been thrown into the atmosphere. This means that, together with the great mass of debris thrown out by nuclear explosions, there is a large quantity of radioactive material in the earth's atmosphere. Unfortunately, most of the fallout descends on the northern hemisphere. This is probably due to the location of test sites, weather, air currents, and conditions in the stratosphere. It has been estimated that by 1965 all the fallout produced prior to 1958 will finally reach the earth

[18]. However, the intensive testing program of 1962 will prolong the fallout hazard for years to come. Let us examine the facts.

WHAT IS RADIATION AND HOW HARMFUL IS IT TO MAN?

Radiation is not something that has been recently created. It is as old as the universe. It is around us in various forms. Light from the sun is radiation we can see. Heat is radiation we can feel. Even the rocks and the earth are mildly radioactive. For purposes of this discussion, radiation can be said to be a fast-moving stream or wave of flying particles coming from very small units of matter, called *atoms*. Atoms from a single element may vary in weight. These variations, called *isotopes*, may be stable or unstable. It is the unstable varieties that are radioactive and are harmful to man [11]. (See pages 505–508 for additional information on radiation.)

Up to 1895 radioactive substances occurred only in nature. In 1895 man-made radiation in the form of the X ray was first discovered. A few years later with the isolation of the element radium, three new forms of radiation were discovered, namely, alpha, beta, and gamma rays. All these rays have the power to penetrate into the deep tissues of the body. If exposure to these rays is long and deep enough, the nuclei of body cells can be seriously altered. It is encouraging to note that man has lived with the natural sources of radiation since he has been on earth with no major threat to his health. However, now that he has been able to intensify the exposure, there is always the threat of too much exposure to X rays or radioactive substances. At this point the scientist asks a very important question: How much radiation can the body stand without harmful effects?

The unit commonly used to measure radiation is the roentgen (r). When a physician X rays a person's chest, the patient receives about 0.3 roentgens. This is thought to be a harmless exposure [11]. If, however, the exposure should be several hundred roentgens, all received at the same time, which, of course, is most unlikely, the cells of the body would be seriously altered.

A team of scientists working with the United Nations lists the *average* world-wide exposure of a person to radiation during a year as 1/10 roentgen from natural sources, 3/10 roentgen from medical or dental radiation, and less than 2/100 roentgen from fallout. From these figures it appears that our chances of being overexposed to radiation are slight [18].

Fallout from atomic-bomb explosions contains hundreds of radioactive materials. One of the most potentially dangerous to man is strontium-90. Heavy or prolonged exposure to it can cause cancer of the bone. Strontium-90, as a radioactive isotope, follows the same metabolic process as calcium when it enters the body. Fortunately, when both are present, the body discriminates against

600 r or more	
Severe radiation sickness with death of up to 100% of exposed individuals. Rapid emaciation and death as early as 2d week with possible eventual death of up to 100% of exposed individuals.	
300-600 r	
Severe radiation sickness with death of up to 50% of exposed individuals. Some deaths in 2 to 6 weeks. Possible eventual death to 50% of the exposed individuals for about 450 r.	
200-300 r	
Moderate radiation sickness. Recovery likely in about 3 months unless complicated by poor previous health, superimposed injuries, or infection.	
100-200 r	
Slight radiation sickness. Blood changes with delayed recovery. Delayed effects may shorten life expectancy by 1%.	
25-100 r	
No radiation sickness expected. Slight temporary blood changes. Exposed individuals should be able to resume usual duties.	
0-25 r	
No radiation sickness. No detectable clinical effects. The exposed person would not be aware of any biological damage.	

External radiation dosages. The shaded portion of each bar represents the level of dosage responsible for the conditions described under each bar. (*Peacetime Radiation Hazards in the Fire Service*, U.S. Department of Health, Education, and Welfare and U.S. Atomic Energy Commission, 1961, p. 15.)

strontium-90 in favor of calcium. The danger from strontium-90 arises when an accumulation in the bone becomes excessive. If the actual exposure to fallout radiation remains less than 2/100 roentgen per year per person, it is not likely that during our lifetime we will receive a dangerous dose of this element.

To safeguard the health of the public, the World Health Organization and allied groups are constantly on the alert for signs of excessive fallout. The U:S. Public Health Service has checking stations in strategic places throughout this country to measure radiation in food and

HOW TO BE A SURVIVOR: CHARACTERISTICS OF NUCLEAR-WEAPON RADIATIONS							
Name and symbol	What is it ?	How does bomb produce it?	Initial velocity	Penetration in air	Penetration in tissue	What will stop it ?	Human hazard in wartime
α Alpha	Helium nucleus	Emitted from unfissioned uranium and plutonium. Is part of fallout debris	.05 c	5 cm	.005 cm (first layer of skin)	Paper / Clothing	A negligible hazard. Not enough gains entrance to body. Can be ignored
β Beta	High-speed electron	Emitted by fission products. Important only as a residual or fallout hazard	.95 c	200 cm	0.125 cm (several layers of skin)	Paper / Clothing	Nuisance only. With military clothing damage will be minimal
γ Gamma	Electromagnetic wave (like visible light)	Emitted by fission products. Important in both prompt and residual radiation	c	Very penetrating. Thousands of meters	Very penetrating. Exit dose for man = 60% of entrance dose	Several feet of concrete or earth	Can be serious. Many casualties possible under certain circumstances
n Neutron	Electrically neutral body	Emitted only during the instant of fission or fusion	.1 c	Very penetrating. Somewhat less than gamma	Very penetrating. About the same as gamma rays	Several feet of concrete or earth	Can be serious. As a prompt hazard to those in foxholes or other blast shelter

The various kinds of nuclear radiation, some of the sources of protection, and aids to survival. *(What's New*, Abbott Laboratories, North Chicago, Ill., 1961.)

drink. Should a dangerous concentration develop, the public would be instantly alerted.

IS IT POSSIBLE TO LIMIT EXPOSURE TO RADIATION?

If you should be working in an area close to radioactive materials, you can limit exposure by staying in the area as short a time as possible, by keeping a safe distance from the source of the radiation, and by wearing protecting or shielding equipment. You need have little fear of the alpha ray, as it can be stopped by clothing; ¼ inch of wood or ⅛ inch of metal will shield from the beta ray. However, it will require a thick layer of cement or lead to protect against the gamma ray. For those working near radioactive substances there is a danger of contaminating clothing; in fact, any exposed part of the body can be contaminated. If this should occur, harmful isotopes can then gain entrance to the body by way of food eaten, or by a cut, or even by smoking. Anyone working near radioactive material should always wear protective outer garments, which should be removed before leaving the area. In addition, all exposed parts of the body should be washed with soap and water and the entire body checked by instrument counters for possible contamination [11].

Fallout shelters

Fallout shelters appear to be a far cry from the realities of everyday living in the United States; but survival in a nuclear attack may be a matter of great concern to millions of Americans in matters of minutes—possibly seconds. With this thought in mind, let us consider the subject of fallout shelters.

The Office of Civil and Defense Mobilization emphasizes the following points: Twenty-four hours after a nuclear attack the entire nation could be covered with fallout, thus necessitating shelters everywhere.

Satisfactory shelters can be built in basements with concrete block, above ground with concrete blocks, or underground using cement reinforcements.

If an attack finds you without shelter and you have no basement available, the best protection is on the ground floor of a house or apartment. If there is a basement, seek the corner least exposed to windows and the deepest below ground level [9].

This agency also lays stress on the importance of family education and cooperation in case of a nuclear attack. For example, they suggest the following precautions:

At the sound of the first alert signal, the family should assemble and get started on emergency assignments.

Long before an alert is necessary, a fallout shelter should be constructed.

Each family should appoint a member to serve as fire marshal to lead all members of the family in a systematic search for home fire hazards.

Each family should provide home fire-fighting equipment and train the family in its use.

As many members of the family as possible should be trained in the emergency care of the injured.

Training should also include finding a missing member of the family lost in the confusion of the emergency.

There should be the equivalent of at least 7 gallons of safe drinking water and other fluids on hand for each member of the family.

It is important that one or more members of the family take a course in the care of the sick and the injured.

These points are but a few of many things that a family can do to meet the emergencies arising from a nuclear attack [17].

The Stanford Research Institute, Menlo Park, California, points out that in an area of heavy fallout it is best to stay in a shelter for at least two weeks. If a person is caught away from his shelter in the emergency, he should seek the best protection available, such as a cul-

A local plan for Civil Defense. (Los Angeles City Health Department.)

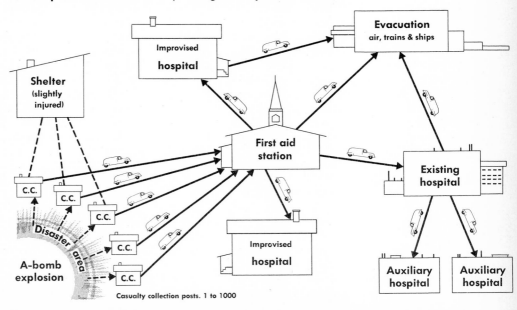

Casualty collection posts. 1 to 1000

vert, a deep hole with some kind of a cover over it, or a cave if one is handy. Emergency supplies for the family shelter should be carefully selected. Supplies for cooking and serving, infant care, sanitation, sleeping, recreation, first aid, and spiritual comfort should be included among them.

When it is reasonably safe to leave the shelter, everything should be decontaminated, including people, shelter, and the area outside the shelter. For example, it is important that people wash, yes,

scrub the body, and thoroughly wash all clothing. The inside of the shelter should be vacuum cleaned. The area outside the shelter should be washed with hose and water, starting with the house and ending with the grounds [5].

A nuclear attack is not a happy thought, but it lies within the realm of possibility and that is sufficient reason to be prepared. Authorities agree that well-constructed shelters offer the populace excellent chances to survive nuclear fallout.

Civil defense (disaster preparedness)

In 1945 the Federal government began setting up a pattern of civil defense. This plan was designed to save lives and property in war-caused or natural disasters by organizing the efforts of citizens, community organizations, and the government. Congress outlined the responsibilities for war-caused disasters in Public Law 920, and for natural disasters in Public Law 875 of the 81st Congress. The Federal government encouraged states and local groups to establish appropriate legislation for the organization of defense and disaster relief. This has been accomplished, and civil-defense programs are in operation throughout the nation.

The President of the United States heads the United States Civil Defense Corps. In July, 1961, President Kennedy urged the adoption of the following plan to increase the efficiency of the Civil and Defense Mobilization Agency:

Conduct a Defense Department survey; mark and make available shelters in all public and private existing buildings.

Construct shelters in existing Federal buildings and in all new Federal buildings.

Make available FHA loans for shelter construction.

Provide a "matching program" to provide money for construction of under-

ground control centers protected from blast and fallout, from which city, county, and state governments can operate in the event of an attack.

Develop and make available to the public radiologic and biologic monitoring devices.

Provide at least 300 million dollars to finance the program.

During the summer of 1953 the U.S.S.R. began constructing both the atomic bomb and the hydrogen bomb. The wide publicity given to this scientific accomplishment and to the more recent intercontinental ballistic missile development has served to stimulate an increased interest in national and local civil defense. The constant threat of attack and war with nuclear weapons has sparked the development of improved civil-defense operations. Federal, state, county, and city organizations are responsible for civil-defense program, equipment, and supplies such as rescue trucks, communications equipment, and medical supplies in stockpile quantities.

The functions of civil defense include the following:

Educating citizens to recognize the siren signals, to understand their meaning, and to know what to do when they are sounded

Teaching citizens how to save lives

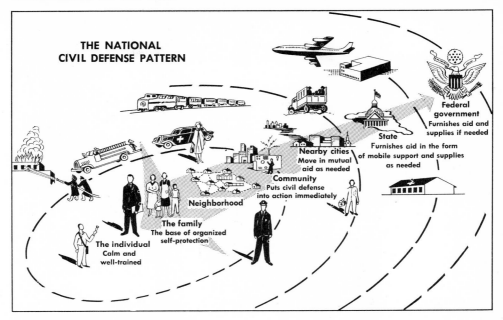

THE NATIONAL CIVIL DEFENSE PATTERN

Federal government Furnishes aid and supplies if needed

State Furnishes aid in the form of mobile support and supplies as needed

Nearby cities Move in mutual aid as needed

Community Puts civil defense into action immediately

Neighborhood

The family The base of organized self-protection

The individual Calm and well-trained

(Los Angeles City Health Department.)

through first aid, fire fighting, and provisions for shelter, food, and clothing

Preparing volunteers for rescue and aid in time of disaster

Preparing leaders and leadership groups to direct such operations as medical, transportation, communications, radiological monitoring, rescue, engineering, welfare, fire, and police

Organizing and coordinating the material resources of government, industry, and commerce to care for the victims of disaster and reduce the effects of disaster

Working cooperatively with all governmental offices so that all services will be provided during emergencies

The effectiveness of the civil-defense program depends upon the extent of citizen participation. Volunteer participation is based on the "minute man" concept of 1776. Each person must protect himself, his family, and his property and must assist others. Such action is designed to minimize casualties and property losses in the event of an actual attack. There are at least 10 major volunteer services which citizens can join:

WARDEN SERVICE. To prepare citizens for emergencies and offer leadership in case of attack.

FIRE SERVICE. To teach householders how to fight fires in the emergency.

POLICE SERVICE. To assist local police in controlling traffic, etc., and maintaining law and order.

HEALTH SERVICE. To assist in first aid, transport the wounded, repair equipment, and prevent radiologic contamination.

WELFARE SERVICE. To provide housing, food, clothing, and money and to assist in locating missing persons.

ENGINEERING SERVICE. To restore damaged installations and clear away debris after an attack.

RESCUE SERVICE. To rescue trapped persons.

TRANSPORTATION SERVICE. To move the injured and also food and medical supplies.

STAFF SERVICE. To keep records, send out

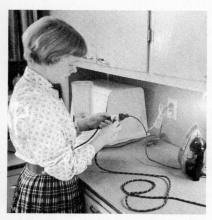

Safety begins in the home or in college housing facilities. Avoid overloading electric circuits.

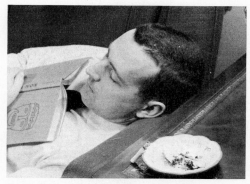

Don't let a live cigarette put an end to your life by fire and asphyxiation.

To all drivers of automobiles and their passengers, the question today is no longer why wear seat belts, but why not wear them and take advantage of the greater margin of safety they afford.

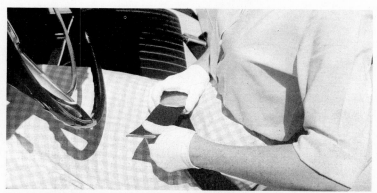

The action of children riding bicycles on the highway is highly unpredictable. When you are approaching bicycle riders, use extra caution.

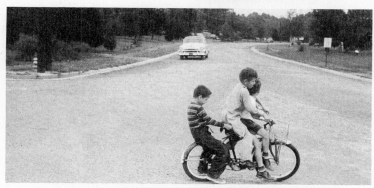

This careless individual is headed for the hospital or the morgue unless the driver has good brakes on his automobile and is able to stop in time.

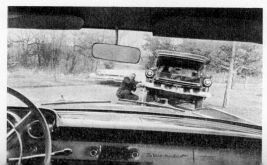

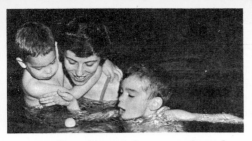

Dispelling fear of the water through games is the first step in teaching children to swim.

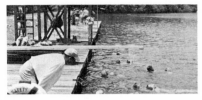

Knowing how to swim is a wise safety precaution, and knowing how to save the lives of others is most commendable.

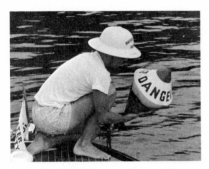

It is important to respect danger signs posted for your protection.

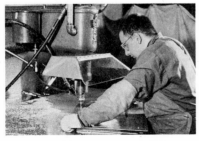

Safety in industry or at the work bench includes protecting eyes and hands. This operator of a metal cutting machine is protected from flying metal shavings by a plexiglass shield, elbow-length gloves, and an air-blast hose which blows the metal chips away from him.

printed materials and letters, do typing, and operate switchboards.

COMMUNICATION SERVICE. To communicate through radio, television, telegraph and telephone.

Safety education

There is little need to speculate on the importance of education as a factor in controlling and preventing accidents. It has been shown repeatedly that where there is cooperative action in safety education, whether it be in school, community, home, or industry, an improved record of accident prevention has been achieved.

Education has at least three unique teaching opportunities, which have a significant bearing on the prevention of accidents: cooperation in all its aspects, assuming of civic responsibilities, and developing a creative attitude. These three need not be confined to the course in health education but can be employed with great profit throughout the total curriculum. For example, authorities in safety education agree that a safety rule or a safe environment cooperatively planned has great potential strength. This is the democratic way of putting purposeful action to practical ends.

Some time ago a large university campus was bisected by a busy city street. Numerous accidents occurred. Some were fatal. During a discussion of the situation in a health education class it was determined to make a critical study of the problem. After two weeks of day and evening observations by students and faculty, facts were assembled and presented to the proper authorities. The result was permanent closing of the street and prevention of further accidents and possible deaths. The study required the cooperative efforts of students, professors, president, board of trustees of the university, and city government officials. It was a cooperative venture, and the university and community at large shared in the profit. Cooperation need not be confined to the campus. The student who believes in safety, both for himself and others, cooperates with authorities and associates in his community, during activities at the beach and swimming pool, on hunting or fishing trips, at the theater, on the highway—in fact, everywhere he goes. He is willing to assume the role of a responsible citizen whether he is under authority or acting under his own control.

The study of political science and allied subjects presents a unique opportunity for broadening the student's concept of government and for creating a feeling of pride in and responsibility for a safe environment in his community. It is a worthy extension of these courses when students and others become actively interested in keeping the immediate environment safe. They may express their interest by calling attention to safety hazards in the community and by working for rules, city ordinances, and state and national laws that both eliminate hazards and widen the areas for safe living for all.

The essence of creativeness is freedom —freedom to think, to feel, and to move according to one's sense of values and the compulsion of both extrinsic and intrinsic disciplines. Too often the word "creative" has been reserved for the fields of literature and the fine arts. It is commendable when one originates a work that adds to the culture and pleasure of his fellow men. Likewise, it is commendable when one originates a plan or constructs a vehicle or machine that breaks through the barriers of routine and imitation and provides the community with a safer and freer way to make a living and to spend leisure time. For example, it was a college student who conceived the idea of equipping all four wheels of an automobile with brakes. Another developed the small light reflectors one finds on most highway curves. The college student moves in an environment conducive to such creative work. Many of the answers to major problems in safety lie within the scope of creative effort.

Causes and prevention of accidents

In explaining the cause of a poor grade to his father, a college freshman began, "Well, Dad, it was this way. I . . . ," etc., etc. After patiently listening to the lengthy defense, the father interrupted, "Now, son, what was the real cause?" All too often the basic cause of accidents is obscured by lengthy rationalization. For every accident there is a fundamental cause, and until that cause is discovered and corrected, accidents and their multiple "reasons" will continue to fill the record books (see Table 14.1).

Determining the cause of accidents by place and related data is simplified when a program of adequate reporting is in force. Developing preventive measures is slower and more difficult.

Authorities in safety education agree that the majority of accidents involve persons who are emotionally unstable, socially maladjusted, selfish, or careless or who have some physical anomaly. When to one or more of these conditions is added excessive speed, inattention, poor judgment, discourtesy, intoxication, or fatigue, there is likely to be an accident.

One must not lose sight of the fact that the prevention of accidents under supervision is easier and probably more effective than it is without supervision. In other words, it is easier to prevent an accident in a controlled environment such as a school, a factory, or a patrolled highway than in the home, where the individual is king and is acting under his own orders.

Table 14.1. Causes and prevention of accidents

Kind of accident	Causes	Prevention
Occupational:		
Mechanical (manual skills)	Occur most frequently when employee is handling objects, working with machinery, working with vehicles, or using hand tools or falls on slippery surfaces or from heights	Less likely to occur when employee is adequately trained and proficient in skills of his trade and is protected from dangers, including falls
Personal	Likely to occur when an employee is fatigued or ill, is upset emotionally, disobeys safety rules, has physical disabilities, is maladjusted socially, is ignorant of job to be done, or lacks recreational skills	Less likely to occur if employee has adequate psychological counseling and medical services, receives precise pre-employment screening by personnel office, practices sound discipline both on and off job, helps plan rules of safety, understands requirements of job, and has opportunity to engage in wholesome recreational programs
Traffic:		
Mechanical (manual skills)	Occur most frequently when motor vehicles collide with pedestrians, with each other, or with trains, streetcars, animals, or fixed objects or when they overturn or run off highway	Less likely to occur if operator of motor vehicle possesses up-to-date license to drive, understands driving techniques, knows and obeys traffic regulations of state and community, respects rights of others, and is skillful in operating vehicle
Personal	Likely to occur when pedestrian or operator of vehicle, or both, are under influence of alcohol, fatigued, sleepy, careless, discourteous, upset emotionally, or ignorant of traffic regulations or have serious physical disabilities	Less likely to occur if pedestrian and vehicle operator keep off highway when under influence of alcohol and when physically, mentally, or emotionally incapable of good judgment
Aquatic:		
Mechanical (manual skills)	Likely to occur when one falls out of boat or canoe and is unable to swim, collides with objects in water, dives or steps into unknown depths, lacks adequate training in water-rescue techniques, or lacks skill in handling boat or canoe	Less likely to occur if one is skilled in handling boats and canoes, knows skills of swimming and diving, knows where these skills can be practiced safely, and is trained in techniques of water rescue
Personal	Likely to occur when one is overfatigued or under influence of alcoholic beverages, becomes frightened while swimming, ignores safety rules, or has uncompensated physical disabilities	Less likely to occur if one stays out of water when overfatigued or when one has been drinking alcoholic beverages, obeys rules established for safety, recognizes physical strengths or handicaps, and stays within safe limits while swimming, diving, or boating
Home, firearms:		
Mechanical (manual skills)	Most likely to occur when one lacks skill in handling a gun (cleaning, pointing, etc.) or knowledge of correct ways to handle a gun while hunting	Less likely to occur if one possesses skill in handling firearms (cleaning, shooting, etc.) and never points a gun at another person when on a hunting trip or elsewhere

Table 14.1. Causes and prevention of accidents (continued)

Kind of accident	Causes	Prevention
Personal	Likely to occur when one leaves an unused gun loaded, is upset emotionally, is careless in handling a gun, is ignorant of or disregards laws of his state governing hunting, or uses firearms while under influence of beverage alcohol	Less likely to occur if one makes sure unused firearms are left unloaded, never looks down barrel of a gun, never lets snow get into muzzle of gun, never gets into an automobile with loaded gun, never moves about in boat with loaded gun, understands regulations governing hunting in his state, and avoids using firearms when under influence of beverage alcohol
Home, burns:		
Mechanical (manual skills)	Likely to occur when one smokes in bed or while lying down, is careless or ignorant of safe manner of handling fireworks, or lacks skill and understanding of safe ways to handle flammables	Less likely to occur if one does not smoke in bed or while lying down, if only skilled operators are permitted to handle fireworks, and if there is skilled and safe use of flammables
Personal	Likely to occur when an individual working with fire or flammable chemicals is overfatigued, has been drinking beverage alcohol, is upset emotionally, or is careless about an open fire	Less likely to occur if smokers who are intoxicated are kept under supervision, if proper safeguards are used around open fires, and if there is constant protection of children against misuse of fire or flammable materials
Home, falls:		
Mechanical (manual skills)	Most likely to occur when good housekeeping techniques are lacking, floors are slippery, passageways and stairs are poorly lighted, or an unstable support is used in reaching for high places	Less likely to occur if good housekeeping techniques are practiced, floors and stairs are not slippery, all passageways are kept free from articles, steps are in good repair, steady hand rails are available on stairways, ladders and other articles used for climbing to high places are made secure and are appropriate for bearing desired weight, and a white line is painted on top and bottom steps
Personal	Likely to occur when one is careless or lacks proper safety attitudes, is intoxicated, or is not alert to environmental hazards	Less likely to occur if one has proper safety attitudes, if intoxicated persons are kept under control, and if members of household receive sound instruction on home safety
Home, poisonous gases:		
Mechanical (manual skills)	Likely to occur when gas appliances are defective, when gas heaters are burning with windows of room closed, when coal-burning furnace is defective, when carbon monoxide is not permitted safe escape, or when one searches for gas leaks with lighted match or candle	Less likely to occur if all heating and cooking appliances are correctly installed and inspected regularly, if room heated by gas has fresh supply of oxygen, and if flashlight is used when searching for gas leaks

Table 14.1. Causes and prevention of accidents (continued)

Kind of accident	Causes	Prevention
Personal	Likely to occur when there is carelessness or ignorance about safe heating and cooking facilities in house, about importance of fresh air in room heated by gas, or about importance of protecting against fatal monoxide gas or when one is careless in determining source of gas leakage or is overfatigued or intoxicated and unable to use gas appliances properly	Less likely to occur if members of household receive adequate instruction on safe use of all gas appliances and individuals realize dangers of carbon monoxide (as in working on running motor with garage door closed)
School-campus: Mechanical (manual skills)	May occur in physical education program when pupils engaged in body-contact sports and games use improper and unsafe equipment or play on slippery surfaces or in unprotected and unsafe areas May occur in shops, laboratories, and classrooms when pupils are not properly instructed in use of hand tools, fast-moving machinery, explosives, and other dangerous chemicals	Less likely to occur if there is proper instruction in skills, if adequate and safe equipment is used, if playing areas are made safe, if there is intelligent supervision of all physical activities, if proper instruction and supervision in use of dangerous equipment is provided in all shops, laboratories, and classrooms, and if dangerous machinery and chemicals are properly safeguarded
Personal	May occur in physical education program when pupil lacks game and sport skills, is overtense, has uncompensated bodily disabilities, is overfatigued or careless, or uses inadequate or unsafe equipment May occur in shops, laboratories, and classrooms when pupil lacks skill and understanding about proper use of assigned materials and equipment, fails to exercise proper safeguards while working with dangerous materials, or is fatigued or sleepy	Less likely to occur if there is adequate medical examination and counseling of all students, if recreation program is provided for entire student body, and if pupils are properly instructed in the skills and safeguards necessary for safe use of dangerous equipment in shops, laboratories, and classrooms

Source: Data from National Safety Council, *Accident Facts* (annual publication); and H. J. Stack and others, *Education for Safe Living*, Prentice-Hall, Inc., Englewood Cliffs, N.J., 1957.

Accident prevention must take all these facts into consideration. Prevention that saves lives as well as provides for safe living is a matter of raising a generation of healthy people and providing them with adequate laws on safety, sound safety engineering, and purposeful safety education.

Safety in recreation and sports

The frequency of injuries occurring in athletic activities can be substantially reduced. In fact, the concept of safety can be so well integrated with the recreation and sports program that players are seldom conscious of safety per se. For example, in baseball, dropping the bat as one starts for first base is as easy as hurling it. Protecting oneself while tackling or being tackled in football is as easy as are undisciplined movements. Leaving a game before one is over-fatigued can be taught as a safe and correct form of participation. Learning to fall without injury is a desirable skill and is applicable to all sports. By a thorough understanding of what to do and what to avoid, by using only acceptable equipment, by seeking the advice of skilled leaders, by staying within the limits of one's ability, by maintaining a sound physical body, and by avoiding hazardous playing conditions, the individual can make safety so much a part of participation that it is thought of only when its absence is apparent.

The following action taken cooperatively by the students and the faculty can be helpful in bringing about a reduction of athletic injuries:

All members of the student body have a periodic health examination followed by appropriate medical care.

All students are properly equipped for the physical activities in which they engage.

Adequate safety precautions are required of all participants in all play areas. This also includes safe playground surfaces and facilities.

All students are properly trained and conditioned for the games and sports in which they participate.

Athletic competition between students is based on reasonably equal skill and strength.

Officials for all athletic competitions are approved by the college faculty.

Only qualified personnel are permitted to give first aid to injured students.

An adequate follow-up is made by school health service personnel of all students injured in games or sports.

A safe-conduct code is developed by students and faculty for all physical education activities conducted on the campus.

All participants in athletic sports are protected by athletic injury insurance.

WATER SAFETY

Being safety-minded when participating in aquatic activities is a desirable attitude. When this attitude, fortified by knowledge, becomes functional through sound behavior, safety in and on the water can be assured. Safety practices will eventually eliminate a high percentage of tragic swimming and boating fatalities and make secure the fun inherent in aquatic games and sports.

The American Red Cross, a leader in safety education, suggests many practical water safety precautions. For example, they emphasize:

Learn to swim and never swim alone.

After eating a meal, do not engage in competitive swimming for three or four hours.

Avoid swimming when fatigued.

If you are caught in a current, attempt to swim diagonally across the current and in the direction of the flow.

When muscle cramps occur in the legs, grasp the cramped area and squeeze until the muscle relaxes.

A person with stomach cramps will need the assistance of a lifeguard or swimming companion to help him to safety.

Skin and scuba diving are increasing rapidly in popularity. This is in large part because the diver immediately passes into an environment totally different from life on land. When the diver respects the new environment and learns to live comfortably in it, he is reasonably safe. If he disregards it, he is in trouble. Following are a few conditions that may be encountered if the skin and scuba diver is uninformed or careless: "thoracic squeeze," a painful lung congestion; hemorrhage of the eyes and eyelids; middle ear injury; nitrogen narcosis; oxygen poisoning; carbon dioxide intoxication; unconsciousness. These conditions can be avoided by exercising safety precautions in matters of equipment and underwater work.

In giving first aid for skin- and scuba-diving accident victims, send for a rescue squad and medical help at once; administer artificial respiration if needed, and get the patient into a decompression chamber as soon as possible.

Lifesaving. Saving the life of another human being is a satisfying experience. All swimmers, in fact, anyone who has contact with streams, lakes, or the ocean, should be trained in water rescue. The American Red Cross offers such train-ing. It is well to remember that rescuing an actively drowning person requires skill. If possible, avoid direct contact with the struggling person. Reach him with a life buoy, a paddle, an oar, a pole, a log, a board, or any object that the drowning person can grasp; then haul him to safety. For a detailed discussion of direct and indirect lifesaving methods, see the American Red Cross textbook on the subject [3].

The five steps in the back-pressure—arm-lift method of artificial respiration: (1) position of subject, (2) position of operator, (3) compression phase, (4) release of pressure, (5) expansion phase. The entire cycle should be repeated 12 times per minute at a steady rate. (American National Red Cross.)

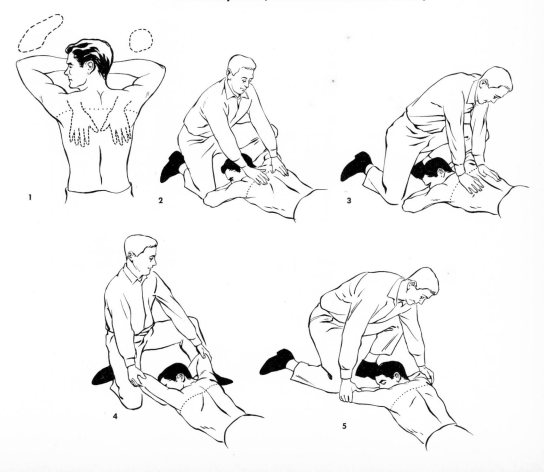

Automobile safety

The daily carnage along city streets and on the open highways presents a major health problem to the American public. It stems from the speed and ease with which Americans travel to and from business and pleasure. It is expressed in annual figures of over 38,000 persons killed and more than 1 million injured in automobile accidents. Preventing these accidents and saving lives is as much a problem for the college student as it is for the law-enforcement officer and the specialist in safety.

For those interested in statistical data the following facts about traffic accidents may be enlightening. From 1950 through 1960 over 413,000 persons were killed in vehicle accidents in the United States. In 1960 alone, the death toll reached 38,200. From 1950 to 1960, the number of persons injured in automobile accidents was 13,500,000 with a resulting economic loss from both death and injury of 45 billion dollars [1].

The major cause of death on the highways is by collision between automobiles. Over 55 per cent of the accidents occurred after dark. Speed is the chief contributing factor in 30 per cent of collisions.

Over 7,000 of those killed in automobile accidents in 1959 were within the college age bracket. The greatest number of fatal automobile accidents occurred on Saturdays, in December, and on rainy days [1].

These are formidable facts, which call for more than passing attention. Our streets and highways can be made safe if the driving public wants to make them safe. This is not entirely a matter of law and engineering. In the final analysis the deciding factor is the individual driver. It is up to him to decide whether he wants safety on the highway or not. There is no security for anyone if he decides to take chances and be half safe. It is primarily the skill, satisfactory physical and mental condition of the driver, and his desire to be safe that will give us the protection we have a right to expect.

The following tips on good driving are recommended by drivers with thousands of miles of safe driving: Before starting on a trip, whether it is 1 mile or 3,000 miles, think through what you are about to do, how you are going to do it, and by what route you are going to travel. In short, get a "mental picture" of the trip and the safety factors involved and then start early enough to arrive on time.

Make sure that your automobile is in

They didn't die. This chart is a different kind of chart. Instead of showing the number of people killed in accidents through the years, it shows the number who were not killed—the number who were saved from accidental death by organized attack on this social problem. (National Safety Council.)

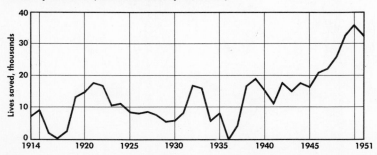

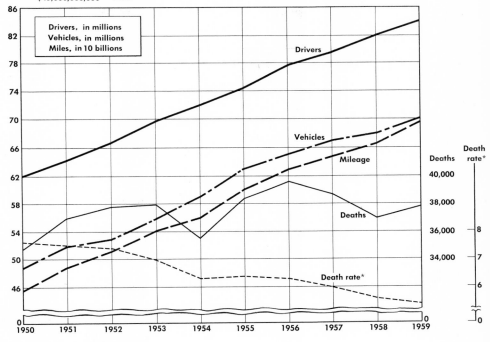

375,000 — Deaths
13,500,000 — Injuries (disabling beyond the day of accident)
580,000,000,000,000 — Motor-vehicle mileage
$45,000,000,000 — Costs

Drivers, in millions
Vehicles, in millions
Miles, in 10 billions

Drivers

Vehicles

Mileage

Deaths

Death rate*

*Deaths per 100,000,000 vehicle miles

A ten-year summary of motor vehicle accidents. During the 1950s, drivers, vehicles, and mileage continued their sharply rising trends, as follows: drivers +42 per cent, vehicles +57 per cent, mileage +68 per cent. Deaths moved irregularly higher, but the over-all increase of 19 per cent was only about one-third that for vehicles and mileage; in three of the years, deaths decreased. The mileage death rate decreased 28 per cent, reaching the lowest level on record in 1959. Accidents during the ten-year period are estimated at 100,000,000, in which about 13,500,000 persons suffered disabling injuries; probably twice this many suffered minor injuries. The economic loss from all these accidents was at least $45,000,000,000. (*Accident Facts*, National Safety Council, Chicago, 1960, p. 41.)

good mechanical condition to complete the journey safely. When you know the mechanical condition of your automobile, and stay within the limits of good performance, you increase your margin of safety.

Many drivers make it a rule to take their automobiles to a garage for periodic inspections and have needed repairs made at once. Doing it yourself can be satisfying, but unless you are a mechanic and have the proper tools, it will pay to

have the job done by a trained person.

Know the recommended inflation for your tires and keep them properly inflated. It is a good plan to have all the tires checked each time you go into a filling station. Underinflation can cause sidewall wear and tear, eventually lowering your margin of safety [19].

Safety engineers strongly urge all owners of automobiles to install seat belts in their cars. The California State Department of Public Health estimates that

1,500 traffic deaths in that state could be prevented annually if automobiles were equipped with seat belts. Since 1952, the Automotive Crash Injury Research Project, conducted at Cornell University, has been studying injuries and fatalities involving passenger automobiles. These studies have produced significant facts regarding speed of the vehicles involved in the accidents, nature of the impact, ejection of the passengers, and internal structure of the automobile. In relation to seat belts, the studies point out that, when similar accidents were compared, the frequency of injury of all degrees was 2½ times greater among passengers without seat belts than among those with seat belts. This means that there was a reduction of 60 per cent in risk of injury among the wearers of seat belts. When injuries sustained by ejected persons not wearing seat belts were compared with injuries sustained by nonejected persons wearing seat belts in similar types of accidents, the death rate was 8 times greater in those who were ejected. This means an 87 per cent reduction in mortality among the wearers of seat belts. To all drivers of automobiles the question is no longer, *Why* wear seat belts? *Why not* wear them and take advantage of the greater margin of safety [14]?

Avoid, if possible, the "gang," or "bunch," driving seen so frequently on expressways, freeways, or throughways. Always allow enough distance between you and the car ahead for a quick stop. Safe drivers allow a car length between them and the car ahead for every 10 miles of speed they are traveling. At 60 miles an hour there should be at least 6 car lengths between cars. In fog, rain, or snow, on slippery highways, or at night it is wise to increase this margin of safety. Exercise extra caution when approaching or passing a truck. They are large and may deceive you regarding the speed at which they are traveling [19].

When driving, take a relaxed position with both hands on the wheel, keep awake, keep alert, and obey the traffic laws and you are quite likely to enjoy the trip and arrive safely.

Fire prevention

Over 6,000 persons die each year by fire, and of this number 300 are in the college age group [1]. A regrettable factor is that most of these deaths result from careless use of fire, and carelessness is a preventable cause. Fatality and accidents by fire could become unimportant items in causes of death if users of matches and tobacco and others would faithfully practice the following:

Avoid smoking in bed, or when sleepy, or while lying down.

Put out every live cigarette or cigar butt before discarding it.

Always break a match in half before throwing it away.

Keep intoxicated smokers under constant surveillance.

Keep matches in covered containers, inaccessible to children and rodents.

Avoid carrying loose matches in pockets of clothing.

Safeguard young children against fire at all times.

Pouring kerosene or gasoline on an open fire; standing too close to an open fireplace or gas heater; or looking for the source of a gas leakage or determining the amount of gasoline in the tank with a lighted match may result in serious, even fatal, burns.

The number of accidents and deaths among college students because of fire is statistically insignificant. Most fatal fires and serious burns involve young children. This fact is a challenge to adults to accept the responsibility of providing a safe environment for children and to educate them in the wise use of fire.

CHECK YOUR RESIDENCE BUILDING FOR FIRE SAFETY

CONSTRUCTION

1. Is building of fire-resistant material?

2. Are vertical openings (i.e. stairways and dumb-waiter shafts) enclosed?

3. Are there several stairways leading from each floor?

4. Are stairways well lighted?

5. Are they marked by exit lights?

MAINTENANCE

6. Are outside doors equipped with panic bar hardware?

7. Are proper size fuses used (not exceeding a 15-ampere capacity)?

8. Are periodic inspections made of all electrical appliances?

9. Are oily rags and flammable liquids stored in tight metal containers?

10. Are fire doors checked regularly to be sure they are kept free of obstructions?

11. Are doors to stair enclosures kept closed at all times?

HAZARDOUS ACTIVITIES AND SITUATIONS

12. Are provisions made for safe smoking?

13. Is ironing restricted to utility rooms?

14. Are irons equipped with pilot warning lights?

15. Is spotting of garments done only in utility rooms?

16. Are only non-flammable cleaning fluids used?

17. Does one double wall receptacle serve no more than two electrical appliances?

18. Are extension cords listed by Underwriters' Laboratories?

19. Are extension cords six feet or less, in length?

20. Are provisions made for safe disposal of trash?

FIRE PROTECTION EQUIPMENT

21. How good is your alarm system?

    A. Is alarm system automatic?

    B. Does the alarm system warn the fire department and building occupants simultaneously?

    C. If the alarm is electric, is there a substitute device for sounding an alarm to building occupants?

    D. Is the alarm system used only for drills or fire?

22. Is your fire-fighting equipment adequate?

    A. Is the building equipped with automatic sprinklers which begin operating when a certain temperature is reached?

    B. Is the building equipped with an adequate number of operable fire extinguisher, located in accessible place?

    C. Do building occupants know how to operate the extinguishers?

    D. Are hoses in good condition and nozzles free of obstructions?

BUILDING EVACUATION PROCEDURE

23. Are unannounced exit drills held at regular intervals?

24. Are blocked exit drills held?

25. Are speed and efficiency of evacuation of the building evaluated and discussed after the drill?

Source: From "Check list," Fire Safety for College Residence Buildings, National Education Association, Washington, 1952.

First aid

Rendering first aid to all who are sick and injured is a timely expression of compassion. When there is an accident and someone receives an injury, those first on the scene, whether stranger or friend, stop to render aid. Sometimes the assistance is good, and sometimes it is unwise. For many years organizations such as the American Red Cross have been instructing people in the proper methods of first aid. A complete and comprehensive understanding of first aid to the sick and injured can be obtained by studying the *American Red Cross First Aid Textbook* or by enrolling in the first-aid classes taught by the American Red Cross.

When an individual is trained in skills of first aid and educated to the concept of accident prevention, he tends to become safety-minded. He acts with poise and confidence in an emergency and demonstrates his willingness to cooperate in the area of living safely.

The following general directions are given to enable one to approach the first-aid problem confidently and intelligently [2]:

Keep the injured person lying down in a comfortable position, his head level with his body, until you know whether the injury is serious.

Immediate first aid must be given for severe hemorrhage, stoppage of breathing, and poisoning. Be sure you examine the victim to locate all his injuries. Give other first aid as needed.

Keep the injured person warm.

Send someone to call a physician or an ambulance.

Keep calm and do not be hurried into moving the injured person unless it is absolutely necessary.

Never give water or other liquid to an unconscious person.

A person skilled in giving immediate and temporary assistance to the sick or injured until the services of a physician are obtained can help meet the following selected emergency conditions.

SHOCK

Shock means that the body is not functioning properly because of improper blood circulation. Shock accompanies all injuries, mild or severe. General weakness together with pale, cool, moist skin are the obvious symptoms of shock. Severe shock is dangerous, and unless it is properly treated, the patient may die.

Keep the victim lying down.

Cover him lightly; if he is on the ground, place a blanket under him.

Do not neglect to give first aid to the injury that caused the shock.

Summon medical help.

WOUNDS

The four most common forms of wounds are *abrasions*, in which the skin has been scraped or rubbed off; *lacerations*, caused by tearing of the flesh; *incisions*, made by a sharp instrument; and *punctures*, made by a sharp-pointed object.

For wounds with light bleeding, first aid includes washing your hands with clean water and soap before giving aid and then washing the wound repeatedly with clear tap water and clean soap, using a sterile pad if possible. Place a dry sterile dressing over the wound and bandage. It is important to let the patient know that this is only a first-aid dressing and that he should see his physician.

Severe *hemorrhage* must be stopped quickly. This can be acomplished by direct pressure over the wound or by pressure applied to blood vessels nearest the wound. If the bleeding cannot be controlled by this method, it may be necessary to use a tourniquet. *This is a last resort procedure and should be used only in extreme emergency.* The tourniquet is a bandage that can be tightened about a limb. A necktie, cloth, or any soft material about 2 inches wide may be used. The band should be placed above the wound and twisted sufficiently to stop the bleeding. A tourniquet patient should be placed under medical care as soon as possible. Wounds that need special care include the following:

In *internal bleeding* the symptoms are similar to shock. Keep the patient lying down. If he has difficulty in breathing, raise his head and chest. Do not give him any form of stimulant. Obtain medical aid at once.

Puncture wounds should be cleaned, a dressing applied, and the victim taken to a physician.

Animal bites should be cleaned and dressed and a physician should be summoned at once. If it is possible, confine the animal and make a report to the police or the public health department.

Do not pinch or attempt to open an *infected wound*. If possible, raise the infected area, apply wet, warm dressings, and seek medical aid.

Bites from *poisonous snakes* usually cause pain, swelling, and discoloration. However, the bite of the coral snake produces only slight pain and there is little swelling; nevertheless, it can be a fatal bite. If the venom from the snake is absorbed by the body, it will produce a fast pulse, difficulty in breathing, weakness, visual disturbance, dizziness, and regurgitation. The victim is in immediate need of medical care. First aid, recommended by the American Red Cross, for a person bitten by a poisonous snake includes the following: [1]

1. Have the victim stop muscular activity at once.
2. Tie a constricting band firmly above the bite if it is on an extremity. This band should be tight enough to prevent the return flow of blood in the surface ves-

sels, but not enough to shut off the surface vessels. If properly adjusted, there will be some oozing from the wound.
3. Sterilize a knife blade with a match flame and make incisions. Try with one of them to get into the venom deposit point, remembering that the snake strikes downward and the fangs retract. Crosscuts, about one-fourth inch long, may be made at each fang mark and over the suspected deposit point. Make shallow cuts through the skin in the crossways direction; longitudinal cuts may be deeper. Muscles and nerves run in a longitudinal direction and a deep crosscut may sever them. Beware of cutting muscles and nerves of the fingers, hands, or wrist for they lie immediately below the skin and their injury may cause much disability.
4. Apply suction, using the mouth or suction cup. The venom is not a stomach poison, but it is advisable to rinse the fluid from the mouth. Some poison might be absorbed along an infected gum margin, but the effects would be mild and local. Continue suction for an hour or more.
5. Get medical care. If transportation is necessary, keep the victim lying down, with the injured part somewhat lower than the rest of the body. During relief-from-suction periods, apply ice or cold water, if possible, to the part involved. This gives some relief from pain and may slow the absorption of poison into the system.

POISONING

First aid for gas poisoning includes removing the victim from the danger area, sending for a rescue squad, and notifying the police. If the victim is not breathing or is having difficulty breathing, give artificial respiration.

Speed as well as skill is essential in administering first aid to a person who has taken poison by mouth. If a universal antidote is available, give it at once (it can be purchased from a drugstore). If this antidote is not at hand, administer the following antidote: 1 part strong tea, 1 part milk of magnesia, and 2 parts crumbled burned toast. It is obvious that this is for a conscious person only. If the victim is unconscious and it is known that he has taken poison, send for medi-

[1] *American Red Cross First Aid Textbook*, rev. ed., Doubleday and Company, Inc., New York, 1957, p. 150.

cal aid and keep him warm. Do not force him to drink.

ASPHYXIATION

Stoppage of breath resulting from asphyxiation is an emergency that demands fast, skillful action. Artificial respiration must be started as soon as the victim has been placed in a safe environment. Medical aid is essential for this emergency.

ARTIFICIAL RESPIRATION

Because the victim of an accident may be within seconds of death and artificial respiration may save him, appropriate action should begin immediately. The three most effective methods of artificial respiration are the back pressure–arm lift method, which is illustrated on page 433; the mouth-to-mouth method which is described on page 441; and the chest pressure–arm lift method, which is used when the patient has to lie on his back. In fact, this method, together with an external heart massage technique, may well be the preferred method of artificial respiration in the future. In all cases requiring artificial respiration, send for a rescue squad and medical help.

The American Red Cross has in the past taught two methods. It now presents a new technique for administering artificial respiration. It is called the mouth-to-

The oral technique (mouth-to-mouth or mouth-to-nose). This can be used on an individual of any age and requires no equipment. (American National Red Cross.)

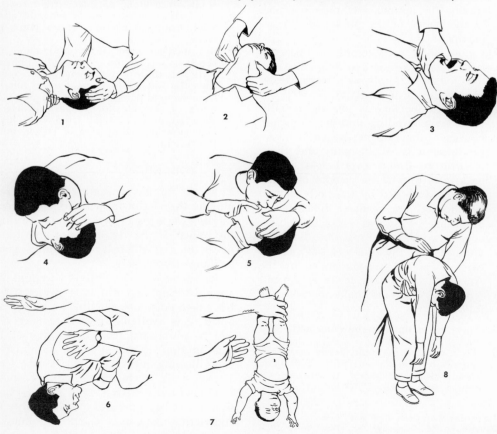

mouth technique. The steps recommended in executing this form of artificial respiration are as follows: [2]

Artificial respiration should be started immediately that the rescuer determines, or has reason to believe, that breathing has stopped.

If there is foreign matter in the patient's mouth, quickly wipe it out with your fingers. Then, with one hand, lift the nape of his neck; with the other hand, tilt his head sharply backward so that his chin points directly upward (see Figure 1). Or grasp his lower jaw at the angles and lift upward (see Figure 2). *CAUTION. Do not press your fingers into the soft tissue of his throat.*

If the patient's mouth is open, insert your thumb between his teeth; hold the rim of his lower jaw with your fingers and lift upward (see Figure 3).

These actions should open an airway by moving the base of the patient's tongue away from the back of his throat. With one of your hands, close the patient's nostrils (see Figure 4). Open your mouth as wide as possible and place it tightly over the patient's mouth (as in Figure 4) so that there is a seal as leakproof as possible.

Then breathe into the patient. After the first blowing effort, remove your mouth, and listen for the return rush of air. If the patient's teeth are clenched, use the nasal route by placing your mouth over his nose and blowing into it (see Figure 5).

For an adult patient, blow vigorously at the rate of about 12 times a minute. If the patient is a child, blow gently about 20 times a minute.

If you are not immediately able to get air into the patient's lungs, recheck the position of his head and jaws. If that is correct, something may be lodged in his throat. To remove it, promptly turn an adult on his side and slap him sharply between his shoulder blades (see Figure 6). Quickly reposition him and at once resume breathing into him again at 12 times a minute.

If the patient is a child, a rescuer of *less* than full size and strength should turn the child also on his side and *pat* him vigorously between his shoulder blades (see Figure 6), reposition him, and promptly start breathing into him gently at about 20 times a minute.

An adult rescuer may suspend a small child very briefly by the ankles (see Figure 7); he may invert a somewhat larger child over one arm (see Figure 8), patting him sharply two or three times between his shoulder blades.

Breathe into the patient until the lower part of his chest starts to rise. Continue breathing until he can breathe regularly on his own. Then stop, but watch the patient carefully and be ready to resume artificial respiration, if necessary.

If vomiting occurs, turn the patient on his side without delay and wipe out his mouth. Then reposition him quickly and at once resume breathing efforts.

After the patient revives, he should be kept as quiet as possible and treated otherwise for shock. If he starts to shiver, cover him according to his needs.

A number of disturbances may follow the stopping of breathing and, therefore, a doctor should always care for the patient during his recovery.

Accident insurance and liability

Liability is based on negligence, and negligence is the absence of prudent action. An individual who successfully appraises dangers inherent in an anticipated act and who uses precautionary measures to avoid a possible accident is acting prudently. The circumstances of an accident determine whether or not one has been negligent.

There are at least three rules determining liability in some states: [3]

A person who negligently or willfully commits an act which proximately causes injury to an innocent party is liable to the latter.

In the event a person injured by the negligence of another is likewise guilty of negligence contributing to his injury, such injured person cannot recover.

[2] *American Red Cross First Aid Textbook*, rev. ed., Doubleday and Company, Inc., New York, 1957, pp. 122-125. By permission, The American National Red Cross, Washington.

[3] Suggested by the general counsel of the Automobile Club of Southern California, 1953.

In the event there is no negligence on the part of any person for the injury of a particular person, the latter has no right of recovery.

Although the aim of safety education is to prevent or reduce accidents, it is wise to be protected against possible liability action resulting from accidents. This can be done by carrying liability insurance.

From the point of view of the college student who drives an automobile, carrying automobile liability insurance is a necessity. Such a policy provides insurance, subject to policy agreement, conditions, and exclusions, against claims arising from accidents resulting from ownership, maintenance, or use of the insured automobile.

If one multiplies the actual cost of protection by his life expectancy, the total will in all probability not be as large as the amount of an average judgment against him. The fee for an attorney to represent one in a damage suit is likely to exceed the amount of the premium for several years. In short, a judgment rendered against a defendant, plus attorney's fees, could prove an economic disaster both to him and to his family. Few student drivers of automobiles can afford to take this risk. It may be of interest to the college group to know that automobile insurance rates are much higher for those under twenty-five than for older persons. This is due in part to the high accident rate incurred by the fifteen- to twenty-four-year-old age group. The record shows that this group has the highest number of collisions between motor vehicles, collision with railroad trains, collisions with fixed objects, and noncollision accidents, such as overturning and running off the highway.

Realizing the importance of carrying liability and accident insurance, many states are making it compulsory for all drivers of automobiles to have this protection.

Summary

To live safely in the Space Age, we must be better informed about the hazards that surround us and be prepared to meet emergencies inherent in a nuclear attack as well. Radiation is a formidable health hazard. Alpha, beta, and gamma radiation can be extremely dangerous, even fatal. However, adequate safety precautions such as fallout shelters ensure reasonable protection against these harmful rays.

A team of scientists working with the United Nations relieve some of our concerns about daily exposure to radiation by the statement that the average worldwide exposure of radioactive material received by a person during a year is $\frac{1}{10}$ roentgen from natural sources, $\frac{3}{10}$ roentgen from medical and dental radiation, and less than $\frac{2}{100}$ roentgen from fallout. Judging from these figures, it would appear that at present our chances of receiving an overexposure of radiation are slight.

In case of a nuclear attack, fallout shelters offer the best means of protection from radiation. The Office of Civil and Defense Mobilization provides a variety of plans to the public for the construction and use of these shelters.

The civil defense program is largely a voluntary project. Its effectiveness depends upon citizen participation. You can have an active part in the program by serving in any one of the following areas: warden, fire, police, health, welfare, engineering, rescue, transportation, staff, or communications.

The practice of safety requires a willingness on your part to cooperate in protecting others as well as yourself, active participation in making the environment in which you live free from hazards, and exercising your creative talents in doing something constructive about safety in your home and your community.

Safety in sports and games is enhanced by sound coaching, skillful performance, participation within the limits of your skill and endurance, maintaining a sound body, and avoiding hazardous playing conditions.

Safety on the highway is primarily a matter of sound legislation, of effective highway engineering, of well-constructed automobiles, and of skillful drivers who know and obey the laws, who are sound physically, mentally, and emotionally,

and who desire to be safe at all times.

The introduction of seat belts in automobiles as a safety measure has been highly effective in reducing injuries and death due to collisions.

First aid to the sick and injured includes such measures as keeping the patient lying down in a comfortable position, giving immediate aid in case of severe hemorrhage, stoppage of breath, and poisoning, keeping the patient warm, and sending for a physician.

Accident and liability insurance is a wise and timely investment.

Suggested readings

1. *Accident Facts,* The National Safety Council, 425 N. Michigan Ave., Chicago 11, Ill.; published yearly.
2. *American Red Cross First Aid Textbook,* rev. ed., Doubleday and Company, Inc., New York, 1957.
3. American Red Cross: *Lifesaving and Water Safety,* Doubleday and Company, Inc., New York, 1956.
4. Barcella, Ernest L.: "Is Reckless Driving a Disease?" *Today's Health,* 38:28, December, 1960.
5. Cannell, Roger S.: *Live,* Stanford Research Institute, Menlo Park, Calif., 1960.
6. Florio, A. E., and G. T. Stafford: *Safety Education,* 2d ed., McGraw-Hill Book Company, Inc., New York, 1962.
7. Gagen, J. Wilfred: "Seat Belts," *Today's Health,* 38:26–29, July, 1960.
8. Halsey, Maxwell, *Skillful Driving,* Doubleday and Company, Inc., New York, 1960.
9. *Home Protection Exercises,* Office of Civil and Defense Mobilization, Washington, 1959.
10. "Is 'Fallout' a False Scare?" (Interview with Lauriston S. Taylor), *U.S. News and World Report,* 51:72–79, Nov. 27, 1961.
11. Kinsman, Simon: "Radiation Simplified," *California's Health,* Jan. 15, 1961.
12. Leonard, Alvin R., Alberta W. Parker, and Barry Miller: "Introduction to Seat Belts," *Public Health Reports,* 75:313–316, April, 1960.
13. "Medical and Dental X Rays," *Consumer Reports,* 26:493–501, September, 1961.
14. Miller, Barry, and others: "Operation Seat Belt," *California's Health,* 17:1–4, July 1, 1959.
15. Office of Civil and Defense Mobilization, *Fallout Protection,* H6, Washington, December, 1961.
16. "Strontium-90," *Consumer Reports,* 25:289–293, June, 1960.
17. *The Family Fallout Shelter,* Office of Civil and Defense Mobilization, Washington, 1959.
18. Ubell, Earl: "Will Radiation Harm Your Child?" *Parents' Magazine,* 25:35, July, 1960.
19. Ward, Roger: "It's Meant to Be Fun," *Sports Illustrated,* 14:37–41, Jan. 30, 1961.
20. Young, Warren R.: "Group Shelters Are a Start—The Facts Require Much More," *Life,* 52: 38–43, Jan. 12, 1962.

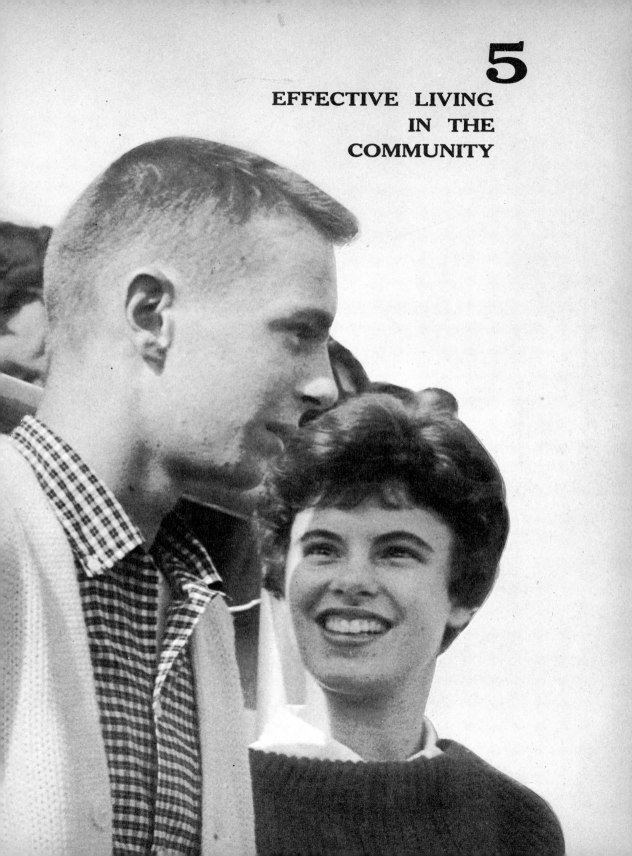

FIFTEEN

Participating in the community health program

No doubt you have a deep affection and sincere loyalty for your "home town" regardless of its size or fame. When one is away from home, especially at the other end of the country, it is a great thrill to meet someone from the home town; immediately a strong bond is established. A similar loyalty exists for one's home state.

Next to individual loyalties, such as those for parents, sweethearts, wives, and husbands, are those pertaining to groups. This is true also of larger groups making up a community, a state, and a nation. For example, during World War II several thousand men volunteered to work on battle-damaged ships in the Navy

Yard at Pearl Harbor, Honolulu. Though they lived together in large housing areas in comfortable quarters and were furnished an extraordinary recreation program in terms of a variety of activities and fine equipment, they were nevertheless not happy. After a few months one recreation leader thought of organizing them into groups according to some natural common bond. Hence state clubs were formed, representing almost every state in the Union, from Maine to Texas and from Florida to Washington. It was not long before the men were happier on the job, enjoyed more thoroughly their leisure time, were engaged in civic enterprises in a new land, and were showing eagerness to make their housing area a better place in which to live.

National loyalties are even stronger. Citizens of the United States are positive that no land compares with theirs, symbolized by the Statue of Liberty. Canadians argue that their part of North America is superior to any other land. Across the sea the British Isles are home to the British; and it is difficult, if not impossible, to dispute the French when they extol the wonders of their native land. These individual and group loyalties are the result of the personal experiences of the individual interacting in his own environment. They represent the individual's interest in his community, both small and large.

What is a community?

Most people today live in a community, if the word "community" is used in its broadest sense to mean a group of people living in a given area under the same unit of government. The community may be a neighborhood, a rural district, a small town, a city, the state, and even the country. More specifically, a community is a group of people living together in a particular area who have organized to meet common interests and problems.

Regardless of the size of the area, the word "community" implies the idea of shared purposes among its people. In a democracy, a person living in a community has certain civic responsibilities as well as responsibilities to himself personally. This idea is in keeping with the present-day health philosophy that health is both an individual and a group responsibility.

There is widespread interest today in community health. This interest, stimulated by World War II, has resulted in a number of organized groups. Each such group promotes one part or another of the total community health program. Most communities have a program already in existence. For these communities the pertinent questions are these:

How effective is the program?

Is it serving the needs of the people?

Are the total resources of the community utilized? If not, why not?

Is there adequate coordination of functions?

How can the present program be improved?

A number of communities, particularly in rural areas, are getting along without much of an organized program. The questions for these communities, then, are these:

How can a community health program be developed?

With what groups can cooperation be achieved in order to obtain services and activities to promote and protect the health of all the people?

In our changing society new communities are springing up almost overnight. Such communities must "start from scratch" in developing a health program. Whatever the situation in a given community, it is necessary to examine critically whatever constitutes a community health program in order to understand the individual's civic responsibilities.

The community health program in the Space Age, whether at the Federal, state, or local level, must be geared to cope with the present changing conditions of society. These conditions are similar to those expressed in Chapter 1 in the description of the college scene.

We must give consideration then to the facts that in our society:

The population is increasing rapidly (estimated to expand as much as one-third in the next 20 years).

The shift of the population continues to the suburbs, increasing many community health problems as a result.

The population is becoming, and will continue to be, a population heavily weighted by older persons.

Our people are continuing to strive for an even higher standard of living for a larger portion of the population.

Raw materials are being consumed faster than ever, and as a result, many natural resources are being depleted.

Technological advances are creating more leisure time.

Our people are in the midst of a period of changing values, characterized by highly materialistic patterns of life.

New problems of outer space, together with the cold war, have brought forth great insecurities.

The increased pace of modern living has brought along with it greater stress on individuals and families.

A portion of the population, due to the above-mentioned conditions, is indifferent toward health.

Modern community health programs must face these social conditions if they are to prove successful. All groups in the community can be mobilized to build better community health programs with better leadership from more highly trained health workers and improved cooperative action among community groups and agencies, including interested community leaders (opinion makers) and average citizens. Such a program is envisaged as one that requires more personal participation of individuals. In the remainder of the chapter, the following questions are considered:

What makes a good community?

What is community organization for health?

What are the principles of a community health program?

What are the components of a community health program?

How do these components function?

What are the functions of state and national health agencies?

How do state and national health agencies relate to local communities?

How can the student participate in activities for improving community health?

What are the health-career opportunities for the college student?

What makes a good community?

Sanders[1] believes that four factors go to make up a good community. First, there is a relatively stable economic base with respect to occupational opportunity, diversity of industry, and amount of taxable property to provide essential governmental services, including health services.

[1] Irwin T. Sanders, *Making Good Communities Better*, University of Kentucky Press, Lexington, Ky., 1950, p. 7.

Second, there is strong community loyalty. Community loyalty is demonstrated by an interest in civic affairs. It is high where there is understanding by members of the community of the projects undertaken and where there is democratic organization. Third, there is a constructive approach to problem solving. Since communities are composed of people, all communities have problems.

A good community finds a democratic way of attacking its problems, that is, by means of community organization. Fourth, there are leaders who see the community as a whole. Such leaders are able to do sound planning and engage in community activities for the welfare of the total group, as well as representing their own professions, institutions, or businesses. Thus they produce more agreement than disagreement. According to Sanders,[2]

> A whole community is also a well community in which sore spots are increasingly being healed and in which a unity of purpose pervades the members. . . . There is a happy medium between a wailing Jeremiah and an unrealistic Pollyanna, between the doleful "this place has gone to the dogs" and the boosterlike "best little town in Michigan."

Community organization for health

Community organization is essential in every neighborhood and community, regardless of size or kind. In a community the individual alone is powerless to make significant changes for effective group living. However, as a member of a planning group or organization, his influence, with group support, can result in tangible improvements for better living. It must be remembered, too, that health is only one value or one problem confronting society. Through community organization, health is given due recognition along with other existing social values.

Community organization provides a medium by which leaders can view the total community and enables them to work with unity of purpose. Health is not to be considered by itself in isolation; rather it is an integral factor in the total life of the community.

THE MEANING OF COMMUNITY ORGANIZATION

Community organization attempts to unite the individual members and groups of an area into one group with a common purpose. It stems from the people themselves and enables individuals and groups to meet their common needs. It involves action and implies that those people who participate in the action are changed. Community organization is an educational process that favorably influences behavior.

Community organization for health is a process of welding together individual members of the community and the health agencies of an area into one group for the purpose of determining health needs and finding ways and means to meet those needs and improve the total health of the community [20]. The uniting of individuals and groups for the building of a much-needed hospital in a local community is an example of action through community organization.

Another example of community organization for health is the mobilization of numerous forces to prevent paralytic poliomyelitis throughout a community. As indicated in Chapter 11, pages 341–342, the effective Salk and Sabin vaccines are contributing greatly to solving the medical problem of this disease. The major problem remaining is education of the public to overcome its apathy. This can best be accomplished by means of community organization, following the adage: "Your health and mine are the result of community planning and work."

San Diego, first in the nation to inoculate first- and second-grade pupils in 1955, also became the first city in California to launch a local community-wide program for vaccinating adults. This city's program began in February, 1957. The San Diego Medical Society opened public clinics for vaccination. The physi-

[2] *Ibid.,* p. 13.

cians volunteered their time to man the clinics. They also made it possible for persons to be vaccinated by their own physician in his office if this procedure was preferred.

Back of the clinic program was a total community effort to motivate and educate citizens to turn out for their vaccinations. This educational part of the program was launched as a result of active community committees with wide representation from geographical and organizational parts of the city. Community, civic, and service organizations; the medical profession; churches; labor; industry and commerce—all worked cooperatively with public health personnel to reach the mutual objective of protecting the citizens of this city against paralytic poliomyelitis. This is truly a community organization endeavor.

What is needed is many more such examples of community effort taking place in communities all over the country until poliomyelitis is stamped out completely.

The community health program

A number of parts make up a total community health program. All these parts together, coordinated and integrated, compose a complete, functional program. This program is designed to promote healthful, effective living for all the people living in the community. A discussion of the components of the program is basic to understanding the individual's role.

THE BASIC PURPOSE OF THE COMMUNITY HEALTH PROGRAM

The purpose of a community health program grows out of the beliefs or point of view of the people. The major purpose of the community health program is similar in most states and is often expressed in the laws of the states and of local communities. The 1869 statute establishing the Massachusetts State Board of Health formulated this mandate as "to take cognizance of the interests of health and life among the citizens." Anderson,[3] in his presidential address to the American Public Health Association at its eightieth annual meeting in Cleveland, Ohio, October, 1952, eloquently presented this objective of public health as the concept that charted the evolution of public health. He pointed out that, at the present time, it also defines its scope of activities. Furthermore, it directs the formation of a community health program, one that "preserves the health and the life of the people" and "keeps people well, not simply keeps them alive." [4] Implied in this objective is the social concept that "society has a responsibility to provide those necessities and protections which individuals cannot provide for themselves." [5]

Anderson [6] developed this point of view still further in the following significant statement:

Public health is an organized community program designed to prolong efficient human life. It has no artificial limitations that would restrict its activities to certain types of problems. It must deal with and endeavor to combat those forces that tend to impair or to shorten efficient human life and must meet each problem according to its particular needs. The essence of democracy is the concept of rule by the people, who have a right to protect themselves against all forces that lead to illness or to death.

Pauline N. Brimhall [7] presents a

[3] Gaylord W. Anderson, "Public Health—A Mandate from the People," *American Journal of Public Health*, 42:1368, November, 1952.

[4] *Ibid.*, p. 1368.
[5] *Ibid.*
[6] *Ibid.*, p. 1373.
[7] Pauline N. Brimhall, in Macoupin County Health Improvement Association, *What's the Health Situation in Macoupin County, Illinois?* The Association, Carlinville, Ill., 1960, p. 97.

modern point of view in her statement of community health education. She writes:

Our task today is to develop sound community health programs to meet the growing public health and social problems of our modern society.

Our opportunity lies in the mobilization of all community forces to move rapidly toward our most important health goals.

Our plans must be based on the study of community needs and problems, and effected by local community action.

Our progress depends upon professional leadership of the highest quality, and the understanding, support, and active participation of every citizen.

Our accomplishments—today and tomorrow—ultimately rest in dedicating ourselves to the tasks before us, and our faith in the fundamental principles of the democratic process.

The above statements adequately express the modern concepts of the community health program and point out the direction for its development.

PRINCIPLES OF A COMMUNITY HEALTH PROGRAM

The principles of community health guide the development of the program [6, 15, 19, 20]:

Access to the means for the attainment and preservation of health is a basic human right.

The most valuable resource in any community is the people who live there. It is necessary, therefore, to understand the people in the community—the kinds of people, their health status, their health behavior, the types of groups, and their characteristics.

Responsibility for health is a joint one, with the individual citizen and local, state, and Federal governments each having major contributions to make to its fuller realization.

Plans begin with people and center in their needs and interests. A study of people and identification of their needs and interests precede a program of action. Successful projects and programs are based on the problems of a specific community not those of a distant community or land.

Community action is needed to strengthen the total life of the community. Community organization for health leads to community action by mustering all the resources of the community, human and otherwise.

Some form of organization is needed to solve problems and to expedite the use of the scientific method. A health committee or council—some planning body that facilitates fact finding, problem solving, and coordination of functions—is needed to assist in developing a community health program.

Problems are best solved by using the scientific method. The procedure for solving community problems follows this method: identify the problem, define it, formulate a hypothesis, gather the facts, classify them, test the findings, draw conclusions, and make interpretations from the data.

People learn best when they participate in solving problems. This is the principle of learning by doing. It also includes the principle of involvement. A plan which one has had a hand in making is not quickly cast aside.

The American people desire and deserve comprehensive health service of the highest quality, and in our dynamic, expanding economy the means can be found to provide it.

The same high quality of health services should be available to all people equally.

A health program must take into account the progress and experiences of the past and the realities of the present and must be flexible enough to cope with future changes.

COMMUNITY HEALTH NEEDS

Community health needs include the desires of the people, plus the lacks and inadequacies or the problems pertaining to effective living. Communities, more and more, are determining their own

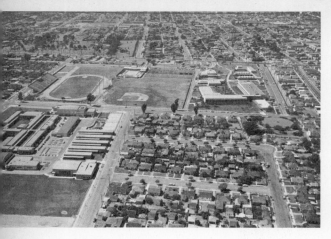

Those within a community—a group of people living in a given area under the same unit of government, whether a neighborhood, town, or larger unit—find that their personal health depends to a large extent on the health of the entire group.

Through community organization, they form a health council. Leaders representing many occupational and professional groups view the needs of the total community. Under the local government . . .

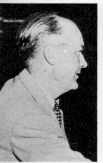 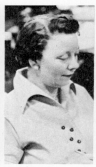 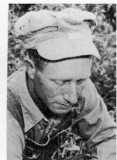 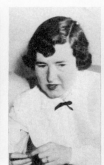 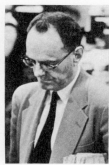 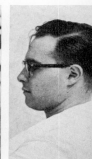

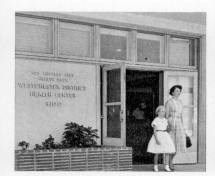

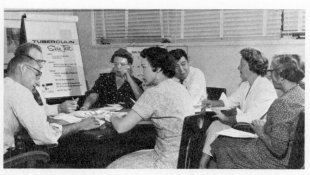

the health department is organized to protect and promote the health of all members of the community. Independent of the government . . .

voluntary health agencies are organized by individuals. These agencies concern themselves with community health education . . .

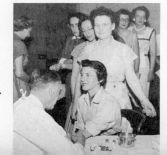

with service to patients and case finding . . .

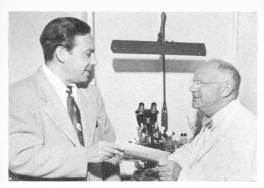

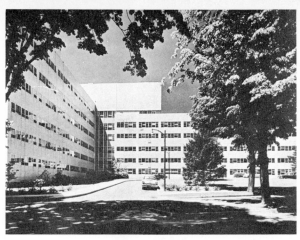

and with medical research projects for the prevention and control of disease. Vital as a health resource of the community . . .

is the community hospital, which provides care for the sick, advanced knowledge for doctors, and health education for citizens. Through these agencies our health is protected in a variety of ways . . .

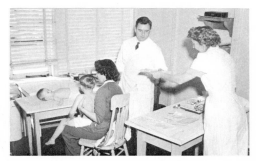

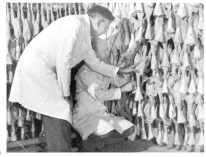

by well-baby conferences at child care clinics . . .

inspection of the food supply . . .

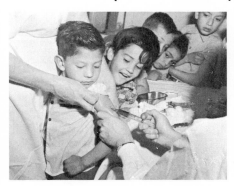

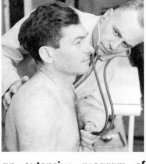

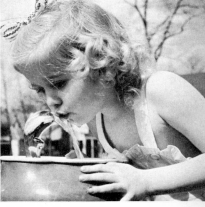

community-wide immunization against diseases . . .

an extensive program of medical checkups . . .

Within these highly organized health activities are the areas of service in which the individual may participate as a volunteer aide to trained personnel.

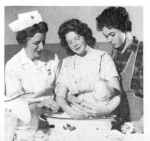

and protection and fluoridation of the water supply.

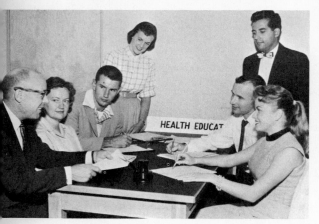

Students may contribute to community health through planning and conducting a health survey. After making a door-to-door canvass of the residents, recording their views on health problems and their knowledge of available health services . . .

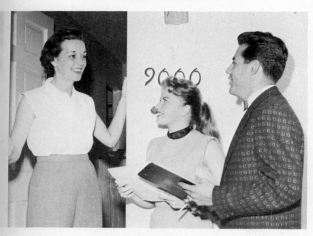

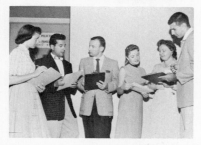

the students correlate their findings and present them to the community health educators. Determining health needs is fundamental to planning a community health program.

needs as a basis for planning constructive health programs. In addition, they are studying the health needs of the nation as a means of understanding their own problems. The evidence from studies on the health needs in the United States shows a common pattern of health needs. For example, the need for health personnel and improved programs of mental health and dental health are consistent problems throughout the country. Each community contributes to this common pattern. At the same time, the needs of the community in many ways are unique and call for individual study. For these reasons, it is important to determine the health needs of the community and to examine examples of local and national health needs.

The specific needs of the community may be determined through a professional survey or through a community self-survey. By the first method, one or more experts in public health evaluation are employed to make the study. The second approach is one in which the citizens themselves, with the leadership of health authorities, make the study. Either method is useful in determining community needs.

An example of the first method on the national level is the U.S. National Health Survey. In 1956, the President signed a bill authorizing a continuous survey of the health of the general population of the United States. This led to the development of the National Center for Health Statistics, of which the National Office of Vital Statistics is an important component along with the National Health Survey.[8] This center makes it possible to assess constantly the needs of the nation. The U.S. National Health Survey began with a program to produce statistics on disease,

[8] "The National Center for Health Statistics," Reprint, Part VIII of Final Report on Mission and Organization of the Public Health Service, U.S. Department of Health, Education, and Welfare, Washington, June, 1960.

injury, impairment, disability, and other aspects of the health of the nation as a whole. The Act of 1956 permitted health surveys to be made cooperatively with other agencies and state health departments. An example of this procedure on the state level is seen in the Hawaii Health Survey.[9] This was a cooperative study of health needs by the U.S. National Health Survey, the Hawaii State Department of Health, the Oahu Health Council, and other local health and welfare agencies, foundations, and industries. The survey found, for example, that the rate of dental visits in Hawaii was considerably higher than on the mainland United States; that asthma–hay fever was the most frequent type of chronic condition, followed by sinusitis, both with a higher rating than on the mainland; and that the incidence of persons injured who required medical attention was approximately 20 per cent higher on Oahu than on the mainland.

A second example of using an expert to conduct a health survey is noted in "Report of a Health Inventory," by Ira V. Hiscock. This is a report of the fourth comprehensive survey of the health situation in Hawaii. Previous studies were made in 1929, 1935, and 1950. Hawaii as a territory, and now as a state, appears to be a favorite area for health investigations. One reason is that the people of the islands are interested in evaluation and in making continued progress in community health. Another reason is that investigators find this a pleasant land in which to work. The 1960 Hiscock survey provides data on what is bad, what is good, and what is needed in Hawaii's program of prevention of preventable diseases [16].

Another example of having our needs pointed out by authorities is the identification of present-day health problems by Nelson A. Rockefeller. Speaking to the American Public Health Association, Governor Rockefeller said: [10]

From all these various contacts with your field of public health, I have formed certain definite impressions about the major health problems which we face at the dawn of the Space Age. . . . These problems are: first, the menace of chronic diseases, and especially the diseases of old age; second, the need for evaluating how our public health dollar is being spent; third, the blight of mental illness and the new major techniques and drugs which have started what may become a major breakthrough in our attack upon this threat to the careers and happiness of one out of every eight Americans; and finally, the emergence of new problems in environmental health, such as radiation exposure and pollution of our air and water resources. . . . I am convinced that dirty air and water need not be the price for expanding our cities and industries if we take effective control measures. And I am convinced of the necessity of providing physical protection for our populace against the hazards of nuclear warfare and of radioactive fallout from this nuclear warfare. . . . It is estimated that without . . . preparation 75 per cent of the casualties—up to 100 million Americans—could result from fallout alone. No area of our country is immune from this silent killer. Protection cannot be improvised after an attack begins.

The second method of evaluation enlists the citizens as members of the health team, which tends to make them supporters and boosters for public health. An example of the findings of this second type is illustrated in the West Los Angeles Health Committee Survey [11] to determine health needs. The needs of this community were studied jointly by citizens and health authorities, and the following problems were identified from the project:

Dental health—40–80 per cent of school children needed dental care. . . .
Health education—need for health education

[9] Public Health Services, U.S. National Health Survey, *Health Statistics: The Hawaii Health Survey*, U.S. Department of Health, Education, and Welfare, Washington, May, 1960.

[10] Nelson A. Rockefeller, "Present-day Health Problems," *American Journal of Public Health*, 50:9, January, 1960.
[11] West Los Angeles Health Committee, *Survey*, Los Angeles County Tuberculosis and Health Association, 1956.

about health facts, health agencies and their services, and for community organization. . . .

Mental health—need for more psychiatric clinic services and better preventive mental health services. . . .

Tuberculosis—need for more intensive education about tuberculosis, greater use of x-ray facilities, additional local facilities. . . .

School health—need for improved health education and health services in all schools. . . .

Problems of aging—need for readily available medical services. . . .

Hospital and clinic facilities—need for increase in both general and county hospital beds . . . part-pay clinics to meet dental, mental and chronic illness. . . .

Health center—urgent need for space, personnel, and more flexible program. . . .

Sanitation—need for increased education of volunteer food handlers in non-commercial gatherings and intensified educational programs within commercial food establishments. . . .

Maternal and child health—need for improved planning of all groups concerned to achieve sound program of education and services for mothers and children. . . .

Family life and sex education—need for improved parent education, improved teaching in schools, in churches, by physicians, health department workers and other groups. . . .

Communicable disease control—need for education regarding basic immunizations and maintenance through adult life. . . .

Housing and community redevelopment—need for blueprint for community redevelopment. . . .

Occupational health—need for an industrial health survey. . . .

Hood and Pence[12] report an example of a community self-survey in a Kansas rural county. The study revealed that the population was old (about twice the national average), that income was low, and that there was almost no medical care, few health services and facilities, no health department, no school health program, no dentist, and no hospital. After the study a young physician and dentist were attracted to the county, a

clinic building was built, and an immunization program was started, along with vision and hearing testing of school children. These and other results were attributed to mobilizing citizens for cooperative action and to their spirit.

From the authoritative study by the President's Commission on the Health Needs of the Nation, several selected findings are listed to illustrate the major health needs of the wider community—the health needs of the United States. For complete information refer to volumes of the Commission's report (see Suggested readings No. 6). Some specific needs are as follows:[13]

Health personnel—physicians, dentists, nurses, and others

Health facilities—general hospital facilities, health centers, beds for mental disease, chronic disease, tuberculosis, rehabilitation, and research facilities

Improving health and medical services for all people

Research

Immunization against communicable diseases

Rehabilitating the handicapped

Concerted attack on chronic disease

Prevention of mental illness

Dental health programs, including dental health education, dental care, scientific fluoridation of community water supplies

Improved environmental health—water, air, food, shelter

Prevention of accidents

Improved maternal and child health

Improved industrial health to extend medical-care plans for workers and their families, and to create more healthful working environments

The Study Group on the Mission and Organization of the Public Health Serv-

[12] Thomas R. Hood, and Virginia Pence, "Community Health Studies in Kansas," *American Journal of Public Health*, 50:1566, October, 1960.

[13] *Building America's Health*, A Report to the President by the President's Commission on the Health Needs of the Nation, vol. II, *America's Health Status, Needs and Resources*, Government Printing Office, Washington, 1952.

ice[14] succinctly identifies the next great areas of national health efforts.

The next great nationwide health efforts may be expected in two broad areas: the physical environment and comprehensive health care. During the present decade, 1960–1970, major national efforts, comparable with the great expansions of medical research and hospitals in the 1950's, will be required in each of these areas. . . .

Effective action for environmental health and comprehensive health care in the present decade requires:
1. For the purpose of environmental health that the private use of water, atmosphere, and land be limited in the public interest. Those who might create environmental hazards should be primarily responsible for averting or abating them.
2. That comprehensive health care, which comprises a continuum of preventive, curative, and restorative services, depends upon personnel with varied technical skills under both private and public auspices. . . .
3. Steady progress in the areas of environmental health and comprehensive health care will depend in large measure on a clearer definition of the respective roles of the principal private and public interests in these areas.

HEALTH PERSONNEL

The most important component of a community health program is the health personnel who make it function. Many programs look promising on paper but are ineffective because of poor personnel. A functional program, one in which health needs are being met successfully, has sufficient, competent personnel.

Health officers, physicians, dentists, nurses, research workers, health educators, classroom teachers, hospital administrators, executive secretaries of voluntary agencies, social workers, and other health workers possess the skills that provide health services, educational experiences, and research findings. Lay citizens join the health personnel in developing a community health educa-

tion program. Space does not permit a discussion of each type of health worker. A brief description of the contributions of five—health officer, physician, dentist, nurse, and health educator—serves as an illustration of the members of the health team.

Health officer. The health officer is a doctor of medicine (M.D.) with special preparation in public health. Usually he is, in addition, a master of public health (M.P.H.) or a doctor of public health (D.P.H.), though not all health officers hold such degrees. However, the trend throughout the country is to highly trained personnel well qualified in both the field of medicine and the applied field of public health. The health officer has a unique leadership function in the community health program. He is responsible for the development and maintenance of the health of the general population and for the prevention and control of communicable disease. He cooperates with all agencies and with the public to improve effective living in the community.

Private practitioners—physicians and dentists. The physicians and dentists are considered to be the authorities on health within a community. These men and women are graduates of accredited medical and dental schools. They are licensed to practice within the state in which they reside. They belong to local, state, and national professional societies. They are members of staffs of approved hospitals and clinics in the community. Every few years they enhance their skill and extend their knowledge through postgraduate studies. The cost for the service they render is usually scaled to the mutual advantage of both patient and practitioner. The doctor is the pivotal person in the health team. He is concerned with the total health program, as well as with medical care. The dentist, too, is concerned not only with meet-

[14] Public Health Service, *Final Report of the Study Group on Mission and Organization of the Public Health Service*, U.S. Department of Health, Education, and Welfare, 1960.

ing the dental health problem but with improving all aspects of healthful living.

In addition to providing medical and dental services, doctors and dentists contribute their time and effort by serving on planning committees and community councils. They take active leadership in formulating and developing programs of action. Through counseling and guidance of patients they educate for better health. Through research they aid in the solution of problems. Their professional associations, the American Medical Association and American Dental Association, provide health education material and individual and group guidance.

Nurse. The supply of nurses, who constitute the largest group of health workers, is limited. The need for additional nurses is even greater today than the need for doctors and dentists. The skilled nurse relieves the doctor, permitting him to perform duties for which only his training and experience qualify him. She carries out the doctor's orders, enabling the patient to regain his health. The bedside nurse is noted for providing physical care and mental comfort for her patients.

One type of nurse considered essential in the community health team is the public health nurse. This nurse provides nursing service and health education in the health department or school where she is employed, as well as in the home. By visiting the home she discovers individual and family health needs, gives demonstrations on maternal and child care to members of the family, and teaches classes for community groups. She works on a family-centered basis for individuals and groups, at home, at work, at school, and in public health centers [13, 15]. The nurse serves as a counselor in individualizing health education and as an interpreter of health needs and a source of information and medical care.

Health educator. The health educator in the community, as a staff member of a health department or voluntary agency, plays an important role in the community health program. He is an interpreter to the people and the members of the agencies of the services and activities of the community health program. He assumes leadership, both direct and indirect, in community organization. Primarily, he assists people in solving their own problems. He plans, stimulates, promotes, organizes, teaches, coordinates, guides, and evaluates activities and programs [32]. Often he is considered the right-hand man of the health officer or of the executive secretary of a voluntary health agency.

In well-organized state or local health departments there are frequently other professional members on the health team: the sanitarian, nutritionist, medical social worker, laboratory technician, public health dentist, preventive mental hygiene personnel, statistician, industrial hygiene engineer—all who promote and protect the health of the community. Information about their functions can be obtained from the suggested readings or through a visit to a health department.

HEALTH SERVICES AND ACTIVITIES

The actual community health program is planned carefully on the basis of health needs. This program consists of health services and educational and other activities as follows: [15]

PROMOTION OF HEALTH. Services and activities contributing to the attainment of health:
1. An adequate, safe food supply and distribution
2. Proper housing
3. A healthful working environment
4. Safety outside the home and workplace, as well as inside
5. Education for health
6. Recreation

[15] President's Commission on Health Needs, *op. cit.*, p. 12.

7. Security, including access to health services

PREVENTION OF DISEASE. Preventive services:
1. Immunization against communicable disease
2. Individual and family health guidance, such as maternity care and infant care
3. Aggressive, early detection of disease, with follow-up to ensure diagnosis and treatment

DIAGNOSIS AND TREATMENT. Personal health services for cure or alleviation of disease:
1. Diagnosis of disease before and after symptoms have appeared
2. Treatment in the home, office or clinic, and general hospital
3. Treatment in specialized institutions, e.g., mental hospitals, tuberculosis sanatoria, nursing and custodial homes, teaching and research centers

REHABILITATION. Services for the restoration of handicapped to total usefulness within their capabilities:
1. In the course of ordinary treatment
2. In special rehabilitation centers

The responsibility for developing such a comprehensive program rests with the local health department, the medical, dental, and allied professions, the hospitals, the schools, the voluntary agencies, and, of course, the public in general.

COMMUNITY HEALTH RESOURCES

Health resources are health agencies and facilities engaged in health endeavors, as follows:

The official agency: the health department. The local health department or center is a unit of the local government. It is commonly referred to as the official health agency in the community. In keeping with the basic mandate of public health, its purpose is to promote and protect the health of the total community.

The functions of a modern health department include activities relating to:
Vital statistics
Sanitation
Communicable disease control
Laboratory services
Maternal and child health
Health education
Control of chronic disease
Accident prevention
Hygiene of housing
Industrial health
School health services
Mental health
Medical rehabilitation
Medical-care administration.

The first six are minimum functions of any local health department, and all constitute present-day optimal services [1]. Examples of these services are discussed below.

Through vital statistics, the health officer keeps his hand on the pulse of the community. The bureal of vital statistics records and analyzes statistics on births, deaths, services, and facilities; many of the health needs of a community health program are found through keeping such data. Any deviation from the normal pattern in the community, such as an increase in deaths in a particular location or an increase in number of cases of one disease, is a significant sign. At once public health officials are alerted to prevent a serious disease epidemic. The charting of health problems on a daily basis through vital statistics enables the health department personnel and others to plan for an optimum community health program.

The listing of common community health needs shows that environmental sanitation is an important need in any community. This is community housekeeping. Well-trained sanitarians, important members of the health team, provide supervision and regulatory services. They promote the maintenance of clean public eating places, markets, hotels, apartment houses, homes, hospitals, rest homes, swimming pools, camps, public rest rooms, bars, and places of employment. They ensure safe milk and water supplies, prevent rat invasions, and control diseases spread by mosquitoes and flies. They enforce regulations and make recommendations for the sanitary disposal of wastes and control of pollution.

The health department administers a variety of personal health services. For example, communicable-disease control is initiated through immunization. Medical diagnosis for communicable disease is offered frequently. Any suspected case of communicable disease may be referred for diagnosis. Some health departments provide clinics for tuberculosis, venereal disease, scalp ringworm, and other infectious diseases. X-ray service is a valuable part of the case-finding program in tuberculosis control. Premarital blood tests illustrate a laboratory service provided by the health department.

Personal services also are provided in maternal and child health clinics and child health conferences. Public health nurses conduct adult classes for fathers and expectant mothers. Prenatal examinations and guidance are given for the protection of the mother and unborn child. At least one home visit is made by the public health nurse to all mothers registered in the prenatal conference. Additional visits are made if necessary. Among the helpful services the public health nurse renders are home demonstrations of infant bathing and preparation of a formula [13, 15].

A public health dentist provides preventive dental service for expectant mothers and young children. Also, a medical social worker provides services of guidance and counseling to those who need help with social problems arising out of medical-care needs.

Many health departments are providing partial or total support of centers for the detection of such chronic diseases as heart disease, cancer, and diabetes. The health department is interested, too, in programs for mental health and for the rehabilitation of persons afflicted with disease or victims of accidents. Such programs enable these people to live useful, productive lives again.

Educating the public for effective living is an important function of the local health department. Citizens need to be informed about the services rendered by their health department. They need to understand how they may prevent diseases and defects and how they may live more effectively. The work of the public health educator has been discussed previously.

According to the modern concept of public health, the health department has a community responsibility in the successful operation of its health facilities. It becomes a center for health personnel and citizens interested in the community health program. The practicing physician officially registers his license with the city or county health department. At the time of registration, he receives information about laws, ordinances, regulations, and policies. This procedure serves as a medium for future cooperation between the physician and the department. The two-way cooperative relationship between the private physician and the health department helps to build the health department into a functional health center. An auditorium, classroom, or both assist in bringing the citizen of the community into the health center. In large communities, several well-equipped health centers with administrative offices, clinic facilities, and auditorium space are essential in promoting and protecting community health.

The health department has a major responsibility in the coordination of the total community health program. The public health personnel must take an active part in coordinating the functions of all agencies and citizen activities to prevent overlapping and duplication of effort. One illustration of coordination is the health department's function in the civil-defense activities. It coordinates these activities, and volunteer personnel maintain a corps ready to serve in any natural disaster or enemy attack. A second example is cooperative planning with school authorities in developing a school health program.

Malcolm Merrill,[16] former President of the American Public Health Association, and California State Director of Public Health, defines the responsibility of the public health department according to the modern concept of public health as follows:

. . . The local health department should assume responsibility for defining, clarifying, and assessing the total health needs of the community. The local department of public health should be the catalyst, the organizer, the planner, the expediter, and the demonstrator. It must see to it that the health services in the community, whether they be preventive, diagnostic, therapeutic, rehabilitative or otherwise, are actually available to the people.

A full-time health department with full-time, adequately prepared personnel can provide a community with the above services and assume the responsibilities for health promotion and protection. Health departments must receive community support. A community of 50,000 people or several neighborhoods or communities banded together can receive at least minimum services for $1.50 per year per person. Additional protection can be obtained for a slightly higher per capita cost. It is estimated that some 40 million Americans live in communities or areas without full-time local public health services [9].

In 1945, a committee of the American Public Health Association [9] proposed a plan that would make available adequate health services throughout the country. The basis of this plan was to consolidate smaller city and county health departments into large enough units to maintain essential health-department functions and at the same time serve the needs of the people. The committee's plan was to effect the organiza-

tion of 1,197 units of local health administration that would cover the 3,070 counties and their contained cities throughout the country. Some consolidation has taken place, and new units have been developed. However, progress has been slower than expected. As a result, public health authorities are looking for new ways of providing needed services for the local level. Malcolm Merrill [26] reports efforts in California to provide counties with less than 40,000 population who are without services to obtain them by contracting them with the State Health Department. This has been worked out so the local area has needed health services and still maintains local responsibility and essential autonomy. This contractual plan has served to cut down the number of counties without any services. Also, it is hoped, since this seems to be successful, that it may spread to yet other counties now without services so that in the near future the whole state of California will have health services at the local level. This approach and other solutions should make possible the strengthening of local health services to needed areas.

The provision of adequate local health services remains a problem and poses a challenge to citizens for community action for good health for all.

Voluntary health agencies. A voluntary health agency is an organization operated by private persons without tax-supported funds for the purpose of improving health. Such agencies usually are concerned with alleviating one particular disease or defect. The voluntary health agencies stem from the American tradition of freedom and individual initiative and the desire of people to relieve suffering [7]. They represent the spirit of the American people, who believe in fostering better health through private means over and above their official health agencies. The number and

---

[16] Malcolm Merrill, "Community Health—Challenge and Opportunity," *American Journal of Public Health,* 51:364, March, 1961.

scope of activities of these agencies are peculiar to the United States.

Voluntary health agencies fall into the following three major classifications:

Agencies devoted to the alleviation of particular diseases, for example, the American Cancer Society, the National Tuberculosis Association, and the National Foundation

Agencies devoted to prevention and rehabilitation of bodily defects, such as the American Heart Association and the National Society for the Prevention of Blindness

Agencies concerned with health and welfare of special groups; for example, the American Red Cross, the National Safety Council, and the National Association for Mental Health

Sliepcevich and Beyrer[17] have compiled a comprehensive list of national voluntary health agencies as follows:

Alcoholics Anonymous, P.O. Box 459, Grand Central Annex, New York 17, N.Y.

Allergy Foundation of America, 801 Second Ave., New York 17, N.Y.

Allied Youth, Inc., 1709 M St., N.W., Washington 6, D.C.

American Cancer Society, 521 West 57th St., New York 17, N.Y.

American Diabetes Association, 1 East 45th St., New York 17, N.Y.

American Hearing Society, 919 Eighteenth St., N.W., Washington 6, D.C.

American Heart Association, 44 East 23d St., New York 10, N.Y.

American Institute of Family Relations, Inc., 5287 Sunset Blvd., Los Angeles 27, Calif.

American National Red Cross, Office of Publications, 17th and D Sts., N.W., Washington 6, D.C.

American Social Health Association, 1790 Broadway, New York 19, N.Y.

Arthritis and Rheumatism Foundation, 10 Columbus Circle, New York 19, N.Y.

Association for the Aid of Crippled Children, 345 East 46th St., New York 17, N.Y.

Association for Family Living, 32 W. Randolph, Suite 1818, Chicago 1, Ill.

Damon Runyon Memorial Fund for Cancer

Research, Inc., 730 Fifth Ave., New York 19, N.Y.

Family Service Association of America, 215 Fourth Ave., New York 3, N.Y.

The Federal Association for Epilepsy, Inc., 1729 F St., N.W., Washington 6, D.C.

Leonard Wood Memorial, American Leprosy Foundation, 1 Madison Ave., New York 10, N.Y.

Leukemia Society, Inc., 27 William St., New York 5, N.Y.

Maternity Center Association, 48 East 92d St., New York 28, N.Y.

Muscular Dystrophy Associations of America, 1790 Broadway, New York 19, N.Y.

The Myasthenia Gravis Foundation, Inc., 155 East 23d St., New York 10, N.Y.

National Association for Medical Research, 920 S. Michigan Ave., Chicago, Ill.

National Association for Mental Health, 10 Columbus Circle, New York 19, N.Y.

National Council on Family Relations, 5757 South Drexel Ave., Chicago 37, Ill.

National Cystic Fibrosis Research Foundation, 1616 Walnut St., Philadelphia 3, Pa.

National Epilepsy League, Inc., 208 North Wells St., Chicago 6, Ill.

National Foundation, 800 Second Ave., New York 17, N.Y.

National Foundation for Neuro-Muscular Diseases, 250 West 57th St., New York 19, N.Y.

National Hemophilia Foundation, 175 Fifth Ave., New York 10, N.Y.

National Kidney Disease Foundation, 143 East 35th St., New York 16, N.Y.

National Multiple Sclerosis Society, 257 Fourth Ave., New York 10, N.Y.

National Organization for Mentally Ill Children, Inc., 171 Madison Ave., New York, N.Y.

National Parkinson Foundation, Inc., 135 East 44th St., New York, N.Y.

National Safety Council, 425 Michigan Ave., Chicago 11, Ill.

National Society for Crippled Children and Adults, Inc., 2023 West Ogden Ave., Chicago 12, Ill.

National Society for the Prevention of Blindness, 16 East 40th St., New York, N.Y.

National Tuberculosis Association, 1790 Broadway, New York 19, N.Y.

Planned Parenthood Federation of America, 501 Madison Ave., New York 22, N.Y.

Public Affairs Committee, Inc., 22 East 38th St., New York 16, N.Y.

Sister Elizabeth Kenny Foundation, 2400 Foshay Tower, Minneapolis 2, Minn.

United Cerebral Palsy Association, Inc., 321 West 44th St., New York 36, N.Y.

[17] Courtesy of Elena Sliepcevich and Mary Beyrer, Professors of Health Education, The Ohio State University, 1961.

The telephone or city directory should be consulted for local or state offices of the voluntary health agencies.

The functions of voluntary health agencies. The functions of the voluntary health agencies include [13]:

PIONEERING. Discovering needs and new ways of meeting existing needs.

DEMONSTRATION. Assuming a public health function or subsidizing a project and demonstrating its worth to the citizens, the city council, or county supervisors until the official agency can take over the function.

EDUCATION. Educating for health is considered one of the functions, if not the most important function, of the voluntary health agencies.

SUPPLEMENTATION OF OFFICIAL AGENCIES. Providing funds and/or activities which the official agencies could not provide because of politics, budgetary limitations or legal action.

GUARDING OF CITIZEN INTEREST IN HEALTH. Supporting good official agency health programs and criticizing poor programs, in either case serving the public interest for community health.

PROMOTION OF HEALTH LEGISLATION. Supporting legislation for measures improving health conditions, working for the defeat of legislation detrimental to public health.

GROUP PLANNING AND COORDINATION. Participating in planning a total community health program, assisting in coordination of efforts to avoid duplication and overlapping.

DEVELOPMENT OF WELL-ROUNDED COMMUNITY HEALTH PROGRAMS. Subordinating a vested interest for the welfare of the total community health program.

In most cases the voluntary health agencies are meeting an important need. They make an extensive contribution to education, research, and service relating to the community health program. Since they are responsible only to their own boards of directors, their programs are flexible and they can adapt readily to changing needs. There is evidence to show that they are broadening their scope of activities. For example, the Tuberculosis Association in Los Angeles and in other communities is called Tuberculosis and Health Association of Los Angeles County, denoting functions besides the fight against tuberculosis. The personnel of the voluntary agencies are doing increasingly more work to promote and protect the health of the total community group rather than attempting to alleviate the one particular disease or defect for which their organization was founded. This is an important new trend. A further essential factor is the cooperative relationship between the official agency and the voluntary agency, in which both are working together for the health of all the people.

The community hospital. The community hospital plays an important role in the community health program. Especially is this true as the quantity and quality of medical care increase. People, today, naturally expect to go to the hospital if they are seriously ill, regardless of their economic status. The increase in prepayment health insurance has made it easier for many to pay hospital bills, which in itself has been a factor in increased patronage of hospitals.

The major objectives of hospital care for the patient are to render diagnosis and treatment and restore him again to a productive life. The hospital contributes to both individual and community health through restoration and rehabilitation of the sick or handicapped person. Many persons are served through the outpatient clinics of the modern hospital.

The hospital contributes to community health also by serving as a facility for the physician as well as for the patient. The modern hospital is a vital part of the physician's medical practice. Actually it is a facility that broadens his skill and medical practice. Not only does the hospital offer the physician equipment that otherwise he might not possess, but it gives him an affiliation with the hospital medical staff and physicians in a number of specialties. This professional association is essential if the physician is to keep up to date and in touch with modern developments in medical practice. Furthermore, the hospital provides a medium by which the physician continues his medical education. For example, he may engage in advanced study for a specialty by fulfilling a hospital residency.

In the past, hospitals were looked upon as "receptacles for the sick." Today the hospital is considered to have a responsibility to the total community health program in fostering and promoting public health and preventive medicine. For illustration, it is considered sound practice for a hospital to have a diagnostic clinic in which physicians employ health examinations as a means of keeping people well. George Bugbee, President, Health Information Foundation,[18] expresses this concept thus:

The hospital is acknowledged not only as the best and safest place for the care of many illnesses, but also as the most comfortable and convenient. In just 50 years it has changed its function from terminal care for the unfortunate individual without resources to a highly complex organization designed to bring to all the dramatic potentials and wonders of modern medical science. . . . The hospital at its best, then, in addition to being the center of medical knowledge, is an extension of home care, providing along with its skills, kindly and sensitive personal attention.

However, over and above that, the physician and the hospital staff are interested in the reasons for the patient's illness. They are concerned with ways and means of restoring him to health so that he can better meet his daily needs after leaving the hospital.

An important modern concept in hospital planning is regional planning and distribution of hospital care. Each area cannot meet all the requirements for hospital care. However, needs can be met by the regional method. The idea is to develop in each region facilities as nearly adequate as possible. The regional center contains the largest hospitals, most complete facilities, and most specialized medical personnel. General hospitals, community hospitals, and health centers send their specialized cases to the regional center. Each region has its share of general hospitals, tuberculosis hospitals, chronic-disease hospitals, and mental hospitals.

It is essential for good community health that cooperative planning and action take place with the health department, the hospital, the medical societies, the voluntary agencies, the schools, and citizens serving as active participants. One of the responsibilities the student or any other citizen has as a community member today is to work with community agencies to obtain adequate hospital facilities.

The schools. Some people have never thought of the school as a health agency in the community; yet without a doubt it is one of the important agencies responsible for the health of the people. The opportunity to educate for health is greatest in the schools. The schools constitute the largest organized group. Pupils spend years in school, at a stage in life when behavior is more easily changed than at any other period. Educators recognize health as a major educational objective. To achieve this objective, a health education program is planned and maintained for all school-age children and youth.

Harnett and Shaw[19] have identified eight broad areas of pupil needs:
A home and family

[18] George Bugbee, "Hospitals and the Challenge of Our Times," *Progress in Health Services*, Health Information Foundation, 5:5, October, 1956.

[19] Arthur L. Harnett and John H. Shaw, *Effective School Health Education*, Appleton-Century-Crofts, Inc., New York, 1959, p. 54.

Opportunity for optimal physical growth and development

Emotional adjustment

Protection against disease and illness

Development of physical skills

Reasonable protection from hazards and injury

Sex adjustments

Dental health

The school health program planned, organized, and conducted to meet these needs includes administrative divisions of healthful school living—the environmental factors, health service to appraise and improve health status, physical education and recreation for healthful activities, and health instruction—planned, direct instruction consisting of meaningful activities to develop scientific knowledge, wholesome attitudes and practices for healthful living.

Health education furnished in the schools establishes the foundation for health behavior that provides improved living for the individual and strengthens the total community. A successful school health program utilizes the health resources of the community to broaden its scope and increase its activities and personnel. Not only does the school contribute to the health of the community, but the community health program strengthens the school endeavors for health.

The community health council. The reason for a community health council is apparent if one understands human nature. It is only natural that each community agency, like each individual, has its own special interest. This is true even though its over-all stated objective is to promote and protect the health of the community. The health council, however, fosters unselfish action by all its members. It serves as a structure to promote democratic action in planning, fact finding, problem solving, and coordination of functions. It makes possible a total program for the health of all the people. The council is a form of community organization that welds together agencies and individuals into one group with united purposes.

The council is a representative group composed of members from the various agencies and organizations interested in community health. It brings together the health department, the voluntary agencies, the county medical and dental societies, the service clubs, women's clubs, parent-teacher associations, and other groups. It reaches the people directly by admitting citizens without group affiliation as members at large. It is a clearing-house for the solution of community health problems.

The council may be called by a variety of names, such as "community health council," "health council," "health division of the community welfare council" [23]; but its functions are the same:[20]

To coordinate as far as possible the thinking and planning of all organizations concerned with the public health.

To work to prevent overlapping and duplication.

To study health needs of the community through appraisals, inventories, and other fact-finding activities.

To develop a community health program related to those needs.

To stimulate public interest in health problems and their solution.

To express itself with strength and authority on matters of health legislation to further sound measures, defeat objectionable ones.

To render to members common services in the field of statistics and research and community health education.

There is no reason for a council unless it has some specific task to perform. The health committee of the West Los Angeles Coordinating Council illustrates the actual work of a council. A new health officer was assigned to this district. The

[20] S. S. Lifson, "The Role of the Community Health Council," *Public Health News*, July, 1948.

citizens and the health officer wanted to assess the health needs of West Los Angeles and to acquaint the people in the district with the health department's services, personnel, and needs. The West Los Angeles Coordinating Council assisted in setting up a health committee to serve as a community health council. The group included representatives from the health department, Tuberculosis and Health Association of Los Angeles County, Nora Sterry Elementary School, Emerson Junior High School, University Senior High School, University of California, Westwood Business Men's Association (including medical and dental representatives), parent-teacher association, Bureau of Public Assistance, and other community organizations, and citizens serving as members at large.

The group voted to make a survey of the area to determine the health needs of West Los Angeles, as previously cited. This survey was a first step in planning a community health program. Evaluation forms were developed. Available data on health needs were obtained from sources such as the vital statistics office of the health department. Additional information was obtained and evaluation instruments refined in a pilot study of 100 families. This study was carried on by the health committee with the assistance of health education students from the University of California. After the pilot study, plans were made for a large-scale survey of 1,000 families as a sampling of the total community population. Volunteers were enlisted and trained to conduct house-to-house interviews. The survey was made. Considerable publicity in the local papers was given the health department and the survey itself. People were made aware of health department activities. Volunteer workers became part of the community health team. The findings of the study have been analyzed and interpreted. It is known that a basis of planning for future

action has been laid. The development of a total community health program has been initiated, and directions for the next steps have been charted.

EVALUATION OF SERVICES AND ACTIVITIES

Evaluation is the process of appraising the progress made toward the achievement of established purposes, objectives, or goals. Self-appraisal of community health program objectives is as important as the self-appraisals the individual makes to determine progress in improving his own health. People want to know how effective the community health program is and how well it is meeting the established health needs. Continuous evaluation of health services and activities makes it possible to utilize existing resources and brings to light the strengths and weaknesses, which stimulates improvement of the program. Evidence of progress is the best means of demonstrating to the public the values of a community health program.

Community appraisals are accomplished by persons making the evaluations, using inventories, schedules, survey forms, or questionnaires. One of the best community health appraisal forms is the American Public Health Association's *Evaluation Schedule,* with its accompanying *Guide to a Community Health Study, 1960,* and *What's the Score?* published by the association. Health-department personnel and lay citizens together can use these materials in determining the effectiveness of their program. The California State Department of Public Health has developed a community self-study form, *Inventory of Local Health Problems, Resources, and Facilities* (Berkeley 4, California). By using this form health personnel and lay citizens can determine how much health protection they have, what their problems are, and what available resources they have. Some communities prefer to develop their own evaluation instruments. For example, the citizens of Clinton County, Ohio, decided to make a survey. They developed their own questionnaire to discover their problems. The results of their survey are available in their publication of the Health Council of Clinton County's *Clinton County Health Survey* (Wilmington, Ohio). An excellent self-study guide for communities is the Hogg Foundation's *So You Want to Make a Community Study* (Austin, Texas, University of Texas Press). An excellent report of a community self-study is *What's the Health Situation in Macoupin County, Illinois,* Macoupin County Health Improvement Association (Carlinville, Illinois).

Evaluation is one of the best means to interest citizens in the program, to awaken their concern about health affairs, and to stimulate action for an improved program. The Missouri State Health Council has published a one-page appraisal form called *Yardstick for Measuring Health Standards of Our County.* This survey form is designed to interest local people in learning more about the general health situation in their own communities or county. An evaluation form designed to appraise the effectiveness of the local health department is *How to Gauge Your Public Health Department,* published by the Health Publications Institute, Inc., Raleigh, North Carolina.

The type of community health program which has been described above pertains to any local area, whether it is a district, a village, a town, a city, or a county.

State and national health agencies

The broad definition of a community presented earlier in the chapter included the state and the nation as community areas. These large geographical and governmental units constitute the wider community. The over-all public health structure includes the programs organized at the Federal, state, and local levels in order to promote and protect the health of the individual citizen and the group. Mountin and Flook compare the public health organization to a government building. The ground floor is composed of the local official and voluntary agencies and the private practitioners; the second floor includes the state official and voluntary agencies and professional societies; and the third contains national official and voluntary agencies and professional societies [27].

Since each level of organization is working to improve the health of the individual and the group, an effective working interrelationship must exist, from the national level, through the state, to the local community, and vice versa.

STATE HEALTH ORGANIZATION

The state department of public health plays the chief role in public health at the state level, for its responsibility is greater than that of other agencies. Its functions differ considerably from those of the local health department. The local health department is concerned with rendering direct services. The state health department, on the other hand, is furnishing advisory and consultant services. Some of its functions are regulatory, depending upon the specific state legal requirements. The state health department plays a vital role in administering financial assistance to the local health departments from both state and Federal sources. It fosters research projects which the local health department is unable to carry out. It serves as the middleman between the Federal agencies and the local unit. It lends needed personnel to local units for special assignments. Also, it assumes active leadership in coordinating the various other agencies, voluntary and professional, functioning at the state level. Assisting the local health departments is its major responsibility [13].

The voluntary agencies and professional organizations operating at the state level, together with the other state governmental agencies, play a contributory and supplemental part in the state health program.

Many states have even more agencies interested and active in health work than has the local community. These range from the department of agriculture, with its extension services, to the state cancer society or the state medical society. As a result, a number of states have organized state health councils to plan, co-

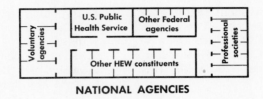

NATIONAL AGENCIES

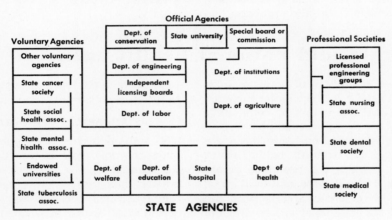

STATE AGENCIES

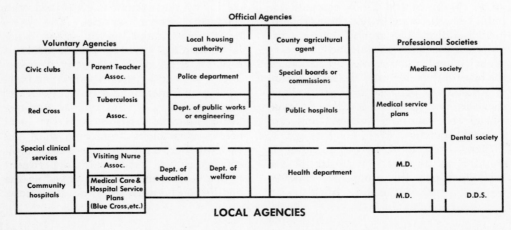

LOCAL AGENCIES

ordinate, and assist in developing health programs.

NATIONAL HEALTH ORGANIZATION

Official, voluntary, and professional health agencies and organizations are active also at the national level. The organization of these agencies is more complicated than at the lower levels, although recent organizational plans enacted by Congress are attempts to improve the organizational structure.

THE DEPARTMENT OF HEALTH, EDUCATION, AND WELFARE

On April 11, 1953, a Department of Health, Education, and Welfare became a legally established executive department. This gave new administrative status to Federal health activities under the direction of a Secretary with cabinet rank. Mrs. Oveta Culp Hobby became the first Secretary of Health, Education, and Welfare, since she was former President Eisenhower's appointee as Federal Security Administrator. President Kennedy appointed Abraham A. Ribicoff as Secretary of Health, Education, and Welfare in 1961. Personnel in the new Department also include an undersecretary; two assistant secretaries; a Special Assistant Secretary on Health and Medical Affairs, who is a medical leader charged with the responsibility of reviewing health and medical progress; the General Counsel; and an Administrative Assistant Secretary.

The operating agencies and bureaus of the Department under the direction of the Secretary are as follows:

PUBLIC HEALTH SERVICE
  Office of the Surgeon General
  National Center for Health Statistics
  Bureau of Medical Services
    Freedmen's Hospital
  Bureau of State Services
  National Institutes of Health
  National Library of Medicine
OFFICE OF EDUCATION
SOCIAL SECURITY ADMINISTRATION
  Office of the Commissioner
  Bureau of Federal Credit Unions
  Bureau of Old-age and Survivors' Insurance
  Bureau of Public Assistance
  Children's Bureau
OFFICE OF VOCATIONAL REHABILITATION
FOOD AND DRUG ADMINISTRATION
SAINT ELIZABETH'S HOSPITAL

The Federal government contributes

The complete health structure on three levels: Federal, state, and local. The local level shows co-ordinated activities among the official agency, the voluntary agencies, and private practitioners. (U.S. Public Health Service.)

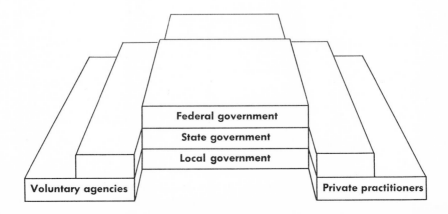

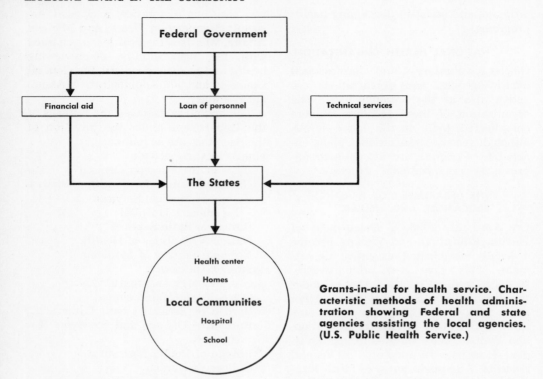

Grants-in-aid for health service. Characteristic methods of health administration showing Federal and state agencies assisting the local agencies. (U.S. Public Health Service.)

to individual and group health in a variety of ways through its several agencies.

The U.S. Public Health Service. The chief public health agency in the Federal government is the Public Health Service. This agency is under the direction of the Surgeon General, who is charged with protecting and improving the health of the people of the United States. Luther L. Terry, M.D., assumed the office of Surgeon General in 1961, replacing Leroy E. Burney, M.D., who had served in this capacity since 1956.

The major functions of the Public Health Service are to: (1) conduct and support research and training in the medical and related sciences, and in public health methods and administration; (2) to provide medical and hospital services to persons authorized to receive care from the Service, to aid in the development of the Nation's hospital and related facilities, and to prevent the introduction of communicable diseases into the United States and its possessions; and (3) to assist the States and other governments in the application of new knowledge for the prevention and control of disease, the maintenance of a healthful environment, and the development of community health services.[21]

The activities of the Public Health Service are organized into the Office of the Surgeon General, the Bureau of Medical Services, the Bureau of State Services, and the National Institutes of Health; there is also the National Library of Medicine.

The Public Health Service has staff in eight of the nine regional offices of the Department of Health, Education, and Welfare. These staffs maintain contact with state and local officials and with the field officers of other Federal agencies, as well as with other organiza-

[21] Office of the Federal Register, General Services Administration, *United States Government Organization Manual 1961–62*, Government Printing Office, Washington, June 1, 1961, p. 347.

tions concerned with health. A medical director heads each regional office. The medical director represents the Surgeon General in carrying out the policies of the Public Health Service and in interpreting these policies to officials and the public within the region. The regional staffs work with state authorities in planning, programing, and budgeting to carry out Federal-state cooperative action.

The total staff of the Public Health Service at the end of the 1960 fiscal year consisted of 26,430 full-time employees. Some 1,666 were members of the regular Commissioned Corps of the Service, and 2,034 were members of the Reserve Corps on active duty. There were 116 members of the Commissioned Reserve on temporary training duty, and the remaining number comprised 22,614 full-time Civil Service personnel. Members of the Commissioned Corps are comparable to commissioned officers of the armed services [44].

The Office of the Surgeon General is a bureau comprised largely of staff services to assist the other three operating bureaus. It is concerned primarily with studying national health needs, providing leadership, coordinating and managing affairs, and analyzing and publishing health statistics.

The Bureau of Medical Services is the medical arm of the Public Health Service. It is chiefly concerned with developing, promoting, and directing medical-care and health service programs. Medical care is provided for those authorized to receive care, such as coastguardmen. A program of therapeutic and preventive care is established for Indians and Alaska natives. Medical examinations are administered to immigrants and prospective immigrants to prevent mentally and physically defective aliens from entering the country.

The Bureau of State Services is the main operating bureau for Federal-state and interstate health programs. It gives direction to the health programs designed to aid states and local communities. The Bureau is responsible for grants-in-aid to states for their programs, and provides consultation and technical assistance. Recently, consultants on school and college health have been added to the staff of this Bureau. The Bureau aids in training personnel and implementing effective health procedures and practices.

The National Institutes of Health constitute the research arm of the Public Health Service. The purpose of the institutes is to extend basic knowledge of health problems, and discover ways in which these problems may be solved or coped with. The seven institutes are located in Bethesda, Maryland. They are as follows:

National Cancer Institute

National Heart Institute

National Institute of Allergy and Infectious Diseases

National Institute of Arthritis and Metabolic Diseases

National Institute of Dental Research

National Institute of Mental Health

National Institute of Neurological Diseases and Blindness

A clinical center provides patient facilities and makes possible clinical investigations for the seven institutes. More than half of the medical research throughout the nation was government-supported during the fiscal year 1960 [44].

The institutes conduct both laboratory and clinical research to discover better methods for preventing, diagnosing, and treating serious diseases. Emphasis is placed today on research relating to the chronic diseases, since these have become increasingly significant; the infectious diseases are declining in comparison with the past. Much of the research is conducted outside the institutes in non-Federal institutions such as medical schools, universities, hospitals, and other research agencies. In 1960, 80 per cent of the total appropriation for research went out in grants-in-aid to non-Federal institutions. In addition, several hundred fellowships are awarded each year as financial support from the institutes to young scientists to ensure future research manpower [44].

The National Library of Medicine houses the greatest collection of medical literature in the world. The collection is in excess of a million items. The library was developed to aid in the advancement of medical and related health sciences. Books, periodicals, and other materials are organized, catalogued, indexed, and made available to help disseminate and exchange scientific information in medicine and public health. Bibliographical guides to medical literature are published, and reference and research assistance is provided by the library staff [29].

In 1959, Surgeon General Leroy E. Burney, M.D., appointed a Study Group on the Mission and Organization of the Public Health Service. The Study Group, composed of 12 eminent career specialists in the Public Health Service, reviewed the present functions and responsibilities of the service; identified the national trends in health problems, manpower, and facilities; and studied the methods available for dealing with health problems as well as investigations made by other groups on health problems and needs. The final report of this group of experts recommends a new structure for the Public Health Service to enable it to meet the health problems of the future. A chart of the recommended organizational plan is presented below.

The recommended organization is developed around six major operating areas and the Office of the Surgeon General. These areas, with the proposed organization of services, are as follows:

Environmental health—Bureau of Environmental Health

Health services and resources for the nation—Bureau of Community Health

Medical services for legally designated beneficiaries—Bureau of Medical Services

New organization of the Public Health Service recommended by the Study Group on Mission and Organization of the Public Health Service in its *Final Report*. (U.S. Department of Health, Education, and Welfare, 1960.)

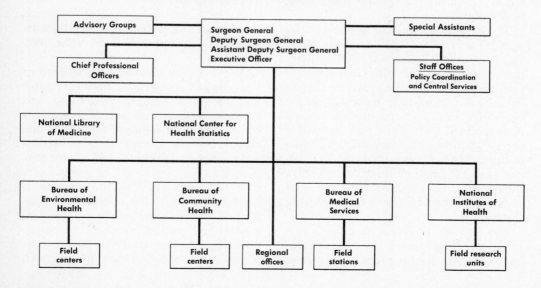

NEW ORGANIZATION OF THE PUBLIC HEALTH SERVICE, 1960

Medical and biological research—National Institutes of Health

National health statistics—National Center for Health Statistics

National Library of Medicine—National Library of Medicine

Careful consideration and administrative efforts are under way to implement the recommendations of the Study Group as changes can be made in the Public Health Service structure. It appears that keen foresight, wise planning, and creative effort has and will continue to be expended by the service administration and staff to protect the health of citizens of the United States.

The U.S. Office of Education. Although the Office of Education is not a direct Federal health agency, it makes an important contribution to public health. Emphasis is placed on school health education by promoting and improving school health programs throughout the country. Specialists in health education offer consultant services in school health to state officials, local school districts, and school health education personnel. The collection, interpretation, and reporting of data on school health programs throughout the country are functions of the Office. Studies on the types of health instruction and the extent, type, and organization of health services in the public schools are sample reports developed by specialists in health education. The Office also administers programs under the National Defense Education Act of 1958 including, for example, Federal participation in college and university student loan funds, fellowships for graduate study, and research in modern communication media for educational purposes.

The Children's Bureau. This Bureau is one of several under the Social Security Administration, now a part of the Department of Health, Education, and Welfare. The purpose of the Children's Bureau is to provide opportunities for the full development of all children by promoting their health and social welfare. It administers vital health services for mothers and children through grants-in-aid. The Children's Bureau investigates and reports upon all matters relating to the health and welfare of children. A bimonthly publication, *Children,* is produced for the professions serving children. The Bureau also works to extend and improve service for children in rural areas and in areas of special need. The Bureau staff is particularly interested in improved programs for crippled children. The Children's Bureau, the Office of Education, and the Public Health Service work cooperatively in promoting school health programs.

The Food and Drug Administration is discussed briefly in Chapter 10.

Sliepcevich and Beyrer[22] have prepared an extensive list of professional associations at the national level concerned with health.

American Academy of Pediatrics, 636 Church St., Evanston, Ill.

American Association of Marriage Counselors, 104 East 40th St., New York 16, N.Y.

American College Health Association, c/o Gannett Clinic, Cornell University, Ithaca, N.Y.

American Council on Education, 1785 Massachusetts Ave., N.W., Washington 6, D.C.

American Dental Association, 222 East Superior St., Chicago 11, Ill.

American Dental Hygienists' Association, 100 East Ohio St., Chicago 11, Ill.

American Dietetic Association, 620 North Michigan Ave., Chicago 11, Ill.

American Genetic Association, 1507 M St., N.W., Washington 5, D.C.

American Home Economics Association, 1600 Twentieth St., N.W., Washington 9, D.C.

American Hospital Association, 840 North Lake Shore Drive, Chicago 11, Ill.

American Medical Association, 535 North Dearborn St., Chicago 10, Ill.

[22] Courtesy of Elena Sliepcevich and Mary Beyrer, Professors of Health Education, The Ohio State University, 1961.

American Nurses' Association, Inc., 10 Columbus Circle, New York 19, N.Y.

American Optometric Association, Council on Optometric Education, 4030 Chouteau Ave., St. Louis 10, Mo.

American Osteopathic Association, 212 East Ohio St., Chicago 11, Ill.

American Pharmaceutical Association, 2215 Constitution Ave., N.W., Washington 7, D.C.

American Physical Therapy Association, 1790 Broadway, New York 19, N.Y.

American Podiatry Association, Council on Education, 3301 Sixteenth Street, N.W., Washington 10, D.C.

American Public Health Association, 1790 Broadway, New York 19, N.Y.

American School Food Service Association, P.O. Box 8811, Denver 10, Colo.

American School Health Association, 515 East Main St., Kent, Ohio

American Speech and Hearing Association, 1001 Connecticut Ave., Washington 6, D.C.

Association for Childhood Education International, 1200 Fifteenth St., N.W., Washington 5, D.C.

Child Study Association of America, Inc., 132 East 74th St., New York 21, N.Y.

National Association of Chiropodists, Council on Education, 3301 Sixteenth St., N.W., Washington 10, D.C.

National Biology Teachers Association, c/o Paul V. Webster, Bryan City Schools, Bryan, Ohio

National Council on Alcoholism, New York Academy of Medicine, 2 East 103d St., New York 29, N.Y.

National Council on Family Relations, 1219 University Ave., S.E., Minneapolis 14, Minn.

National Education Association, 1201 Sixteenth St., N.W., Washington 6, D.C.
  American Association for Health, Physical Education and Recreation
  American Association of School Administrators
  American Driver and Safety Education Association
  Council for Exceptional Children
  Department of Classroom Teachers
  Department of Elementary School Principals
  Department of Rural Education
  National Association of Secondary School Principals
  National Commission on Safety Education
  National School Boards Association
  National Science Teachers Association

National League for Nursing, Inc., 10 Columbus Circle, New York 19, N.Y.

Society of Public Health Educators, 1790 Broadway, New York 19, N.Y.

NATIONAL VOLUNTARY HEALTH AGENCIES

The voluntary health agencies at the national level fulfill many of the functions that the state and local agencies do; education, service, and research are their primary concerns. However, some differences exist, since they serve at the national level and, in many instances, are the parent organizations. For example, the national agencies make every effort to strengthen the state and local agencies.

They offer them advisory and consultant services. They promote inservice education of workers at the three levels. They prepare educational materials that are generally distributed to the public by the state and local organizations. Some of the functions of the national agencies are directed toward advancing themselves and "selling" their own organizations. They conduct and sponsor more research than is possible at the lower levels. They work to improve national legislation for health. In general, they strive for better health of the public. See the list of National Voluntary Agencies, page 462.

THE NATIONAL HEALTH COUNCIL

The coordinating body at the national level is the National Health Council. It provides the structure that welds together all efforts for health at the national level.

The Council has three principal functions —helping member agencies work more effectively together in the common interest; helping identify, call attention to, and promote solutions of national health problems; and promote better state and local health services, whether governmental or voluntary.[23]

A continuing work of the Council is the promotion of state and local health councils, similar in action to the national council. It is through these councils that

[23] Philip E. Ryan, "The National Health Council," *National Tuberculosis Association Bulletin*, 47:11–12, January, 1961.

groups can work together, identify needs for services, and carry out effective planning.

The functions of the National Health Council include promoting health education, serving as a clearinghouse for public health information, developing new state and local health councils and assisting old ones, promoting full-time local health departments, offering a consultant service on community health and other services to individuals and groups, and coordinating the activities of the national health agencies.

One of the most significant recent contributions is the sponsorship of the Health Career Horizons Project and the distribution of health-career publications. This project is discussed below under Health Careers. The National Health Council is the medium for community organization at the national level.

Health careers

Each community health need study has indicated the lack of qualified health personnel as a major concern throughout the United States. This situation is due to the American people demanding higher health standards plus a large increase in total population with only a slight proportionate increase in the working age group. Howard Rusk,[24] commenting on the demand for high-level medical, dental, and other health services, states: "Today the demand in these fields outstrips the supply. . . . The outlook for many years to come, in spite of expanding educational facilities, is for continuing shortages."

This existing need may be viewed as a lifetime opportunity for many college students, both men and women, who as yet have not decided upon a career. Some 156 opportunities in health occupations are awaiting individuals interested in careers of service to protect and promote the health of families, communities, and the nation.

Forward steps have been taken to meet the need and to recruit young people into the health fields. The Health Career Horizons Project has been sponsored by the National Health Council and developed with the cooperation of professional associations and national agencies in the fields of health, educa-

tion, and counseling. Two important publications giving detailed information on health careers developed from the project: *Health Careers Guidebook* and *Partners for Health*. These are distributed by the National Health Council and supported by Equitable Life Assurance Society. The *Health Careers Guidebook* is a complete reference on health occupations for the college student and the vocational counselor or health educator. *Partners for Health*, a briefer story than the *Guidebook*, is valuable for class discussions and use by community agencies and groups. A new publication, *Health Careers Exchange*, is a newsletter to keep people up-to-date on recruitment information.

HEALTH-CAREER OPPORTUNITIES

A number of health vocations have been described throughout this chapter as well as in Chapter 10. In addition, a classification of the 156 health-career opportunities described in the *Health Careers Guidebook* is presented below, organized into thirty categories:[25]

22 IN ADMINISTRATION OF HEALTH SERVICES. Admitting officers, assistants for public health administration, business and maintenance workers, comptrollers, hospital administrators, per-

[24] Health Career Horizons Project, *Factsheet*, National Health Council, New York, September, 1955, p. 7.

[25] *Partners for Health*, National Health Council, New York, 1955, p. 40. This grouping of health occupations is based on the Briefings in the *Health Careers Guidebook*, National Health Council.

HEALTH CAREERS CALENDAR

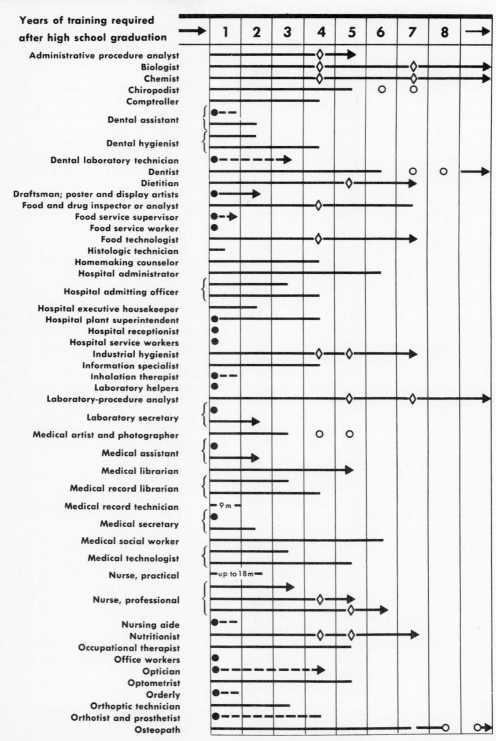

Years of training required after high school graduation

	1	2	3	4	5	6	7	8	

- Administrative procedure analyst
- Biologist
- Chemist
- Chiropodist
- Comptroller
- Dental assistant
- Dental hygienist
- Dental laboratory technician
- Dentist
- Dietitian
- Draftsman; poster and display artists
- Food and drug inspector or analyst
- Food service supervisor
- Food service worker
- Food technologist
- Histologic technician
- Homemaking counselor
- Hospital administrator
- Hospital admitting officer
- Hospital executive housekeeper
- Hospital plant superintendent
- Hospital receptionist
- Hospital service workers
- Industrial hygienist
- Information specialist
- Inhalation therapist
- Laboratory helpers
- Laboratory-procedure analyst
- Laboratory secretary
- Medical artist and photographer
- Medical assistant
- Medical librarian
- Medical record librarian
- Medical record technician
- Medical secretary
- Medical social worker
- Medical technologist
- Nurse, practical
- Nurse, professional
- Nursing aide
- Nutritionist
- Occupational therapist
- Office workers
- Optician
- Optometrist
- Orderly
- Orthoptic technician
- Orthotist and prosthetist
- Osteopath

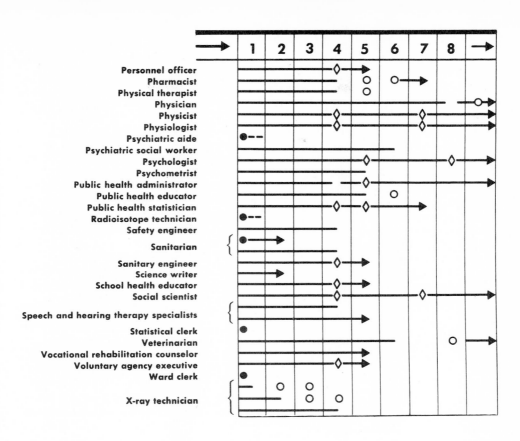

	1	2	3	4	5	6	7	8	

Personnel officer
Pharmacist
Physical therapist
Physician
Physicist
Physiologist
Psychiatric aide
Psychiatric social worker
Psychologist
Psychometrist
Public health administrator
Public health educator
Public health statistician
Radioisotope technician
Safety engineer

Sanitarian

Sanitary engineer
Science writer
School health educator
Social scientist

Speech and hearing therapy specialists

Statistical clerk
Veterinarian
Vocational rehabilitation counselor
Voluntary agency executive
Ward clerk

X-ray technician

● This kind of work requires no special training beyond what you can usually get in high school.

●--- After starting, you serve an apprenticeship or get organized on-the-job training.

——— Lines and symbols used with them indicate full years. To start, requires special training in college, in a hospital or special school, or in a professional school after 1-4 years of college.

{ — Special training is required, but you have a choice, each type of training taking a different number of years.

◇ First symbol means you can get beginner's job after college, but will usually need more study, as well as experience, for advancement. Graduate training ordinarily goes to or beyond master's or doctor's degree.

➤ Your planning should look beyond minimum requirements; continuing study after entering professional practice is important to further advancement.

○ Though the line shows minimum to qualify, more preprofessional years in college often lengthen the total training time.

— 9 m — Special course or on-the-job training is shown in number of months.

Source: Reprinted by permission from *Health Careers Guidebook*. Courtesy of the National Health Council and the Equitable Life Assurance Society of the United States.

sonnel officers, voluntary health agency executives

25 IN BASIC SCIENCES RELATED TO HEALTH. Physical and social scientists, laboratory secretaries, helpers

1 IN CHIROPODY.

12 IN DENTISTRY. Dentists and dental specialists, industrial and public health dentists, dental assistants, hygienists, laboratory technicians

6 IN DIETETIC AND NUTRITIONAL SERVICES. Dietitians, nutritionists, food service workers

2 IN THE ENVIRONMENTAL HEALTH SERVICES. Sanitary engineers, sanitarians

3 IN FOOD AND DRUG PROTECTIVE SERVICES. Food technologists, food and drug inspectors and analysts

2 IN HEALTH EDUCATION. Public health educators, school health educators

6 IN HEALTH INFORMATION AND COMMUNICATIONS. Writers, artists, photographers

2 IN HEALTH STATISTICS. Public health statisticians, statistical clerks

1 IN MEDICAL LIBRARY SCIENCE.

21 IN THE MEDICAL PROFESSIONS. Physicians in general practice and in the medical specialties

2 IN MEDICAL RECORD KEEPING. Medical record librarians, medical record technicians

2 IN MEDICAL-OFFICE SERVICES. Medical secretaries, medical assistants

6 IN MEDICAL TECHNOLOGY. Medical technologists, histologic technicians, blood-bank technologists

15 IN NURSING AND RELATED SERVICES FOR PATIENTS. Professional nurses and nurse specialists, practical nurses, inhalation therapists, ward clerks, orderlies

2 IN OCCUPATIONAL HEALTH SERVICES. Industrial hygienists, safety engineers

2 IN OCCUPATIONAL THERAPY.

3 IN OPTOMETRY, OPTICIANRY, AND ORTHOPTICS.

2 IN ORTHOPEDIC AND PROSTHETIC APPLIANCE WORK.

1 IN OSTEOPATHY.

3 IN PHARMACY. Retail pharmacists, hospital pharmacists, manufacturing pharmacists

1 IN PHYSICAL THERAPY.

4 IN PSYCHOLOGY. Clinical psychologists, social psychologists, counseling psychologists, psychometrists

1 IN RADIOACTIVE ISOTOPE WORK.

2 IN SOCIAL WORK. Medical social workers, psychiatric social workers

3 IN SPEECH AND HEARING THERAPY.

2 IN VETERINARY MEDICINE. Private practitioners, public health veterinarians

1 IN VOCATIONAL REHABILITATION COUNSELING.

1 IN X-RAY EQUIPMENT OPERATION.

The "Health Careers Calendar" presented on pages 476 and 477 gives a quick, easy check on the amount of preparation and training required after high school for specific health careers. The Calendar shows a number of careers calling for one, two, or three years of college. However, a majority require four years of college and a degree. A number of the careers specify advanced graduate preparation leading to a master's or doctoral degree. The *Guidebook* gives more detailed information on each career than can be shown on the Calendar.

VARIETY OF ABILITIES AND SKILLS NEEDED

Modern health services require all types of people working together in partnership to serve individuals, families, and communities. There is a place in the health field [26]

For those who enjoy doing things with their hands, running machines, handling equipment

For the good mixer who likes to work with people and for those who have a special gift of understanding and sympathy

For the rugged individualists and for those who like to work entirely on their own

[26] Reprinted by permission from the *Health Careers Guidebook*, p. 10, published by the National Health Council and supported in the public interest by the Equitable Life Assurance Society of the United States. Copyrighted.

For the "big brain" and the whiz at math or science

For those with a special knack at typing or at other clerical skills

For the business-minded, the good manager, and the executive type

For those who have a flair for food or an easy way with household chores and housekeeping management

For the born teacher and for those whose talents lean toward the arts or toward newspapers, magazines, radio, TV, and movies

The unifying focus in health work regardless of which occupation chosen is *people*—providing them a chance to live healthy, more effective, satisfying lives. The *Health Careers Guidebook* [27] states, "In health—if you so choose—you will make service your career, helping others, as well as yourself, to make the most out of life itself."

A health career demands more from a person than an ordinary job. It calls for a point of view that places others above personal interests, and it demands work and service often "beyond the call of duty." However, rewards are achieved in working with others in a cause that is greater than oneself, in service to humanity.

In so far as the matter of monetary reward is concerned, one may not get rich, but neither should one lack for necessities. Most salaries in health occupations enable one to raise a family comfortably and enjoy an interesting life with them. Since many careers are in health departments, hospitals, schools, colleges, and other essential institutions, they offer better-than-average job security.

Summary

A community is a group of people living together in a particular area who have organized to meet common interests and problems. There is widespread interest today in community health. You, as a college student and as a citizen, have a role to play in community endeavors for better health.

Community organization is necessary today in order to unite the individual members and groups of an area into one group with a common purpose, the development or improvement of a community health program. A functional health program at the local, state, and national levels comprises health services and educational activities organized and conducted by competent personnel. Many opportunities exist for the citizen to participate actively in the community health program, thus assuming part of his civic responsibilities.

A modern point of view of community health is that a community health program preserves the health and life of the people and is designed to keep people well so they may live more effective lives. The scope of community health programs is broadened to meet the growing public health and social problems of modern society. Progress depends upon the professional leadership together with the understanding, support, and participation of the citizenry.

A discussion of health personnel at the local, state, and Federal levels describes the roles of various types of leaders essential in community health activities.

A new organizational plan is presented, which was recommended by an expert Study Group to streamline the Public Health Service and enable it to function more effectively in the years ahead.

The activities of the official, voluntary, and professional agencies are described as they are organized at the local, state, and national levels. Coordinating bodies —a local or state health council and the

[27] *Ibid.*, p. 39.

National Health Council—weld together all efforts toward improved community health at each particular level.

The Health Career Horizons Project, sponsored by the National Health Council and its affiliated organizations, is a forward step in recruitment of young people into health careers. Some 156 health-career opportunities are outlined and the attention of the student is called to these for a possible choice of a life-long vocation.

Suggested readings

1. American Public Health Association: "The Local Health Department: Services and Responsibilities," *American Journal of Public Health,* 41:302–307, March, 1951; an official statement of APHA.
2. Baumgartner, Leona: "Public Health in an Affluent Society," *American Journal of Public Health,* 50:1521–1528, October, 1960.
3. Breslow, Lester, "Health Effects of Air Pollution," *American Journal of Public Health,* 48:913–917, July, 1958.
4. Buell, Bradley, and associates: *Community Planning for Human Services,* Columbia University Press, New York, 1952.
5. Bugbee, George: "The Hospital: Progress and Change," *Public Health Views,* 4:1–7, 1956.
6. *Building America's Health, A Report to the President by the President's Commission on the Health Needs of the Nation,* vol. I, *Findings and Recommendations;* vol. II, *America's Health Status: Needs and Resources,* Government Printing Office, Washington, 1952.
7. Carter, Richard: *The Gentle Legion: A Probing Study of the National Voluntary Health Organizations,* Doubleday and Company, Inc., New York, 1961.
8. Ehlers, Victor M., and Ernest W. Steel: *Municipal and Rural Sanitation,* 5th ed., McGraw-Hill Book Company, Inc., New York, 1958.
9. Emerson, Haven, and Martha Luginbuhl: "1,200 Local Public Health Departments for the United States," *American Journal of Public Health,* 35:898–904, September, 1945.
10. Freeman, Ruth: *Administration of Public Health Services,* W. B. Saunders Company, Philadelphia, 1960.
11. Freidson, Eliot, and Jacob J. Feldman: *The Public Looks at Hospitals.* Research Series, No. 4, Health Information Foundation, New York, 1958.
12. Halderman, J. G., and Evelyn Flook: "The Development of Community Health Services," *American Journal of Public Health,* 49:10–21, January, 1959.
13. Hanlon, John: *Principles of Public Health Administration,* 3d ed., The C. V. Mosby Company, St. Louis, 1960.
14. *Health Careers Guidebook,* National Health Council, New York, 1955.
15. Hiscock, Ira V.: *Community Health Organization,* The Commonwealth Fund, New York, 1950.
16. Hiscock, Ira V.: "*Public Health in Hawaii, 1960:* Report of a Health Inventory," *Hawaii Medical Journal,* 20, January-February, 1961.
17. Hood, Thomas R., and Virginia Pence: "Community Health Studies in Kansas," *American Journal of Public Health,* 50:1560–1569, October, 1960.
18. Hope, Malcolm C., and B. Cowles Mallory: "An Approach to Metropolitanism," *Public Health Reports,* 75:859–863, September, 1960.
19. Johns, Ray, and David F. Demarche: *Community Organization and Agency Responsibility,* Association Press, New York, 1951.
20. Kooz, Earl L.: "Community Organization for Health: Practice and Precept," *Public Health Reports,* 68:86–87, January, 1953.
21. Kooz, Earl L.: *The Health of Regionville,* Columbia University Press, New York, 1954.
22. Larimore, Granville W.: "The Elements of Health Education in Good Public Health Programs, *Public Health Reports,* 75:933–936, October, 1960.
23. Lyons, Yolane: *Stepping Stones to a Health Council,* rev. ed., National Health Council, New York, 1952.
24. Maisel, Albert Q.: *The Health of People Who Work,* National Health Council, New York, 1959.
25. Macoupin County Health Improvement Association: *What's the Health Situation in Macoupin County, Illinois?* The Association, Carlinville, Ill., 1960.
26. Merrill, Malcolm H.: "Community Health—Challenge and Opportunity,"

American Journal of Public Health, 51:359–367, March, 1961.

27. Mountin, Joseph W., and Evelyn Flook: *Guide to Health Organization in the United States,* Public Health Service Publication 196, Government Printing Office, Washington, 1953.

28. National Conference of Social Welfare: *Community Organization: 1958.* Columbia University Press, New York, 1958.

29. Office of the Federal Register, National Archives and Records Service, General Services Administration: *U.S. Government Organizational Manual 1961–1962,* Government Printing Office, Washington, June 1, 1961.

30. Osborn, Barbara: *An Outline for Community Health,* Department of Health and Safety, Los Angeles State College, Los Angeles, 1960.

31. *Partners for Health,* National Health Council, New York, 1955.

32. Patterson, Raymond S., and Beryl J. Roberts: *Community Health Education in Action,* The C. V. Mosby Company, St. Louis, 1951.

33. Poston, Richard W.: *Democracy Is You,* Harper & Brothers, New York, 1953.

34. Prince, Julius S.: "A Public Philosophy of Public Health," *American Journal of Public Health,* 48:903–912, July, 1958.

35. Public Health Service: *Health of the Nation,* reprinted from *Annual Report,* U.S. Department of Health, Education, and Welfare, Washington, 1958.

36. Public Health Service, U.S. National Health Survey: *Health Statistics: Origin and Program of the U.S. National Health Survey,* U.S. Department of Health, Education, and Welfare, Washington, May, 1958.

37. Public Health Service: *National Institutes of Health,* Public Health Service Publication 81, rev. ed., U.S. Department of Health, Education, and Welfare, Washington, 1960.

38. Public Health Service: *Final Report of the Study Group on Mission and Organization of the Public Health Service,* U.S. Department of Health, Education, and Welfare, Washington, 1960.

39. Public Health Service, U.S. National Health Survey: *Health Statistics: The Hawaii Health Survey,* U.S. Department of Health, Education, and Welfare, Washington, May, 1960.

40. Rockefeller, Nelson A., "Present-day Health Problems," *American Journal of Public Health,* 50:8–13, January, 1960.

41. Rosen, George, and Edward Wellin: "A Bookshelf on the Social Sciences and Public Health," *American Journal of Public Health,* 49:441–454, April, 1959.

42. Sanders, Irwin T.: *Making Good Communities Better,* University of Kentucky Press, Lexington, Ky., 1950.

43. Smolensky, John, and Frank Haar: *Community Health,* W. B. Saunders Company, Philadelphia, 1961.

44. U.S. Department of Health, Education, and Welfare: *Annual Report,* Government Printing Office, Washington, 1960.

45. West Los Angeles Health Committee: *Survey,* Los Angeles County Tuberculosis and Health Association, Los Angeles, 1956.

46. Yahraes, Herbert, *What's in Your Future—A Career in Health,* Public Affairs Pamphlet 281, Public Affairs Committee, New York, 1959.

SIXTEEN

Solving international health problems

Health is a world-wide problem. The 3 billion persons living in an increasingly closer relationship with each other in the international community provide ample evidence to substantiate this statement. Diseases have no respect for geographical boundaries, either between local neighborhoods or between the nations of the world. As has been stated in Chapter 15, the public itself is responsible for its own healthful environment. In addition, the concept of health as something more than freedom from disease is being recognized, and a more positive outlook is developing among the peoples of the world. The relation of health status to poverty and ignorance becomes increasingly evident as improvements in one condition result in like improvements in the other.

Individuals in all nations of the world must become increasingly aware of the nature of world health problems in order to cooperate in solving them. College students may be able to make valuable contributions, now or in the future, to the solution of international health prob-

lems if they understand the factors involved. Such an understanding involves a consideration of the following questions:

What is the significance of health in the world today?

What are the outstanding health problems that are confronting the peoples of the world?

How are organizations contributing to the solution of international health problems?

Significance of health in the world

No nation is free from the threat of epidemics when diseases are permitted to run rampant in other countries. Modern transportation has many advantages, but it also provides for the rapid movement of insect vectors, as well as human carriers, of many communicable diseases. Breakfast in England, lunch in North America, and back to England for tea is now possible. Even greater speeds are forecast as "jet," "rocket," and "atomic" become commonplace adjectives in a discussion of transportation and as man extends his explorations of space. Such rapid movement adds immeasurably to the problem of controlling the spread of communicable diseases.

HEALTH STATUS INFLUENCES AND IS INFLUENCED BY OTHER FACTORS

The health status of the people and the economy of a country are closely allied. In Ceylon, for example, it is estimated that the elimination of malaria produced a saving of 30 million dollars per year. Malaria-eradication programs in Thailand cost approximately $500,000 per year between 1954 and 1958 to control a disease that was responsible for 50 million agricultural worker-days lost each year—the equivalent of a rice harvest of 15 million dollars [10].

The significance of the interrelationship of health, education, and nutritional

status is demonstrated by the close working relationship between FAO (Food and Agriculture Organization), UNESCO (United Nations Educational, Scientific, and Cultural Organization), and WHO (World Health Organization). A person who is hungry and ill is not able to benefit fully from educational opportunities and is more likely to be an economic liability than an asset. The fact that more than half the people in the world are seriously underfed—that upward of 1½ billion persons are not getting enough food for proper physical development, for resistance to disease, or for profit-producing labor—suggests the immensity of the problem.

The problem of the interrelationship between socioeconomic conditions and health is further illustrated by the economic cycle of disease, shown in the figure on page 484.

These less fortunate people of the world are trapped in a whirlpool from which they find it extremely difficult to escape. Illiteracy and poverty contribute to their poor health status. Their poor health in turn decreases their ability to improve economically. Low income means there is not enough money to pay for even a limited education or, for that matter, to purchase food needed for survival. The improvement of health status is both dependent upon and essential to

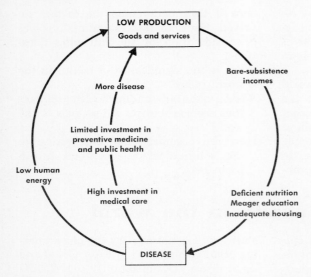

LOW PRODUCTION
Goods and services

Bare-subsistence
incomes

More disease

Limited investment in
preventive medicine
and public health

Low human
energy

High investment in
medical care

Deficient nutrition
Meager education
Inadequate housing

DISEASE

The economic cycle of disease. (Abraham Horwitz, On Health and Wealth, Pan American Sanitary Bureau, Washington, May, 1960.)

higher standards of living and increased opportunities for education.

WHAT DOES HEALTH MEAN TO THE PEOPLE OF THE WORLD?

The importance of health has been recognized by mankind for thousands of years. Calder[1] notes an ancient reference by Buddha to the desirability of health and comments about the attainment of health by the peoples of the world:

Arogya Parama Laba ("health is the greatest blessing of all"). . . . Health may be the greatest blessing, but half of the people of the world do not know what it means. They only know it by its reverse as disease, ill-health and misery. They have no means to know that sense of well-being which is something quite different from not being ill. Health is not just the absence of disease.

No doctor can prescribe health; no government can ordain health by statute; no international agency can administer health. A community, for instance, may provide houses; it cannot provide homes. A "home" is what a family makes of a house. So with health; all that a community, local, national or international, can do is provide the means

and the services—social conditions, public-health measures, sanitation, better treatment of diseases—by which the individual can enjoy the well-being and happiness which only he can create.

Unfortunately, there are too few healthy individuals who appreciate the health they enjoy and too many individuals who never have the opportunity to experience the state of health suggested in the preceding statement.

As indicated in Chapter 1, the nations represented in the World Health Organization have agreed on a definition of health. They suggest that it is both a right and a duty of all individuals. Their concept of health is expressed in the following pattern:[2]

HEALTH. A state of *complete physical, mental and social well-being* and not merely the absence of disease or infirmity.

A RIGHT. One of the *fundamental rights of every human being* without distinction of race, religion, political belief, economic or social condition.

A DUTY. The health of ALL peoples is fundamental to the attainment of PEACE AND SECURITY and is *dependent upon the fullest co-operation of individuals and states.*

[1] Ritchie Calder, *The Lamp Is Lit: The Story of the World Health Organization,* World Health Organization, Geneva, 1951, p. 1.

[2] *World Health Organization: What It Is, What It Does, How It Works,* 5th ed., World Health Organization, Geneva, 1956, p. 1.

Development of world organizations for health

Many early efforts by nations to control disease and promote world health were doomed to failure because of the effect of control measures in limiting trade. However, in 1902 a permanent organization created for multilateral international action relating to public health was established by the nations in the Americas. The meeting in Washington of the First International Sanitary Conference of the American republics in that year resulted in the establishment of the Pan American Sanitary Bureau, which has contributed extensively to improvement of health conditions in the Americas.

The primary concern of the Pan American Sanitary Bureau was to control the spread of diseases between nations. In 1909 the International Office of Public Health was established, with headquarters in Paris, for the same purpose but on a world-wide scale. Forty-six countries were included in the membership of this organization.

The need for improving health conditions within, as well as between, countries was recognized, and the Rockefeller Foundation established an International Health Commission to aid in developing cooperative action for building up sound programs for disease control and health promotion within individual countries.

In 1923 the League of Nations, which was established following World War I, formed its Health Organization. This organization provided the first machinery for an effective approach to the solving of world-wide health problems. The accomplishments of the Health Organization of the League of Nations were outstanding until its functions were disrupted by World War II. The Service of Epidemiological Intelligence, which collected data on the prevalence and movement of communicable diseases and provided for extensive distribution of this information, was one of the most valuable functions of the League organization. Other services were provided by such groups as the Commission on Biological Standardization, the Malaria Commission, the Commission on Housing, and groups making nutrition studies.

The World Health Organization was developed from the background of international experiences with the Pan American Sanitary Bureau, the International Office of Public Health, the International Health Commission of the Rockefeller Foundation, and the League of Nations Health Organization.

At the United Nations meeting in San Francisco in 1945, delegations from Brazil and China introduced a resolution calling for a special meeting to establish an international health organization. The Economic and Social Council of the United Nations called for such a conference to meet in New York in July, 1946. At this New York meeting, the representatives of 61 nations drew up and adopted a constitution for the new organization. The representatives appointed an Interim Commission to function until the constitution was ratified by 26 nations. The Interim Commission was composed of representatives from 16 nations selected by the conference.

The slow process of ratification by member nations delayed the final establishment of the organization but did not prevent the Interim Commission from functioning. In 1947 a cholera epidemic in Egypt provided an opportunity for international action, and the Commission accepted the challenge. Through the efforts of this world organization, medical supplies were gathered from all over the world and rushed into Egypt to assist the Egyptian health workers in vaccination and treatment necessary to control the epidemic. One month after the onset of the epidemic it had spread throughout the country, and in a single day 1,000 new cases and 500 deaths were recorded [25]. In another six weeks the epidemic had been brought under control, and the battle was won. Many lives were saved and much misery was avoided as a result of the cooperation of many nations to assist the Egyptians.

Despite this evidence of the value of coordination of effort in solving health problems, the nations were slow in ratifying the constitution. The Interim Commission called a meeting for June 24, 1948, even though there were not enough signatory nations when the meeting date was set. With the stimulus of the call to meeting, many nations signed in order to be eligible for this first meeting of the World Health Assembly. On April 7, 1948, the twenty-sixth nation signed the constitution, and as a result April 7 is now celebrated each year as World Health Day. The United States became the forty-second nation to accept membership by ratifying the constitution on June 14, 1948. By the first meeting 54 nations had ratified the constitution and by 1961 membership had reached 102.

Since the first meeting in 1948, the World Health Assembly has met each year for the purpose of planning and establishing over-all policies.

Officially, the World Health Organization was recognized on Sept. 1, 1948. The work of this organization in helping nations to solve their health problems has been outstanding. The National Citizens' Committee on World Health was organized in the United States in 1951 to support activities of WHO. The function of the World Health Organization is discussed in greater detail later in the chapter.

In addition to the World Health Organization, which represents nations of the world, other international health organizations are contributing to the health status of people throughout the world.

The Pan American Health Organization has been closely aligned with the Pan American Sanitary Bureau, Regional Office of WHO, and has conducted a variety of health activities to improve health conditions in the western hemisphere [20].

The International Union for Health Education of the Public (IUHEP) is a nongovernmental organization established in 1951 to contribute to the development of health education on a world-wide basis. Active membership in IUHEP includes national committees, societies, associations, or similar national voluntary health agencies. IUHEP works cooperatively with WHO and UNESCO and has representation at the WHO Assembly. The theme of their 1959 meeting in Dusseldorf, Germany, was "Health Education of Children and Youth." The theme of the 1962 meeting in Philadelphia was "Health Problems and Health Education of the Public." The national committee for IUHEP in the United States is the American National Committee for Health Education of the Public, which was organized in 1958.

A study was conducted, and an international conference on "Child Health and the School" was held, by the WCOTP (World Confederation of Organizations of the Teaching Profession) in 1960. Reports from 40 countries and resolutions coming from the Assembly in Amsterdam are guides for improving the health of children in schools throughout the world [5]. Organized within the structure of WCOTP is the International Council for Health, Physical Education, and Recreation.

Among other international health organizations that have been making significant contributions to improved health status of peoples throughout the world are MEDICO, HOPE, and the World Medical Association.

Health problems throughout the world

Themes for World Health Day, which is April 7 each year, illustrate some significant health problems: "Healthy Surroundings Make Healthy People"; "Safe Water"; "Food and Health"; "Malaria Eradication—A World Challenge." The importance of the problems suggested by the themes is indicated in the following paragraphs.

It has been estimated that approximately 2 billion babies will be born in the world in the sixteen-year period ending in 1975 and that 80 per cent of them will be born in the less well-developed countries [23]. When this figure of nearly 125,000,000 births per year on the average is considered in relation to the following statement by Eastman in 1956— and little improvement in personnel has been made on a world-wide basis—the enormity of this problem is almost beyond comprehension: [3]

The number of babies born in the world each year is in the general order of eighty million. Of this number, the great majority, certainly more than three of every four, are delivered not by doctors, nor by nurses, nor by trained midwives, but by a vast army of untrained attendants who, for the most part, are also illiterate, steeped in superstition, and abysmally ignorant of the veriest rudiments of clean and safe maternity care. . . .

Although the figure I am about to cite may seem incredible, the evidence suggests that if every umbilical cord in the world could be handled with just ordinary cleanliness, the number of neonatal lives saved thereby each year would exceed a million. . . . Of the three great causes of maternal death, hemorrhage, infection, and toxemia, the majority of women now dying in economically underdeveloped countries from these causes could be saved by the application of just a few elementary principles of prenatal care and cleanliness.

The lot of many of the children who survive the birth process is far from encouraging. It has been said that most children of the world face a short life, a sick life, and a hungry life [13]. Infant mortality rates in the developed and less-developed countries of the world show vast differences between chances for survival.

Life expectancy for the average newborn child tells an equally grim tale when comparisons are made: in the United States, the infant's expectation of life is seventy years; in India, thirty-two years; in Sweden, more than seventy years; in Egypt, thirty-eight years.

Accidents are a major problem facing children in most nations of the world where the communicable diseases have been decreasing as a primary threat to children and young persons. In 15 European countries accidental deaths among the 1- to 19-year age group accounted for a low of 14.4 per cent to a high of 38.4 per cent of the total deaths. The eight most dangerous accidents for boys and girls were motor vehicles, other transport, poison, falls, fire and explosion, heat and radiation, firearms, and drowning [17].

Water is one of man's most pressing problems. The amount of water required to provide for the needs of people in both developed and less-developed countries is of growing concern as population increases by leaps and bounds. The quality of water is of primary concern to most people in the less-developed countries. The World Health Organization estimates that one-fourth of the world's hospital beds are occupied by persons ill because of poor water and that 39 per cent of the people in Latin America living in towns of more than 2,000 inhabitants are without water service [26].

The task of meeting the nutritional needs of the rapidly expanding population of the world is enormous. When one considers that half the present popula-

[3] Nicholson J. Eastman, "Global Aspects of Midwifery," *American Journal of Public Health*, 46:310–311, March, 1956.

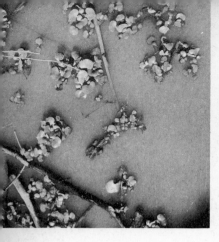

In a country like Argentina, a river or even a small stream, so still and calm, may be a breeding place for mosquitoes, the carriers of malaria.

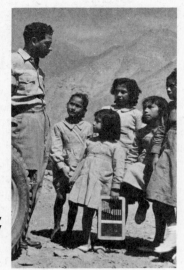

In the valleys and in the hills, malaria is a constant threat, particularly to the children, who seem to be constantly swatting mosquitoes.

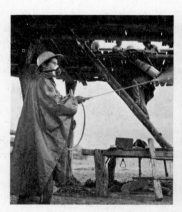
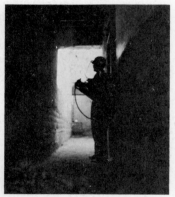

With the help of the United Nations World Health Organization and the United Nations Children's Fund, the governments of malaria-infested countries have launched an all-out effort to eradicate the disease. The campaign begins with spraying DDT on the dwellings, as a protection against the malaria-carrying mosquitoes.

The attack is carried to the home of the mosquito larvae, the streams and rivers.

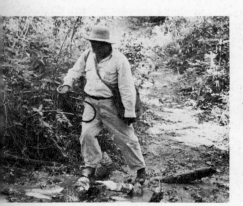

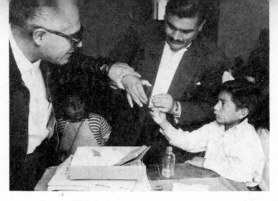

The campaign extends to the schools, where blood tests are made . . .

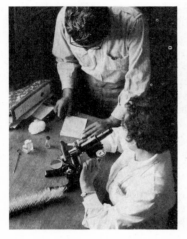

then analyzed in laboratories. Frequent and accurate reports give an over-all picture of the progress being made throughout the country . . .

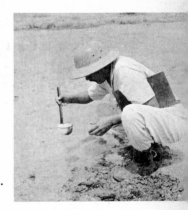

from the coastal swamps . . .

to the hills . . .

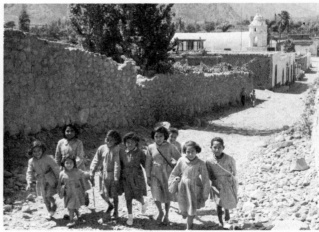

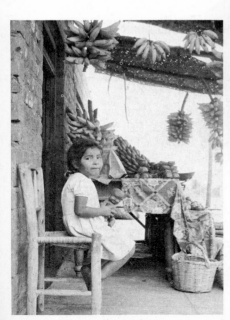

so that children like five-year-old Gladya can be free from the sickness that brings apathy, lethargy, and death.

tion of the world is underfed and that the population, at the present rate of increase, will be double in another 35 years, nutrition problems appear to be almost insurmountable. Man's ingenuity will be tested to the fullest to increase production of food to the point where needs can be met. Unfortunately, the answer to the problem is not transporting surplus foods from one part of the world to another.

Kwashiorkor (protein malnutrition) continues to be a pressing nutritional-deficiency disease in many of the less-developed countries of the world. In some areas vitamin deficiencies, such as riboflavin, thiamine, or ascorbic acid, are the primary problem; in other areas it may be iron deficiency, resulting in anemia, or iodine insufficiency, resulting in goiter.

Despite tremendous advancements, malaria continued to be a threat to the health of more than 1 billion human beings in 1960. The tragic consequences of an epidemic of malaria are illustrated by the 3 million victims of the disease in Ethiopia in 1958. Of this number, 100,000 died. In the malaria areas of this country, with a population of approximately 18 million, it was estimated that half the people were infected with the disease [12].

The African Congo achieved worldwide political attention during 1960. Another problem confronting the Congolese received considerably less attention: the health problem. In 1960 there was not one Congolese doctor, and it was estimated that there would be no more than twenty by 1965. In 1958 there were 703 doctors, all European, for the 14 million Congolese people and the foreigners living in the Congo [6]. The shortage of qualified medical personnel in the less-developed countries of the world is a serious obstacle to progress.

World Health Organization at work

Fortunately, the leaders of the World Health Organization have realized that this group cannot solve the health problems of nations by sending in an army of workers to kill insects, immunize individuals, or provide penicillin injections. Improvements in health status cannot be imposed from outside; rather, improvements must result from the combined effort of an enlightened population, assisted, if necessary, by trained personnel and equipment from other nations.

The influence of the World Health Organization is exemplified by the statement by Dr. H. B. Turbott, President of the Thirteenth World Health Assembly: [4]

As national health men we all experience the frustrations inherent in national control of finance, where competing interests delay that progress in national health which we see so clearly could be achieved so quickly

[4] "The Price of Health," WHO Chronicle, 14:271, July, 1960.

if only we had the means. Enter the World Health Organization, with its supplemental offer of the merest modicum of finance, but of real substantial help in planning, training and action aspects of programmes for health betterment. From this stimulation—for that is all it is—stems our success. The country being helped responds, participates in greater degree than previously thought possible by the Government, is caught up in teamwork with other countries to safeguard its newly envisaged achievement. . . .

ORGANIZATIONAL STRUCTURE OF THE WORLD HEALTH ORGANIZATION

The organizational structure of the World Health Organization is illustrated in the accompanying chart. Leadership is vested in the Health Assembly, which meets annually. The Assembly is composed of representative delegations from each member nation. This body is responsible for determining the policies of the WHO program.

The executive board is composed of

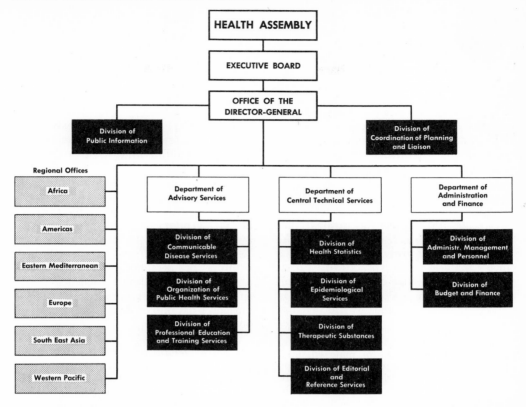

Organizational structure of the World Health Organization. (By permission of World Health Organization.)

24 members selected by the Health Assembly. This group is responsible for putting into effect the decisions reached by the Health Assembly and for initiating emergency action necessary between meetings of the Assembly. This technical and nonpolitical group meets at least twice each year.

The working section of WHO is the Secretariat, headed by the director-general. This group is composed of both technical and administrative personnel.

The functions of WHO are allocated to the regional offices of the organization as much as is possible, with the Geneva headquarters serving to coordinate all the activities of the regional offices and the many divisions shown in the structural chart.

ACTIVITIES OF THE WORLD HEALTH ORGANIZATION

The activities of WHO are numerous and varied. Some are general in nature for the benefit of all nations, and others are more specific to assist a particular nation in solving a health problem. The activities are carried on by the several divisions shown in the accompanying chart and discussed in the following paragraphs.

Advisory services. The function of the Department of Advisory Services is to assist countries in developing health administration. Its purpose is accomplished by such means as public health demonstration teams, consultants from professional training centers, and a fellowship program. The effectiveness of the World Health Organization during its relatively short period of existence since 1948 provides ample evidence of its value.

Malaria has received special attention from WHO, and the benefits from isolated campaigns against this widespread illness resulted in an all-out effort, starting in 1960, to eradicate the disease completely. Some of the victories over malaria are its eradication in Ceylon, and a resulting annual saving of 30 million dollars; a decrease of over 50 per cent in infant mortality in French Guiana following large-scale antimalaria operations; and an increase of 4 to 5 centimeters in the average height of army recruits in Greece since malaria has practically been eliminated from that country. The project initiated in 1960 is described in figures quoted by the World Health Organization: [5]

Thousands of teams, tens of thousands of vehicles, millions of tons of material, hundreds of millions of houses to spray, hundreds of millions of blood samples to be examined, drugs to be transported by the ton, maps to be drawn by the thousands, the movement of millions of migrants to be observed.

Success of this vast malaria campaign would mark a milestone in man's progress toward a happier, healthier, more productive life.

Progress against numerous other diseases is also being made. Smallpox is slowly being eliminated as a health problem. From 242,000 cases reported in 1958 there was a reduction to 72,000 cases in 1959. Even with an immunization procedure that could eliminate the disease completely, progress has been slow. The complacency of many persons permits the disease to be a problem even in the more highly developed nations. There were 19 cases reported at Heidelberg, West Germany, for example, in 1959. Ad-

ditional cases and some deaths were reported in West Germany in 1961 and in England early in 1962.

A mass campaign to overcome yaws has been highly successful in Indonesia. By the end of 1958 approximately 45 million persons had been examined and almost 6½ million persons treated with a form of penicillin that heals yaws lesions in a few days. Approximately 37 tons of penicillin were used during this period of time.

An estimated 12 million victims of leprosy (Hansen's disease) throughout the world have new hope as the mystery of this legendary disease is being stripped away and effective treatment undertaken [8]. Expanded efforts in case finding, training of personnel, leprosy control units, and outpatient treatment with sulfone drugs have gradually changed the outlook from one of dread and secrecy to one of hope.

Central technical services. The functions of Central Technical Services Department produce results less spectacular than the activities of the Advisory Services Department but equally significant.

The contributions of Technical Services include [1, 28]:

Publishing the first international pharmacopoeia, which contains formulas for making up medicines to ensure uniform strength of the preparations in the different nations

Standardizing biological substances such as the antibiotics, serums, and vitamins in order to provide an added margin of safety in treatment of diseases in the various nations

Broadcasting up-to-the-minute information on epidemic diseases to all national health services as well as to ships at sea and to aircraft in flight

Maintaining a library service available to various nations and publishing materials for world-wide distribution

Collecting, interpreting, and publishing statistics

[5] "Malaria, a Gigantic Enterprise," *World Health*, 13:3, March–April, 1960.

Among the publications of WHO are: *Bulletin of the World Health Organization, International Digest of Health Legislation, WHO Chronicle, Weekly Epidemiological Record, World Health, Epidemiological and Vital Statistics Report,* a monograph series, and a technical report series.

Cooperation with other international agencies. The program of the World Health Organization is carried on in close cooperation with other international agencies whenever the opportunity arises. UNICEF (United Nations Children's Fund) has numerous activities to improve the health status of children throughout the world. In 1960 the UNICEF program included child health and welfare projects in more than 100 countries and territories, including projects in India to buy equipment to produce larger quantities of edible peanut flour to supplement the protein diet of undernourished children and in Indonesia to expand production of saridele, a vegetable milk made from soya beans; basic health services for mothers and children, including safe-water programs; malaria-control aid projects representing the expenditure of $3,100,000; and other disease control projects for leprosy, tuberculosis, venereal diseases, bilharziasis, trachoma, yaws, typhus, and smallpox [9, 13, 15].

The joint efforts of UNICEF, WHO, and FAO in distributing dry skim milk have provided a ray of hope for millions of malnourished persons [3]. The FAO officially launched a campaign in July, 1961, to run through 1965, with campaign activities planned in three categories: information and education, research, and action programs [15].

A contribution of international activities conducted during the past years has been increased understanding of the most effective ways to accomplish objectives. Spurgeon M. Keeny, Director, Asia Region, UNICEF, in discussing successes and failures of ten years of work in Asia, listed things that have been learned:[6]

The latest discoveries can be put to use in Asia as soon as mass production brings prices to a reasonable level.

Western methods may have to be drastically modified to meet Eastern conditions.

Western technical help is often necessary, but it is useless unless there is competent national leadership.

Plans of operation must be drafted well in advance with precision and in detail so that each branch of the government knows what it needs to do and when.

Good timing is essential, especially in operations that must be completed within reasonable time limits, such as those against malaria.

Targets at all levels, from the national plan to the individual worker, must be set, and the morale created to attain them.

The ordinary people in the villages must be told what the program hopes to achieve. If they understand, they will cooperate.

Care must be taken not to offend the customs of the country.

Thoroughness is essential. In mass programs such as yaws and malaria eighty per cent success is failure.

Results must be tested objectively, and plans constantly revised accordingly. For an expert the greatest merit is humility.

Altogether, it has been an interesting and certainly a lively ten years. But one child in five in Asia still dies in its first year of life; in the United States, one in forty. There is still much to do; but in the last ten years we have learned much about how to do it. The harvest the next ten years will be better.

Some of the additional sources of funds for international activities in health include the United Nations Expanded Program for Technical Assistance to Underdeveloped Countries, the United States Agency for International Development, the British Commonwealth Technical Assistance Plan (the Colombo plan), the CARE Organization of the United States of America, national and religious relief and welfare organizations, the International Committee of the Red Cross, and the League of Red Cross Societies.

[6] Spurgeon M. Keeny, "Asia's Health: A Ten Year Look," *United Nations Review,* 6:20–23, February, 1960.

Bilateral international health programs of the United States

In addition to the multilateral international health programs, which pool the resources of many nations, there are numerous cooperative agreements between pairs of nations to assist in solving the health problems of one or both of the countries. The bilateral health programs in which the United States participates are in addition to the activities of the World Health Organization.

In 1960, the United States was working with over 50 nations and dependent territories in technical cooperation activities, which involved nearly 5,000 U.S. technicians overseas. In Turkey, tens of thousands of young men are learning to write; in Guatemala, the U.S. Operations Mission, in cooperation with the Guatemalan government, fostered a rural redevelopment program to resettle 10,000 rural familes on tracts of about 50 acres; in Somaliland, with the cooperation of Italy, the United States has a program to drill or dig approximately 500 wells to supply the nomadic dwellers with adequate water; in Taiwan, the United States has assisted in constructing a needed highway; in Yugoslavia, United States assistance has increased the yield of the corn crop; and in Ethiopia, a program for the development of an Agricultural Technical School has done much to improve the nation's agricultural program [27].

One of the most significant developments has been the stimulus provided to education in foreign countries through the International Cooperation Administration: [7]

Schools have been built and equipped, teachers trained, and technical advice provided in dozens of countries. Ethiopia progressed from less than 500 qualified teachers, 72,000 students, 718 makeshift classrooms to about 5,000 teachers, 210,000 students, and 4,000 classrooms. Jordan, which had no organized teacher training education programs before ICA assistance in 1952, now has preservice training facilities for about 500 and inservice training and summer school programs for about 200 to 2,500 teachers annually. Turkey under an ICA program every year teaches about 65,000 military recruits to read and write. From 1952 to 1959, about 2,156 elementary school classrooms and 192 secondary school classrooms were built for the 750,000 to 1 million Vietnamese children not attending school because of lack of facilities. . . . ICA helped start land-grant colleges in 19 countries.

Education for economic stability has also been supplemented by education for specific health responsibilities. Examples of such cooperation are the University of Minnesota helping National University of Seoul, in the Republic of Korea, to strengthen medical and nursing programs, the State University of New York aiding public health education in Israel, Indiana University helping the University of Peshawar, in Pakistan, to develop a basic science curriculum for the Khyber Medical College, and the University of California associating with the University of Indonesia to develop medical education.

The ICNND (Interdepartmental Committee on Nutrition for National Defense) was established in early 1955 to assist in solving nutrition problems of technical, military, and economic importance in foreign countries. By July, 1961, the program carried on by the committee had extended to 16 countries in the Far East, Near East, South America, Africa, and Europe and also into Alaska. Results of surveys in 14 countries had shown that despite numerous similarities in nutrition problems in these countries, each country, and areas within the coun-

[7] *Foreign Aid: Facts and Fallacies.* Bureau of Public Affairs, U.S. Department of State Publication 7239, Washington, 1961, p. 51.

try, have special problems. Among the most commonly discovered nutritional problems were inadequate amounts of vitamin A, riboflavin, thiamine, vitamin C, protein, and calories. In addition, goiter and anemia were problems in some areas [14].

In Bolivia, which had the highest smallpox attack rate in the hemisphere, a joint Bolivian–United States control program was undertaken in 1958. After an intensive immunization program, smallpox cases decreased from 1,310 in 1957 to 193 during the first six months of 1958 and no cases between July, 1958, and June, 1959.

Other examples of successful bilateral health programs are the reduction of yaws in Ecuador and Colombia; reduced incidence of trachoma in Iran and Libya; case finding and vaccination for tuberculosis in Taiwan; development of a sanitary engineering specialty in Brazil over a fifteen-year period to prepare qualified personnel to overcome major environmental health problems; improvements in water supply and sewage disposal systems in Honduras, Venezuela, Jordan, Ecuador, and Korea; and expanded rural health services in Taiwan, in Peru, in the Philippines, and in Iran [16].

A healthy world population benefits all mankind

The relatively small amount of money being invested in health projects throughout the world is paying dividends well beyond expectations. That these benefits are not merely those experienced by the people in underdeveloped nations of the world is suggested by the following quotation:[8]

Whereas about two-thirds of the world is struggling in poverty, owing to low productivity per man, the other third is anxiously wondering how to secure markets for all the goods it manufactures. As the underdeveloped nations begin to raise their standards of living so will the market for the goods of the technically advanced steadily expand.

The present unbalance between prosperity and impoverishment is a constant source of human suffering; it is also a threat to the stability of the world. The urgent need is that more shall be done more quickly to redress the balance. Nor is that all. The mastery of ill-health is only half the story. Beyond that is the ideal of establishing positive health throughout the world and so releasing in all their abundance the creative powers of man, the powers he needs to tackle and surmount his problems—and to savour the full joy of living. A vigorous, peaceful, happy, productive world can arise from the abundant health and vitality of men and women; it can never grow under the existing burden of sickness, malnutrition, and poverty.

Summary

Developing and maintaining health is an important individual problem. In addition, it is a community problem of worldwide scope. Individuals of all nations must assume added responsibilities for assisting others to attain a quality of life that enables them to live effectively.

The establishment of the World Health Organization dedicated to the im-

proved health status of all people, was helped by a number of other international organizations which preceded it, such as the Pan American Sanitary Bureau and the League of Nations Health Organization. Some of the most significant international health problems are indicated by themes for World Health Days, which are celebrated on April 7. Three of the most indicative themes have been "Safe Water," "Malaria

[8] James Hemming, *A Strategy for World Health*, World Health Organization, Geneva, 1955, p. 34.

Eradication—A World Challenge," and "Food and Health."

The World Health Organization has been highly effective in stimulating nations to improve health conditions. In addition to the functions of the World Health Organization, numerous multi-lateral and bilateral health activities are carried on between nations. The significance of improved health status on the economic well-being of nations is being more widely accepted, and the sincere desire of the people of one nation to assist people of other nations is illustrated more frequently with each passing day.

Suggested readings

1. Calder, Ritchie: *The Lamp Is Lit: The Story of the World Health Organization,* World Health Organization, Geneva, 1951.
2. Cambournac, F. J. C.: "Health in Africa," *American Journal of Public Health,* 50; part II: 13–19, June, 1960.
3. Cambournac, F. J. C.: "Milk and Malnutrition," *WHO Chronicle,* 14:390–393, October, 1960.
4. Cassels, Louis: "They Save Lives on a Global Scale," *Today's Health,* 39:28–31, January, 1961.
5. *Child Health and the School,* World Confederation of Organizations of the Teaching Profession, Washington, 1960.
6. "Health in the Congo," *World Health,* 13:27–31, November-December, 1960.
7. Keeny, Spurgeon M.: "Asia's Health: A Ten Year Look," *United Nations Review,* 6:20–23, February, 1960.
8. "Leprosy Demystified," *World Health,* 13:14–21, July-August, 1960.
9. Lyon, Peter: "A Better World for Children," *Holiday,* August, 1960.
10. "Malaria," *World Health,* 13:1–40, March-April, 1960.
11. "Malaria: A Gigantic Undertaking," *World Health,* 14:12, January-February, 1961.
12. "Malaria Epidemic Strikes in Ethiopia," *World Health,* 13:39, May-June, 1960.
13. Pate, Maurice: "UNICEF Goals in Maternal and Child Health," *American Journal of Public Health,* 50; part II: 8–12, June, 1960.
14. Schaefer, Arnold E., and Frank B. Berry: "U.S. Interest in World Nutrition," *Public Health Reports,* 75:677–686, August, 1960.
15. Sen, B. R.: "For Freedom from Hunger to Assure the Triumph of Human Dignity," *United Nations Review,* 6:6–9, April, 1960.
16. *Technical Cooperation in Health,* International Cooperation Administration, Washington, 1959.
17. "The Child's Enemy No. 1: Accidents," *World Health,* 13:17–21, May-June, 1960.
18. *The First Ten Years of the World Health Organization,* World Health Organization, Geneva, 1958.
19. "The Most Powerful Weapon," *International Journal of Health Education,* 2:131–134, July, 1959.
20. The Pan American Health Organization: *PAHO: What It Is, What It Does, How It Works,* Pan American Sanitary Bureau, Washington, 1960.
21. Thompson, John M.: "Teachers Accept the Challenge," *International Journal of Health Education,* 4:22–26, January-March, 1961.
22. Thompson, Warren S.: "World Population and Food Supply," *Journal of the American Medical Association,* 172:159–162, Apr. 9, 1960.
23. "UNICEF Broadens Its Program for the World's Children," *United Nations Review,* 6:33–35, June, 1960.
24. *UNICEF: What It Is, What It Does, How It Works,* United Nations Children's Fund, Geneva, 1960.
25. United Nations Office of Public Information: *Everyman's United Nations,* 6th ed., United Nations, New York, 1959.
26. "Water," *World Health,* 13:22–23, May-June, 1960.
27. *Working with People: Examples of U.S. Technical Cooperation,* International Cooperation Administration, Washington, 1960.
28. *World Health Organization: What It Is, What It Does, How It Works,* 5th ed., World Health Organization, Geneva, 1961.
29. Yamaguchi, Masayoshi: "The Population Problem and Its Relation to the Public Health," *American Journal of Public Health,* 50, part II: 83–87, June, 1960.

SEVENTEEN

Health in space

Man, through his preliminary explorations of space, has added new dimensions to the attainment of health for effective living. Space travel has been brought to the public attention through the exploits of the American astronauts and Russian cosmonauts. Life on the earth is becoming reasonably well understood, and health problems are gradually being resolved. However, before man has achieved success in overcoming many health problems on earth, new hazards involving man in space have been added. Man's efforts to solve health hazards confronting him in space may help resolve problems he now faces on earth.

Some health problems in space are the following:

Weightlessness

Meeting nutritional needs in a different environment, with limitations of storage space and weightlessness

Danger of solar energy damage to the eyes

Artificial provision of oxygen and elimination of carbon dioxide

Exposure to wide variations in temperature and to extreme variations in pressure

Danger from radiation both from the power plant of the space vehicle and from sources in space

Elimination of body waste

Possible harmful organisms that might be brought back to earth from other planets or might affect persons who eventually land on other planets

Loneliness and boredom due to confinement in a limited environment for long periods of time

Noise and vibration associated with the propulsion of the vehicle

Stress due to rapid acceleration and deceleration

Adaptation to a new daily work-eat-sleep-rest cycle in place of day and night as we know it

Weakness due to inactivity

Danger from collisions between space vehicles and meteoroids

Some results of space exploration are good for human health. As a result of the research related to space travel, a whole new concept of human-factor engineering to fit the machine to the man has been established. In addition, medical instrumentation has been improved; extensive studies of cause and effect of stress, fatigue, and tension are under way; chemicals effective in treatment of diseases and disorders are being discovered; and new concepts in nutrition are evolving.

In order to gain insight into the concept of health in space, let us answer the following questions:

What is space?

What are potential health problems associated with space travel of short duration?

What are health problems associated with space travel to other planets?

How can the health of the space traveler be protected from the hazards of space?

A concept of space

When space travel is mentioned, most individuals think of man coming and going between planets or picture the "man from Mars" landing on our planet. Few people have given much thought to the medium through which space travelers must pass. Distance in space seems almost impossible to grasp in comparison with our everyday concepts of distance and our conventional means of travel. The hazards of space have not received much attention from the average individual because he has little chance of becoming a space traveler. In the following paragraphs a brief discussion of space is presented as a basis for the later consideration of space health problems.

There is no complete agreement as to where space starts. According to some authorities, the top of the atmosphere is where space begins; others think of space as beyond the gravitational pull of the earth; still others believe that approximately 120 miles from the earth, where appreciable friction from passage through the atmosphere disappears, is where functional space begins [31]. In any event, space is the area through which man hopes to travel to reach other planets. Table 17.1, showing problems of space flight to be overcome at various altitudes, gives some clues as to the nature of space.

Space is often referred to as a void, but in actuality it is composed of matter and energy: meteoroids of all sizes;

dust particles—neutral and electrically charged; molecules and atoms, i.e., corpuscular particles, mostly hydrogen—neutral and charged; electromagnetic radiation—X rays, ultraviolet, infrared, and radio; magnetic field forces; and gravitational field forces. This space environment is never uniform but fluctuates with time. Meteoroids, described as orbits of disintegrated comets, are usually concentrated in streams in space. In addition, charged particles that crisscross space are found to be concentrated in magnetic fields, such as the Van Allen belt. This double layer, or zone, of radiation encircles the earth, but apparently some pathways through the radiation areas are safer than others. The inner belt extends from approximately 1,400 to 3,400 miles above the earth's surface, with the peak intensity somewhere near 2,400 miles. The outer layer extends from approximately 8,000 to 12,000 miles out from the earth, with peak intensity at about 10,000 miles [20]. The two zones were named after Dr. James Van Allen, planner of the satellite radiation research program. Findings from the NERV (nuclear emulsion recovery vehicle) indicate that there are more low-energy protons in the lower Van Allen belt than was originally believed. Table 17.2 shows the radiation dose from the two belts along with other information on radiation [19, 32].

Solar radiation also shows tremendous differences, depending upon distance from the sun. In addition, there are occasional variations as the sun emits huge jet streams of solar plasma and the radiation intensity increases [32]. K. A. Anderson has developed prediction

Table 17.1 Problems of space flight

Altitude	Problem
600 miles	(limit of the atmosphere)
400,000 feet	Darkness of space
	Silence of space
	Weightlessness
140,000 feet	Ultraviolet radiation
120,000 feet	Cosmic radiation
63,000 feet	"Boiling" of body fluids
50,000 feet	Anoxia
23,000 feet	Aeroembolism
0 feet	(sea level)

Source: David G. Simon: "Space Medicine," *Therapeutic Notes*, 65:174, July-August, 1958. Courtesy of Parke, Davis and Company.

theories regarding solar protons activities that are so accurate that undue exposure could be avoided by good timing. This is significant because inadequate knowledge of the biological effects of protons from solar flare is one of the most serious deficiencies blocking extended manned flight into space [21].

Strughold, in a discussion of space, gives the following description: [1]

Interplanetary space itself is an extremely hard vacuum. It contains about 16 atoms of matter, mostly hydrogen, per cubic inch and about one dust particle per 10 cubic yards. It also contains some meteoric material, electromagnetic rays, and, from the sun and galaxies, particle rays made up of fragments of atoms.

Additional information is being accumulated as unmanned vehicles explore space and either send or bring back data. In the next few years, as man himself ventures further out into space, a great deal more will be learned about this new medium.

Potential health problems in space

WEIGHTLESSNESS

Careful study indicates that weightlessness in itself is harmless. Nevertheless, it does pose problems for man in space,

and the possible danger associated with readjustment to body weight after long periods of time under conditions of no

[1] Hubertus Strughold, "The Challenge of Medicine in the Space Age," *Today's Health*, published by American Medical Association, 38:39, March, 1960.

Successful space travel by man is preceded by extensive testing of the space vehicle in both unmanned flights and in static tests.

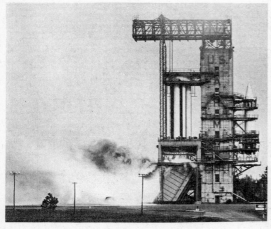

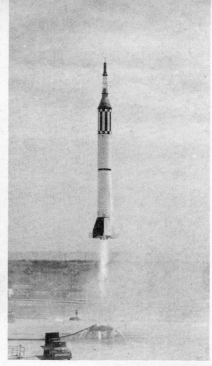

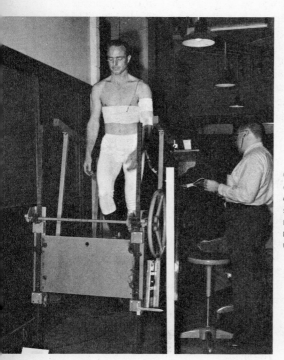

Careful selection and preparation of the space traveler, or astronaut, includes stress testing on a treadmill and testing to determine ability to function under the stress of heat.

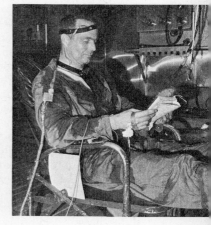

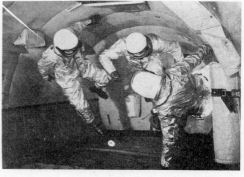

The astronaut is also exposed to conditions of weightlessness under controlled circumstances to determine his reaction to this unusual state.

gravitational pull is not yet well understood. The problems of weightlessness differ in short manned flights in which man is maintained in position and in long flights or in artificial satellites where he must be free to move about in the space vehicle. The successful orbital flights of Glenn, Gagarin, and Titov and the suborbital flights of Shepard and Grissom showed that for periods of time up to a day weightlessness is not a serious problem.

Some aspects of weightlessness are best described by one who has experienced them. An astronaut, in a discussion of tests during weightlessness, related how his attempt to press on a screwdriver to force a screw into the wall resulted in his being pushed backward across the room. His attempt to turn a bolt on the wall resulted in his going head over heels while the monkey wrench and bolt stayed still. The astronaut also indicated that after completing two short periods (a few minutes) of *g* pull testing in a centrifuge he fell asleep while reading— the same effect as a full day's work in a few minutes [17].

Handling food in a state of weightlessness provides problems. Utensils float in space and liquids under zero *g*'s break up into droplets and cannot be poured. Danger of inhaling the droplets and food particles is greatly increased.

Studies of weightlessness are providing new information on blood flow and on action of the bladder. More detailed studies of receptor organs of the central nervous system, particularly portions of the inner ear and the skin, extend studies of weightlessness. Reference to the nerve endings as *gravireceptors* and the related reflexes as *gravireflexes* has been suggested.

A series of studies conducted by the Air Force, Army-Navy, the U.S.S.R., von Beckh, and MIA (Mouse in Able) indicate that stresses due to acceleration and episodes of weightlessness encountered in aircraft and in biological missile flights were well within tolerance range of both human and animal organisms. Prolonged and fluctuating tachycardia (rapid heartbeat) was observed in early states of weightlessness, and decreased cardiac activity was noted later. This would seem to indicate a functional adaptation of the heart to decreased mechanical load under weightlessness [7].

PRESSURE AND TEMPERATURE

Because the atmosphere diminishes as man travels away from the earth, pressure becomes a problem. Rapid movement into thinner atmosphere can cause *aeroembolism*, in which nitrogen comes out of solution and forms bubbles in the blood and body fluids. As the air becomes thinner, man is unable to make use of oxygen available in the air because of insufficient pressure. Air pressure at sea level is 14.7 pounds per square inch; at 35,000 feet it drops to 3.4 pounds per square inch, and at 60,000 feet to 1 pound per square inch. Man cannot survive above 45,000 feet without an artificially pressurized environment [32].

If the air pressure, which can be readily controlled with equipment now available, was to decrease suddenly in a space vehicle, due either to a structural failure or to a collision with a meteoroid, man would perish in a few seconds, unless he was wearing a full-pressure space suit. Unless repairs could be made in the hull of the vehicle, the pressure suit would not protect him indefinitely in space.

Temperature control is likewise a problem due to the extremely high temperatures generated when a space vehicle must reenter the atmosphere at very high velocity. It is estimated that speeds as high as 25,000 miles per hour will be reached by vehicles returning from other planets. Fortunately, there are some effective ways to relieve the heat problem. The blunt nose of the Mercury capsule, for example, creates a shock wave, which diverts about 99 per cent of the heat energy and furnishes about 98 per cent of the decelerating force; and new ablation materials reduce the temperature to a level that the astronaut can tolerate [1, 3].

OXYGEN AND CARBON DIOXIDE SUPPLY

Man cannot survive without oxygen and with too much carbon dioxide. In space travel, therefore, it is necessary to provide an oxygen supply artificially and to limit the accumulation of carbon dioxide. Some potentially feasible plans have been developed, but experimentation is continuing.

For short space flights the problem is relatively simple. Oxygen under pressure can be carried in sufficient quantity to meet the needs of the individual without adding excessive weight, and chemicals can be used to absorb carbon dioxide. For longer flights out into space the problem becomes much more complicated.

Chemical sources of oxygen and means of eliminating carbon dioxide fall under two categories. *Demand chemicals,* such as alkali and alkaline peroxides, superoxides, and ozonides, release oxygen when they react with water or carbon dioxide. They provide a means of making the oxygen supply self-regulating because the waste carbon dioxide is used up in the reaction that releases oxygen. *Controlled-supply chemicals,* such as the sodium chlorate candle, which burns to supply oxygen, are the second possible source. Combinations of the two, with demand chemicals serving for most purposes but controlled-supply chemicals available for emergency, are a distinct possibility. One major drawback to chemicals of this type as the source of oxygen is the weight of chemicals and the space required for storage for long trips [5].

Experimentation suggests that a closed-circuit system may be part of the food supply plan as well as providing for elimination of human waste. Experiments with a closed-circuit system in which algae uses man's carbon dioxide and releases oxygen into the air offers a great deal of hope. Man has survived without ill effects for more than twenty-four hours in such a closed-circuit system. It is possible that the algae could also serve as the primary source of food for man, or for an animal that man could eat, and that his waste material could be processed to serve as the source of nourishment for the algae. The sun, when available, could be a source of energy for the system. Otherwise a nuclear power plant might serve the purpose [32, 37].

MEETING NUTRITIONAL NEEDS

Meeting nutritional needs of people on the earth has its complications. Doing so in space has many more. Procedures must be developed for concentrating food to save space, packaging to reduce weight, and at the same time facilitating use in a state of weightlessness and producing food in the limited space of the vehicle. The estimated requirements of food per man per day soon adds up to a sizable amount for a long period of time. More effective processing and packaging could reduce the weight of the food needed.

Some of the projects under way to solve the problem of food supply include making use of algae, dehydration of foods, new packaging procedures, and making synthetic foods that will meet nutritional needs.

The algae system is reasonably feasible except that this would mean a single-food diet of food that at present is not highly palatable. Psychological aspects of food but a few steps removed from one's own waste are not known, and acceptability by the crew for prolonged periods is questionable. Algae are a potentially nourishing food in that they are approximately 50 per cent protein, 15 per cent carbohydrate, 25 per cent fat, and 10 per cent ash, and they supply some B vitamins, carotene, and ascorbic acid [37].

As a result of studies in food packaging, it is suggested that perhaps squeeze tubes made of aluminum, which have been most successful in tests, may solve the problem of feeding during weightlessness. Procedures for feeding the traveler during prolonged space trips have not yet been successfully resolved.

If food and water are carried in the vehicle, it is suggested that the water be carried as ice, primarily because of the problem of containers. Containers for water would need to be watertight and strong enough to withstand high-acceleration stresses, whereas ice could be enclosed in lightweight plastic [23].

A possible solution for water supply is a recycling system. One such system developed by the General Electric Space Sciences Laboratory requires only one day's supply of water and oxygen and is recycled endlessly from man's metabolic waste. One subject was tested six days in 1960 on this recycling system and suffered no ill effects from his experience. Tests showed that the water recovered is as palatable, or more so, than that of many cities. Water in the cabin is also retrieved by use of lithium chloride desiccant or by dew-point condensation or freezing. A system for eliminating carbon dioxide and producing oxygen is also part of the recycling system [13]. In a sealed cabin experiment reported in 1961, two men used a combination of stored water and recycled water (from urine, wash water, and water from atmosphere) for a 30-day period without ill effects [36].

ELIMINATION OF BODY WASTES

Closely allied with the problems of feeding the space traveler and providing him with oxygen is the need to remove excess carbon dioxide and dispose of human waste material. The problem of carbon dioxide control was discussed earlier. One suggestion for the elimination of human waste was indicated in the discussion of the closed system using algae, in which the waste would be used as a source of nourishment for the plants.

Other possibilities suggested for elimination of waste material are to send it back to earth by a service vehicle (if orbiting satellites or space stations are developed and can be serviced) or shoot it out into space. One possible disadvantage of the latter proposal is the requirement for fuel to eject the container with the waste material. It appears that some system of using the waste effectively is most logical for closed-vehicle travel for prolonged periods, although waste could be stored in space formerly occupied by food if food is carried and not produced on board.

ACCELERATION AND REENTRY

Normal g pull refers to the pull of the earth's gravity on a human body; the force of this pull is equal to the weight of the body. When a body experiences a g pull greater than 1, the force exerted on the body is equal to the g pull times the weight of the body. Both the strength of the g pull and its duration are important to the health of the astronaut because of the powerful forces exerted on his internal organs.

The effect of the force of gravity can be modified greatly by the clothing and type of seat prepared for the astronaut. The g-load tolerance can be increased by several hundred per cent by improved seats, which are available. John MacDonald, of the Wright Air Development Division, makes this comparison: [2]

On an ordinary seat, a pilot begins having visionary trouble at about four times gravity. With a g suit on, the pilot can withstand a force up to 8 times gravity for a few seconds before blacking out. Sitting in our new seat, however, just about anyone with normal health can ride in shirtsleeve comfort at

[2] Louis Chester, "A Machine to Fit the Man," *Space World*, 1:50, January, 1961.

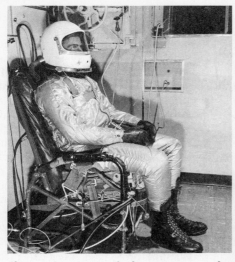
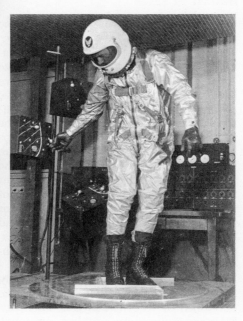

The environment of the space traveler makes it necessary to provide him with a space suit which offers protection against such hazards as pressure changes and at the same time enables him to perform required duties.

about twelve times gravity, and a trained rider can withstand 17 *g*'s and still turn out useful work without fear of blackout.

Extensive tests on the effect of acceleration indicate that man, with proper equipment, can tolerate without serious consequences the stresses due to acceleration and reentry; the flights of Shepard, Gagarin, and others proved this [34].

OTHER FORMS OF LIFE

Scientists are concerned about microorganisms from the earth seriously contaminating the planets before evidence is conclusive concerning life on these planets. They are likewise concerned with the threat of probes returning from space with organisms dangerous to life on the earth.

Officials of the National Aeronautics and Space Administration expressed fear, for example, that a Soviet probe might contaminate Venus if the vehicle was not sterilized. They are concerned that contamination might render the planet useless for further study in search of extraterrestrial life, that organisms might multiply and make it impossible to determine forms of life that originally existed on the planet, or that organisms might thrive and eliminate native life [12].

Sterilization of vehicles is being studied and conducted on the basis of radiation procedures, the use of heat, and the use of chemicals. A combination of the three may be the best solution. Ethylene oxide used in a plastic bag enveloping the space vehicle appeared to be most effective procedure available early in 1961. It has been pointed out that potential contamination from the surface of a space vehicle is relatively minor compared with potential contamination in the intestines and organs of animals. Experiments at the Walter Reed Army Institute of Research to raise germ-free animals may provide an answer to this problem. From the standpoint of contamination being brought back to the earth, the National Aeronautics and Space Administration has been working on a project to develop a means of sterilizing returning space vehicles by means of a built-in antiseptic factor [12].

Interest in possible life on other planets has been heightened by the successful growth of soil bacteria in laboratory containers simulating conditions on Mars [32].

ADJUSTING TO DAILY RHYTHMS

Man, accustomed to night and day on the earth, will find that life in space is different. It has been suggested that space travelers may work more effectively and sleep better if the 24-hour cycle is discarded and longer rhythms are established. On the basis of experiments with longer rhythms, it has been found that there is a greater range in body temperature and a greater degree of alertness as well as more effective relaxation [24].

Simulated tests of six men for a seven-day period in a two-compartment chamber with definitely assigned tasks during the confinement have illustrated the adaptability of the human and resulted in recommendations that routine tasks be made more complex so that they require a higher level of behavior [15]. More evidence is needed to clarify the work-eat-sleep-rest cycle of the man in space.

VISION PROBLEMS

Early flights into space by the astronauts posed some vision problems against which future space travelers must be protected. Among these are a hindering of aerial perspective due to the lack of dust particles beyond the earth's atmosphere, which interferes with the scattering of light; temporary nearsightedness, which causes visual disturbance; and the effect of gravitational forces on eyesight due to reduction in the blood supply to the eye [30]. The danger to vision posed by radiation is discussed later.

RADIATION HAZARDS

Radiation hazards are one of the more recent serious health problems of man because of the increased amount of exposure to radioactivity through diagnostic and therapeutic uses of X rays and radioactive substances (which are essential); through atomic tests and the resultant fallout; through nuclear power plants, in use and planned; and through projected travel into space with its radiation hazards. This discussion concerns nuclear power plants in space travel and

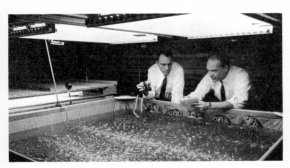

Experiments are being conducted to determine the most effective means of converting human waste to drinking water and providing a medium for growing food such as algae to sustain the space traveler on long trips for which adequate storage space for food and water is unavailable.

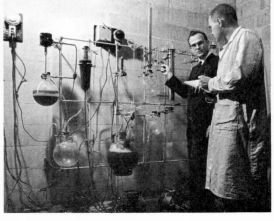

the radiation in space through which vehicles must travel.

Connor aptly stated the problem: [3]

As with almost every previous instrument of cultural advancement, nuclear power brings an attendant price. This price may be met by: man's absorbing large (and therefore unacceptable) amounts of ionizing radiation; or completely shielding and containing all radiation sources (and thereby negating their usefulness); or adopting a compromise whereby an acceptable, biologically insignificant amount of radiation may be tolerated while deriving the manifest benefits of this revolutionary source of energy.

Connor was optimistic in his appraisal of the attendant risks, as he judged them to be no more, or perhaps less, than the risks associated with the progressive development of electric power, the airplane, the automobile, or even fire [9].

Effects of radiation. Radiation hazards to human beings fall into two categories. The potential dangers are *genetic* or *somatic*. In either case the damage is to individual cells. It is considered that there is no threshold level for genetic effect. The least exposure will cause some genetic effect, and this is undesirable because of possible mutations [22]. It was noted in Chapter 14 that man has been exposed to some natural radiation since the beginning of time. This should dispel undue alarm about relatively small exposures but at the same time should suggest caution about long-range genetic effects.

The amount of radiation an individual can tolerate without serious somatic effect is more clearly understood, although much remains to be learned. It is apparent that damage to cells is dependent upon the radiation dose and the specific tissues involved. Cells most vulnerable are those with relatively small amounts of cytoplasm and those in process of multiplying most rapidly. The blood-forming tissues of the bone marrow, tissues of the reproductive system and embryonic tissue are examples of the most vulnerable cells [18].

It should be noted that the passage of ionizing radiations through the body are not felt by the individual, even though the dose may be lethal. The damage is due to ejection of electrons from atoms through which the ionizing radiation passes. The molecule containing the ionized atom undergoes change. It is the chemical change, which occurs as a result of ionization, that produces biological effects. The ions (atoms positively charged) produced and the way they are distributed in cells determine the damage [22].

When an astronaut reaches space beyond the light-scattering region of the earth's atmosphere, the sun will appear as a brilliant disk in a field of blackness. Adjusting to the brilliance after looking into darkness may cause severe retinal damage to the eye. It has been estimated that ten seconds' exposure to solar radiation at a point just beyond the earth's atmosphere will result in retinal burn. The size of the burn will increase as one approaches the sun, but the critical time of exposure will be approximately the same [33].

Protection for the astronaut is essential. It is likely to be accomplished by means of light-absorbing glasses with automatically adjusting attenuation, by retractable light-scattering visors, by light-scattering ceilings, and by education regarding solar hazards [33].

Radiation in space. The radiation in space that appears to be a problem to the traveler comes from the sun or from cosmic rays. The sun emits light rays, heat rays, and X rays, which in outer space, beyond the protection of the atmosphere, must be considered as a serious threat to man unless protection is

[3] Joseph A. Connor, "Aerospace Nuclear Safety," *Aerospace Medicine*, 31:805, October, 1960.

Table 17.2   Maximum allowable radiation doses and some typical levels

	Roentgens
Maximum per week	0.3
Maximum per quarter	3
Maximum annual	5
Maximum emergency	25
Normal sea-level background	0.001 per day
Normal interplanetary space	5–12 per year
Heart of inner belt	24 per hour
Heart of outer belt	200 per hour
Solar flare	10–1,000 per hour
Total for flare	2–4,000

Source: Jay Holmes: "NERV Data Alters Thinking on Shields," *Missiles and Rockets*, 8:29, Feb. 20, 1961.

provided. Cosmic rays also pose a serious threat to man in outer space. Included in the cosmic rays are alpha particles, heavier nuclei, protons, and hydrogen nuclei. The effect of primary rays on matter can be devastating.

In the earlier discussion of space, the higher concentration of radiation danger in the Van Allen belts was discussed. Prolonged exposure in the areas of greatest concentration of these belts would present serious problems in protecting a space traveler. Experimental flights of animals through these belts has indicated that the radiation danger can be reduced by limiting time of transit and selecting safer paths through the belts.

Protection from radiation. One approach to radiation protection has been research to discover protective drugs to reduce the biological effects of radiation. With animals, drugs have cut in half the damage from radiation doses up to 400 roentgens. The damage-reducing pills being used experimentally with humans at the Walter Reed Army Institute of Research have been derived from protein-bonding materials, which are readily available in nature. The drugs used in early experiments protected only from gamma rays and protons [11]. Further research with drugs is under way, and other means of reducing damage are being considered.

In addition to protecting the individual who is actually exposed to radiation, extensive research has been directed at means of shielding, or preventing the rays from reaching the individual. Ultraviolet rays can be absorbed by materials used for space suits and the hulls of vehicles.

Effective shielding will be required, on the basis of present thinking, to protect solar cells and electronic components as well as the human occupants. There is some evidence, however, that heavy shielding may even be harmful in some instances. In trips of less than fifty hours it may be better to allow radiation to pass through the individual's body rather than have the primary radiation stop in his body and/or permit him to be exposed to secondary radiation produced [6].

The extent and the type of shielding depends upon the type of radiation. A thin layer of lead is effective against X rays, a thin layer of shielding will stop high-energy electrons, protons require a heavier layer of shielding, and aluminum may be more effective for solar flares. High-energy protons, more prevalent during solar flares, interact with lead and gold and create X rays that can be harmful. It is suggested that the best shielding in the outer Van Allen belt might be a light layer of material to stop electrons with a thin layer of lead on the inside to stop X rays [6, 19].

Another suggestion is magnetic shielding. With the possibility of solar power and nuclear auxiliary power showing promise, the idea of developing a magnetic shield around the space vehicle to deflect energy particles in much the same way that the magnetic field shields the earth is receiving considerable attention [21].

Testing living human cells and animals

in unmanned flights into space furnishes additional information to those planning for long-range space flights by man.

Radiation, with many unanswered questions, is a major obstacle in interplanetary space travel plans.

Space equipment and health

The vehicle that takes a man into space and the suit he wears illustrate a new man-machine complex in which the vehicle and clothing are designed to protect the occupant to the utmost instead of forcing the human to adapt to the machine. This new human-factor engineering is a departure from considering how much radiation a man can take to considering how to protect him from radiation; from considering how much sudden acceleration man can stand to considering how to propel the vehicle within the occupant's normal limits; and from considering how much temperature he can withstand to considering how to develop a temperature level he can tolerate [8].

The U.S. Navy's Mark IV full-pressure suit for use by Alan Shepard, the first American astronaut, is an example. This suit, weighing approximately 20 pounds, was designed to protect individuals at altitudes above 45,000 feet from the effects of low ambient pressure as well as rapid or slow decompression of pressurized chambers. In tests wearing this suit a man survived 7 hours at temperatures lower than —60°F without suffering physical discomfort. The suit not only protects; it also enables the individual to carry on required functions. Under full pressure an individual is able to pick a tiny straight pin off the floor [29].

Vehicles must do more than take an occupant to the selected destination; it must also protect his health and maintain his ability to function effectively. Progress is being made in developing vehicles that will take a man to distant places in the world of space and bring him back as healthy as when he departed.

The astronauts

The selection of the group of astronauts from which the passenger in the first American manned space flight was chosen involved, among other criteria, a thorough check on health. From the original list of 100 pilots who met general qualifications, 69 were interviewed and 80 per cent of the group volunteered for the assignment. Thirty-two volunteers were tested extensively, and seven were finally selected. After thorough preparations and further testing, three among the seven were named for consideration as the first man in space. The first astronaut, Commander Alan B. Shepard, Jr., U.S.N., met all the demands most successfully.

Included in the screening of the thirty-two volunteers was a seven-day and three-night medical check including X-ray examination of almost every part of the body. Sperm cells were collected and studied in order to establish base lines for assessing the threat to fertility of cosmic radiation as a result of space travel. Also included in the screening were tests for claustrophobia, isolation, and stress (acceleration, humidity, pressure breathing, immersion of feet in ice water, reaction under extremely high altitude), psychological and psychiatric tests, simulated flight tests, and equilibrium tests [2, 10, 25].

The seven astronauts who were finally

selected underwent further tests to determine their ability to perform under stress conditions. The stress loads they were subjected to included those listed below [28]:

ACCELERATION. A maximum of 18 g's with light profiles flown to 16 g's to simulate abort—time above 4 g's was limited to about ninety seconds.

WEIGHTLESS FLIGHT. An average of thirty minutes with a sixty-second experience at zero g's on each flight and free-floating experience in fifteen-second flights.

REDUCED PRESSURE. In full pressure suit to simulated 65,000 feet altitude at 5 pounds per square inch.

HEAT. For ninety minutes at 105°F and 40 per cent humidity and 85°F and 85 per cent humidity.

DISORIENTATION. An average total experience of thirty minutes in the Navy's disorientation room at Pensacola.

TUMBLING EXPERIENCE. At the Lewis Research Center in the multiple-axis test facility up to 54 cycles per minute of random tumbling to simulate capsule tumbling.

CARBON DIOXIDE INCREASE. To simulate malfunction of the environment the normal 0.3 per cent earth environment was increased to 3 per cent over a four-hour exposure with no observable effects.

NOISE AND VIBRATION EXPOSURE. Up to 140 decibels as compared with an anticipated 105 to 110 decibels in the Mercury capsule.

Health was an important criterion in selecting the astronauts for manned space flight. The effectiveness of the selection procedures has been demonstrated by the success of Shepard, Grissom, and Glenn in withstanding the stresses to which they were exposed. The orbital flight of astronaut John H. Glenn, Jr., which lasted nearly five hours, illustrated dramatically the ability of man to maintain a high level of health and to function efficiently in space.

Space medicine

Space medicine (aerospace medicine), along with human-factor engineering, space nutrition, astromicrobiology, bio-astronautics, and other new fields of scientific endeavor, has made remarkable progress during the few years of its existence. It has been said that the end of traditional therapeutic medicine is approaching and that an era of true constructive and preventive medicine is being entered, with the Space Age providing impetus for the change.

The current task of getting patients well enough to go back to their work takes up so much of the physician's time that he can devote little time to preventive medicine. When medicine improves to the point where evaluations of the dynamic response of the body and mind to total stress situations can be made with speed and accuracy through sure and simple tests, then preventive medicine will have arrived [14]. Space medicine studies will speed its arrival.

Space medicine is concerned with the health of individuals in situations where many stresses are not yet clearly understood. In the process of determining both the stress situations and the means of protecting individuals from them, space medicine is making many contributions to medical care for those of us who are earth-bound as well as the potential space travelers. The future health status of man appears to be much more favorable as a result of the research that has been and is being conducted to protect man in space flight.

Summary

Health problems of man in space present a new frontier in the everlasting struggle to develop and maintain optimum health. Man has not yet solved many of the health problems that confront him on earth, and yet he is discovering new problems through his explorations of space. At the same time he is resolving problems related to space travel and applying some of his findings to improve health conditions on earth.

Among the problems receiving the attention of research workers are weightlessness, extreme pressure and temperature variations, oxygen supply and carbon dioxide control in a sealed cabin, meeting nutritional needs within the limitations of the space vehicle, exposure to solar and cosmic radiation, rapid acceleration and deceleration and the resultant gravitational pull exerted on the space traveler, unknown forms of life that may exist on other planets, psychological factors associated with confinement in a space vehicle for long periods of time, and adapting to a new daily work-eat-sleep-rest cycle in place of day and night as we know it to be on earth.

The successful orbital flights of Glenn, Gagarin, and Titov and the suborbital flights of Shepard and Grissom demonstrated that man is able to function efficiently in a limited venture into space. Human factor engineering in the preparation of machines and equipment enabled man to make these early explorations safely. The thorough appraisal of the potential astronauts' health status as a basis for selection as an astronaut reemphasizes the importance of health.

Few individuals alive today are likely to become space travelers, but many of us may owe our lives and well-being to new information about developing and maintaining health discovered as a result of research related to space travel. Space medicine is a new area of specialization that offers hope that man will someday more effectively control factors enabling him to achieve a personally satisfying and socially useful life.

Suggested readings

1. Arnheim, Wolf: "The Problem of Re-entry," *Space World,* 1:29–31, January, 1961.
2. "Astronauts: How Seven Were Chosen," *Newsweek,* 53:64–65, Apr. 20, 1959.
3. Becker, John V.: "Re-entry from Space," *Scientific American,* 204:49–57, January, 1961.
4. Benson, Otis O., Jr., and Hubertus Strughold: *Physics and Medicine of the Atmosphere and Space,* John Wiley & Sons, Inc., New York, 1960.
5. Bovard, Robert M.: "Oxygen Sources for Space Flights," *Aerospace Medicine,* 31:407–412, May, 1960.
6. Bulban, Erwin J.: "Anti-radiation Shielding May Be Reduced," *Aviation Week,* 74:40–41, Jan. 2, 1961.
7. Burch, George E., and Siegfried J. Gerathewohl: "Observations on Heart Rate and Cardiodynamics during Weightlessness," *Aerospace Medicine,* 31:661–669, August, 1960.
8. Chester, Louis: "A Machine to Fit the Man," *Space World,* 1:14–16, January, 1961.
9. Connor, Joseph A.: "Aerospace Nuclear Safety," *Aerospace Medicine,* 31:797–806, October, 1960.
10. Cooley, Donald: "Man in Space," *Today's Health,* 36:31–37, May, 1958.
11. David, Heather: "Drugs May Halve Radiation Damage," *Missiles and Rockets,* 7:39–40, Sept. 26, 1960.
12. David, Heather: "Experts Fear Venus Contamination," *Missiles and Rockets,* 8:30, Feb. 20, 1961.
13. David, Heather: "Endless Recycling of Water and Oxygen," *Missiles and Rockets,* 8:22–24, Mar. 31, 1961.

14. Flickinger, Donald D.: "From Outer Space: New Concepts in Medicine," *Today's Health,* 37:50–55, September, 1959.

15. Hanna, Thomas D., and John Gaito: "Performance and Habitability Aspects of Extended Confinement in Sealed Cabins," *Aerospace Medicine,* 31:399–406, May, 1960.

16. Hanrahan, James Stephen, and David Bushnell: *Space Biology: The Human Factors in Space Flight,* Basic Books, Inc., New York, 1960.

17. Henry, Frank: "The Life of the Astronauts," *Science Digest,* 47:38–43, January, 1960.

18. Hollander, Alexander, and George E. Stapleton: "Ionizing Radiation and the Living Cell," *Scientific American,* 201: 94–100, September, 1959.

19. Holmes, Jay: "NERV Data Alters Thinking on Shields," *Missiles and Rockets,* 8:28–29, Feb. 20, 1961.

20. Kinney, William A.: *Medical Science and Space Travel,* Franklin Watts, Inc., New York, 1959.

21. Kolcum, Edward H.: "Apollo Will Avoid Solar Radiation Hazards," *Aviation Week,* 74:32–33, Jan. 9, 1961.

22. Konecci, Eugene B., and Robert Trapp: "Calculations of the Radiobiologic Risk Factors in Nuclear-powered Space Vehicles," *Aerospace Medicine,* 30:487–506, July, 1959.

23. Ley, Willie: "Living in Orbit," *Space World,* 1:21–23, January, 1961.

24. "Longer Days Proposed for Space Travelers," *Science News Letter,* 77:382, June 11, 1960.

25. Pape, Max A.: "Man in Space," *Health Education Journal,* 24:14–16, March, 1961.

26. "Planned for Space Risks," *Science News Letter,* 79:373, June 17, 1961.

27. "Progress in Missiles Has Advanced Medicine," *Science News Letter,* 78:312, Nov. 12, 1960.

28. "Project Mercury Stress Data Emphasizes Pilot's Active Role," *Aviation Week,* 74:91, Jan. 30, 1961.

29. Rublowsky, John: "Dress for Space," *Space World,* 1:24–27, January, 1961.

30. "Sight Protection Major Problem for Space Travel," *Wise Owl News,* National Society for the Prevention of Blindness, No. 40, Winter, 1961.

31. Simon, David G.: "Space Medicine," *Therapeutic Notes,* 65:174–177, July-August, 1958.

32. Strughold, Hubertus: "The Challenge of Medicine in the Space Age," *Today's Health,* 38:36–41, March, 1960.

33. Strughold, Hubertus, and Oskar L. Ritter: "Eye Hazards and Protection in Space," *Aerospace Medicine,* 31:670–673, August, 1960.

34. "U.S. Spaceman A-okay," *Science News Letter,* 799:307, May 20, 1961.

35. Warren, Shields: "Ionizing Radiation and Medicine," *Scientific American,* 201:165–176, September, 1959.

36. Welch, B. E.: "Sealed Cabin Experimentation," Review of January, 1961, Lectures in Aerospace Medicine at the USAF School of Aviation Medicine, by E. B. Konecci, Missiles and Space Systems Engineering, Douglas Aircraft Company, Santa Monica, Calif., Feb. 13, 1961.

37. "What Will Spacemen Eat," *Science Digest,* 47:80–84, January, 1960.

IN CONCLUSION

MENS SANA IN CORPORE SANO IN SOCIETATE SANA

GLOSSARY

Accident-prone. Tending to have accidents.

Acetylcholine. An acid which is present in many parts of the body. It may assist in nerve impulses crossing a synapse.

Acne. An inflammation of the sebaceous glands which occurs frequently on the face, neck, chest, and back of young people.

ACTH. The adrenocorticotropic hormone from the anterior pituitary. It stimulates the adrenal cortex to secrete its entire set of hormones.

Adjustment. The attainment of a satisfactory relationship between the individual and his environment and/or between his needs and his desires; meeting the demands of a situation.

Adjustment, therapeutic. Chiropractic adjustment including manipulation and treatment of the spinal column to restore normal function of the nervous system.

Adulteration. The addition of inferior substances to foods or drugs illegally, with a resultant reduction in quality of the product.

Aeroembolism. A condition produced by a rapid decrease of pressure and characterized by the formation of nitrogen bubbles in the blood and body tissues.

Agglutination. The clumping together of cells in a suspension by action of a specific antibody.

Alcohol addict. A person with an uncontrolled desire for beverage alcohol.

Alcoholic addiction. Uncontrolled consumption of beverage alcohol.

Allergen. Any agent capable of producing an allergic reaction.

Amblyopia. A dimness of vision.

Amino acids. The basic constituents of proteins.

Analgesic. A substance that relieves pain.

Anemia. A condition resulting from decrease in normal blood volume due to hemorrhage or to a deficiency in the number of red cells or in the amount of hemoglobin.

Antibody. A specific chemical protective substance formed in the body in response to the stimulation of an antigen.

Antigen. A substance, usually a foreign protein, which when introduced into the body stimulates the production of specific antibodies; an antibody-generator.

Antiseptic. A substance that will prevent the growth of microorganisms without necessarily destroying them.

Appraisal. An accurate determination of values; the synthesizing and interpreting of data.

Arteriosclerosis. Thickening of the inner lining of the arteries which causes loss of ability to expand and contract.

Artificial respiration. A substitution for natural breathing.

Aseptic. Completely free from infectious material.

Astigmatism. A defect of the refractive surface of the eye which distorts light rays so that they cannot focus at a single point on the retina.

Atherosclerosis. A type of arteriosclerosis characterized by the deposit of fatty materials along the inner lining of the arteries.

Atrium. The chamber of the heart which receives blood from the veins.

Attenuation. The weakening of the toxicity or virulence of a disease-producing organism.

Auditory acuity. Keenness of hearing; usually measured by an audiometer.

Ballistocardiogram. A device for recording the stroke volume of the heart and means of determining the cardiac output.

Barbiturate. A salt of barbituric acid which produces sleep.

BCG. Bacillus Calmette-Guérin or the vaccine prepared from this organism. An immunization against tuberculosis.

Behavior. The observable external responses of an individual such as knowledge, attitudes, and practices.

Behavior, health. All observable health activities in terms of the individual's knowledge, attitudes, and practices.

Benign tumor. A tumor or growth which is not malignant.

Blackhead. Dried waste products in the pore of the skin.

Bromide. A sedative.

Buerger's disease. A serious disease of the blood vessels of the extremities. It may lead to gangrene.

Caffeine. An alkaloid found in coffee, tea, cola beverages, and maté. It is a stimulant to the heart and the nervous system.

Calorie (large calorie). The amount of heat required to raise the temperature of 1 kilogram of water from 0° to 1° centigrade.

Carbohydrate. An organic substance belonging to the class of compounds represented by sugars, dextrins, starches, and celluloses.

Carcinogen. Any cancer-producing substance or agent.

Cardiovascular. Pertaining to the heart and the blood vessels.

Carrier. An individual who harbors and may transmit pathogenic organisms but shows no symptoms of disease.

Cataract. A condition in which the crystalline eye lens or its capsule loses transparency.

Cerumen. Earwax; a secretion from glands in the outer auditory canal of the ear.

Cervix. The narrow end of the uterus; the part which connects with the vagina.

Cholesterol. A fatty substance found in all animal fats and oils.

Chromosomes. Segments within the reproductive cell which transmit hereditary traits.

Chronic alcoholism. A state in which an individual is not able to control his desire for alcoholic beverages.

Chronic disease. A disease which persists but is not communicable.

Circumcision. Surgery to free the foreskin of the penis.

Cirrhosis. A fibrosis caused by the excessive formation of connective tissue.

Collateral circulation. Secondary or accessory circulation which may result when primary blood circulation is impaired.

Colorblindness. Inability to distinguish differences of color.

Communicable disease. A disease transmissible from person to person, either directly or indirectly.

Community. A group of people living in a given area under the same unit of government who have organized to meet common interests and problems.

Community health council. A fact-finding, problem-solving, coordinating body composed of representatives from various health agencies and organizations welded into one group working for better community health.

Community organization. The process of welding together individuals and groups of one area into a single group with a common purpose of identifying and meeting local needs.

Compulsory medical care. A plan to provide medical care for all people, required by law and administered by state or national government. Payment for services would be deducted from salaries or paid by taxes. The English medical-care system is an example.

Conception. The impregnation of the ovum by the sperm.

Conflict. The simultaneous presence of opposing impulses, desires, or tendencies.

Congenital. Existing at birth.

Constitutional Theory of Personality. Sheldon's theory that temperament and physical constitution are correlated.

Consumer health. The part of health or health education concerned with health products, health services (including medical care), and scientific health information.

Contact lenses. A thin curved shell of plastic or of glass fitted to the front of the eyeball for the purpose of correcting refractive errors.

Convalescence. The gradual recovery of health from illness, accident, or surgery.

Cosmetic. A preparation for beautifying or conditioning the complexion.

Cosmic radiation. Extremely high energy radiation consisting of both particles and rays which originate in space and bombard the earth.

Dental caries, tooth decay. A disease process that destroys the structure of the teeth, thus producing cavities.

Dental plaques. Gelatinlike material that clings to the teeth and affords protection for bacteria.

Dentifrice. A preparation—powder, paste, or liquid—used for cleaning the teeth.

Deodorant. A substance which has the power to mask or destroy an odor.

Depilatory. A preparation used to remove unwanted hair from the body.

Depressant drug. A drug which when taken internally reduces functional activity and vital energies of the body.

Deterrent. That which deters or prevents action.

Diabetic coma. The result of an excess amount of sugar in the blood stream due to lack of insulin.

Diastolic pressure. Lowest blood pressure recorded when the ventricle of the heart is relaxed and dilated.

Digestion. The process of converting food into substances which the body can assimilate.

Disease agent. An organism causing disease.

Diuretic. An agent which increases the volume of urine.

Dynamics. Moving moral or physical forces of any kind.

Dysmenorrhea. Painful or difficult menstruation.

Ectomorph. One who is slender and tall, with small fragile bones.

Edema. Swollen tissue due to an abnormal effusion of water.

Ejaculation. Discharge of semen from the penis during orgasm.

Embolism. The blocking of an artery by any bit of foreign matter in the blood stream; e.g., blood clot, cancer cells, fat.

Endemic. Pertaining to the constant occurrence of disease in a community.

Endocardium. The membrane lining the interior of the heart.

Endocrine glands. Ductless glands whose secretions, hormones, pass directly into the blood stream.

Endometrium. Tissue lining the uterus.

Endomorph. A person who is generally fat, with undeveloped muscular tissue.

Energy. The capacity for doing work.

Enrichment. The addition of essential nutrients to food during commercial preparation.

Environment. The sum total of activities and stimuli acting on the individual.

Enzymes. Substances which serve as catalysts to promote chemical change.

Epidemic. An unusual number of cases of a disease in a given area.

Epidemiology. The study of occurrence and distribution of disease. It is most commonly applied to epidemic and endemic disease.

Epilepsy. A chronic functional disease characterized by fits or seizures and attended by convulsive motions of the muscles and loss of consciousness.

Erythroblastosis fetalis. Condition of a baby shortly before or after birth in which there is an excessive destruction of red blood cells.

Erythrocyte. A red blood cell.

Ethyl alcohol. Ordinary alcohol found in intoxicating drinks.

Etiology. The study of the cause of any disease.

Fallopian tubes. Tubes through which the egg passes from the ovary to the uterus.

Fatigue. A temporary diminution of the capacity of the body for work.

Fatty acids. The end products of fat digestion.

Feces. The waste material excreted from the intestinal tract.

Fertilization. Union of sperm with ovum to begin a new human life.

Field Theory. Lewin's "structured organism-environment" field theory of behavior. The structured elements include the relation between the person, his psychological environment, and his life space. The life space is the person plus his psychological environment which contains all the facts that determine his behavior. The psychological environment includes everything in the life space except the person. Differences in psychological environments or in persons create differences in behavior. The Field is dynamic in that the person and his psychological environment change as forces play upon them. Little weight is given to fixed traits, so emphasis is placed upon resolving conflicts and making adjustments.

Fitness. A desirable state of physical, mental, emotional, social, and spiritual well-being.

Fixation of complement test. The entering of a complement into combination with an antigen-antibody aggregate so that it is fixed and not available for subsequent reaction. The basis of the Wassermann, Reiter-protein, and other serologic tests.

Flocculation. The coagulation of finely divided particles or colloidal particles into larger particles which precipitate.

Fluoridation of water. The addition of one part of fluoride per million parts of drinking water.

Food additive. A substance, not a basic foodstuff, which is intentionally added to a food as a result of production, processing, storing, or packaging.

Fraternal twins. Twins which result from the fertilization of two eggs. They may be of the same or of opposite sex.

Gamma rays. Electromagnetic waves emitted from radioactive material that have great penetrating power.

Genetic damage. Damage to genes, such as that produced by exposure to radioactivity.

Genitalia. The reproductive organs.

Geriatrics. The branch of medicine concerned with old age and its diseases.

Germs. Infectious agents; disease-producing microorganisms.

Gerontology. Scientific study of the phenomena of old age.

Gingivitis. A periodontal disease in which the gums are inflamed.

Glaucoma. A disease of the eye, marked by intraocular pressure, atrophy of the retina, and blindness.

Glycogen. The form in which carbohydrate is stored in the body.

g pull. The force of the pull of gravity on the human body.

Hair follicle. A small sac which extends from the epidermis into the subcutaneous tissue and which contains the individual hair root.

Health adviser. A competent professionally prepared person, associated with appropriate professional associations, who is skilled to counsel and/or treat the individual. A medical doctor and a reputable dentist are examples.

Health education. The process of providing learning experiences which favorably influence knowledge, attitudes, and practices relating to individual, family, and community health.

Health status. The health condition of an individual.

Hemoglobin. Pigment of red blood cells which has the ability to combine with and release oxygen.

Hemolytic streptococcus. Organism which destroys red blood cells and allows hemoglobin to escape.

Hemorrhoids. An enlarged and varicose condition of the veins of the lower portion of the rectum and the tissues about the anus.

Herpes. An inflammatory reaction of the skin characterized by the formation of small groups of vesicles.

Hobby. An activity, voluntarily selected, which permits self-expression with a recreative purpose.

Hormone. A regulatory substance produced by an endocrine gland.

Host. Any individual, animal, or plant harboring a parasite or a disease-producing microorganism.

Huntington's chorea. An hereditary disease of adults marked by irregular movements, speech disturbances, and dementia.

Hymen. Membrane found at the opening of the vagina.

Hypertension. Excessive tension, usually referring to high blood pressure.

Hypertension, essential. Hypertension for which there is no known organic cause.

Hyperthyroidism. Overactivity of the thyroid gland.

Hypothyroidism. Underactivity of the thyroid gland.

Hysterectomy. Total or partial removal of the uterus.

Identical twins. Results of a single fertilized egg which divides to form two independent and separate individuals of the same sex.

Immunity. A high degree of resistance sufficient to protect the individual against specific invading organisms. Immunity may be active, artificially conferred (passive), or inherited.

Inflammation. The condition of the tissues as a result of injury characterized by pain, heat, redness, and swelling.

Inoculation. The introduction of substances (microorganisms, infected material, serums, etc.) into the tissues of man or animal for the purpose of producing an immunity.

Insomnia. A state in which an individual is unable to go to sleep.

Insulin. A hormone secreted by the islets of Langerhans in the pancreas. Insulin is essential to normal oxidation of sugar by the body cells.

Insulin shock. The result of an overdose of insulin.

Integration. The coordination of specific responses into unified patterns.

Interaction. A relation between independent entities in which reciprocal influences of one upon the other are possible.

Intercourse. Act of sexual relations in which the penis is inserted into the vagina.

Interest, health. An expression of a desire to learn more about some aspect of healthful, effective living.

Irradiation. Treatment of diseases by means of radiant energy, such as by roentgen, radium, ultraviolet, infrared, or other rays.

Kwashiorkor. A protein-deficiency disease.

Leukemia. Cancer of the blood-forming organs.

Leukorrhea. A whitish discharge from the female genital canal.

Maladjustment. The inability of an individual to adjust to everyday situations. The condition may range from minor to severe.

Malaise. A general feeling of illness. It may be characterized by restlessness, lack of appetite, and decreased energy.

519

Malignant tumor. A tumor which will continue to grow and spread to other parts of the body.

Masturbation. Self-stimulation or manipulation of the genitalia to produce orgasm.

Menarche. The time when the first menstruation occurs.

Menopause. The cessation of menstruation, usually between the forty-fifth and fiftieth years. The term commonly refers to symptoms associated with the cessation of menstruation and the end of the childbearing period.

Menstruation. Periodic discharge of lining tissue from the uterus, occurring when the ovum has not been fertilized and implanted in the wall of the uterus.

Mesomorph. A person of the athletic type, with hard, firm muscles.

Metabolism. The sum of all physical and chemical processes by which living organized substance is produced and maintained.

Metastasis. The transfer or spread of disease from a primary point to distant points through the blood vessels or lymph channels.

Microorganisms. Microscopic plants or animals.

Monogamy. Marriage with only one mate at a time.

Morbidity. The presence of disease; or the ratio of the number of sick persons to the total population of a community.

Mortality. Death; or the death rate.

Multiple birth. Birth of more than one baby at a time.

Muscle tone. A tension or slight contraction of the muscle.

Naïve. Unaffected.

Needs, health. The health demands, both internal and external, made upon an individual as he seeks to adjust to his environment.

Neonatal. Newborn.

Nephritis. Inflammation of the kidney.

Nephrons. The filtering units in the kidneys.

Nephrosis. A noninflammatory disease of the kidney.

Nocturnal emission. Orgasm which occurs while the male is asleep.

Normal. Common, typical, or standard.

Nostrum. A medicine prepared and/or sold by a quack.

Nutrient. A nutritive ingredient.

Obesity. Excessive storage of fat in the body.

Opiate. A drug derived from opium which induces sleep.

Orgasm. Intense excitement occurring as a result of sexual stimulation; the culmination or climax of the sexual act for both male and female, accompanied by ejaculation of seminal fluid from the male.

Orthodontics. A specialized field of dentistry which includes the detection, study, prevention, and correction of irregularities in tooth position.

Ovary. Sex gland in the female, producing ova and hormones.

Ovulation. The maturation and release of an ovum from the ovary.

Ovum. Female reproductive cell, produced in the ovary.

Pandemic. A widespread epidemic affecting many countries or world-wide in scope.

Paranoia. A chronic, slowly progressive psychotic disorder marked by systematized delusions.

Parasite. A plant or animal (usually disease-producing) which lives upon or within another living organism at whose expense it derives gain without compensation.

Patent medicine. The common term for a nostrum, usually of secret composition, advertised directly to the public.

Patented medicine. A medicine whose manufacture is protected by letters of patent.

Pathogen. A disease-producing agent.

Pathogenic. Capable of producing disease.

Periodontal diseases. Diseases of the gum

and other supporting structures of the teeth.

Peristalsis. A progressive wave of contractions by the muscles in the walls of the intestines to force material through the intestinal tract.

Peritonitis. Inflammation of the peritoneum, the membrane lining the interior of the abdominal cavity.

Personality. The total of the individual's behavior as he makes personal and social adjustments while participating in life activities.

Personality emergence. The development of the personality from an obscure condition into a state of well-being recognized by others.

Pertussis. Whooping cough.

Phagocyte. A white blood cell capable of ingesting disease-producing microorganisms.

Piles. See hemorrhoids.

Postnatal. After the birth of a child.

Posture. Bearing or the position of the body as a whole.

Pregnancy. A state in which a woman has a child in her uterus.

Premature birth. A birth which occurs after the sixth month but before the end of the normal term of pregnancy.

Prenatal. Before the birth of a child.

Procreation. The act of begetting offspring.

Progesterone. Hormone produced by the corpus luteum of the ovary to stimulate the lining of the uterus to prepare for a fertilized ovum.

Promiscuity. Indiscriminate sexual relations.

Proprietary medicine. Any chemical or drug used in the treatment of disease that is protected against free competition as to name, product, composition, or process of manufacture by secrecy, patent, copyright, or other means.

Protein. One of a group of complex nitrogenous substances which are required for normal growth and repair of body tissues.

Psychoneurosis (neurosis). A personality disorder, less severe than a psychosis, characterized by incapacity to make satisfactory adjustments or to cope with frustration and anxiety.

Psychosis. A severe or major mental disorder involving the total personality. The patient's mental functions are so disturbed that he is incapable of participating in everyday activities.

Psychosomatic. Pertaining to bodily symptoms that arise from psychological factors.

Psychosomatic medicine. An approach to the sick individual as a whole person rather than as one with a localized disease.

Puberty. The period at which the generative organs become capable of exercising their reproductive function, indicated in the male by discharge of semen and in the female by the appearance of menses.

Pyorrhea. A disease of the periodontium —the structure of soft tissues, gums, and bone which supports the teeth. It is characteristic that the gums withdraw from the teeth, forming pockets that become filled with pus.

Quack. A faker or incompetent person fraudulently practicing the art of healing the sick; one who, without special education or professional affiliation, attempts the practice of medicine. His dominant motive is to make money.

Rad. Unit of measurement for energy absorbed from radiation in a given amount of tissue (100 ergs absorbed per gram of tissue).

Radioactive. The giving off of atomic energy in the form of radiations such as alpha, beta, or gamma rays.

Radioactive material. Substance which emits alpha, beta, or gamma rays.

Radioisotopes. Radioactive materials.

Recreation. Any type of activity, voluntarily engaged in, which refreshes the participant and is a source of joy to him.

Regimen. A systemic course of action.

Reservoir. The source of infection. Man, animal, or the environment are sources

521

of infection, since they harbor disease-producing organisms.

Residual. Remaining.

Resistance. The ability of the body to ward off disease.

Rheumatism. A family of diseases which produce an inflammation of body tissues.

Rh negative. Having no Rh factor in the blood.

Rh positive. Having Rh factor present in the blood.

Roentgen (r). A unit of measurement for ionizing radiation.

Saturated fat. A fat which cannot add more hydrogen, as opposed to unsaturated fats which can add more hydrogen.

Scuba. An abbreviation for self-contained underwater breathing apparatus.

Semen. The fluid produced by the male reproductive organs and carrying the sperm cells.

Shock. A state of the body in which there is an acute peripheral circulatory failure.

Siamese twins. Identical twins who have not completely separated.

Skeletal muscle. Contractile tissue characterized by cross striations.

Sociopathic personality. A person exhibiting antisocial or dyssocial reactions.

Spectrum. A range; any series of entities arranged according to the quantitative variation of a given common property.

Sperm (spermatozoon). Mature male germ cell.

Sphygmomanometer. An instrument for measuring blood pressure.

Sterile. Not capable of reproduction.

Stillbirth. The birth of a dead child.

Stroke volume of the heart. The amount of blood passing from each ventricle of the heart during a systole.

Strontium-90. A radioactive element found in fallout from atomic explosions.

Subclinical deficiency. A deficiency of a substance so mild that the deficiency is not recognized by ordinary visual or clinical means.

Susceptibility. The opposite condition to immunity. Like immunity, it may be acquired, familial, individual, inherited, racial, and species.

Symbiosis. The growth of two or more organisms in a mutually helpful relationship.

Systole. The contraction of the heart muscle, emptying the chamber of the heart.

Systolic pressure. Highest blood pressure recorded when the ventricle of the heart is contracted.

Testicle. Sex gland in the male, producing sperm and hormones.

Thrombus. A blood clot formed within the heart or blood vessels.

Tension. A state of readiness to meet a real or imaginary situation.

Theobromine. A stimulant closely related to caffeine.

Toxic. Pertaining to a poison, usually that of a disease-producing organism.

Toxicity. The degree of being poisonous; the degree of violence of a disease-producing organism or of a poison.

Toxoid. A modified toxin which has lost its poisonous properties but has retained its power to stimulate antitoxin formation.

Trachoma. A serious disease of the mucous-membrane lining of the inner surface of the eyelids.

Tranquilizing drugs. Drugs used in the treatment of mental illness and emotional states, characterized by their calming effect on the patient.

Treponema pallidum immobilization (TPI) Test. Nelson's specific test using living treponemes mixed with the serum of a patient immune to syphilis. Organisms become fixed in the presence of complement. Very valuable for confirming a biological false positive reaction.

Tumor. A new growth of cells or tissues.

Universal antidote. An antidote composed of one part strong tea, two parts crumbled browned toast, and one part milk of magnesia.

Urinalysis. Analysis of the urine to determine its composition.

Uterus. A hollow muscular organ of the female reproductive system in which the embryo and fetus grow and develop prior to birth.

Vaccine. Material for preventive inoculation, particularly prepared bacterium or its products, which when introduced into the body stimulate specific antibody formation.

Vector. A carrier, such as the insect or animal carrier of disease-producing organisms from one host to another.

Ventricle. Chamber of the heart which forces blood out into the arteries when it contracts.

Vertigo. Sensation that the world is revolving about one or that one is moving in space.

Vincent's infection. A periodontal disease involving the gums, mouth, and throat.

Virulence. The strength or ability of an organism to overcome the body defenses and cause disease.

Viscosity. State of being viscous or sticky.

Visual acuity. Keenness of sight.

Voluntary medical-care plan. A plan in which the individual voluntarily subscribes for partial or total medical and hospital expenses. Usually these plans are based on a prepayment procedure whereby the individual pays a certain amount each month whether sick or well. Health insurance and Blue Shield and Blue Cross plans are examples.

Weightlessness. The condition resulting when an object has no gravitational pull exerted upon it, such as the state to which man is subjected in space.

Zygote. The fertilized ovum before cleavage.

THE
HUMAN
BODY

THE HUMAN BODY

An accurate knowledge of the architecture of the human body is of great importance to students in hygiene, nursing, and physiology. The anatomical plates on the following pages have been specially prepared and included in this text to provide a ready reference source not only of the various structures of the body, but also of their relationships to one another.

The various body systems are shown in the natural color of healthy tissues, and special attention has been paid to labeling the structures and organs that are usually discussed in college-level courses. It is suggested that frequent reference to this section will prove invaluable in helping the student visualize more clearly the body as a functional organism. To facilitate their use, certain illustrations have been placed on facing pages for easier comparison, and the same general body outlines have been used throughout. Furthermore, all structures are shown in proportionate size to afford a clearer understanding of their size and the space they occupy in the body.

These illustrations were prepared by Robert J. Demarest, Medical Illustrator, in consultation with a number of medical authorities.

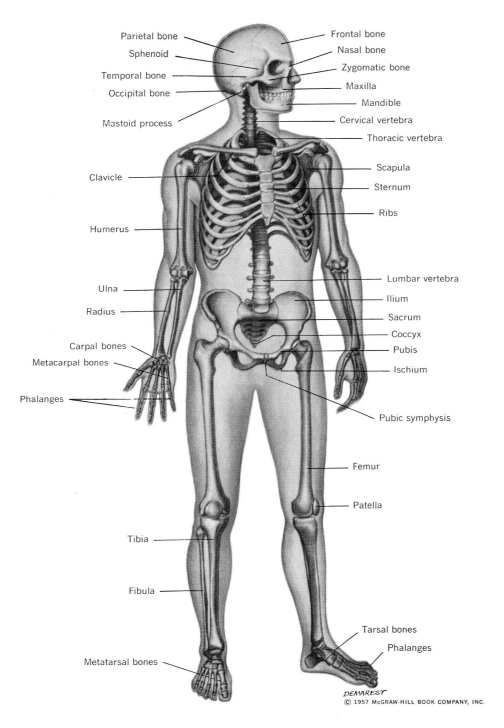

Parietal bone

Sphenoid

Temporal bone

Occipital bone

Mastoid process

Frontal bone

Nasal bone

Zygomatic bone

Maxilla

Mandible

Cervical vertebra

Thoracic vertebra

Clavicle

Scapula

Sternum

Ribs

Humerus

Ulna

Radius

Carpal bones

Metacarpal bones

Phalanges

Lumbar vertebra

Ilium

Sacrum

Coccyx

Pubis

Ischium

Pubic symphysis

Femur

Patella

Tibia

Fibula

Tarsal bones

Phalanges

Metatarsal bones

DEMAREST
© 1957 McGRAW-HILL BOOK COMPANY, INC.

PLATE A SKELETAL SYSTEM (anterior view)

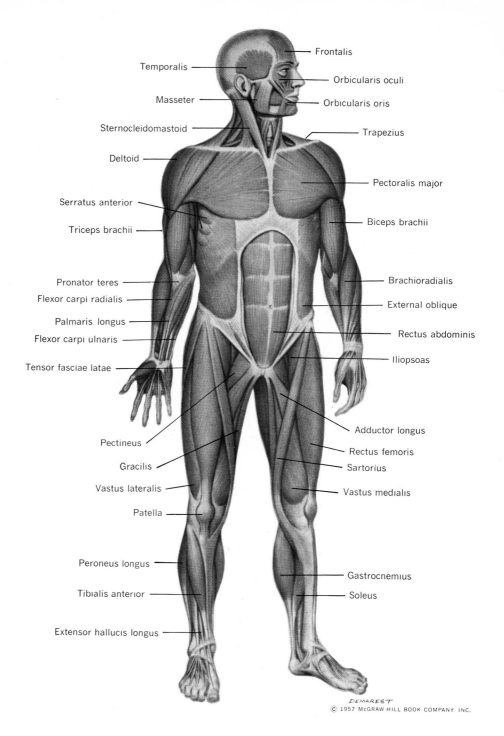

Frontalis

Temporalis

Orbicularis oculi

Masseter

Orbicularis oris

Sternocleidomastoid

Trapezius

Deltoid

Pectoralis major

Serratus anterior

Biceps brachii

Triceps brachii

Pronator teres

Brachioradialis

Flexor carpi radialis

External oblique

Palmaris longus

Rectus abdominis

Flexor carpi ulnaris

Iliopsoas

Tensor fasciae latae

Adductor longus

Pectineus

Rectus femoris

Gracilis

Sartorius

Vastus lateralis

Vastus medialis

Patella

Peroneus longus

Gastrocnemius

Tibialis anterior

Soleus

Extensor hallucis longus

DEMAREST

© 1957 McGRAW HILL BOOK COMPANY INC.

PLATE B MUSCULAR SYSTEM (anterior view)

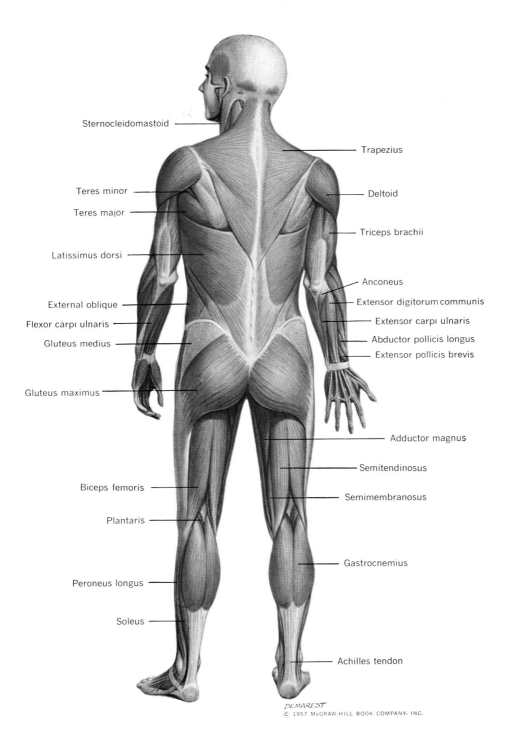

Sternocleidomastoid

Teres minor

Teres major

Latissimus dorsi

External oblique

Flexor carpi ulnaris

Gluteus medius

Gluteus maximus

Biceps femoris

Plantaris

Peroneus longus

Soleus

Trapezius

Deltoid

Triceps brachii

Anconeus

Extensor digitorum communis

Extensor carpi ulnaris

Abductor pollicis longus

Extensor pollicis brevis

Adductor magnus

Semitendinosus

Semimembranosus

Gastrocnemius

Achilles tendon

DEMAREST
© 1957 McGRAW-HILL BOOK COMPANY, INC.

PLATE C MUSCULAR SYSTEM (posterior view)

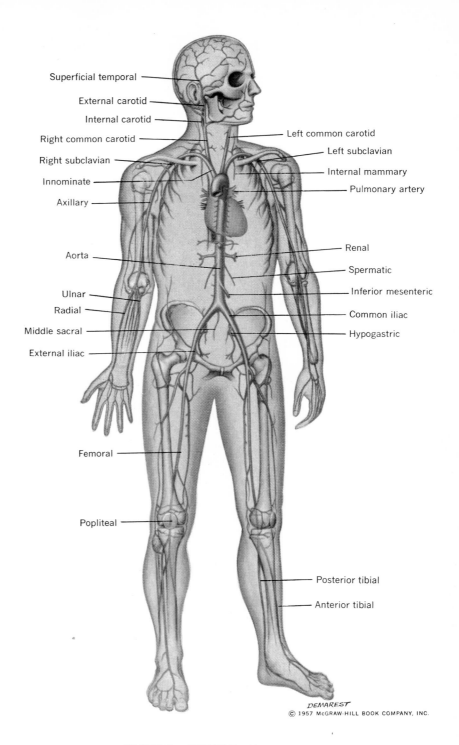

Superficial temporal

External carotid

Internal carotid

Right common carotid

Right subclavian

Innominate

Axillary

Left common carotid

Left subclavian

Internal mammary

Pulmonary artery

Aorta

Renal

Spermatic

Ulnar

Radial

Middle sacral

External iliac

Inferior mesenteric

Common iliac

Hypogastric

Femoral

Popliteal

Posterior tibial

Anterior tibial

DEMAREST
© 1957 McGRAW-HILL BOOK COMPANY, INC.

PLATE D ARTERIAL SYSTEM

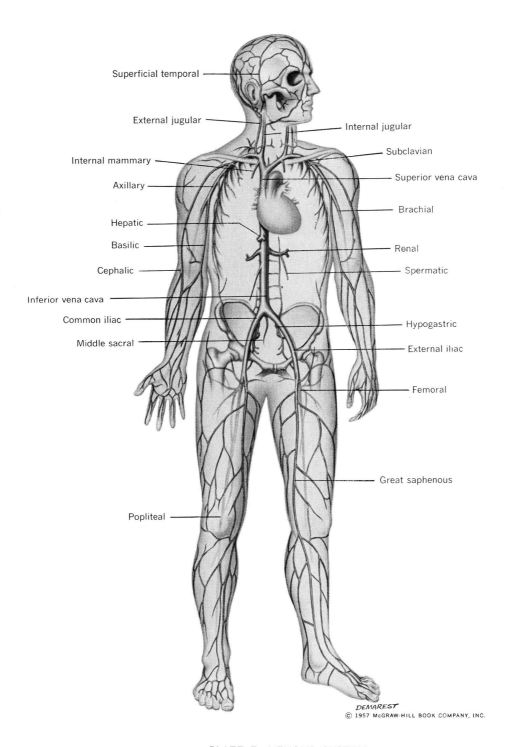

Superficial temporal

External jugular

Internal jugular

Internal mammary

Subclavian

Axillary

Superior vena cava

Hepatic

Brachial

Basilic

Renal

Cephalic

Spermatic

Inferior vena cava

Common iliac

Hypogastric

Middle sacral

External iliac

Femoral

Great saphenous

Popliteal

PLATE E   VENOUS SYSTEM

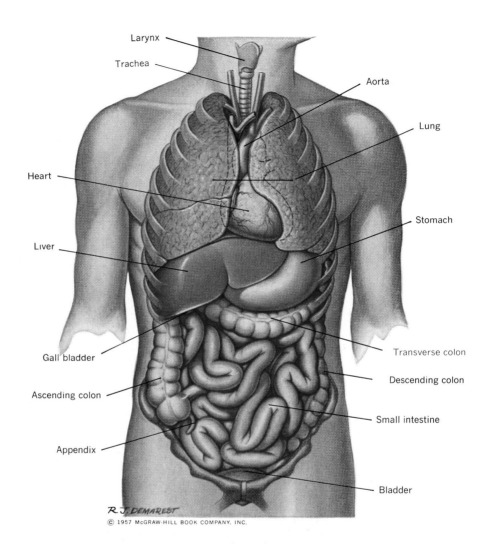

Larynx

Trachea

Aorta

Lung

Heart

Stomach

Liver

Gall bladder

Transverse colon

Descending colon

Ascending colon

Small intestine

Appendix

Bladder

R J DEMAREST

© 1957 McGRAW-HILL BOOK COMPANY, INC.

PLATE F VISCERA

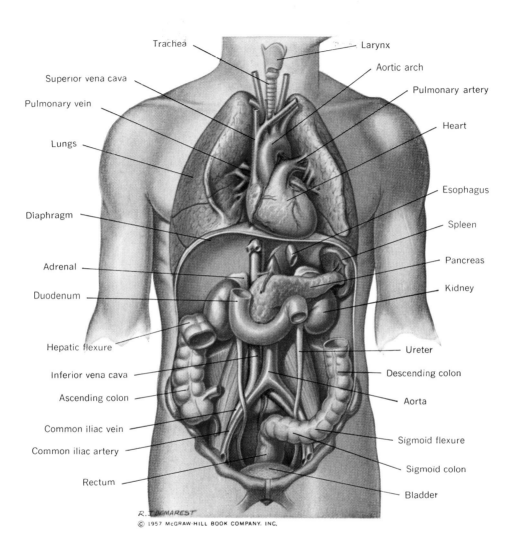

Trachea — Larynx

Larynx

Aortic arch

Superior vena cava

Pulmonary artery

Pulmonary vein

Heart

Lungs

Esophagus

Diaphragm

Spleen

Adrenal

Pancreas

Duodenum

Kidney

Hepatic flexure

Ureter

Inferior vena cava

Descending colon

Ascending colon

Aorta

Common iliac vein

Sigmoid flexure

Common iliac artery

Sigmoid colon

Rectum

Bladder

R. J. DEMAREST

PLATE G   VISCERA (deep structures)

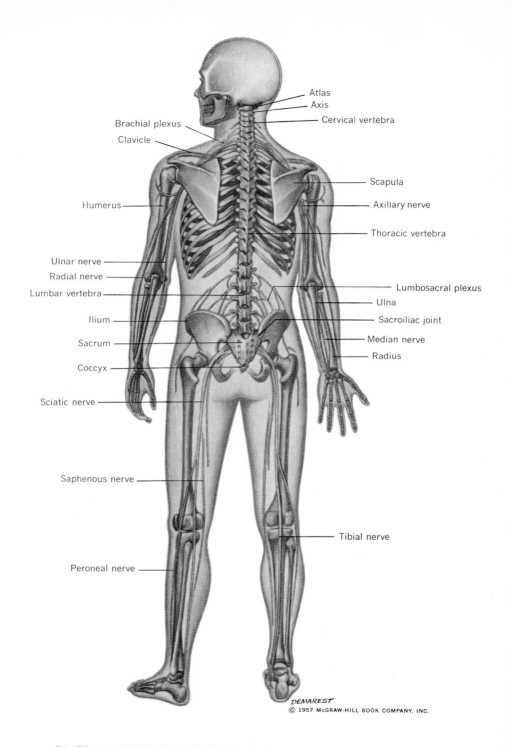

Atlas

Axis

Cervical vertebra

Brachial plexus

Clavicle

Scapula

Axillary nerve

Humerus

Thoracic vertebra

Ulnar nerve

Radial nerve

Lumbar vertebra

Lumbosacral plexus

Ulna

Ilium

Sacroiliac joint

Sacrum

Median nerve

Coccyx

Radius

Sciatic nerve

Saphenous nerve

Tibial nerve

Peroneal nerve

DEMAREST

© 1957 McGRAW-HILL BOOK COMPANY, INC.

PLATE H SKELETAL SYSTEM (posterior view showing spinal nerves)

INDEX

ABOUT THE ARTIST

ROBERT J. DEMAREST'S medical illustrations have appeared in many texts and medical journals as well as in several popular weekly magazines. Such a variety of uses clearly indicates the appeal of the life-like medical illustrations this young artist does. Trained at the Art Students' League and the School for Medical Illustrators, Demarest on graduation was honored as the recipient of the Saunders' Fellowship in Medical Art at the University of Pennsylvania. Mr. Demarest is currently associated with the College of Physicians and Surgeons, Columbia University.

INDEX

American Dietetic Association, 272
American Heart Association, 235
American Home Economics Association, 272, 273
American Hospital Association, 190, 289
American Institute of Family Relations, 150
American Medical Association, 114, 285
  on depressants and stimulants, 405–409
  Journal, 271
  protection against fraud, 262, 264, 271, 272, 278, 279
  voluntary health insurance, 289
  on water fluoridation, 189
American National Committee for Health Education of the Public, 486
American Osteopathic Association, 284
American Public Health Association, 4, 25, 321, 373, 455, 461, 466
American Red Cross, 433, 439–441, 462
American Social Health Association, 114, 124, 128
American Temperance Society, 402
Amino acids, 236
Anderson, K. A., 499
Anemia, 242, 360
Angina pectoris, 364, 365
Angiotensin, 363
Antibodies, 317
  definition, 317
  types, 317
Antibiotics, 317, 318, 329
Antigen, 318
  allergies and, 383
Antihistamines, 385
Antimetabolites, 375, 378
Anxiety neurosis, 92, 366
Apoplexy, 365, 366
Appendicitis, 253
Appraisal devices, 122–125
Arteries, 359, 364
Arteriosclerosis, 364
Arthritis, 381, 382
  quackery, 261, 262
Arthritis and Rheumatism Foundation, 261
Artificial respiration, 440
  back-pressure–arm-lift, 433
  chest-pressure–arm-lift, 440
  mouth-to-mouth, 440, 441
Asia, health work in, 493
Asphyxiation, 440

Aspirin and arthritis, 382
Asthma, 383–385
Astigmatism, 192
Astronauts, selection of, 508, 509
Ataxia, 387
Atherosclerosis, 236, 364
Athetoid palsy, 387
Athlete's foot, 346, 347
Atrioventricular node, 358
Atrium, 358
Attitudes, 6, 23
  definition, 87
Automobile Club of Southern California, 441
Automobile Crash Injury Research Project, Cornell University, 436
Autonomy, 64, 67

Baby, 158
  birth, 161–163
  breast-feeding, 163, 165
  care of newborn, 165
  multiple birth, 163, 164
  place for birth, 161
  postnatal care, 162, 165
  premature, 164
  sex, 158, 162
  (*See also* Children)
Baby-sitting, 170
Bacon, Seldon, 403
Bacteria, description, 305–307
  diseases caused by, 306
  drawing, 306
Baldness cures, 264
Barbituric acid, 410, 417
Basal metabolism, 231, 232
Basic Seven food groups, 230
Behavior, health, formula for changing, 6, 31
Benign tumors, 370
Benzedrine, 415, 417
Beriberi, 244
Better business bureaus, 272, 273, 278
Beyrer, Mary, 462, 473, 474
Bilateral International Health Programs of the United States, 494, 495
Births, annual, in world, 487
Bjerver, K., 401
Blood, Robert O., Jr., 132, 135, 138, 140, 142
Blood composition, 359

537